Tl   )F
V   H

Sixth Edition

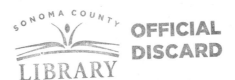

THE NEW A TO Z OF WOMEN'S HEALTH

Sixth Edition

Christine Ammer

Foreword by
JoAnn E. Manson, M.D., Dr.P.H.,
Professor of Medicine
and
Elizabeth F. Brigham
Professor of Women's Health, Harvard Medical School,
Chief of Preventive Medicine, Brigham and Women's Hospital

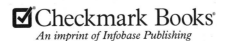
✓Checkmark Books®
An imprint of Infobase Publishing

The New A to Z of Women's Health, Sixth Edition

Checkmark Books
An imprint of Infobase Publishing
132 West 31st Street
New York NY 10001

The Library of Congress has cataloged the hardcover edition as follows

Ammer, Christine.
The encyclopedia of women's health / Christine Ammer ; foreword by JoAnn E. Manson. — 6th ed.
p. cm.
Includes bibliographical references and index.
ISBN-13: 978-0-8160-7407-5 (hardcover : alk. paper)
ISBN-10: 0-8160-7407-0 (hardcover : alk. paper)
ISBN-13: 978-0-8160-7408-2 (pbk. : alk. paper)
ISBN-10: 0-8160-7408-9 (pbk : alk. paper)
1. Women—Health and hygiene—Encyclopedias. 2. Women—Diseases—Encyclopedias. I. Title.
RA778.A494 2009
613'.0424403—dc22   2008013641

Checkmark Books are available at special discounts when purchased in bulk quantities for businesses, associations, institutions, or sales promotions. Please call our Special Sales Department in New York at (212) 967-8800 or (800) 322-8755.

You can find Checkmark Books on the World Wide Web at http://www.checkmark.com.

Text design by Cathy Rincon
Cover design by Alicia Post
Illustrations by Dale Dyer

Printed in the United States of America

VB Hermitage 10 9 8 7 6 5 4 3 2 1

This book is printed on acid-free paper and contains 30 percent postconsumer recycled content.

CONTENTS

Foreword   vii

Author's Note   ix

Acknowledgments   xi

How to Use This Book   xiii

Entries A–Z   1

Appendix: Resources   447

Index   456

AUTHOR'S NOTE

The underlying assumption of this book is that every woman wants to take responsibility for her own health. The only way she can act intelligently and safely in her own best interest is to understand the workings of her body and to know what kinds of care and treatment are available. Medicine is not yet a "hard" science; indeed, it may never be one, and certainly not for many years to come. An enormous number of things about our bodies still are not known or are at best imperfectly understood. Therefore it is especially important to know the various options and to choose among them with the fullest possible information. There is more than one way to deal with breast cancer, more than one way to treat a vaginal infection, more than one way to practice birth control.

We women are the major consumers of health care. We live longer than men and see doctors more often. Moreover, our bodies are different from men's in more than the obvious ways. True, we outlive men by about eight years on the average, but our immune systems turn on us far more often: We are three times more likely than men to develop one or more autoimmune disease, such as multiple sclerosis or rheumatoid arthritis. We are twice as likely to contract a sexually transmitted disease and 10 times more likely to contract HIV, the AIDS virus, during unprotected sex with an infected partner. We are more likely than men to die from a first heart attack, and more likely to suffer a second one within a year. We are two to three times more likely to suffer from clinical depression. Those of us who smoke are at greater risk of developing lung cancer than are men smokers, and those of us who drink tolerate far smaller amounts of alcohol. We are entitled to the best care, but we must learn to recognize it and know how to obtain it.

The body of medical knowledge is growing constantly. This sixth edition has been completely updated with new findings and the addition of new entries and tables. The rapid medical and technical advances of recent years required careful vetting of each entry, both to include new advances and to delete material that is outdated or obsolete. While great care has been taken to make sure that the information in this book is accurate, new facts are constantly coming to light and new treatments and procedures are being developed. For any serious health problem, therefore, the reader is urged to consult her clinician and, if there is still doubt in her mind, to follow the practice recommended throughout this book, and by all reputable professionals, to *get a second opinion*. No book can be a substitute for clinical examination, diagnosis or treatment. If something seems to be wrong, check it out.

The entries in this concise encyclopedia cover a broad range, from the anatomy of the female and male reproductive systems to the basic workings of the endocrine system, from the events of puberty through those of the child-bearing years to menopause and old age. They cover the functioning and malfunctioning of the sexually active woman, the decisions involved in whether to bear children, how to prevent pregnancy and how to overcome infertility. They cover all aspects of normal and abnormal pregnancy and birth as well as some of the common problems that occasionally arise for either mother or baby after birth. Included also are articles pertaining to the maintenance of good health, to diet and exercise, to weight control, drinking, smoking, drug use. They describe what a woman should expect (and demand) during a thorough medical checkup, what tests and procedures are necessary and when. And finally, they include the principal diseases and disorders that affect women's bodies and minds, their diagnosis, their treatment (including home and herbal remedies as well as prescription drugs and surgery), their outlook and, in the case of chronic diseases, their effect on a woman's sexuality and childbearing.

Despite the technical nature of some of the material, every effort has been made to present subjects simply and clearly, in everyday language. For this reason comparatively complex subjects, such as the menstrual cycle or the different kinds of mastectomy, are treated at greater length than other equally important subjects; the space allotted reflects only the practical considerations of adequate explanation. With controversial questions or issues, every attempt has been made to present all sides, including all the known alternatives, and the advantages and disadvantages of each.

A word of caution: Nearly four out of 10 Americans who use the Internet mine it for medical information. But not all the information can be trusted. Among the 350+ medical sites, you can find profit-driven, misleading or just plain erroneous data. The best online site is the one driven by the National Institutes of Health, www.nih.gov. Through it one can get information about many diseases as well as links to other government sites, such as www.clinicaltrials.gov; www.medlineplus. gov, run by the NIH and the National Library of Medicine; www.healthfinder.gov, run by the Department of Health and Human Services; and www.cancer.gov, run by the National Cancer Institute. For nongovernment sites, the Mayo Clinic's www.mayoclinic.com has good information. For drug information, look on www.PDRHealth.com. The patient advocacy groups for whatever disease one is interested in can be very useful, but some of their information may be biased, so use them with caution. (See also Resources in the Appendix.) Further, buying prescription drugs online may be cheaper than in a local drugstore but also may be hazardous. Many of the sites are legitimate and operate according to strict government and drug industry standards, but others may be unregulated, unprincipled, unreliable and potentially dangerous. It is advisable to buy only from sites that require a physician's prescription, that verify each prescription before dispensing a medication, and that provide access to a licensed pharmacist who can answer questions.

Many women, even those who are well educated and well informed, are reluctant to assert themselves during a visit to a doctor. They may be afraid to ask questions, or they may unwittingly put up with a "There, there dear, doctor knows best" approach. On the other hand, they may confront the physician with many pages of research from the Internet, which is not always reliable. They may try to diagnose themselves, often with mixed results. This book attempts to give readers the confidence they need to obtain good care.

ACKNOWLEDGMENTS

I am deeply grateful to the many experts and friends who have answered questions and made valuable suggestions, criticisms and corrections. Special warm thanks go to the many women who have shared with me their personal experiences concerning health, disease and medical care. Thanks also are due to the women who expressed and explored their concerns in special workshops, consciousness-raising groups and other discussion groups. The common ground of our experiences gave the original impetus to this book.

Finally, gratitude and appreciation must go to the practitioners in many fields who have critically read relevant portions of this encyclopedia. They include Cynthia P. Anderson, A.C.S.W., American Association of Sex Education Counselors and Therapists, sex and family therapist; Karyn Kai Anderson, Ph.D., MPH; Vincent W. Ansanelli, Jr., M.D., F.A.C.S., P.C., Department of Surgery, Columbia University; Shiva Barton, N.D., R.A.C., President, Massachusetts Acupuncture Society; Elisabeth Bing, cofounder, American Society for Psychoprophylaxis in Childbirth, author and childbirth educator; Peter T. Bruce, M.D., F.R.C.S., Senior Lecturer in Urology, Melbourne University; Ann Burnham, M.D., Lexington Eye Associates; Laura C. Fine, M.D., Ophthalmic Consultants of Boston; Katherine Gulick Fricker, Ed.M., science teacher and naturalist; Stephen Fricker, M.D., Massachusetts Eye and Ear Infirmary; A. Gordon Gauld, M.D., formerly obstetrics-gynecology staff, Boston Hospital for Women; Renee Goldberg, M.D., F.A.C.O.G., Medical Director, Obstetrics and Gynecology, Beth Israel Deaconess Healthcare; George Grady, M.D., Assistant Commissioner of Public Health, Chief State Epidemiologist, Commonwealth of Massachusetts; Nancy Greenleaf, R.N., Ph.D., Professor, University of Southern Maine School of Nursing; Joseph A. Grocela, M.D., Director, Urodynamics Laboratory and Continence Center, Massachusetts General Hospital; Adolph M. Hutter, M.D., Department of Cardiology, Massachusetts General Hospital, Associate Professor of Medicine, Harvard Medical School; Young Bae Kim, M.D., Division of Gynecologic Oncology, Beth Israel Deaconess Medical Center, Boston, Assistant Professor of Obstetrics, Gynecology, and Reproductive Biology, Harvard Medical School; Cheryl E. Kraley, M.S., R.N., R.N.C., certified nurse-practitioner in obstetrics-gynecology, Harvard Community Health Plan; Arleen Kulin, R.N., doula; James Gavin Manson, M.D., Chief Orthopedic Surgeon, Mt. Auburn Hospital; Edward C. Mun, M.D., Director, Bariatric Surgery, Beth Israel Deaconess Medical Center, Boston, Assistant Professor of Surgery, Harvard Medical School; the late Esther Rome, Boston Women's Health Collective and Ananda Health Collective, author, nutritionist and masseuse; David Satcher, M.D., Ph.D., Chairman, Department of Community Medicine and Family Practice, Morehouse College School of Medicine; Nathan T. Sidley, M.D., Fellow, American Psychiatric Association and President, American Academy of Psychiatry and the Law; David Singer, M.D., American Diabetes Association and private practice; Vincent R. Sites, M.D., Teaching Associate in Radiology, Massachusetts General Hospital and private practice; Louis R. Slattery,

M.D., Acting Director of Surgery, Bellevue Hospital; the late Samuel Stein, M.D., Assistant Director, M.I.T. Health Service; and Alan Ziskind, M.D., M.P.H., Fellow, American Academy of Pediatrics. This book has been vastly improved through their expertise. Its errors and shortcomings remain my own responsibility.

HOW TO USE THIS BOOK

The terms in this encyclopedia, whether they consist of one word or several words, are listed in alphabetical order, letter by letter, up to the comma in case of inversion. Identical or related terms with different meanings are defined under a single heading in a series of numbered definitions.

Terms that are mentioned in one entry but are further explained in another, where the reader is advised to seek them out, are printed in large and small capital letters, for example, PAGET'S DISEASE, or LABOR, or CANCER, BREAST.

For terms that have several common names or both common and scientific names, all the important versions of the term are included. In the case of herbs, common usage varies considerably, the same name sometimes being used for several different herbs, so to avoid confusion every herb mentioned is identified by its botanical name.

Readers seeking advice and more information about specific subjects are advised to look at Resources, in the Appendix.

In addition, readers may consult the comprehensive Index.

ENTRIES A–Z

abnormal presentation In childbirth, any position in which a part of the baby other than the crown of its head will emerge first (see CEPHALIC PRESENTATION). The principal kinds of abnormal presentation are breech, brow, face, posterior and shoulder; there is a separate entry for each of them.

abortifacient A drug, herb or other chemical agent that dilates the cervix and/or causes the uterus to contract, resulting in the ending of a pregnancy before the fetus can survive on its own. Plants of various kinds have been used for this purpose since ancient times. Among the most effective for cervical dilation is LAMINARIA, a marine plant whose stem gradually expands when it is moist. Dried laminaria, when inserted into the cervix, causes it to open and, over a period of hours, gradually stretches the cervical canal. It does not, however, induce uterine contractions.

A number of herbs are said to be EMMENAGOGUES, that is, they allegedly induce menstruation delayed by illness or emotional stress, and sometimes also by pregnancy. As abortifacients they supposedly work best when taken very soon after conception, even before the next menstrual period is due, and generally they must be brewed to a fairly concentrated strength. When effective, they then induce abdominal cramps and uterine contractions, ending in abortion. This procedure also tends to be accompanied by pain, vomiting and diarrhea; indeed, some herbalists warn that an herb-induced abortion is more traumatic than a medical procedure performed in early pregnancy, such as VACUUM ASPIRATION. Further, some vegetable compounds so used are toxic in large doses, and the oil of at least two plants, pennyroyal (or squawmint; *Mentha pulegium*) and Eastern red

cedar (*Juniperus virginiana*), has caused a number of deaths. Among the herbs said to be effective abortifacients are blue cohosh or squaw root (*Caulophyllum thalictroides*), common rue (*Ruta graveolens*), black cohosh or black snakeroot (*Cimicifuga racemosa*) and tansy (*Chrysanthemum* or *Tanecetum vulgare*). The last two are toxic in large doses, and black cohosh should be avoided if a woman has low blood pressure. An abortifacient long used in the American Deep South is cotton bark (*Gossypium herbaceum*), which brings on uterine contractions when chewed. The cotton tree often is a host to ERGOT, a parasitic fungus whose derivatives have long been used in childbirth under medical supervision to strengthen uterine contractions.

Other substances that stimulate uterine contractions and may effectively terminate pregnancies of 4 to 20 weeks are PROSTAGLANDINS, compounds naturally occurring in various animal tissues, including human, that have been synthesized in the laboratory. They are used in a vaginal suppository, causing uterine contractions to begin a few hours after insertion. If these drugs are to be effective, however, women must take such high doses that they suffer nausea, vomiting, diarrhea and severe abdominal cramps. Their use therefore requires either pain-killing medication or anesthesia.

A newer abortifacient, RU-486 (mifepristone, or Mifeprex), administered together with prostaglandins, is about 95% effective in inducing abortion during the first three months of pregnancy. Developed in France, it works by blocking progesterone, a hormone needed to maintain pregnancy. (See CONTRAGESTIVE for more detailed discussion.) In 1994 the U.S. Food and Drug Administration approved trials using two different drugs to induce miscarriage, first an injection of methotrexate (which is used to inhibit tissue growth in some cancers, ectopic pregnancies and other conditions), followed four days later by tablets of misoprostol (used to prevent ulcers and hasten labor) inserted into the vagina.

Currently, the medications are administered orally, in pill form. Up to 49 days after the start of the last menstrual period (some say up to 63 days), the woman takes 600 mg. of Mifeprex; two days later she takes 400 mcg. of misprostol (brand name Cytotec). For a time, women could insert misoprostol vaginally at home two to three days after taking Mifeprex, which allowed for smaller dosages, fewer office visits and quicker results. However, after a few deaths were reported in 2006, mainly due to serious infection, providers returned to recommending only oral pills. Some pain and cramping is normal, indicating the pregnancy is terminating, but heavy bleeding, severe abdominal pain and nausea and fever indicate the woman should contact her practitioner without delay. (See also CONTRAGESTIVE.)

In pregnancies of 16 weeks or longer, the replacement of some of the amniotic fluid with a strong solution of salt, urea or prostaglandins brings on labor (see AMNIOINFUSION).

Where therapeutic abortion has not been available, women have used a variety of ineffective but often life-endangering agents to try to end a pregnancy. Among them are concentrated soap solution used as a douche, the insertion of suppositories of potassium permanganate and the ingestion of quinine pills, or of castor oil or other strong laxatives. None of these is an effective abortifacient. Some authorities point out that intrauterine devices and some oral contraceptives are actually abortifacients, since they do not prevent the fertilization of an egg by a sperm but rather prevent the implantation of the egg in the uterine wall, with the result that it is expelled during the next menstrual period.

See also ABORTION.

abortion   The interruption or loss of any pregnancy before the fetus is viable (capable of living). In common usage, however, a *spontaneous* or *natural abortion* is usually called a MISCARRIAGE, and the term "abortion" is reserved for *induced* or *elective abortion*, that is, the intentional termination of a pregnancy. A *therapeutic abortion* is an elective abortion that is legal; a *criminal abortion* is an illegal abortion. The procedures used for elective abortion depend on the length of pregnancy. For pregnancies of 12 weeks or less, an ABORTIFACIENT such as mifepristone (RU-486) or methotrexate may be used, or MENSTRUAL EXTRACTION (def. 2) or VACUUM ASPIRATION (def. 2), which have largely replaced surgical dilation and curettage (D AND C). For pregnancies of 13 to 20 weeks, DILATATION AND EVACUATION are used, and for 18 to 24 weeks, AMNIOINFUSION or HYSTEROTOMY. (For RU-486, see CONTRAGESTIVE.)

Unlike most medical procedures, abortion has long been the subject of moral and legal controversy, owing to disagreement about what constitutes a living human being and when life actually begins. Those who believe that a life is created at the moment of conception regard abortion as equivalent to murder. Many other views have prevailed, ranging from the idea that life begins when a fetus's movements first are felt (St. Thomas Aquinas), to a particular time period after conception (Aristotle said 40 days for boys and 90 days for girls), to after delivery (the ancient Hebrews). In the late 19th century Pope Leo XIII declared that all abortion is a sin, even if it is performed to save the mother's life, and the present-day Roman Catholic Church has retained this view. During the course of the 19th century most countries of the Western world made abortion illegal. This did not prevent women from seeking abortions, often from unskilled persons who performed the procedure for money alone and frequently botched the job. These criminal abortions often were *septic abortions*, that is, serious complications (usually infection and/or hemorrhage) resulted from them. The women who survived them often could not bear subsequent children, either because of scar tissue blocking their tubes or because the only way their lives had been saved was by hysterectomy (removal of the UTERUS). In the 1960s increasing pressure from women in the United States and Canada relaxed some of the laws in those countries. In the United States abortion is governed by state rather than federal law. In 1973, in a decision called *Roe v. Wade*, the U.S. Supreme Court declared that under the Constitution a woman was

OVERVIEW OF STATE ABORTION LAW

STATE	MUST BE PERFORMED BY A LICENSED PHYSICIAN	MUST BE PERFORMED IN A HOSPITAL IF AT:	SECOND PHYSICIAN MUST PARTICIPATE IF AT:	PROHIBITED EXCEPT IN CASES OF LIFE OR HEALTH ENDANGERMENT IF AT:	"PARTIAL-BIRTH" ABORTION BANNED	PUBLIC FUNDING OF ABORTION — Funds All or Most Medically Necessary Abortions	Funds Limited to Life Endangerment, Rape and Incest	PRIVATE INSURANCE COVERAGE LIMITED TO LIFE ENDANGERMENT
AL	X	Viability	Viability	Viability*	▶		X	
AK	X				▶	X		
AZ	X		Viability	Viability	▶	X	X	
AR	X		Viability	Viability⁺	▶		X	
CA	X			Viability		X		
CO	X						X	
CT	X	Viability		Viability		X		
DE	X			▶‡			X	
DC							X	
FL	X		24 weeks	24 weeks			X	
GA	X		3rd trimester	3rd trimester	Postviability		X	
HI	X					X		
ID	X	Viability	3rd trimester	Viability‡	▶		X	X
IL	X		Viability	Viability	▶	X		
IN	X	2nd trimester	Viability	Viability*	X		X*	
IA	X			3rd trimester	▶		XΩ	
KS			Viability	Viability	Postviability		X	
KY		2nd trimester		Viability	▶		X	X
LA	X		Viability	Viability	X		X	
ME	X			Viability			X	
MD	X			ViabilityΩ		X		
MA	X	12 weeks		24 weeks	▶	X		
MI	X		▶	Viability‡			X	
MN	X	2nd trimester		▶		X		
MS	X				X		XΩ	
MO	X	Viability	Viability	Viability	▶		X	X
MT	X		Viability	Viability*	Postviability	X		
NE	X			Viability	▶		X	
NV	X	24 weeks		24 weeks			X	
NH	X			24 weeks	▶		X	

(continues)

OVERVIEW OF STATE ABORTION LAW (CONTINUED)

STATE	MUST BE PERFORMED BY A LICENSED PHYSICIAN	MUST BE PERFORMED IN A HOSPITAL IF AT:	SECOND PHYSICIAN MUST PARTICIPATE IF AT:	PROHIBITED EXCEPT IN CASES OF LIFE OR HEALTH ENDANGERMENT IF AT:	"PARTIAL-BIRTH" ABORTION BANNED	PUBLIC FUNDING OF ABORTION — Funds All or Most Medically Necessary Abortions	PUBLIC FUNDING OF ABORTION — Funds Limited to Life Endangerment, Rape and Incest	PRIVATE INSURANCE COVERAGE LIMITED TO LIFE ENDANGERMENT
NJ	X	14 weeks			▶	X		
NM					Postviability	X		
NY			24 weeks	24 weeks‡		X		
NC	X	20 weeks		20 weeks	X		X	
ND	X	12 weeks	12 weeks	Viability	X		X	X
OH	X		▶ Viability	▶*	X		X	
OK	X	2nd trimester	Viability	Viability			X	
OR						X		▶
PA	X	Viability	Viability	24 weeks*	▶		X	
RI	X			24 weeks‡	X		X	
SC	X	3rd trimester	3rd trimester	3rd trimester	X		X	
SD	X	24 weeks		24 weeks	X		Life Only	
TN	X			Viability	X		X	
TX	X			3rd trimester			X	
UT	X	90 days		▶*	X		X*,Ω	
VT						X		
VA	X	2nd trimester	Viability	3rd trimester	▶		XΩ	
WA				Viability	▶	X		
WV					▶	X		
WI	X	12 weeks		Viability			X*	
WY	X			Viability			X	
TOTAL	39	19	18	36	14	17	32+DC	4

▶ Permanently enjoined; law not in effect.
* Exception in case of threat to the woman's physical health.
† Exception in case of rape or incest.
‡ Exception in case of life endangerment only.
Ω Exception in case of fetal abnormality.
Source: Guttmacher Institute

OVERVIEW OF STATE ABORTION LAW

STATE	PROVIDERS MAY REFUSE TO PARTICIPATE		MANDATED COUNSELING INCLUDES INFORMATION ON:				WAITING PERIOD (in hours) After COUNSELING	PARENTAL INVOLVEMENT REQUIRED FOR MINORS
	Individual	Institution	Breast Cancer	Fetal Pain Effects	Serious Psychological Effects	Abortion Alternatives and Support Services		
AL	X					X	24	Consent
AK	X	Private				X		▶
AZ	X	X						Consent
AR	X	Religious		X^Φ	X	X	Day Before	Consent
CA	X	X						Notice
CO	X	X						
CT	X							
DE	X	X				X	▶	Notice^ξ
DC	X							
FL	X	X						Notice
GA	X	X		X		X	24	Notice
HI	X	X						
ID	X	X					24	Consent
IL	X	Private		X				Consent
IN	X	Private				X	18	Consent
IA	X	Private						Notice
KS	X	X				X	24	Notice
KY	X	X				X	24	Consent
LA	X	X		X		X	24	Consent
ME	X	X						
MD	X	X						Notice^ξ
MA	X	X					▶	Consent
MI	X	X				X	24	Consent
MN	X	Private	X	X^Φ		X	24	Notice^b
MS	X	X	X			X	24	Consent^b
MO	X	X					24	Consent
MT	X	Private					▶	Notice
NE	X	X				X	24	Notice
NV	X	Private			X			▶
NH	X							▶
NJ	X	Private						

(continues)

OVERVIEW OF STATE ABORTION LAW (CONTINUED)

STATE	PROVIDERS MAY REFUSE TO PARTICIPATE		MANDATED COUNSELING INCLUDES INFORMATION ON:				WAITING PERIOD (in hours) After COUNSELING	PARENTAL INVOLVEMENT REQUIRED FOR MINORS
	Individual	Institution	Breast Cancer	Fetal Pain Effects	Serious Psychological Effects	Abortion Alternatives and Support Services		
NM	X	X						▼
NY	X							
NC	X	X						Consent
ND	X	X				X	24	Consent^P
OH	X	X				X	24	Consent
OK	X	Private		X^Φ		X	24	Consent and Notice
OR	X	Private						
PA	X	Private				X	24	Consent
RI	X					X		Consent
SC	X	Private				X	1	Consent
SD	X	X			▼	X	24	Notice
TN	X	X				X	▼	Consent
TX	X	Private	X			X	24	Consent
UT	X	Private				X	24◊	Consent and Notice
VT	X	Private				X		
VA	X	X				X	24	Consent
WA	X	X						
WV						X	24	Notice^ξ
WI	X	X			X	X	24	Consent^ξ
WY	X	Private						Consent
TOTAL	**46**	**43**	**3**	**6**	**3**	**26**	**24**	**35**

▼ Permanently enjoined; law not in effect
§ Temporarily enjoined; law not in effect
Φ Fetal pain information is given only to women who are at least 20 weeks gestation.
ξ Specified health professionals may waive parental involvement in certain circumstances.
P Both parents must consent to the abortion.
◊ The waiting period requirement is waived if the pregnancy is the result of rape or incest, the fetus has grave defects or the patient is younger than 15.
Source: Guttmacher Institute

entitled to an abortion at any time during the first trimester (three months) of pregnancy; during the second trimester the individual states retained the right to determine where and by whom abortions could be performed. Since then opponents to abortion on moral and religious grounds have waged a powerful "right-to-life" campaign in order to reverse this decision. Extreme holders of this view have engaged in violence against clinics and doctors involved in performing the procedure, leading to a reduction in the number of facilities available. The number of abortion providers declined by one-third between 1982 and 1996, and in 2008, 87% of U.S. counties lacked an abortion provider. Also, a number of decisions by the U.S. Congress and the U.S. Supreme Court have curtailed abortion rights by upholding various state restrictions on the procedure. Among them are banning federal Medicaid funding (for poor women) unless the woman's life is in danger, requiring prior notification of a minor's parents and a 24-hour waiting period before abortion. In 2007 the Supreme Court reversed a previous decision and upheld the federal Partial-Birth Abortion Ban Act. This procedure, also called *intact dilatation and extraction,* involves removing a fetus in an intact condition rather than dismembering it in the uterus. It is only rarely performed, but no exception has been made to allow the procedure when the mother's health is at risk. (See also DILATATION AND EVACUATION.) Attempts have been made to prohibit federally funded clinics from providing information about abortion and referrals. The greatest impact of these restrictions is on poor, rural and minority women. However, Medicaid, a medical insurance program for low-income people, is financed jointly by the federal government and the states. At this writing 32 states and the District of Columbia provide abortions in cases of life endangerment, rape and incest. Four of them also provide state funds for abortions in cases of fetal abnormality, and three of them provide state funds for abortions that are necessary to prevent grave, long-lasting damage to the woman's physical health. One state provides abortions only in cases of life endangerment. Seventeen states use state funds to provide all or most medically necessary abortions; four of them do so voluntarily and 13 do so pursuant to a court order. (See accom-

panying table.) In Canada since 1989 there have been no legal restrictions on abortion but access is limited by poverty, geography and the health care system.

Another drawback for women seeking abortion is the lack of trained practitioners. Most American medical schools avoid the topic entirely, so training is not available. Doctors who provide the procedure have dropped in numbers; in 2001 there were only about 2,000 in the country, and most were in their 50s and 60s. It was not known who would replace them when they retired.

Women who are considering abortion should remember that the earlier it is performed, the safer it is. Many of the facilities (clinics) and physicians performing abortions offer a limited range of services, so it is important to investigate what is available. Such research can be done through local health departments, women's health centers and clinics, and local Planned Parenthood associations, which usually have a referral list for their locality. Factors to consider in choosing a physician or service include preferences as to general or local anesthesia (general anesthesia is advisable only in a hospital), private or clinic care, inpatient or outpatient care, the type of procedure desired, the availability of emergency care should it be needed and aftercare should complications develop.

Prior to performing an abortion, a clinician should review the woman's medical and menstrual history, with special attention to disorders contraindicating abortion in a clinic (such as a cardiac condition or bleeding disorders); administer a pregnancy test and blood tests for anemia and blood type, as well as Rh factor and venereal disease; check blood pressure, temperature, pulse and respiration; perform breast and pelvic examinations; and take a Pap smear and gonorrhea culture. Rh-negative women can have serious difficulties with a later pregnancy if they are not given RHo-D immune globulin (RhoGAM) within 72 hours following an abortion (or delivery or miscarriage; see RH FACTOR). Many abortion facilities provide a trained counselor to discuss the woman's decision with her as well as to explain the procedure in detail and advise her on birth control methods. If there is no such counselor, it is up to the clinician to explain the procedure and discuss subsequent birth control.

Another route taken by opponents of abortion is the establishment of crisis pregnancy centers, or pregnancy resource centers. Typically funded by Christian charities, they offer pregnancy tests, ultrasound and models of fetuses at various stages of development. They do not offer any birth control information. They often give inaccurate information about the dangers of abortion and try to persuade a woman to continue her pregnancy. In 2007 there were an estimated 2,500 such centers in the United States.

See also ABORTIFACIENT.

abortion pill　See CONTRAGESTIVE.

abruptio placentae　Also *placenta abruptio, placental abruption, premature separation of the placenta.* The separation of all or part of the PLACENTA from the uterine wall after the 20th week of pregnancy but before the baby is delivered. Such detachment also can occur before the 20th week and is a frequent cause of MISCARRIAGE. However, the clinical features of early and later detachment differ, the latter having far more serious consequences. Along with PLACENTA PREVIA, abruptio placentae is one of the two most common causes of hemorrhage in late pregnancy, but it is still relatively rare, occurring mostly in women who have borne six or more children. The cause is unknown and the symptoms vary, depending on the degree of placental separation and the amount of blood loss. Bleeding tends to begin just under the placenta, which by the seventh month of pregnancy usually is attached to the fundus (top), front or rear wall of the uterus. Blood accumulates and the placenta begins to break loose from its delicate fastening. In some cases, the blood passes through the cervix and out of the vagina (external hemorrhage); in others it is retained inside the uterus (concealed hemorrhage); in still others some blood is retained and some is expelled. Concealed hemorrhage is the most dangerous because it hides the severity of the condition more than profuse vaginal bleeding does. During this process the uterus becomes tightly contracted, tenderness develops, the patient begins to show signs of shock and there are signs of fetal distress, including absence of a fetal heartbeat.

Abruptio placentae calls for immediate emergency treatment, with transfusions to replace lost blood and to fight shock, and antibiotics to protect against infection. The fetus must be delivered, either vaginally, with labor induced by rupturing the membranes and/or administering OXYTOCIN, or surgically, by CESAREAN SECTION. Most authorities believe the fetus should be delivered within six hours, the method chosen depending on the degree of abruption. Although prompt treatment will nearly always save the mother, the fetus, which depends on the placenta for its oxygen, has much less chance for survival—practically none in severe cases and only 40% to 70% in moderate to mild cases. Many clinicians believe that an immediate Cesarean section yields the best results for mother and baby.

abscess　**1.** An accumulation of pus in a well-circumscribed area, resulting from acute bacterial infection. Abscesses can occur in many parts of the body, both internally and externally.

2. pelvic abscess. An abscess inside the genital tract, usually following childbirth, abortion or surgery or, more rarely, in the ovaries or fallopian tubes as a result of PELVIC INFLAMMATORY DISEASE. Such abscesses usually are caused by bacterial infection. The bacteria may be already present in the vagina or, more often, are introduced from the outside (by nonsterile instruments, for example). Early symptoms are pain in the pelvic region and development of a fever. With severe infection, high temperature, chills, vomiting and an abnormally fast heartbeat also may occur, singly or in combination. The white blood count will rise markedly, and a softened area becomes discernible in the pelvic mass. Treatment is usually with antibiotic drugs, often a combination of two drugs administered intravenously, the kind depending on what organisms are found to cause the infection. As soon as the abscess has ripened and begun to drain, a soft rubber tube may be inserted into the pelvic area through the abdomen and left in place for several weeks until drainage is complete.

See also PUERPERAL FEVER.

3. breast abscess. Also *submammary abscess.* An abscess that develops most often during breast-feeding if the nipples become dry and cracked. These cracks, or fissures, give access to bacteria, often staphylococci, present on the skin or in the baby's mouth. The area around the fissure becomes red, swollen and tender. Fever and chills may occur, and soon a large hard lump is palpable. Treatment consists of antibiotics, and when the abscess ripens surgical drainage may be performed. Breast abscess was once a very common occurrence after childbirth, especially with a first baby, but today early antibiotic treatment frequently cures such infections before an abscess can form.

See also MASTITIS.

absolute contraindication   See CONTRAINDICATION.

abstinence, periodic   See NATURAL FAMILY PLANNING.

abuse   See DOMESTIC ABUSE.

acini   Also *acinus* (sing.). The milk-producing glands in the breast. Each lobe inside the female BREAST is made up of many smaller lobules, which in turn contain anywhere from 10 to 100 acini. Each acinus is made up of glandular cells spherically arranged around a central space, or lumen. The cells secrete milk into the lumen, which is connected to a collecting duct. The acini and ducts are surrounded by a layer of cells having the ability to contract. When they contract, they produce a milking action, that is, they express milk from the lumen into the collecting duct. From there it is forced through other ducts into the terminal duct for each lobe, which exits on the surface of the nipple.

See also LACTATION.

acne   A common inflammatory skin disease, most often affecting the face, neck, chest and upper back. It is characterized by lesions called comedones (pimples), pustules (pus-filled lesions) and sometimes cysts. Contrary to older thought, acne is not the result of eating certain foods, such as chocolate or fats, nor of overindulging in sexual fantasies or masturbation. Rather, it is caused by a complex interaction among hormones, sebum (produced by the sebaceous or oil glands of the skin) and bacteria. Acne usually begins at PUBERTY, when the increase in androgens—male hormones produced in girls by the adrenal glands and in boys by both the testes and the adrenals—causes an increase in the size and activity of the sebaceous glands. Hereditary predisposition also plays a role. The glands secrete more oil, some of the tiny follicles on the skin become blocked and comedones form. A simple blockage, called a *blackhead* or *open comedo,* is an oil-blocked pore, part of which is exposed to the air and turns dark, or black. A *closed comedo,* or *whitehead,* forms in the same way except that the pore has no opening to the air, the oil cannot drain and a small cyst forms under the skin. Bacterial action causes pus to form, seen on the outside as a small white area; often the area around the whitehead is painful. Occasionally acne will erupt later in life, particularly premenstrually (sometimes flaring up before each menstrual period), while taking oral contraceptives or after discontinuing them. In these instances, too, the triggering mechanism seems to be changed hormone levels, though the culprit then is thought to be progesterone, which apparently is somewhat similar to the androgens. A recent study of teenagers with mild to moderate acne showed that in times of high emotional stress, such as before a major exam, students were 23% more likely to break out. Apparently levels of sebum production did not vary with stress, so it was presumed that stress triggered inflammation, which has been true in other circumstances.

With post-Pill acne the condition usually clears up within six months of stopping oral contraceptives. At menopause, acne may develop when the ovaries produce less estrogen and progesterone but the adrenal glands continue to produce androgen. Severe cystic acne that develops suddenly in middle age or later may be a symptom of ovarian or adrenal malfunction and therefore should be investigated by a physician.

Treatment for acne, basically palliative, depends on the severity of the case. With superficial acne, washing the face thoroughly two or three times a day with either a mild toilet soap or one containing special drying agents (resorcinol, salicylic acid or benzoyl peroxide) is recommended. Greasy lotions and cosmetics, which in some women actually trigger acne, should be avoided. The hair should be kept clean—shampooed two or three times a week—since oily hair can aggravate the eruptions. Sunlight (in moderate doses) and topical irritating agents, which cause dryness and scaling, may dry up superficial lesions. Tretinoin (vitamin A acid), in liquid, cream or gel form, may be effective but must be used with caution; it is applied nightly or less often for several weeks, during which time exposure to sunlight and other medications must be avoided. It usually takes several weeks to become effective. Sold under the brand name Retin-A, tretinoin appears to be able to counter the effects of sun-damaged skin, such as fine wrinkles, brown spots and scaly patches, and sometimes to halt or reverse the progress of early skin cancers. This "antiaging" value was discovered accidentally, among middle-aged patients being treated for acne. However, the drug's benefits do not appear for some months and last only as long as it is used. Furthermore, its long-term effects are not known, and most physicians caution pregnant women about its safety. Accutane, a closely related drug, can cause very severe birth defects in babies exposed to it during fetal life, even if the exposure is limited to a few days. In 2002 the U.S. Food and Drug Administration imposed strict rules for patients taking Accutane, and in 2004 a federal advisory board recommended mandatory enrollment in a registry for all who take the drug or its generic equivalent (isotretinoin) to ensure that they receive regular pregnancy tests and use two forms of birth control. Several newer drugs applied topically (as creams or gels) are less likely to irritate the skin than Accutane but also are to be avoided in pregnancy. Among them are tazarotene (Tazorac) and adapalene (Differin).

Other topical irritants used for acne include benzoyl peroxide, which kills bacteria, and various sulfur-resorcinol combinations, which cause the skin to dry and peel. Squeezing and other manipulation of the comedones and pustules, except with a special extractor, should be avoided because they can produce permanent scars. For severe acne a course of oral antibiotic therapy lasting several months, usually with tetracycline, may be helpful, but it should be noted that this drug makes women more prone to vaginal infection, especially YEAST INFECTION. Topical antibiotics avoid this side effect. Cryotherapy (freezing skin to make it peel) sometimes helps. X-ray therapy, topical application of corticosteroids and the use of hormones in general are not recommended. No matter how severe the case, acne nearly always clears up by itself after puberty when hormone levels subside; this is the only real cure.

acquired immunodeficiency syndrome   See AIDS.

acromegaly   Overproduction of the pituitary growth hormone marked by excessive body growth, especially of the hands, feet, nose and lower jaw. Laboratory tests will reveal the presence of an increase in the pituitary hormones and usually a decrease in sex hormones, resulting in amenorrhea (no menstruation) in young women. Acromegaly may be caused by a pituitary tumor, which is usually treated with radiation therapy or surgery.

acrosin test   A test that measures the enzyme activity of sperm. Such activity is required for them to penetrate the outer layer of the egg and effect fertilization.

acupressure   See ACUPUNCTURE.

acupuncture   A system of diagnosis and treatment based on the idea that disease, injury and the pain and discomfort they cause are disturbances in the body's normal flow of bioelectric energy, called *qi* or *chi*. Treatment therefore is directed at correcting obstructions, imbalances or other adverse changes in the pathways of that flow. These pathways have been mapped as a system of 14 major "meridians" passing over points associated with specific organs and body functions. To restore the body's natural balance, the principal method of treatment is the insertion of hair-thin needles of surgical steel at one or more of almost 2,000 points on the body (361 lie along the meridians; the rest are nearby) to stimulate them so as to affect the particular problem being treated. The technique varies, in some cases not even involving insertion under the skin, but merely touching it, and in others, inserted to a depth of up to an inch. Usually 10 to 12 needles are used at the same time. In one common technique, the inserted needles remain in place for 15 minutes to an hour at a time; usually a series of treatments—5 to 20 on the average—is required. The precise duration and number of treatments depend on the patient's age and general health as well as the nature of the problem. The needles, of surgical steel, are carefully sterilized. About 2 inches long and as fine as a strand of hair, they rarely cause bleeding or pain. The sensation varies, depending on the depth and angle of insertion and one's pain threshold. It may resemble a slight tingling or mild electric shock, or a vague tugging or aching feeling. Acupuncturists sometimes also use heat or electric stimulation (applied via the needles) and/or special herbal medicines and Oriental massage.

A new use of acupuncture is for cosmetic purposes. Like other cosmetic surgery, it aims to erase wrinkles and unsightly lines. Although evidence shows that acupuncture is an effective adjunctive treatment for hypertension, chronic pain, headache, and back pain, it still has not been proved that acupuncture reduces wrinkles.

Originating hundreds of years ago in China, acupuncture has become increasingly available in the West. There it is best known for treating pain, especially musculoskeletal conditions (back pain, neck pain, bursitis, sciatica, arthritis, sports injuries, etc.), in which it is believed not only to relieve discomfort but to promote healing. Some women have found it effective for such conditions as premenstrual syndrome and other kinds of dysmenorrhea, vaginal and urinary infections, endometriosis, fibrocystic breast disease, morning sickness and hot flashes. In these conditions acupuncture is believed to afford relief by restoring the hormonal balance. It also has been used with some success for drug addiction. In theory, at least, acupuncture is useful for a wide variety of complaints, ranging from the common cold to asthma, arthritis, hypertension,

infertility, substance abuse and emotional disorders (anxiety, depression). In practice, many Western patients try it as a last resort, after conventional medical therapies have failed. (In China and other Eastern countries acupuncture has the same status as Western medicine.) However, acupuncture should *not* be used by a person suffering from hemophilia or other bleeding disorders.

At this writing there are 52 nationally accredited schools of acupuncture in the United States that require three years of training in traditional Chinese medicine and passing a test for certification. They are represented by the American Association of Acupuncture and Oriental Medicine, which can provide names of certified acupuncturists. In addition, physicians who have completed a 200-hour course developed at the University of California at Los Angeles that focuses on acupuncture but does not include the use of Chinese herbs are represented by the American Academy of Medical Acupuncture, which will provide names of local members. At this writing there are an estimated 11,000 licensed U.S. acupuncturists, and this number is growing rapidly. In addition, about 3,000 chiropractors also practice acupuncture. Acupuncture also is taught in some medical schools, and as it gains acceptance by insurance companies and state regulatory agencies, it is becoming more widely available.

Licensing requirements for nonmedical practitioners vary from state to state, and in the 43 states where licenses are required, the practitioner may be called "licensed," "certified" or a "diplomate (of acupuncture)." To find a competent practitioner one should consult either of the two professional organizations listed in the Appendix, under Acupuncture.

Even if an acupuncturist comes well recommended, one should guard against infection by making sure that the needles used either are disposable (for one-time use) or have been properly sterilized (in an autoclave for at least 30 minutes at 250 pounds of pressure). Some practitioners use disposable needles on request, and others keep a particular set of needles for each patient.

A related technique is *acupressure,* in which the relevant points on the body are stimulated by applying pressure rather than by inserting needles.

There are a variety of acupressure techniques. Once a technique has been demonstrated, it can be performed by a friend or family member.

acute Developing suddenly, having severe symptoms and usually (but not always) brief in duration. The opposite of acute is CHRONIC.

addiction Dependence on a mind-altering drug or on alcohol, interfering with the ability to work, study or interact with family and friends, and sometimes leading to lying, stealing or similar behavior in order to obtain the substance. Every addictive substance, whether it is morphine or another pain-killer, cocaine, marijuana, heroin, amphetamines, nicotine or alcohol, induces a pleasant state or relieves distress. Continued use induces adaptive changes in the central nervous system that lead to tolerance, physical dependence, sensitization and craving. Today, addiction is generally regarded as a brain ailment rather than a moral failing. It can be treated and overcome, but not easily. Stopping use generally gives rise to withdrawal symptoms, which can be very serious, so a process of *detoxification* must be instituted. For addicts to opioids (morphine, oxycodone, heroin, etc.) withdrawal symptoms can be eased with clonidine or methadone; the latter, however, is itself strongly addictive and available only in clinics. A newer prescription medication approved in 2002, buprenorphine, also an opiate, is available in pharmacies and does not, like methadone, cloud the mind and allows patients to work or study, as well as to lose all physical cravings for drugs, and many can wean off the drug, sometimes within a year. For mild addiction to prescription drugs, gradual decrease of dosage may overcome the dependency.

See also ALCOHOL USE; DRUG USE AND PREGNANCY; SMOKING, TOBACCO.

adenocarcinoma 1. A cancer involving gland tissue (see CANCER) or one whose cells take the form of gland tissue. Most breast cancers are adenocarcinomas.

2. clear-cell adenocarcinoma. A cancer of the vagina and cervix first noted in the 1960s in daughters of women who had received diethylstilbestrol (DES) while pregnant. In normal women the vaginal lining has no gland tissue, so adenocarcinomas cannot develop there. However, many daughters of women who took DES while pregnant have been found to have many tiny glands in their vagina (see ADENOSIS, def. 1), presumably caused by DES in the developing fetus. Since that discovery and the realization that DES daughters, as they are called, have a much higher risk of developing vaginal and cervical cancer, there has been a widespread effort to locate and warn all such women to undergo frequent examination. Treatment depends on the location of the tumors. Those in the vaginal wall generally respond to radiation, which, however, can cause vaginal stenosis (narrowing); this can sometimes be avoided by surgical means or corrected by grafting.

See also DIETHYLSTILBESTROL.

3. of the uterus. The most common kind of uterine cancer, arising in the endometrium (uterine lining).

See also CANCER, ENDOMETRIAL.

adenofibroma Another name for FIBROADENOMA.

adenomyosis A condition in which fragments of endometrial tissue (from the lining of the uterus) become embedded in the muscular wall of the uterus. Like ENDOMETRIOSIS, it represents a displacement of endometrial tissue. It tends to occur somewhat later in life, between the ages of 35 and 50. The symptoms of adenomyosis include menorrhagia (longer, more profuse menstrual periods) and dysmenorrhea (painful periods), which range from mild pressure and discomfort to severe, colicky pain (caused when the endometrial tissue becomes swollen). Pelvic examination shows the uterus to be enlarged, soft and boggy. For minor symptoms no treatment is required. More severe symptoms may be treated with hormones to interrupt the menstrual cycle, as in endometriosis, or a D AND C to scrape out some of the endometrial tissue. If neither treatment is effective and severe pain persists, hysterectomy (surgical removal of the uterus) may be recommended. Adenomyosis tends to disappear after menopause, when estrogen production is greatly reduced.

adenosis **1.** The presence of abnormal, mucus-secreting gland tissue in the cervix or vagina. It is an extremely rare condition except in daughters of women who took DIETHYLSTILBESTROL (DES) during the first trimester of pregnancy, about 90% of whom have been found to have adenosis. Since it is believed to be a precancerous lesion, which may develop into ADENOCARCINOMA (see def. 2), careful diagnosis and regular follow-up care are urged. Diagnosis involves COLPOSCOPY. If adenosis is found, a PAP SMEAR and pelvic examination should be performed every six months, and colposcopy at least yearly. Some physicians treat the condition with more aggressive methods, ranging from electric cautery (burning) and cryosurgery (freezing) to surgical excision of the abnormal tissue, but most prefer a more conservative approach. Some clinicians recommend avoiding the use of oral contraceptives lest they encourage the growth of the lesions, but others see no connection between the two.
   2. See SCLEROSING ADENOSIS.

adhesion Also *synechia, scar tissue.* A dense layer of connective tissue that forms over a healing abrasion, cut or other lesion. In the pelvic area, especially in the fallopian tubes, uterus and cervix, adhesions can cause infertility (see ASHERMAN'S SYNDROME). Adhesions in the abdominal area can cause intestinal blockage, a serious and potentially fatal condition.

adjuvant treatment Any treatment used in addition to some other treatment in order to enhance its effects. The term is used particularly for additional systemic treatment following surgery for CANCER, such as radiation therapy, hormone therapy, bone marrow transplants and/or chemotherapy.

adnexae Neighboring organs. Gynecologists and obstetricians frequently use this term for the organs adjacent to the uterus, that is, the fallopian tubes and ovaries.

adolescence See PUBERTY.

adolescent nodule A smooth, round enlargement directly under the nipple of the breast, seen most often in girls aged 9 to 11 and in boys 12 to 14. The nipple usually is tender to the touch. The nodule results from hormone stimulation of gland tissue during puberty, a condition that generally subsides after some months. No treatment of any kind is advisable.

adrenalectomy Surgical removal of the ADRENAL GLANDS, a treatment once used for advanced breast cancers whose growth is stimulated by estrogen (see ESTROGEN-RECEPTOR ASSAY). Since the adrenal glands produce some estrogen, their removal reduces levels of that hormone. After such surgery the patient had to receive replacement of the vital adrenal hormones, usually in the form of hydrocortisone, for the rest of her life. However, hormone therapy directed at blocking estrogen production may be just as effective and is reversible. Adrenalectomy also may be performed in aldosteronism (see ALDOSTERONE).

adrenal glands A pair of ENDOCRINE glands that are located on top of each kidney (*ad-* means "on," *renal* means "pertaining to the kidney"). Each gland consists of a *cortex,* a firm outer portion that constitutes most of the gland, and a *medulla,* a soft inner part. The medulla produces the hormone *adrenaline,* while the cortex produces more than 30 different hormones, some of which are indispensable to life. The most important of them are cortisol and corticosterone, both glucocorticoids (cortisol lets the body get energy from carbohydrates, maintains blood pressure and offers protection from physical stress); aldosterone, a mineralocorticoid that keeps the kidneys from losing too much sodium and water (see ALDOSTERONE); and dehydroepiandrosterone sulfate and androstenedione, both androgens (male hormones). The adrenals also produce other steroids such as estrogen, which can in some cases aggravate a disease process (see ADRENALECTOMY) and after menopause may compensate somewhat for diminished estrogen production by the ovaries.

The proportions of hormones produced by the adrenal glands vary with a person's age. The adrenals of the FETUS produce mainly dehydroepiandrosterone sulfate. During infancy and childhood the corticoids are produced in amounts proportional to body size; in puberty and thereafter the androgens are produced in significant amounts, but it is not known whether this is a cause or a result of pubertal changes. In old age corticoid production continues but that of the adrenal androgens may decline, a change that some think may be responsible for OSTEOPOROSIS and other bone changes of old age.

In order to function, the adrenal cortex must be stimulated by another hormone, ACTH (adrenocorticotropic hormone), produced by the pituitary gland. ACTH release in turn is controlled by a release factor produced by the hypothalamus. In the absence of ACTH, the adrenal glands atrophy (shrink) and cease to secrete most hormones; the only exception is aldosterone, which is produced in an outer layer of the adrenal cortex and appears to be stimulated by a substance called angiotensin, formed in blood plasma and activated by complex enzyme changes.

The adrenal glands are subject to a number of diseases, two of which in particular affect women, causing menstrual irregularities and other problems. They are ADRENOGENITAL SYNDROME and CUSHING'S SYNDROME.

adrenal hyperplasia   See ADRENOGENITAL SYNDROME.

adrenal steroid   A steroid HORMONE produced by the adrenal glands.

adrenogenital syndrome   Also *adrenal virilism, congenital adrenal hyperplasia*. A disorder, usually present from birth, that is characterized by overproduction of androgens by the adrenal glands, resulting in the development of male secondary sex characteristics in girls and precocious sexual development in boys. The effects depend on the age of the patient and are more marked in females. The underlying cause is usually either a tumor of the adrenal glands or hyperplasia (overgrowth of gland tissue), which in turn may be caused by an inherited enzyme deficiency that prevents the adrenal glands from synthesizing cortisol. The principal symptom is hirsutism (excess body hair), which appears even in mild cases. Other symptoms include baldness, acne, deepening of the voice, cessation of menstruation, atrophy of the uterus, deformed genitals (especially growth of the clitoris so that it resembles a small penis), decreased breast size and increased muscularity. Treatment with cortisone usually eliminates the condition; in the congenital form of the disease it must be continued for life.

aerobic exercise   See EXERCISE.

AFP   See ALPHA-FETOPROTEIN TEST.

afterbirth   Another name for PLACENTA.

afterpains   Uterine contractions following the delivery of a baby.
See also CONTRACTION, UTERINE.

agalactia   The inability to lactate (secrete milk) after childbirth. True total agalactia is a rare condition. When the quantity of milk secreted is smaller than desired, the condition usually can be corrected by more frequent stimulation of the breasts by suckling.
See also BREAST-FEEDING; LACTATION.

age, childbearing   In theory, the years from the first ovulation following MENARCHE (average age, 12.6) through MENOPAUSE (average age, 50). Physically, the ideal years for childbearing are from the late teens through the twenties. Indeed, any woman who becomes pregnant when she is under the age of 16 or over 34 is considered at risk (see HIGH-RISK PREGNANCY). The risk is to both mother and child. Pregnant women over 34 run a greater risk of developing complications such as pre-eclampsia and placenta previa, although placental complications appear to be linked more to cardiovascular disease than to maternal age. They also are more likely to have diabetes or hypertension, disorders that increase with age. Labor and delivery are likely to be more difficult, especially with a first baby. The rate of premature delivery rises. Labor tends to be prolonged, ABNORMAL PRESENTATION is more common and postpartum hemorrhage (owing to weak uterine contractions after delivery) also occurs more often. Other hazards to the baby, apart from those named above, concern the greater likelihood of BIRTH DEFECTS. One genetic defect associated with older women is DOWN SYNDROME, the risk for which is 10 times higher after the age of 40 than it is for a woman in her 20s. Other chromosomal abnormalities also are related to maternal age, along with nonchromosomal defects such as cleft lip and palate, congenital heart defects, spina bifida, hydrocephalus and cerebral palsy. Since certain defects can be detected by AMNIOCENTESIS or CHORIONIC VILLUS SAMPLING, some clinicians recommend that all pregnant women of 35 and older undergo one of these procedures. Age also affects the capacity of the uterus to sustain a fetus, so that with increasing age there is a higher risk of miscarriage and stillbirth. However, in recent years, by means of IN VITRO FERTILIZATION, a number of postmenopausal women have been impregnated by using eggs taken from younger women and fertilized with sperm from the older woman's husband, and have given birth to healthy offspring. Despite the risks, more and more women are delivering a first baby after the age of 35, and between 1970 and 1990 there was a 50% increase in the rate of first births to women between 40 and 44 years of age.

Young teenagers also are at high risk. They have a higher incidence of pregnancy-induced hypertension, preeclampsia and eclampsia, and their babies tend to have a low birth weight. Anemia also is more common, perhaps as a result of poor nutrition. Statistics indicate that the rate of American

CHROMOSOMAL ABNORMALITY AND MOTHER'S AGE

Mother	Risk
Age 20	= 1 in 525
Age 25	= 1 in 475
Age 30	= 1 in 380
Age 35	= 1 in 180 (approx. 0.5%)
Age 38	= 1 in 105 (approx. 1%)
Age 40	= 1 in 65 (approx. 1.5%)
Age 42	= 1 in 40 (approx. 2.5%)
Age 45	= 1 in 20 (approx. 5%)

teenagers aged 15 to 19 who bear children has been steadily rising, a matter of considerable concern. However, there are important considerations besides physical ones for parenthood, and ideally all factors should be examined and weighed before undertaking a pregnancy.

See also PREGNANCY COUNSELING.

age-parity formula See STERILIZATION.

agoraphobia An irrational fear (phobia) of open spaces, which for most sufferers usually means any place other than their own home. A person with agoraphobia who leaves home (for a store, a street, an airport—almost anywhere) will often experience an *anxiety attack,* that is, a sense of overwhelming panic, with such physical manifestations as nausea, sweating, rapid heartbeat and dizziness. (See also ANXIETY.) Agoraphobia is much more common in women than in men and tends to strike early, often beginning in the late teens or early twenties. It has been variously explained. According to traditional psychoanalytic theory, patients develop phobias in order to avoid certain objects or situations. They often have the feeling that something terrible, but usually nameless, will happen to them. In extreme cases of agoraphobia, fear may keep a person a virtual prisoner in the home, afraid of venturing outdoors at all. Psychoanalytic treatment of agoraphobia, directed at having the patient discover the roots of the fear in her past, has not been very successful. More patients seem to benefit from a behavioral approach, which is less concerned with the source of the fear than with conditioning a person not to be afraid.

AIDS Acronym for *acquired immunodeficiency syndrome,* a fatal condition first diagnosed in 1981 and caused by the *human immunodeficiency virus,* or *HIV,* first identified in 1983 and known in two forms, HIV-1 and HIV-2. The virus attacks the body's immune system so that it becomes vulnerable to infections and cancers ordinarily resisted. These diseases ultimately cause death; at this writing there is no cure for AIDS.

A woman can contract AIDS through intimate sexual contact with an infected person, by sharing intravenous needles with an infected person, or through contact with blood, semen or vaginal or cervical secretions contaminated with HIV. The greatest risk of infection for women is intravenous drug use and/or sex with intravenous drug users. Furthermore, women are 10 times more likely than men to contract HIV during unprotected sex with an infected partner. (See below for more details on how HIV is transmitted.) Moreover, women diagnosed with HIV develop AIDS symptoms sooner and with less of the virus in the bloodstream than men.

An infected woman may infect not only her sexual partner but also her baby during pregnancy or through breast-feeding. The chances of a baby's being infected in utero are 25–30%; the risk can be reduced by giving the mother the drug AZT (see below).

HIV is a retrovirus that can reside in the body for nine years or longer before giving rise to any symptoms. During this period a person carrying HIV can infect others, whose symptoms actually may appear sooner than those in the carrier. Often the earliest symptoms are swollen glands and a brief illness resembling mononucleosis (aches and pains, fever, swollen glands), which subsides; in many patients no such episode occurs.

Eventually the infection progresses to an intermediate stage, at one time called *AIDS-related complex (ARC).* The most common symptom is lymphadenopathy—swollen lymph nodes in the neck, armpits and/or groin, which may be either painless or tender. Other symptoms include loss of appetite and weight loss (very severe, that is, 15% of body weight); intermittent fever and night sweats; fatigue and malaise; persistent unexplained diarrhea; persistent dry cough; oral thrush (candidiasis), a yeast infection characterized by white spots and blemishes in the mouth and throat; shingles; hairy leukoplakia, a precancerous condition characterized by white sores and a thickened mucous membrane in the mouth and vagina; leukopenia (lowered white blood-cell count); and thrombocytopenia (increase in blood platelets).

Full-fledged AIDS is said to exist if the patient has one or more life-threatening opportunistic infections (illnesses taking advantage of the body's lowered resistance) and/or particular cancers known to be associated with HIV infection. (It is also diagnosed by a blood test; see below). The principal opportunistic diseases are pneumocystis pneumonia, a lung infection caused by the parasite *Pneumocystis carinii,* as well as recurrent pneumonia caused by other organisms (pneumonia is the leading cause of HIV-related morbidity and death); cytomegalovirus (CMV) infection, a type of herpes virus that can cause blindness, pneumonia, colitis and esophagitis; candidiasis (yeast infection) of the esophagus, causing pain and difficulty in swallowing; cryptosporidiosis, severe diarrhea caused by the parasite *Cryptosporidium;* cryptococcosis, an infection of the central nervous system or kidneys, bone or skin caused by the organism *Filobasidiella neoformans;* toxoplasmosis, a type of encephalitis caused by the protozoan parasite *Toxoplasma gondii;* Kaposi's sarcoma, a skin cancer; invasive cervical cancer; infection of the brain or lungs (including tuberculosis) caused by *Myobacterium avium intracellulae;* herpes simplex infections of various organs; tuberculosis; and dementia.

In women, certain conditions that persist and seem resistant to treatment are also suspected of becoming opportunistic infections; these include pelvic inflammatory disease, genital warts, yeast infection, genital herpes, chronic vaginitis and any of the SEXUALLY TRANSMITTED DISEASES. Consequently women who have an extensive history of these conditions may be advised to be tested for HIV.

Diagnosis of HIV infection is based on a blood test for HIV antibodies, which, however, is not always wholly accurate. In low-risk individuals who test positive, another, more accurate test is used for confirmation. Further, a negative antibody test may mean that the person was exposed recently but antibodies have not yet developed; that response sometimes takes a few weeks, but in some cases many months or even years. The presence of antibodies indicates that a person will probably develop AIDS but possibly not for 6 to 8 years (the range is 1 to 20 years). Recently scientists discovered a gene variant that is responsible for the very rapid decline of some HIV-infected persons, resulting in death in one to three years. It is present in approximately 10% of all individuals. One in four Americans living with HIV do not know they are infected. Since early diagnosis can mean early treatment and longer lives, the U.S. Centers for Disease Control has recommended that doctors ask all patients between the ages of 13 and 64 whether they want to be tested for the virus.

Anyone with a positive test result, even if no symptoms are present, can infect someone else and therefore is urged not to donate blood, sperm or organs for transplant; any such woman is strongly advised to avoid pregnancy lest she infect her baby. In more advanced stages, when suspicious symptoms have occurred, diagnosis of AIDS is based on measuring the levels of the particular white blood cells that control the body's immune responses to disease-causing organisms that are attacked by HIV—called CD4+ or T-lymphocytes. A count of 200 or fewer CD4+ T-cells per cubic millimeter of blood (as opposed to 800 to 1,300 in healthy individuals) is currently defined as a diagnosis of AIDS. Although these blood cells are HIV's principal targets, the virus also attacks other cells, notably brain cells, and so can cause serious neurologic and psychological problems. (See also HIV.)

AIDS is a bloodborne disease. The virus penetrates through the skin and into the body, not only through cuts in the skin or injections into the blood but through tiny tears or sores in the mucous membranes of the mouth, vagina or rectum. Although it is transmitted most readily through unprotected anal intercourse because rectal tissue is more easily broken than vaginal tissue, it can be transmitted in any contact involving the sharing of bodily fluids in which the virus is present. That includes heterosexual vaginal intercourse, in which the most common pattern of transmission of AIDS is from man to woman (who is especially vulnerable if she is menstruating or has vaginal lesions due to vaginitis, fibroids, pelvic inflammatory disease, herpes, yeast infection, an IUD, a dry vagina or some other cause). Woman-to-man infection also occurs, and although it is rarer, woman-to-woman transmission of HIV is also possible. The exposure of a mucous membrane such as the mouth to vaginal secretions and menstrual blood is potentially infectious.

AIDS also can be transmitted through oral sex, anal sex, fisting, finger insertion, rimming, and sharing uncleaned sex appliances such as dildos and vibrators. It is also readily transmitted through injections with contaminated needles or serum (hemophiliac men, who rely on blood transfusions and consequently were infected with the virus before it was known to present a danger, were an early source of the infection's spread; today blood for transfusion is routinely tested for the virus). Shared needles used for drug use, tattooing or body piercing also present a danger. AIDS can be transmitted through the placenta, and even though transmission to the baby is estimated at about 25 to 35% and can be reduced by some treatments (see below), HIV-positive women who become pregnant are urged to consider terminating the pregnancy. Transmission also can occur through breast milk, but more rarely.

Although AIDS is an infectious disease, it is not highly contagious through superficial contact. One cannot get AIDS by touching or hugging a patient. The virus may be present in an infected person's saliva, but a quick kiss on the mouth probably will not transmit it; a deep, open-mouth kiss, however, might do so. Neither perspiration nor vomit contains the virus, and tears and urine contain only miniscule amounts. It also cannot be transmitted through food preparation, drinking from the same glass, toilet seats or insect bites.

It is believed that HIV originated in African monkeys; by the late 1970s there was a human epidemic in central Africa. In the United States, in the early years since AIDS was first diagnosed, the ratio of infection was 15 men to every woman. However, as diagnosis and testing have become more sophisticated, a larger and larger proportion of women have been found to be infected. In Africa, which in 1994 accounted for 70% of the world's 15 million AIDS patients, the disease seems to affect both sexes equally, and the infection was spreading most rapidly among teenagers and young adults (ages 15 to 24).

At this writing there is no definite cure for AIDS. Four kinds of drug are currently available to treat HIV infection. The oldest is the antiviral agent azidothymidine (AZT; later renamed zidovudine, or ZDU), first approved in 1987. In pregnant women who test positive for HIV, it cut by two-thirds the risk of the mother's transmitting HIV to her baby. Moreover, Cesarean delivery also cuts the risk and combined with AZT, the chance of infecting the baby drops to 2%. In 2004 a new study showed that a single dose of a generic AIDS drug, nevirapine, given to mothers during labor and to babies after delivery, prevented transmission of HIV in four out of five cases. All the mothers were also receiving treatment with AZT and none of the babies was breast-fed. AZT belongs to the class of drugs called nucleoside reverse transcriptase inhibitors. The other three classes are the non-nucleoside reverse transcriptase inhibitors, protease inhibitors, and entry inhibitors. None actually kills HIV, but each prevents the virus from replicating, and all have fairly severe side effects. Also, because HIV usually becomes resistant to any of these drugs when used alone, they are best administered when at least two or three are given together in a "cocktail," which is more powerful than single drugs in reducing HIV levels, helps prevent the development of drug resistance, and in some cases boosts the level of the other drugs. In 2006 the FDA approved a three-in-one antiretroviral pill, to be taken by HIV patients twice a day. It combines the three common first-line drugs: AZT, sold in the United States as Retrovir; 3TC (lamivudine, sold as Epivir); and NVP (nevirapine, sold as Viramune). It does not include another first-line drug, D4T (stavudine, or Zerit), which is more toxic than the others. Another new formulation required taking only one pill a day. In 2007 the FDA approved another new drug, maraviroc (Selzentry), which blocks a crucial doorway, the CCR5 receptor, that the HIV virus uses to enter white blood cells. Also in process of testing are Isentress and GS-9137, which stop HIV from duplicating inside the body. Guidelines from the U.S. Public Health Service recommend starting antiviral treatment when testing indicates there are 10,000 copies of HIV per milliliter of blood, indicating that the immune system is losing ground to the virus; however, studies indicate that women infected with HIV may be at a more advanced stage of infection and at higher risk for developing AIDS than men with identical blood test results. Therefore it is possible that treatment for women should begin earlier than for men.

Treatment has reduced deaths from AIDS considerably; however, by the late 1990s the AIDS virus had at least a dozen strains, some of which had developed resistance to antiviral drugs. Moreover, it was suspected that one individual could harbor several strains of the virus, suggesting even greater difficulties for successful treatment.

Some patients have found relief of symptoms through ALTERNATIVE MEDICINE of various kinds, such as acupuncture or herbs to improve immune system functioning and relieve the side effects of anti-AIDS drugs, relaxation exercises to lessen stress, and nutritional supplements to increase physical energy. All these treatments are basically palliative.

SAFE SEX TO AVOID AIDS

- Avoid multiple partners, unknown partners or partners who themselves may have had multiple and/or unknown partners.
- Avoid receptive, insertive anal intercourse; avoid contact with semen, blood, feces, or urine; if engaging in anal intercourse, use a latex condom and a water-based lubricant.
- Do not share dildos or other insertive objects.
- Avoid sexual contact with intravenous drug users, including open-mouth kissing.
- Avoid oral sex, including oral-anal contact, with an infected or high-risk partner.
- Use a fresh condom and spermicide (nonoxynol-9, which may kill the virus) for each instance of vaginal intercourse; use a condom alone for oral sex; use latex (not "natural") condoms, and throw away after intercourse.
- Do not douche before or after sex.
- Do not use Vaseline or any other oil-based lubricant (they weaken condoms); do not use saliva as a lubricant; use only water-based gels.
- Avoid intravenous drugs; if you do use them, never employ a used needle.

Currently researchers are focusing on various approaches, among them developing an AIDS vaccine, finding a wholly effective vaginal microbicide that would kill the AIDS-causing organism without damaging either the woman's tissues or the man's sperm (lest damage to the latter cause birth defects) and discovering various means of restoring the body's immune function. Gene therapy—attacking the HIV virus at the gene level—is a promising avenue of research but is still in fairly early stages. The development of a vaccine may be even more difficult, since the traditional form of development—treatment with an inactivated or weakened virus—is too dangerous.

Until an effective cure and/or preventive vaccine for AIDS is available, prevention is the only possible protection. The principal means is so-called *safe sex*—in reality only *safer* sex—the recommendations for which are listed in the accompanying chart.

albumin, urinary   Also *albuminuria*. The principal protein found in the urine of persons suffering from a variety of kidney diseases. It is not present in normal urine. In pregnant women it is a warning sign of PREECLAMPSIA, and for this reason testing the urine for albumin is a standard part of each prenatal check-up.

alcohol use   The drinking of alcoholic beverages, which in moderation—a drink or two a day—is generally thought to be harmless for most individuals, but which in larger quantities can be harmful and addictive, so that a person becomes severely dependent on alcohol. Some researchers distinguish between *alcohol abuse* and *alcoholism*. They define the first as drinking-related failure to fulfill one's obligations at work, school, or home, incurring interpersonal social or legal problems due to alcohol use, and drinking in hazardous situations. Alcoholism, on the other hand, is characterized by compulsive drinking, preoccupation with drinking, and elevated tolerance to alcohol. Combined, they affected 17.6 million Americans in 2001–02, up from 13.8 million a decade earlier.

The National Institute on Alcohol Abuse and Alcoholism defines light drinking as less than one drink per day, consisting of 12 ounces of beer or 5 ounces of wine or 1.5 ounces of distilled spirits (whiskey, brandy or the like). Some authorities think one drink a day is not problematic. However, they warn that seven drinks a week or more than three drinks on one occasion may be risky.

While the moderate use of alcohol is actually thought to be of some physical benefit to the heart, heavy drinking can damage the heart and blood vessels. Heavy drinking also is associated with cancer (particularly when combined with heavy cigarette smoking), especially of the mouth, throat, larynx and esophagus, stomach, pancreas and breast, as well as with serious liver disease. Alcohol increases the body's need for two B vitamins, niacin and thiamine, which are used in its metabolism, and for folic acid, with whose absorption and storage it interferes, and it seems to impede calcium absorption. Other disorders associated with alcoholism (alcohol addiction) are peptic ulcer, severe anemia, and depression, eating disorders and other mental illnesses. Combining alcohol with other drugs, even with necessary medications, can have severe and sometimes fatal results. Combining sleeping pills, antidepressants or anti-anxiety medication with alcohol is particularly dangerous, and contrary to popular thought, caffeine can enhance rather than counteract alcohol's effects.

Heavy drinking during pregnancy can cause serious and irreversible birth defects. Babies of alcoholic mothers are at risk for *fetal alcohol syndrome*, a pattern of physical and mental defects that includes severe growth deficiency, heart defects, malformed facial features, a small head, abnormalities of fine motor coordination and mental retardation. Since it is not known exactly how much alcohol intake endangers a fetus, it generally is recommended that a pregnant woman restrict herself to no more than two ounces of table wine a day. Furthermore, some authorities warn that even this amount can be detrimental in some individuals, and to be absolutely safe *no alcohol* should be consumed during pregnancy, an opinion endorsed by the U.S. Surgeon General's Office in 1981.

The causes of alcoholism are not known, but it is a serious health problem that is affecting more and more American women. Until about 1970 male alcoholics were believed to outnumber female alcoholics 5 to 1. Since then studies indicate that the difference is rapidly narrowing, especially among younger persons, including girls in the early teens. Women apparently become drunk more quickly than men, even if they drink the same amount relative to body size, because their stomachs are less able to neutralize alcohol (they have less of the enzyme alcohol dehydrogenase), so that much more alcohol (an estimated 30% more) goes directly into the bloodstream through the stomach wall and thence to the brain. Moreover, the ability to metabolize alcohol declines with age. In alcoholic women the stomach apparently stops digesting alcohol totally, which is not the case with alcoholic men.

Treatment for alcoholism usually involves *detoxification*—recovery from both acute intoxication and withdrawal—and related medical care as well as counseling and/or psychotherapy to gain understanding of the underlying problems and to help change the alcoholic's living patterns appropriately. Local alcoholism treatment clinics usually offer outpatient services, including medical treatment, psychotherapy, Alcoholics Anonymous services and vocational guidance. For the severely ill, inpatient care may be needed in a hospital, detoxification center, residential care facility or alcoholism clinic. The drug disulfiram (Antabuse) has long been used for alcoholism; anyone taking the drug and then drinking an alcoholic beverage becomes very ill (nausea and vomiting, drop in blood pressure, severe headache, etc.). Another drug used to lessen alcohol dependency is naltrexone. It does not make one sick, but it does allow continued drinking, and it cannot be used by a person with liver disease. Approved in 2006, administered in a monthly injection and sold as Vivitrol, it is thought to reduce the euphoria alcoholics feel when they drink. A prescription medication approved in 2004, Campral, blocks cravings for alcohol, and still others are being developed. In China herbal healers have long treated alcohol abuse with a medicine derived from the root of the kudzu vine, which seems to reduce alcohol craving without other side effects. Western scientists who extracted two active ingredients from this plant found they reduced alcohol consumption in hamsters, and it is hoped there will soon be a clinical application to human patients.

aldosterone A hormone secreted by the ADRENAL GLANDS that causes body tissues to retain sodium, and therefore water, and to lose potassium. Overproduction of aldosterone (*aldosteronism*), owing to a tumor or to hyperplasia (overgrowth) of the adrenal glands, is characterized by hypertension (high blood pressure) and muscular weakness as well as fluid and sodium retention combined with potassium loss. Treatment consists of removing the tumor or, sometimes, the entire gland (ADRENALECTOMY).

Secondary aldosteronism, caused by some disorder outside the adrenals, is similar in symptoms and signs to primary aldosteronism and like it is characterized by edema (fluid retention). Some authorities believe that aldosterone may be implicated in the fluid retention associated with premenstrual tension (see DYSMENORRHEA, def. 5).

alopecia See HAIR LOSS.

alpha-fetoprotein test Also *AFP, maternal serum test.* A blood test performed to evaluate the development of the fetus and to look for fetal abnormalities. Alpha-fetoprotein (AFP) is a substance produced by the fetus early in life, present in both the amniotic fluid and the mother's bloodstream. Abnormally high levels are associated with various birth defects, especially NEURAL TUBE DEFECTS such as spina bifida; they also occur when the mother is carrying twins and when the fetus has died. A low level suggests a higher than average risk of Down syndrome. A blood test performed at 16 to 18 weeks screens those women who are likely to be carrying affected fetuses. If a second test confirms a high AFP level, ultrasound or amniocentesis are indicated to determine if birth defects actually are present.

Nowadays the AFP test is often combined with two other tests, giving it the name *triple screen* or *maternal serum alpha-fetoprotein-3 (MSAFP-3) test.* It measures not only AFP but estriol, the dominant estrogen in pregnancy, and human chorionic gonadotropin (HCG), produced by the developing embryo.

alternative medicine Also *complementary and alternative medicine, holistic medicine.* A general name for various forms of treatment that differ from traditional Western medical practice. It includes approaches that rely on the well-established principle that stress and emotions can affect physical health, often called *mind-body therapies;* among them are BIOFEEDBACK, HYPNOTHERAPY, meditation, relaxation training and guided imagery (VISUALIZATION). Mind-body therapies have been particularly useful for easing pain from headaches, arthritis and low back problems, and an estimated 30% of American adults have used them. They often are used in conjunction with conventional medical treatment. Hence the term *complementary medicine,* meaning it is used as an adjunct; for example, AROMATHERAPY might be used to lessen discomfort following surgery, whereas a special diet used to treat cancer instead of surgery, radiation or chemotherapy would be considered *alternative medicine.* Another term is *integrative medicine,* which similarly combines conventional with alternative medicine, but where the latter shows high-quality evidence of both safety and effectiveness. Examples include acupuncture and massage used together with conventional cancer treatment. The term also includes the practice of ACUPUNCTURE, of manipulative therapies such as CHIROPRACTIC and various kinds of MASSAGE therapy, and of therapies relying on the use of alternative medications, such as HOMEOPATHY, NATUROPATHY, HERBAL REMEDIES, aromatherapy, nutritional therapies such as PROBIOTICS and megavitamins as well as numerous substances aimed at treating cancer. Some of these treatments, such as acupuncture, herbalism, yoga and AYURVEDA, have a long and honorable tradition in non-Western cultures. Others, such as biofeedback, are of more recent origin, although their roots usually can be traced to older modalities. In many instances patients turn to such therapies when conventional medicine has failed to relieve their symptoms, but as pointed out, some are used in conjunction with conventional treatment. Long disdained, dismissed or at best ignored by the American medical establishment, alternative medicine has attracted an increasing number of patients, and gradually at least some of these therapies have been acknowledged to be effective. In 1992 the U.S. government's National Institutes of Health opened an Office of Alternative Medicine in order to foster serious research in alternative treatments and evaluate their effectiveness. Meanwhile, it seems prudent to try conventional treatment before turning to alternative medicine (or combining the two). Further, before choosing a practitioner, one should investigate his or her training and certification; the scope of his or her practice and specialties; methods of assessment and treatment; and use of tests, medications and other substances.

Alzheimer's disease An organic disease of the elderly characterized by memory loss, intellectual deterioration, confusion and dementia, ending in death. It may occur in the middle years (40s and 50s) and was long identified only with such early onset (then called *presenile dementia*). Since the late 1970s, however, the name *Alzheimer's* has meant dementia caused by a specific kind of brain degeneration regardless of the patient's age. Alzheimer's is overwhelmingly a disease of the very old, and since women tend to outlive men by a decade or so, it is more prevalent in women.

At this writing, Alzheimer's is incurable and can be definitively diagnosed only by examining brain tissue under a microscope, which reveals plaques of a protein called beta amyloid and tangles inside cells of a second protein called tau. There is also a crippling loss of nerve cells in brain areas involved in cognitive functions, which leads to the main symptom, failure of memory. A brain scan made with positron emission tomography (PET) can show reduced activity in those parts of the brain affected by Alzheimer's and can help diagnose the disease earlier, giving patients time to perhaps start medication and arrange for long-term care. Definitive diagnosis still requires brain biopsy, rarely done because it is difficult and dangerous and consequently performed only at autopsy.

Because numerous other treatable and reversible conditions can give rise to Alzheimer-like symptoms—notably depression, drug intoxication, thyroid imbalance, vitamin B_{12} deficiency, hormonal disorders, hypothermia, various chemical imbalances, small strokes—it is essential to rule these out before accepting a presumptive diagnosis of Alzheimer's. The earliest symptoms, absentmindedness and forgetfulness, are hard to distinguish from normal levels of these characteristics. But as the brain decays, memory loss becomes more severe and personality changes such as paranoia, confusion or belligerence occur. In the final stages, usually 8 to 10 years after diagnosis, patients often cannot control their bodily functions, becoming incontinent, unable to speak, swallow or recognize their families.

The cause of Alzheimer's is not yet known, but scientists have identified five genes as mutations that cause the buildup of amyloid in susceptible individuals. It is now hoped that such findings will enable not only early identification of those at risk but preventive therapy as well. Several recently developed procedures show promise for early diagnosis. One involves an eye test using tropicamide, which dilates the pupils far more in Alzheimer's patients than in others. Another is a blood test to identify three versions of ApoE, a protein, one of which appears to be associated with increased risk and another with reduced risk of developing Alzheimer's. A third uses an imaging technology called SPECT, similar to a bone scan, which measures blood flow to tissues. Comparing the brains of older adults and persons who report mild memory loss, it was found that most who showed abnormal functioning in key brain areas governing memory eventually developed Alzheimer's. At this writing all these tests are still experimental, and more studies are required to verify the results. Among other tools being tried to detect early signs of the disorder is magnetic resonance imaging (MRI) to measure atrophy in key areas of the brain. In one study, individuals with mild cognitive impairment had greater rates of brain shrinkage even before symptoms appeared.

Meanwhile several avenues of treatment are being investigated, among them the use of vitamin E for its antioxidant properties (the damage may result from oxygen-rich compounds released during brain cell activity); estrogen, for a similar effect; and cholinisterase inhibitors, to combat an enzyme that mops up acetylcholine, a chemical that helps nerve cells exchange messages and is deficient in Alzheimer's patients. One study found that intravenous immunoglobulin, a substance used to treat immune disorders, alters amyloid levels in the body, which may slow or even halt

mental decline in cases of mild to moderate Alzheimer's. Cholinesterase inhibitors, medications used to improve memory, judgment and thought, are often prescribed for dementia patients. The principal ones used are donezepil, galantamine and rivastigmine. So far, four acetylcholine enhancers have been approved for treatment—donepezil (Aricept), tacrine (Cognex), rivastigmine (Exelon), and galantamine (Reminyl); they produce improvement for a time in some patients with mild to moderate Alzheimer's. The first drug approved to treat advanced Alzheimer's, memantine (Namenda), blocks excess amounts of glutamate, another brain chemical that can damage or kill nerve cells. The drug does not reverse the disease but can slow the pace of deterioration. Also, preliminary studies of an herbal medication called gingko biloba have shown some benefits. However, considerable further study is needed before any agent is considered a wholly effective treatment. Preventive measures also are being investigated. They include: lowering levels of homocysteine (an amino acid possibly implicated in developing Alzheimer's) by increasing intake of folate and vitamins B_6 and B_{12}; taking a nonsteroidal anti-inflammatory drug such as ibuprofen; taking vitamin E; taking a statin; and a diet rich in omega-3 fatty acids, dark green leafy vegetables, blueberries, green tea and red wine. Exercise increases blood flow to the brain and staying active socially and mentally with adult classes, reading, doing crossword puzzles, playing word games or the like are also believed to be beneficial.

amenorrhea 1. Failure to menstruate at an age when regular menstruation is the norm and in the absence of pregnancy or lactation. *Physiological amenorrhea* refers to lack of menstruation at times when it normally does not occur, that is, before puberty, during pregnancy and lactation, and after menopause.

2. primary amenorrhea. Failure to begin menstruating by the age of 18. Although many adolescent girls worry if they do not yet menstruate when most of their agemates have begun, the course of puberty and the age of MENARCHE vary so widely that there need be no real concern until the age of 16, *provided* there are other signs of early pubertal changes (growth spurt, underarm or pubic hair, breast development). Many clinicians carry out some preliminary tests on a girl who has never menstruated by the age of 16, as much to reassure the patient as to rule out serious disease. One phenomenon that may be ruled out is *crypto-menorrhea*, in which menstrual bleeding does occur but is retained inside the vagina by some anatomical obstruction, such as an imperforate HYMEN. Another is the presence of a pituitary tumor, which can be investigated by means of a skull X-ray. Treatment for primary amenorrhea usually is not undertaken until the age of 18.

Primary amenorrhea is most often caused by some disturbance in the relationship between the pituitary gland and the ovaries (see MENSTRUAL CYCLE for further explanation) and only rarely by some anatomic problem (such as lack of a vagina, uterus or ovaries). Amenorrhea is not a disease but a symptom. However, it may be *idiopathic,* that is, the most thorough examination and extensive tests may uncover no discernible physical or emotional cause. Diagnosis nevertheless is directed at finding an organic cause, usually by process of elimination. It begins with taking a very detailed history, including acute or chronic illness of any kind, the possibility of unsuspected pregnancy, recent weight gain or loss, symptoms of other metabolic disease (thyroid, diabetes, etc.), and both the patient's early developmental history and the family history relating to menstruation, fertility, metabolic disease and tuberculosis. It is followed by a careful physical examination, preferably including a pelvic examination. However, the position, size and shape of the uterus and ovaries often can be determined by rectal examination if a vaginal examination seems difficult or disturbing. A skull X-ray may be taken to rule out pituitary tumors, and tests made of both vaginal and buccal (inside the mouth) smears and of the urine for the presence of hormones and for chromosomal abnormalities. An X-ray of the hands may show whether the long bones of the fingers show pubertal changes indicating that menarche is likely to occur in a few months.

If the physical examination reveals no abnormalities, the laboratory findings are close to normal and there are no symptoms and signs of other disease, the diagnosis probably is *delayed puberty,* a matter of slow maturation that eventually will correct itself. Sometimes it is simply a matter of a girl's attaining the CRITICAL WEIGHT apparently needed for menarche. Many clinicians, therefore, recommend a wait-and-see approach, with follow-up scheduled every 6 to 12 months.

Among the pathologic conditions that can cause primary amenorrhea, most of them relatively rare and many either partly or wholly curable by medication and/or surgery, are ACROMEGALY and other pituitary disturbances; POLYCYSTIC OVARY SYNDROME and other ovarian disorders; disease of the thyroid or adrenal glands; chromosomal disorders such as TURNER'S SYNDROME, HERMAPHRODITISM and ANDROGEN INSENSITIVITY SYNDROME; nutritional disorders such as ANOREXIA NERVOSA and OBESITY; serious illnesses that affect the endocrine system, such as DIABETES, or generally delay growth and development, such as ileitis (Crohn's disease), heart disease and tuberculosis; the adverse effects of a variety of drugs, including some tranquilizers, barbiturates, corticosteroids and progesterone; and emotional stress, ranging in severity from temporary distress to a major psychiatric disorder.

For women with primary amenorrhea who wish to bear children, a variety of treatments are available, depending on the cause. If the uterus and ovaries are normal and hormonal problems are responsible, treatments for restoring hormonal imbalance are available. If the hymen or cervix is closed, minor surgery can correct it. If the uterus is normal but the ovaries are nonfunctional, the woman may be able to nurture a donor embryo in her uterus; her partner's sperm is used to fertilize a donor's egg, and the fertilized egg is transferred to the woman's uterus (see also EMBRYO TRANSFER). If the ovaries are normal but she has no uterus, a surrogate mother may be used to bear the woman's fertilized egg.

3. secondary amenorrhea. Ceasing to menstruate for more than three months after normal menstrual periods have been established but well before the usual age for menopause. It must first be distinguished from *oligomenorrhea*, infrequent periods with intervals of more than 38 days but fewer than 90 days between periods, and *hypomenorrhea*, fewer days of menstrual flow, or scanty flow or both. There is so much variation in cycles among perfectly healthy women, as well as considerable variation in the same woman, that unless symptoms are extreme or there is another problem, such as inability to conceive, there is no pressing need to investigate. Especially during the first months or even years following menarche, many young women have very irregular cycles. Naturally, pregnancy and early menopause both must be ruled out before proceeding with diagnostic tests.

Diagnosis, as in primary amenorrhea, involves a detailed history, physical examination (including pelvic examination), skull X-ray and laboratory tests of urine and vaginal smears. An endometrial biopsy may be indicated if hormone patterns show a high risk for endometrial cancer. If no serious disease is suspected, secondary amenorrhea may need no treatment unless a woman wishes to become pregnant. In that event hormone therapy, particularly stimulating the pituitary gland with progesterone alone or in combination with estrogen to establish bleeding, and then stimulating ovulation by means of a FERTILITY DRUG, often is effective.

Causes of secondary amenorrhea include, *in addition* to those listed for primary amenorrhea (see def. 2 above), damage to the pituitary resulting from postpartum hemorrhage and/or shock (SHEEHAN'S DISEASE); destruction of the endometrium by overvigorous curettage (ASHERMAN'S SYNDROME), radiation therapy or an abnormally adherent placenta in a prior pregnancy; ovarian cysts and/or tumors; and drugs, including oral contraceptives (see POST-PILL AMENORRHEA). Extreme weight loss and/or very vigorous physical activity, such as that of ballet dancers or professional athletes, also may lead to amenorrhea (see also CRITICAL WEIGHT).

A small percentage of women with secondary amenorrhea exhibit an excess of male hormones. This condition, called HYPERANDROGENISM, and amenorrhea can lead to overstimulation of the endometrium, which may signal increased risk of endometrial hyperplasia and cancer. Consequently, it calls for hormone treatment of some kind.

In addition, following childbirth there may be postpartum amenorrhea and lactation amenorrhea (it is considered amenorrhea if it persists for more than three months after delivery in a mother who is not breast-feeding or longer than six weeks after

nursing is discontinued), in which the continued production of PROLACTIN by the pituitary is not inhibited in the normal way by the hypothalamus; this condition may be self-correcting in time or be corrected by hormone therapy.

amenorrhea-galactorrhea syndrome   Also *inappropriate lactation syndrome, lactation amenorrhea*. A disorder characterized by the absence of menstruation, usually after a period of regular menstrual cycles, and the inappropriate production of breast milk. There are two versions of this syndrome, one occurring after a pregnancy (*Chiari-Frommel syndrome*) and the other unassociated with pregnancy (*Ahumada del Castillo syndrome*). Both are caused by the absence of the prolactin-inhibiting factor (PIF) that is normally produced by the hypothalamus. Because this condition can be caused by a pituitary tumor—even a very tiny one—such a lesion must be ruled out before proceeding with treatment. Another common cause is hypothyroidism (underproduction of thyroid hormones) without any other symptoms. Frequently the syndrome is drug-induced by oral contraceptives (the Pill), considered by some to be the leading cause, or by phenothiazines (a class of tranquilizers), tricyclic antidepressants, certain antihypertensive drugs (taken for high blood pressure) or narcotics. The estrogen in oral contraceptives stimulates prolactin production, and when the Pill is discontinued the breast may continue to produce milk. Phenothiazines and tricyclic anti-depressants act on the brain, blocking the neurotransmitter that is believed to stimulate PIF production, thereby allowing unlimited prolactin production. Other causes include excess androgen production, caused by adrenal disease. Sometimes the exact cause cannot be identified. Treatment consists of eliminating the cause (for example, removing a pituitary tumor, giving thyroid supplement) and/or administering the drug bromocriptine, which suppresses prolactin production. Some authorities believe that the Chiari-Frommel syndrome often is self-correcting, although it tends to recur after subsequent pregnancies.

amniocentesis   The procedure of removing fluid from the AMNIOTIC SAC surrounding a fetus in order to detect certain genetic disorders and birth defects (including Down syndrome and Tay-Sachs disease), and RH disease of pregnancy, and to assess the baby's maturity. First developed in 1966, the procedure takes only a few minutes to perform under local anesthetic and usually is done on an outpatient basis in either a hospital or doctor's office. However, it usually is not performed until a pregnancy has advanced to 15 or 16 weeks. Experimentally it has been done as early as 12 weeks, but at least one major study found such early testing led to a large increase in the risk of a foot deformity similar to clubfoot, as well as a slight increase in the chance of miscarriage or stillbirth. Using ULTRASOUND to determine the position of placenta and fetus, a needle is introduced through the abdomen and uterine wall into the amniotic sac and withdraws 10 to 20 ml of amniotic fluid for analysis. Because the fetal cells contained in the fluid must first grow in a special nutrient medium, chromosome analysis usually takes from two to four weeks, and metabolic studies, which require a larger number of cells, may take even longer. It is advisable to undergo amniocentesis with a clinician who is experienced with the procedure and has access to a laboratory accustomed to dealing with fetal cell analysis. Even then, in about 10% of cases the cells do not grow the first time, especially if taken earlier than 16 weeks, so the procedure must be repeated.

The risk of amniocentesis to the mother is minimal. The risk to the fetus is somewhat greater, principally because the test may bring on premature labor, which, however, occurs only in about 0.5% of cases. The procedure does not detect all birth defects. It is useful for discovering chromosomal abnormalities, the most common of which is Down syndrome, some inherited metabolic disorders and certain structural defects of the spine, notably SPINA BIFIDA and anencephaly (absence of the cerebrum, which precludes survival). It does not detect birth defects caused by the mother's exposure to RUBELLA, X-rays, drugs or other harmful substances. Despite its limitations, it is widely recommended as a routine procedure for women carrying a child after the age of 35, when the risk of chromosomal defects is substantially higher; for all women who have a high risk for transmitting a specific inherited

disorder, such as SICKLE-CELL DISEASE; and for all women who previously have borne a child with an inherited or chromosomal disorder. In addition, since amniocentesis also identifies the sex of the fetus, it is useful for women carrying a trait for sex-linked genetic disorders, such as MUSCULAR DYSTROPHY or HEMOPHILIA. Finally, in women who face some special problem in carrying a baby to full term, such as risk of uterine rupture, amniocentesis can help determine the maturity of the fetus, particularly its lungs (see HYALINE MEMBRANE DISEASE), and indicate when a Cesarean section can be safely performed. (See also AMNIOGRAPHY; FETOSCOPY.) In recent years many younger women who are not in any high-risk group have elected to undergo amniocentesis even though their statistical risk of carrying a fetus with chromosomal abnormalities is quite small. Some believe this use of the procedure is unnecessary and adds to medical costs. Others say the procedure's cost is minimal compared to caring for an abnormal child. It probably is best to make the decision on an individual basis.

A test that can be performed earlier is CHORIONIC VILLUS SAMPLING. A newer, noninvasive test that can be done as early as 10 weeks and that combines ultrasound with a blood test is the NUCHAL TRANSLUCENCY-BIOCHEMICAL TEST.

See also PERCUTANEOUS UMBILICAL BLOOD SAMPLING.

amniography A special X-ray procedure whereby structural defects in a fetus can be detected. Usually not possible to perform until late in pregnancy lest the X-ray itself harm the fetus, the procedure involves injecting a special dye into the AMNIOTIC SAC and then taking an X-ray; the dye outlines the shape of the fetus much more clearly than an ordinary X-ray. However, because it must be done so late in pregnancy, abortion of a severely malformed fetus usually is much more difficult, so the technique has limited use.

See also FETOSCOPY.

amnioinfusion Also *amniocentesis abortion, intra-amniotic infusion, medical induction, second-trimester abortion, late abortion, premature* *induction of labor*. A method of ending a pregnancy of 15 to 24 weeks that involves the injection of a foreign substance into the amniotic sac surrounding the fetus, which after several hours induces regular uterine contractions that expel the fetus. The substance injected may be a strong salt solution (*saline abortion*), urea (a nitrogen waste product; *urea abortion*) or prostaglandins (a hormone; *prostaglandin abortion*). Prostaglandins may be administered either by intramuscular injection or vaginal suppositories.

Amnioinfusion can rarely be performed before 15 weeks of pregnancy (counting from the first day of the last menstrual period) and is almost always done in a hospital so that emergency problems arising during the drug injection or during expulsion can be managed with safety. The average time needed for the procedure is 24 hours, but there is considerable variation among women in the time it takes for contractions to begin and for the fetus to be expelled, so one should allow for a hospital stay of at least 48 hours. The procedure begins with administering local anesthetic to a small area in the lower abdomen. The clinician then inserts a slender hollow needle through the abdominal wall into the AMNIOTIC SAC and introduces saline, urea or prostaglandins over a period of 10 to 15 minutes (even more slowly with saline, and then some amniotic fluid always must be withdrawn first). The woman must be fully awake during this procedure so that she can immediately report any sensation of warmth, pain, dizziness or other unusual feeling that might indicate an adverse drug reaction. The needle is then withdrawn and the area covered with a bandage; the patient then waits until contractions begin. Sometimes the cervix is dilated by inserting LAMINARIA, usually 24 hours prior to infusion, to ease the passage of the fetus, and occasionally OXYTOCIN is given intravenously to promote and strengthen uterine contractions. Prostaglandins tend to work faster than saline but may give rise to nausea and/or diarrhea; saline works more slowly (it takes at least 8 to 12 hours for contractions to begin, often up to 24 hours) and may make the patient very thirsty.

The contractions begin gradually and increase in intensity. The cervical canal gradually dilates and eventually the amniotic sac breaks, releasing fluid through the vagina. After 2 to 15 hours, the fetus is expelled. During the last few hours of expulsion painkillers and sedatives may be administered as needed, but general anesthesia is not used. With saline abortion the fetus usually dies while still in the uterus; with prostaglandins it very occasionally emerges alive, and the hospital is then legally obliged to treat it as a premature infant (although its chance of survival is very small). Usually the placenta emerges after the fetus, but in some cases it must be extracted, and in still others portions remain inside the uterus, necessitating a curettage (scraping) for removal.

Medically and emotionally, amnioinfusion is a far more traumatic procedure than other abortion procedures performed earlier in pregnancy. In pregnancies up to 18 weeks, DILATATION AND EVACUATION has largely replaced it. Amnioinfusion requires hospitalization and so is more expensive, and many hospitals refuse to admit patients for this procedure at all. Others may ask the patient to go home after infusion and not return until contractions are well established, a dangerous practice that should be avoided.

The risks to the patient undergoing amnioinfusion are somewhat greater than those of normal childbirth. If saline solution is accidentally injected into a blood vessel, there is danger of shock and even death. The risk of hemorrhage and retained placental material is higher than for earlier abortion. The greater duration of the pregnancy, so that women frequently have felt the movements of the fetus, and the occasional delivery of a live fetus make amnioinfusion emotionally painful. Finally, the similarity of the experience to labor and delivery makes it traumatic for both patient and hospital staff.

There are definite contraindications to amnioinfusion. A saline abortion should *never* be performed on a woman with liver or kidney disease, hypertension (high blood pressure), sickle cell disease or serious heart disease. A prostaglandin abortion should *never* be performed if a woman has a known allergy to this hormone or has hypertension, asthma, heart disease, lung disease, epilepsy, a history of convulsions or glaucoma. Unfortunately, the only alternative to amnioinfusion for terminating a pregnancy of more than 20 weeks is major surgery (see HYSTEROTOMY).

amniotic sac   Also *bag of waters, membranes*. A sac made of a membrane, called the *amnion*, that develops around a fertilized egg about one week after fertilization and eventually surrounds the entire embryo (later called "fetus"). As it grows it fills with a clear fluid called *amniotic fluid* (or *waters*). The amount of fluid increases rapidly to an average amount of 55 ml at 12 weeks, 400 ml at 20 weeks, and approximately 1 liter (about 1 quart) at 36 to 38 weeks (near term). The volume then decreases as term approaches and, if the pregnancy is prolonged, may become relatively scanty. An excess of amniotic fluid, or HYDRAMNIOS, sometimes is associated with fetal malformations, multiple pregnancy (especially identical twins) and maternal diseases such as diabetes.

The makeup of the amniotic fluid changes during the course of the pregnancy. During the first four and one-half months it is made up of much the same components as the mother's blood plasma. Thereafter, however, particles of fetal tissue are shed into the fluid, enabling detection of some abnormalities in the unborn child (see AMNIOCENTESIS).

The amniotic fluid serves several important functions. It provides a medium in which the fetus can readily move, cushions it against possible injury and helps it maintain an even temperature. The fetus also drinks large amounts of amniotic fluid and excretes into it. During labor, if the presenting part of the fetus is not pressing closely against the cervix, as with a BREECH PRESENTATION, the hydrostatic action of the fluid may be important in helping to dilate the cervix.

During the course of labor, usually toward the end of the first stage or early during the second stage, the amniotic sac ruptures by itself and the amniotic fluid gushes out through the mother's vagina. Occasionally the membranes rupture before labor begins, or sometimes they remain intact until the infant has been delivered so that it is born surrounded by them; the portion of membrane covering the baby's head is sometimes called the *caul*. Surgically or manually rupturing the membranes during early labor (or before) is one way of inducing labor (see AMNIOTOMY).

amniotomy   Also *membrane rupture, breaking the bag of waters*. Deliberate rupture of the membranes, or AMNIOTIC SAC, in order to induce or hasten labor. Usually the clinician inserts an index finger or two fingers encased in a sterile glove through the partially dilated cervix until the baby's head is felt. Then, with the aid of an amniohook or other surgical instrument, the protective amniotic membranes are punctured, torn, or stripped from the uterine wall in the area near the cervix. The baby's head is then held up slightly with a finger to allow the amniotic fluid to escape. If the cervix is ready, labor usually begins within an hour or two of amniotomy, although it may take as long as six to eight hours. If labor does not begin within 24 hours, it may be stimulated further with oxytocin administration (see INDUCTION OF LABOR). No anesthesia is needed for amniotomy. The principal risk of the procedure to the mother is bacterial infection; the risk to the baby is loss of the cushioning effect of the amniotic fluid during the early part of labor, and, critics maintain, the procedure can slow the fetal heart rate.

Although amniotomy has been performed for several hundred years, a study published in 2007 that reviewed controlled trials of almost 5,000 women found that amniotomy did not shorten the length of labor, decrease the need for administration of oxytocin, decrease pain, reduce the number of instrument-aided births or lead to serious maternal injury or death. The researchers therefore advised that in women whose labor was progressing normally, their waters be left intact.

anabolic steroids   A group of synthetic hormones that resemble male sex hormones, such as testosterone, in that they increase muscle mass and have other body-building properties. Sometimes used in the treatment of certain endocrine and blood disorders, severe burns and muscle-wasting diseases, anabolic steroids also have been used to build up both men and women athletes, especially in sports requiring considerable strength (such as weight-lifting and wrestling). Not only is this use considered unfair (and illegal in some competitions, such as the Olympics), but it can give rise to serious side effects. In men the side effects include enlargement of the penis, sterility, breast growth and milk secretion, gastrointestinal complaints (nausea, vomiting, appetite loss), jaundice and abnormal retention of fluids and electrolytes. Women athletes who take steroids may develop facial hair growth, voice deepening (sometimes permanent), diminished breast size, acne, clitoral enlargement and menstrual irregularities. Steroids also raise blood cholesterol, depress the immune system and increase the risk of serious liver disease. Further, they can cause temporary mental problems, including mood swings and violent impulses. Because of their increasing use, urine tests to detect the presence of such steroids have been developed, and they are mandatory for athletes entering certain competitions.

Another substance, androstenedione, is a type of steroid that is designed to increase the amount of muscle-building testosterone in the body. An over-the-counter supplement first developed in the 1970s in East Germany, it was introduced commercially in the United States in 1996. It is banned by many sports-governing bodies, including the International Olympic Committee, but can be bought by anyone. Pregnant women and men with prostate problems are specifically warned to avoid the substance. Teenagers also may risk serious side effects, such as shutting off bone growth and stunting height.

See also CHROMOSOME TEST.

anal fissure A deep crack or split in the mucous membrane of the anal canal, which often is extremely painful because it can cause spasm of the anal sphincter (muscle). It is caused by the passage of large, hard stools or may result from anal surgery, anal intercourse or other trauma. The pain is particularly acute when the anus is stretched by a bowel movement or for examination. Anal fissures also cause bleeding and soiling, so that underwear is always stained no matter how thorough a wiping and cleaning follow bowel movements. A superficial fissure usually will heal by itself, but some become chronic. Treatment includes a high-fiber diet, stool softeners and the use of anesthetic ointment before and after a bowel movement. A warm SITZ BATH immediately after a bowel movement may help ease the spasm. Chronic fissures that

do not respond to treatment may require surgical repair.

analgesic Also *painkiller*. Any pain-relieving drug or remedy. Analgesic drugs are either narcotic or nonnarcotic. The principal narcotics are opium and its alkaloids (morphine, codeine) and synthetic narcotics, including meperidine (Demerol), methadone and propoxyphene (Darvon). All narcotics are potentially habit-forming; a person becomes physically and emotionally dependent on using them and experiences severe withdrawal symptoms when they are discontinued. The principal nonnarcotic analgesics, most of which not only relieve pain but also reduce fever and inflammation and therefore are also called nonsteroidal anti-inflammatory drugs (NSAIDs), are the salicylates, such as aspirin; ibuprofen (Advil, Medipren, Motrin, Nuprin), which, like aspirin, prevents the release of prostaglandins; naproxen (Aleve, Naprosyn), similar to ibuprofen but longer-acting; the pyrazolone derivatives, such as phenylbutazone (Azolid, Butazolidin) and indomethacin (Indocin); and three newer drugs, sulindac (Climoril), ketoprofen (Orudis) and diclofenac (Voltaren). In contrast, the aniline derivatives, such as acetaminophen (Tylenol, Datril, Panadol, Liquiprin, Anacin-3), are not anti-inflammatory. Aspirin, acetaminophen and ibuprofen are equally effective in reducing fever and relieving mild to moderate pain. Ibuprofen and naproxen are slightly better for pain from dental work, sprains, strains and similar soft-tissue injury as well as for menstrual cramps. A dose of naproxen lasts twice as long as one of ibuprofen but also is more likely to cause stomach upset and intestinal bleeding than ibuprofen.

All the NSAIDs are mainstays in treating arthritis and other sources of chronic pain, but taken in high doses or over a long period of time they can lead to gastrointestinal bleeding or kidney damage. Aspirin and ibuprofen also impair clotting and are not recommended for women who are pregnant or breast-feeding, heavy drinkers, persons susceptible to ulcers or gout, and those taking anticoagulants. Acetaminophen is considered safer, although it is contraindicated for those with liver and kidney disease and for heavy drinkers. All these analgesics are best taken during or after a meal. Also, they should not be taken in combination with one another. Celecoxib (Celebrex), the first of a new category of drugs called COX-2 inhibitors, was recommended for approval by the U.S. Food and Drug Administration, and others of its kind have followed (Vioxx, Bextra). They appear to relieve pain and swelling as successfully as the NSAIDs do, but without the same serious side effects. The reasons behind this are that the NSAIDs block both COX-1 and COX-2 enzymes, two versions of cyclooxygenase that are both involved in prostaglandin production, but COX-1 protects the stomach lining and regulates blood platelets while COX-2 triggers pain and inflammation. The new drugs block only COX-2, and early studies indicate that they also may protect against some cancers, Parkinson's disease and Alzheimer's disease. In 2004 Vioxx was found to increase the risk of heart attack and stroke, and was withdrawn from the market. As a result, further investigation of other COX-2 inhibitors was begun, and many clinicians advised patients to discontinue these drugs until such studies were completed. Many pharmacies now issue an FDA-approved medication guide for any NSAIDs prescribed, listing warnings about potential risks and side effects.

RISKS AND BENEFITS OF ANALGESICS

- All NSAIDs and COX-2 inhibitors can cause or worsen hypertension, congestive heart failure, swelling, and impaired kidney function.

- No clear difference in pain relief effectiveness among NSAIDs and COX-2 inhibitors.

- Most NSAIDs and COX-2 inhibitors pose similar increased risk of heart attack.

- The NSAID naproxen (Aleve, Naprosyn) carries smaller risk of heart attack than other NSAIDs or COX-2 inhibitors.

- Risks of serious gastrointestinal problems for users of Celebrex are similar to risks for users of Motrin, Advil, Voltaren, and other NSAIDs.

- More evidence needed to compare cardiac and gastrointestinal risks of aspirin at doses effective for pain relief v. other NSAIDs.

- Acetaminophen (Tylenol) generally reduces pain less effectively than NSAIDs but carries smaller risk of gastrointestinal problems. High doses may pose heart attack risk similar to NSAIDs.

Agency for Healthcare Research and Quality, October 2006

It is important not to combine different pain-killing drugs, whether over-the-counter or by prescription, so as not to get too much of a medication. Many prescription analgesics, among them Endocet, Darvocet and Vicodin, contain acetaminophen, which should therefore not be combined with over-the-counter acetaminophen such as Tylenol. Others, among them Celebrex and Percodan, contain NSAIDs, so one should avoid taking over-the-counter NSAIDs such as ibuprofen at the same time. If in doubt, one should check with one's clinician.

Numerous herbs also have been used as analgesics; indeed, opium itself is obtained from the poppy plant. Among HERBAL REMEDIES, a mild analgesic is catnip (Nepeta cataria), drunk as a tea prepared from its leaf sprays and flowers.

Narcotics such as Demerol were long used routinely to ease the pain of childbirth, but these and other analgesics all pass the placental barrier and may affect the baby, making it less able to suck, sleepy and unresponsive to the environment. They also may slow labor or make for weaker contractions and cause nausea and vomiting, grogginess or dizziness in the mother. If these agents are required, the smallest possible doses should be used. However, administration of narcotics such as sufentanyl into the epidural space (see EPIDURAL ANESTHESIA) can be effective and pose less risk to the fetus, as well as enabling the mother to continue to be active during labor (feeling the sensation to push and being able to do so).

anal intercourse, anilingus, anal sex See ANUS.

androgen A general name for any hormone that has a masculinizing effect on either sex. The principal androgen is TESTOSTERONE, in men produced mostly by the testes and in small quantity by the adrenal glands, and in women, in much smaller quantities, by the ovaries and adrenal glands. Other androgens secreted by the ovaries and female adrenal glands are androstenedione and dehydroisoandrosterone, but except in certain diseases the amounts are not large enough to have a masculinizing effect. During pregnancy the placenta converts these two androgens into estrogens (female hormones). Synthetic androgens are used mainly to treat men with disorders caused by failure of the testes to produce androgen. They are not effective in treating sterility or impotence unless these conditions are the result of under-developed testes. Androgens are believed to be responsible in part for the sex drive (see LIBIDO), but the exact relationship is not totally clear.

See also ANABOLIC STEROIDS.

In women testosterone produced by the ovaries fluctuates during the menstrual cycle, the high-est amount being produced, along with estrogen, at ovulation. Because of this link, testosterone is increasingly being prescribed to postmenopausal women and women who have had their ovaries removed to increase their sex drive or to treat other complaints. Side effects associated with this use are lowered voice, facial hair, acne and weight gain.

A greater problem for women is an excess of testosterone, or *hyperandrogenism*, resulting not only in cosmetic problems like acne, balding and excessive facial hair (some women must shave twice a day) and secondary AMENORRHEA, but in such severe complications as infertility (see POLY-CYSTIC OVARY SYNDROME), diabetes, high blood pressure, heart disease and cancer of the uterus. Recent research indicates that the problem has been greatly underestimated and that as many as 15 to 30% of all women may have disorders caused by overproduction of testosterone. Early signs are a tendency to put on weight in the upper body, especially the stomach, rather than on thighs and buttocks; irregular periods; and hair sprouting in great abundance on the face, thighs and in a stripe pattern from pelvis to navel. Treatment consists of birth control pills, spironolactone (an anti-andro-gen drug) and dexamethasone (a synthetic steroid that suppresses adrenal activity).

androgen insensitivity syndrome Also *testicular feminization*. A congenital condition in which girls or women appear to have normal external female genitals except for a swelling or lump in each groin, little or no pubic or underarm hair and a vagina usually not deep enough for sexual intercourse. They also lack a fully developed uterus and fallo-pian tubes, do not menstruate and cannot become pregnant. The condition arises in the fetus when internal masculine organs begin to form but are never completely developed, and their rudimen-tary presence prevents the development of female organs. At puberty the breasts do develop, because the female hormone estrogen is produced by the rudimentary testes (seen as lumps in the groin), and the shape of the body becomes decidedly female. The disorder is named for the fact that it is due to the lack of sufficient androgen-binding protein in the cells; the sex chromosomes are all XY, as in normal men. Women with this condi-tion often can lead normal lives—an operation to lengthen the vagina can be performed to permit vaginal intercourse—except that they cannot bear children.

andrologist A specialist in laboratory evaluations of male FERTILITY.

anemia A shortage of red blood cells, diagnosed by means of a blood count (see under BLOOD TEST). If red blood cells make up less than 37% of total blood volume, or the blood's hemoglobin value is below 12 grams per 100 ml (milliliters) of blood, a woman is said to be anemic. (The normal values are somewhat higher for men.) General symptoms of anemia include undue fatigue, light-headedness, frequent headaches, dizziness, spots before the eyes, ringing of the ears and paleness of the skin under the fingernails. By far the majority of cases of ane-mia are caused by iron deficiency. Other causes are unusual blood loss (through hemorrhage or major surgery, for example), vitamin deficiency (usually of vitamin B_{12} and/or folic acid), bone marrow dis-ease and a group of hereditary blood disorders that includes SICKLE-CELL DISEASE and thalassemia. Also, certain cancers, liver, kidney and thyroid disorders and chronic infection all can cause anemia.

Under certain conditions women in particular are apt to become anemic. Among these are preg-nancy, which makes heavy nutritional demands on the body, particularly for iron and folic acid (also see below); the use of an intrauterine device (IUD), which often causes heavy menstrual flow and may therefore call for supplementary iron (either in the diet or in pill form); and the use of oral contraceptives, which in some women creates a folic acid deficiency. There is disagreement as to whether all menstruating women require supplementary iron. Although some iron is lost with every menstrual period, normally it is restored between periods. Women with poor diets and/or exceptionally heavy periods run a higher risk of iron-deficiency anemia, but most women with average flow who eat well-balanced diets need no supplements. In pregnancy, however, most authorities agree that iron and folic acid supplements are advisable. Other women at risk are long-distance runners, who may lose blood from the circulation while running, and the elderly, whose diet is inadequate for such reasons as bad teeth for chewing iron-rich meat, poor absorption from the bowel or poverty.

One kind of anemia, *megaloblastic anemia,* is specifically caused by folic acid deficiency. Folic acid, or folate, plays an important role in the bone marrow cells that give rise to red blood cells. In the absence of folate, these cells become large and irregular. Called megaloblasts, they do not generate enough red blood cells. The condition occurs mainly in pregnant women, alcoholics and individuals with intestinal malabsorption, and as a side effect of certain drugs, among them methotrexate.

The best dietary sources of iron are lean red meats, liver, egg yolks and dried fruits. Folic acid (and also iron) is found mainly in green leafy vegetables (lettuce, spinach, cabbage, broccoli, watercress, parsley, escarole) and kelp (seaweed). Cooking can deactivate folic acid, so raw green vegetables (salads) are a better source. Vitamin B_{12} is present in liver and organ meats, as well as in beef, pork, eggs, milk and milk products. (See also DIET.) Numerous herbs contain iron, among them red raspberry leaf (*Rubus idaeus*), strawberry leaf (*Fragaria vesca*), burdock root (*Arctium lappa*), dandelion root (*Taraxacum officinalis*) and yellow dock root (*Rumex crispus*).

Both coffee and tea interfere with iron absorption by the gut and therefore should not be drunk *with* meals, while extra vitamin C may increase iron absorption from food. Also, certain cholesterol-lowering medications, vitamin E, any antacids and the antibiotic tetracycline all block iron

absorption. Women who must take these should do so at least three to four hours *after* meals and/or iron supplements.

While it is preferable to treat iron deficiency through an improved diet, occasionally iron supplements may be required. Most contain one of three types of iron: ferrous sulfate, ferrous gluconate, or ferrous fumarate. For maximal absorption they are best taken on an empty stomach, but if they cause diarrhea, constipation or cramps, they should be taken with a meal along with 500 mg of vitamin C. Iron supplements tend to turn the stools dark green or black. Further, too much iron taken for too long a time can be dangerous. Therefore, as soon as the anemia has been corrected, the supplements should be stopped. In cases of anemia linked with kidney disease, heart failure or other serious disorders, production of *erythropoietin,* the hormone that stimulates red blood cell production in the bone marrow, may be insufficient. In those cases erythropoietin therapy may be indicated.

anesthesia   **1.** Loss of feeling induced by chemical agents called *anesthetics,* affecting a limited surface area (*topical anesthesia*), or a specific circumscribed area (*local* or *regional anesthesia*), or with loss of consciousness, the entire body (*general anesthesia*). It is used to block sensations of pain from minor wounds and injury, as well as pain during surgery, dentistry, other traumatic medical procedures and childbirth. Topical anesthetics are available in the form of throat lozenges, eardrops, mouthwash, ointments, rectal suppositories and so on; many of these are very mild and are available without prescription.

Local and general anesthesia, in contrast, must be administered by a physician, licensed nurse-practitioner or dentist. When it is used for procedures major enough to require a hospital or clinic setting, it is preferable to have it administered either by an *anesthesiologist,* a physician with advanced training in its use, or by a specially trained nurse or technician under an anesthesiologist's supervision. General anesthesia, used for extensive surgical procedures, usually involves administering an anesthetic, an analgesic (pain reliever) and a muscle relaxant. The last may necessitate intubation—insertion of a tube into the larynx to assist breathing.

Local anesthesia is always given by injection; general anesthesia is either inhaled or injected (see also under def. 2). For some procedures local anesthesia may be combined with drugs that cause a partial loss of consciousness; this is sometimes called *augment anesthesia.*

The choice of anesthetic agent and of the kind of anesthesia usually is dictated by the condition or operation involved—its nature, how long it takes to perform, the area affected—as well as by the patient's state of health. The major exception is childbirth, in which a woman's preferences also may be taken into account (see below). Before surgery, the anesthesiologist should ask the patient whether she takes any medications, including over-the-counter drugs, herbal remedies and psychoactive drugs (tranquilizers, etc.). Some of these may pose risks during anesthesia. Also, a recent study showed that the foods consumed before surgery (even several days before) could influence the effectiveness of many anesthetics and muscle relaxants. Potatoes, tomatoes and eggplant in particular were implicated.

2. in childbirth. The earliest anesthesia used in childbirth was chloroform, discovered in 1847. The first woman in labor who inhaled chloroform fumes was made unconscious and delivered within half an hour; she herself did not awaken for three days and had no memory of delivering the baby. At first the new method was denounced, but after it was used by Queen Victoria herself for delivery, opposition died down. In time, other kinds of *inhalation anesthesia* came into use, principally ether, cyclopropane and halothane. These *general anesthetics,* as well as thiopental sodium (Pentothal), which is injected intravenously, all have one serious disadvantage in childbirth: They pass through the placenta and anesthetize the baby as well as the mother. They tend to produce sleepy babies with delayed sucking response and weight gain, and sometimes with serious respiratory problems as well. Nor is general anesthesia without risk to the mother. The most serious is vomiting, which may cause material to be aspirated (breathed into the lungs). Also, general anesthesia slows down uterine contractions, so today it is used quite rarely, and then only near the end of labor, just before expulsion of the baby, or for an emergency Cesarean, or if for some reason a spinal injection cannot be given. (Nitrous oxide,

which is inhaled, induces an altered consciousness and pain relief but not loss of consciousness or true anesthesia; it usually is administered together with oxygen in concentrations below 80%.)

Most of the problems of general anesthesia in childbirth have been eliminated with REGIONAL ANESTHESIA, also called *conduction anesthesia,* which does not blot out consciousness but only blocks the conduction of pain sensations to the brain from a specific region of the body. Relatively little of a regional anesthetic is absorbed into the mother's bloodstream or crosses the placenta, so it does not affect the baby and can be used to relieve pain during labor as well as delivery. The anesthetic agents injected for this purpose include procaine (Novocain), lidocaine (Xylocaine) and various related compounds. However, those agents also can create some problems, such as lowered blood pressure in the mother and thereby a lowered fetal heart rate, causing fetal distress, impairment of contractions and, with spinal anesthesia, headache after delivery. Indeed, one such agent, bupivacaine, led to cardiac arrest in some patients when it was used in very high concentrations. Because no anesthetic is totally risk-free, since the 1950s there has been increasing emphasis on various psychological methods of pain control, ranging from hypnosis to breathing exercises (see PREPARED CHILDBIRTH), to replace or supplement anesthetics.

See also ANALGESIC; CAUDAL ANESTHESIA; EPIDURAL ANESTHESIA; PUDENDAL ANESTHESIA; SPINAL ANESTHESIA.

3. in abortion. The kind of anesthesia used in abortion depends on the stage of pregnancy and kind of procedure used. For first-trimester abortions performed by vacuum aspiration (suction), general anesthesia rarely is needed, since a local anesthetic injected into the cervix usually is sufficient to ease cramps. (It does not, however, eliminate the pain of cramps caused by contractions of the uterus during the procedure.) For a second-trimester abortion, with dilatation and evacuation, most often regional anesthesia (with or without augment) may be necessary. As with all medications, anesthesia poses some risk of adverse reaction and, in the case of general anesthesia, increases some of the risk of abortion, such as more bleeding owing to greater relaxation of the uterine muscle.

angina pectoris Also *angina*. Chest pain or a sensation of pressure occurring when the heart muscle does not receive sufficient oxygen owing to a blockage or narrowing of the arteries. The pain may also be felt in either shoulder, or down the inside of the arm. Angina affects women more than men but usually at a later age. It tends to occur during physical exertion or emotional stress, which increases the heart's need for oxygen. If the arteries are narrowed enough, angina can occur even at rest. Diagnosis is based on the reporting of symptoms; an electrocardiogram (EKG) may show no abnormality. Treatment is focused on treating the underlying heart disease (see ARTERIOSCLEROSIS), but immediate relief of pain is generally provided by placing a tablet of nitroglycerin (which dilates blood vessels) under the tongue.

anorexia nervosa A form of self-starvation with both physical and psychological symptoms. It affects mostly white girls and women in their teens and early 20s from a middle-class or affluent background, and it may be fatal in as many as 10 to 15% of cases. Its principal characteristic is the patient's refusal to eat. The eating behavior for any food that is consumed often is bizarre; eating may be followed by repeated self-induced vomiting and diarrhea (see BULIMIA). Consequently, there is extreme weight loss (at least 25% of body weight), accompanied by any or all of the following: secondary amenorrhea (cessation of menstruation), hyperactivity, hypothermia (intolerance to cold), low blood pressure, slowed heartbeat, lanugo (extensive growth of downy body hair), fear of weight gain, an obsessive pursuit of thinness, denial of hunger, sense of ineffectiveness and struggle for control over one's life. Unlike these changes, which can be reversed upon recovery, anorexia impedes normal bone growth. Young girls therefore may never reach their full height, and women lose enough bone mass to put them at great risk for osteoporosis.

Anorexic patients, 90 to 95% of whom are female, have a grossly distorted body image, regarding themselves as obese when in reality they are emaciated. They also may suffer from severe depression and attempt suicide.

The cause of anorexia is unknown but has long been thought to be psychological rather than organic. Numerous factors have been suggested: a desire to avoid sexuality (fear of pregnancy, denial of femininity); a caricature of conventional femininity (desire to conform to social norms by becoming slender; studies indicate that more than half of prepubertal girls try diets and other measures to control their weight); a sense of helplessness when faced with impending adulthood, and thus a means of avoiding independence. Many if not most anorexic patients tend to be meticulous, with very high standards for achievement. The parents of anorexic girls also have been blamed, the mothers for being dominant and intrusive, the fathers for being passive and emotionally withdrawn. Recently researchers have begun to investigate the possibility of organic disease, perhaps in the HYPOTHALAMUS, which controls appetite. Some authorities believe there may be a genetic predisposition for anorexia. A study of identical twins showed that if one twin suffered from anorexia, the odds were high that the other twin did as well. Anorexics who vomit and/or purge themselves should be assessed if they are using oral contraceptives for birth control. Although pregnancy in the anorexic with amenorrhea is unlikely, it must be monitored carefully if it does occur.

With the cause unknown and many patients denying their problems and resisting treatment, what treatment is possible is directed largely at preventing death from starvation; usually it is carried out in the hospital and in conjunction with psychotherapy and antidepressant medication when appropriate. In less severe cases, psychotherapy alone—often family therapy, especially for younger patients—may be tried. In general, the disease is either self-limiting—the girl resumes eating, which after months of starvation may itself cause gastrointestinal and other physical problems—or the patient starves to death. The outlook after recovery also is not entirely promising. More than half repeatedly return to this behavior, and a sizable percentage develop BULIMIA.

anovulatory bleeding Also *anovulation*. Vaginal bleeding, often on a regular basis, without release of an egg (see OVULATION). In a physically mature woman, there is a regular monthly cycle: Estrogen stimulates the buildup of the uterine lining (endometrium); an egg is released from the ovary; the remnant of the egg follicle produces progesterone; and either the egg is fertilized and becomes implanted in the endometrium, or it and the extra endometrial tissue are sloughed off in menstrual flow. (See MENSTRUAL CYCLE for a more detailed description.) Without ovulation, no progesterone is produced and the hormonal feedback system is thrown out of kilter. The extra endometrial tissue built up under estrogen stimulation is eventually shed, but not at the regular rate and time that would have occurred with ovulation. Progesterone regulates the timing of the menstrual cycle, and without it menstruation becomes irregular or may cease altogether, or it may involve heavy, long-lasting menstrual periods.

Anovulatory bleeding is quite common in the first two or three years following MENARCHE and again in the five or so years preceding MENOPAUSE. Also, women on ESTROGEN REPLACEMENT THERAPY or taking oral contraceptives that suppress ovulation have anovulatory cycles, which in their case are regulated by externally administered hormones. During a woman's reproductive years, lack of ovulation usually causes no problems unless she is trying to become pregnant or is distressed by menstrual irregularity. Fertility specialists believe that 20% of ovulation failures are the result of stress (including heavy physical exercise), obesity, diet, excess androgen production, thyroid gland dysfunction or excess PROLACTIN production. The administration of oral progesterone often will stop heavy bleeding but cannot reinstate ovulation. Some authorities maintain that lack of ovulation is responsible for practically all DYSFUNCTIONAL BLEEDING (vaginal bleeding not caused by an organic disease or lesion).

See also ENDOMETRIAL HYPERPLASIA.

anteflexed uterus   The normal forward tilt of the UTERUS.

anteverted uterus   A UTERUS that is tilted forward somewhat more than normal. It requires no treatment.

See also RETROVERTED UTERUS.

antibody   A specific substance in the blood that detects and reacts to a material foreign to the body, called an ANTIGEN, and neutralizes it. Antibodies are one of the body's two chief defenses against invading organisms; the other consists of cells, such as white blood cells, that surround and break up foreign matter. Antibodies are produced only when the appropriate antigens are present; each kind of antibody is effective only against a specific antigen. When an infection (invasion) ends, the blood levels of the appropriate antibodies fall; if the same invader attacks again, antibody buildup is more rapid and effective than the first time. It is this enhanced response that constitutes IMMUNITY.

See also AUTOIMMUNE DISEASE; HIV.

anticancer drugs   See CHEMOTHERAPY.

antidepressants   Also *mood elevators*. A class of drugs used to relieve serious DEPRESSION. Because the majority of American psychiatric patients are women, and depressive illness is far more common in women than in men, they are more likely to be treated with antidepressants than men. There are four main kinds of antidepressant: the tricyclic antidepressants, the monoamine oxidase (MAO) inhibitors, the selective serotonin reuptake inhibitors (SSRIs) and serotonin and norepinephrine reuptake inhibitors (SNRIs). The tricyclics have a mood-elevating effect but generally must be used for two to five weeks before their benefits are felt. They often are effective but do not work in every case. Also, they must be used with great caution in patients with a history of glaucoma, phlebitis, heart disease, thyroid disease, or epilepsy. Moreover, they can cause such unpleasant side effects as dry mouth, drowsiness, blurred vision, constipation and urinary hesitation, although these effects often disappear after a few weeks' use or when dosage is lowered. Finally, they never should be discontinued abruptly; once the symptoms subside, the dose should be reduced very gradually.

The MAO inhibitors, which generally are tried only in severe cases of depression not helped by the tricyclics, are more potent drugs. They both elevate the mood and lower the blood pressure. However, they can have serious side effects and may not be used in the presence of asthma, heart, liver or kidney disease, or in conjunction with some drugs. Also, certain foods and beverages must be avoided when they are taken.

The SSRIs and SNRIs, sometimes called second-generation antidepressants, often are prescribed because the tricyclics can cause intolerable side effects. They increase the levels of serotonin and/or norepinephrine, neurotransmitters (brain chemicals) that appear insufficient in patients suffering from depression. Neurotransmitters, which ferry signals between nerve endings in the body and neurons in the brain, act very briefly and then are broken down by enzymes or reabsorbed by the neurons that released them. The SSRIs block that reabsorption, or reuptake. The best-known of them is fluoxetine (Prozac), but sertraline (Zoloft), fluvoxamine (Luvox), citalopram (Celexa), paroxetine (Paxil), escitalopram (Lexapro) and trazodone (Desyrel) are also in use. The SSRIs' side effects, minor in most patients, include nervousness, nausea, headache, weight loss, loss of libido and a rash accompanied by joint pain and swelling. Occasionally, severe insomnia, impotence and other more serious side effects are reported. Nevertheless, they have become the antidepressant of choice for the elderly and for patients with milder forms of depression, who might not otherwise be treated with medication. However, they do not work for every patient; an estimated 20 to 40% of cases derive no benefit. A new study shows that both SSRIs and the older tricyclic antidepressants result in a significant increase in preterm delivery. Also, full-term infants exposed to SSRIs during the third trimester had an increased risk for respiratory distress syndrome, endocrine and metabolic disturbances and temperature regulation disorders. Neither kind was associated with an increased risk for congenital abnormalities. If discontinued, at least one (Paxil) may cause withdrawal symptoms, so it should be stopped only gradually. A recent study indicated that daily use of SSRIs by adults over the age of 50 doubled their risk of "fragility fractures," that is, fractures caused by falls from beds, chairs, or a standing position. The higher the dose, the greater the risk.

In addition, there are several other drugs: venlafaxine (Effexor), a serotonin/norepinephrine reuptake inhibitor, similar to SSRIs but faster acting, with antianxiety properties, and effective against more severe depression (it can raise blood pressure, which must be monitored, and cause nausea and fatigue); nefazodone (Serzone), a serotonin antagonist reuptake inhibitor, which has antianxiety properties and causes less insomnia, jitteriness and sexual dysfunction than SSRIs but is more sedating and can cause dizziness or faintness; and buproprion (Wellbutrin), with a stimulant effect, which may aid in weight loss and is also approved for helping patients stop smoking (but also has numerous side effects and an increased risk of seizures at higher doses, especially in women with anorexia or bulimia).

In the United States, some SSRIs also have been approved for treatment of BULIMIA, and more recently also to treat obsessive-compulsive disorder. However, because they have a generally mood-heightening effect and seemingly transform personality (enhancing confidence, etc.), there has been some concern about their abuse by individuals simply taking them to "feel good." Moreover, their long-term effects are unknown, since they were introduced only in the late 1980s.

The herb St. John's wort (*Hypericum perforatum*) has been used to treat mild to moderate depression. Its chemical action is not completely understood, although it is thought to affect the reabsorption of serotonin in the brain. Like other antidepressants, it takes about four weeks to have a significant effect. Its side effects, usually mild, include fatigue, dizziness, skin rash and increased sensitivity to sunlight. Much cheaper than the other antidepressants, it is sold over the counter as a dietary supplement, in elixir (liquid) or capsule form. St. John's wort may be effective in mild to moderate depression but is ineffective in treating major depression. Like all herbal remedies, it should be approached with caution. Its long-term effects are not known, and it should not be used together with other antidepressants, nor by women who are pregnant or breast-feeding. Further, St. John's wort appears to interact with a number of other medications, including at least one HIV drug.

No antidepressant should be taken without a careful evaluation of its benefits compared to its risks. Further, women who menstruate are advised to monitor their symptoms over the course of the menstrual cycle. If, as in many cases, their depression worsens premenstrually, they may want to ask their clinician to adjust the dosage of their medication accordingly.

See also TRANQUILIZERS.

antigen   Any substance that stimulates the body to produce antibodies and reacts specifically with them. Such substances include toxins (poisons), foreign proteins, bacteria and foreign tissue.

See also ANTIBODY.

anus   The opening of the rectum to the outside of the body, through which solid body wastes (feces) are expelled. The *anal canal,* a short passage about one and one-half inches long, leads from the external opening to the rectum. The skin around the anus is highly sensitive, both to irritation (as from diarrhea or vaginal discharge) and to erotic stimulation, as in oral-anal sex.

Anal intercourse, with the partner's penis or a dildo inserted into the anus, requires more gentleness than vaginal intercourse, because the anus is not as elastic as the vagina and the delicate mucous membranes inside it may tear. Use of a lubricant (saliva, vaginal mucus or water-soluble jelly) therefore is recommended, as well as a condom for protection against AIDS and other sexually transmitted diseases, which are very readily transmitted in this way. Also, because anal bacteria can cause serious vaginal infection, a penis or finger inserted into the anus during lovemaking should always be washed before being inserted into the vagina (or a condom may be used for anal intercourse and then removed or replaced for vaginal penetration). For the same reason, girls and women are urged to wipe from front to back after a bowel movement to avoid wiping anal bacteria toward the entrance of the vagina or urethra.

Oral-anal contact, called *anilingus* or *rimming,* carries the danger of oral contact with feces, which can lead to several serious infections, among them hepatitis B and HIV (AIDS virus) infections. It is safest to avoid it, but if it is done, use a barrier, such as a rubber dam (latex barrier, used in dentistry) or a portion of a latex glove, to prevent the exchange of fluids between the tongue and the anus. In another practice called *fisting,* the whole hand is inserted into the rectum and balled up into a fist. This is likely to cause tears in the walls of the rectum, with risk of a potentially fatal injury or infection (peritonitis, AIDS). If performed, one should use a rubber glove and then dispose of it immediately. Both LYMPHOGRANULOMA VENEREUM and GONORRHEA can affect the anus, and syphilis and herpes infection are other SEXUALLY TRANSMITTED DISEASES that can give rise to perianal lesions (near the anus).

See also ANAL FISSURE; HEMORRHOID.

anxiety   Also *panic disorder.* An emotional disorder characterized by prolonged feelings of profound fear and apprehension that have no appropriate cause. Everyone feels anxious at one time or another, but the feeling usually is of short duration and is directly related to an external cause; when the cause is removed, the anxiety disappears. Furthermore, if the source of anxiety is repeated again and again (as with stage fright, the fear of appearing before an audience), usually less and less fear is felt as a person gains experience with the situation. With neurotic anxiety, however, a person may feel increasing panic with each repetition, leading her to avoid the situation entirely.

Anxiety disorders affect 19.1 millions Americans, and women have twice the risk of men. They often are not recognized as disorders resulting from an imbalance of brain chemicals. They can take a variety of forms: phobia, obsessive-compulsive disorder, generalized anxiety disorder, panic disorder and post-traumatic stress disorder. A *phobia* is anxiety relating to a specific situation or object; phobias occur twice as frequently in women as in men. The most common include fear of flying; animal phobias; fear of heights or storms; fear of blood, injury or injections; situational phobias, such as fear of riding in elevators or driving on bridges; and fear of leaving home (see AGORAPHOBIA). Another kind is *social phobia,* fear of any situation in which one must interact socially with others, especially if one has to perform (make a speech, play an instrument). Many of these disorders overlap.

Sometimes anxiety takes the form of *obsessive-compulsive behavior*, that is, recurrent persistent ideas or repetitive compulsive actions, such as incessant hand-washing. Men and women are equally afflicted. *Generalized anxiety disorder* is characterized by the constant anticipation that something awful will happen, to oneself or a loved one, while *panic disorder* is an acute attack of the same symptoms. These symptoms include feelings of tension and apprehension, difficulty in making a decision and in concentrating, and sleep disturbances. Physical symptoms, particularly acute during an anxiety attack (or attack of panic), include trembling, twitching, dizziness, palpitations, shortness of breath (panting) and sweating. Nausea and vomiting or diarrhea may occur. *Post-traumatic stress disorder* is persistent anxiety following severe trauma, such as rape.

Although the symptoms of a panic attack frequently resemble those of a heart attack or other serious condition, no organic cause of such anxiety has been identified. This resemblance, however, hampers diagnosis; one study showed that the average patient sees as many as 10 physicians before getting an accurate diagnosis of panic disorder.

Prolonged and debilitating anxiety is usually treated with psychoactive drugs, principally the minor tranquilizers and antidepressants, and psychotherapy, especially cognitive-behavior therapy, which in effect teaches the sufferer how not to become anxious. An herbal anti-anxiety remedy is kava (or Kava-Kava), an extract from the roots of *Piper methysticum*, a species of pepper plant. Used for centuries in South Pacific rituals and long available in European pharmacies, it appears to have a relaxing effect without serious side effects. However, its action is not completely understood, and there are few data concerning interaction with other drugs.

Studies advise against using kava while pregnant or breast-feeding. Like other herbal remedies, it should be used with caution. Moreover, there have been reports of liver damage, sometimes severe enough to require a liver transplant, and sales of the herb have been halted in France and Switzerland and suspended in Britain. Consequently no one with liver trouble or who drinks a lot of alcohol should use kava. Possibly these serious effects are due to overdoses; in Germany 60 to 120 mg of kavalactone (the active ingredient) is considered a reasonable daily dose, but not to be used for more than four weeks.

Apgar score A system of evaluating the physical condition of a newborn infant that is used in many American hospitals. About one minute after birth the baby is evaluated on the basis of five signs: heart rate, respiratory effort, muscle tone, reflex response (to a catheter in the nostril and a foot slap) and color. The baby is graded 0, 1 or 2 for each sign, the best possible score being 10 (a grade of 2 for each sign) and the lowest, 0. A score of 7 to 10 indicates the infant is in good condition, 4 to 6 shows he or she is moderately depressed and needs resuscitation (administration of oxygen and suction) and 3 or less shows such severe depression that survival is in danger. The system is named for Virginia Apgar, an American physician who developed it in the 1950s.

aphrodisiac A substance that stimulates or enhances sexual desire. Over the centuries and in different cultures, plants such as ginseng, foods such as pomegranates, oysters and honey (and royal jelly), and various drugs all have been used

APGAR SCORE			
Sign	**0**	**1**	**2**
Heart rate	Absent	Slow (below 100)	Over 100
Respiratory effort	Absent	Slow, irregular	Good, strong cry
Muscle tone	Flaccid	Some flexion of extremities	Well flexed, active motion
Reflex response	No response	Grimace, weak cry	Vigorous cry
Color	Blue, pale	Body pink, extremities blue	Completely pink

for their alleged aphrodisiac properties, but there is little or no scientific evidence that they do or do not work. Modern researchers have found that certain drugs do increase sexual desire by acting on the hypothalamus, the part of the brain that is its "sex center," especially those that interact with receptors for the neurotransmitter dopamine. Among these are bupropion, an antidepressant; L-dopa and selegeline, anti-Parkinson's drugs; oxytocin, used to stimulate labor; and Estratest, a hormonal combination used for estrogen replacement. On the other hand, those that act primarily on serotonin receptors, such as the antidepressant fluoxetine (Prozac), definitely depress the sex drive, as can such other widely used medications as various remedies for high blood pressure and high cholesterol. The same is true of alcohol and marijuana, which may loosen inhibitions but can impair performance. Regular exercise seems to enhance libido, but probably the most potent aphrodisiacs are mental, particularly psychological intimacy and voyeurism (looking at pictures or films of persons engaged in romantic or sexual interplay).

See also LIBIDO.

apocrine glands   Scent glands in the pubic and axillary (underarm) areas that emit a milky, organic material with an erotically stimulating odor during sexual excitement. The scent is trapped by the pubic and axillary hair. Women have 75% more apocrine glands than men. They develop during puberty and also are present around the labia minora, nipples and navel.

appendectomy   Surgical removal of the vermiform appendix, a small appendage of the cecum, the upper end of the large intestine. It can become inflamed and infected, usually with the bacterium *Escherichia coli*, which is normally resident in the healthy intestine. This condition is called *appendicitis* and calls for removal of the appendix because, should the infection become severe, peritonitis readily develops. *Peritonitis* is inflammation of the membrane that lines the abdominal cavity and constitutes a life-threatening emergency. The appendix serves no vital function, and a healthy

appendix often is removed during other abdominal surgery, especially hysterectomy and Cesarean section, as a preventive measure.

Appendicitis also can develop during pregnancy—in fact, it is the most common acute surgical condition occurring in pregnant women—and then calls for especially prompt treatment. Treated early, it rarely interferes with the pregnancy. Should treatment be delayed and the appendix perforate (burst), labor often is brought on, regardless of the length of the pregnancy.

Pregnancy makes appendicitis more difficult to diagnose. The usual symptoms and signs—pain in the lower right quadrant of the abdomen, an elevated white blood cell count, nausea and vomiting—are similar to some of the sensations of normal pregnancy, and the locus of pain is harder to determine because of the enlarged uterus. Surgery usually is the best course of treatment. If peritonitis has already developed, powerful antibiotics must also be used to control the infection.

areola   The ring of pink or brownish skin surrounding the nipple of the breast. Like the nipple itself, the areola has nerve endings and blood vessels that extend from larger connections within the breast itself. Within the areola are some rudimentary sebaceous (oil) glands, called *areolar glands, tubercles of Montgomery* or *Montgomery's follicles,* arranged in a circular fashion around the edge; during pregnancy these small roundish elevations are somewhat more prominent. Also, during pregnancy the areola's color becomes deeper, and some women develop a *secondary areola,* a circle of faint color that is seen just outside the true areola from about the fifth month on. Following delivery, the secondary areola becomes fainter or disappears.

See also NIPPLE.

aromatherapy   The use of certain aromatic plant oils to treat a variety of ailments. The oils are obtained by steaming, pounding or heating the plants, or by soaking them in alcohol or hot oil. They are administered through massage, baths (a few drops in the water) and skin preparations such as salves, compresses, and steam inhalations. The pleasant-smelling scent of such plants as heliotrope has been used to alleviate anxiety and stress in patients with cancer, and the scent of lavender oil appears to be helpful for insomnia. The scent of rosemary, a plant containing cineole, a central nervous system stimulant, is thought to help prevent memory loss and dementia. Chamomile allegedly promotes relaxation, and eucalyptus and geranium oils may help fight viral infection. Hyssop and garlic oils have been used to treat both high and low blood pressure. However, there is scanty scientific research to back up the claims of aromatherapists, for whom there currently are no licensing standards. One should never take any of these essential oils by mouth (some are very toxic), and it is wise to dilute them before applying to the skin in case they prompt an allergic reaction. Further, some are dangerous. Pennyroyal can cause a miscarriage, and overdoses of saffron can trigger convulsions, delirium and even death.

See also HERBAL REMEDIES.

arteriosclerosis Also *atherosclerotic cardiovascular disease (ASCVS), cardiovascular disease, coronary artery disease, hardening of the arteries.* A group of diseases characterized by thickening and loss of elasticity of the arterial walls, impairing the flow of blood through the arteries. The principal diseases are arteriosclerosis itself, in which there are changes in the small arteries and which usually is secondary to HYPERTENSION (high blood pressure) and, most common of all, *atherosclerosis,* in which the arteries are narrowed by *atheromas,* localized accumulations of fatty substances. Atherosclerosis, also called *atherosclerotic cardiovascular disease,* may begin early in life and usually gives rise to no symptoms for years. Gradually the walls of the arteries become thicker and the flow of blood is restricted. Eventually an atheroma may completely block a major artery, which can, depending on its location, lead to dramatic and sometimes fatal results—a heart attack or cerebral vascular accident, or stroke. (In a heart attack, technically called a *myocardial infarction,* the atheroma blocks the blood supply to the heart muscle, or myocardium; in stroke it blocks the blood supply to the brain.) Atheromas also promote the clotting of blood in arteries, and when

clots create a blockage in a vital artery (supplying heart or brain), a similar crisis may result.

Women tend to get heart disease later in life than men, but as a rule it is more severe; it is the leading cause of death in women over age 66, claiming 6 times the number of lives lost to breast cancer, and the rate is still higher for black women.

Although the causes of atherosclerosis are not known, there are definite predisposing factors. Chief among them are hypertension, high blood levels of cholesterol and triglycerides, lack of physical activity, cigarette smoking (especially in conjunction with birth control pills), diabetes, obesity and possibly stress. Recent studies indicate that high levels of an amino acid, HOMOCYSTEINE, also are linked with an increased risk of heart disease. The risk increases with a family history of early atherosclerosis and also with age. Recent findings also indicate that women whose waist measurement exceeds 30 inches, or who have a waist-to-hip ratio greater than .88, run a higher risk of a heart attack or death from heart disease. Even if such women are not overweight, their "apple shape," as opposed to a "pear shape," puts them at higher risk. (A similar risk exists for men.) The reason is not known, but it is speculated that abdominal fat is more dangerous than fat elsewhere. There are two kinds of abdominal fat: visceral, which surrounds the abdominal organs and appears in the apple shape, and subcutaneous, lying between the skin and abdomen. Apart from bringing weight under control, the best approach to reducing abdominal fat is moderate-to-intense physical activity at least 30 minutes a day and an hour of weight training twice a week. Research is underway to develop drugs that target abdominal fat.

The name *metabolic syndrome* has been given to a cluster of problems that appear to predict heart attack risks. A patient with three or more of the following is considered at risk: obesity centered around the waist; high blood pressure; low levels of HDL (the "good cholesterol"); high levels of triglycerides; and difficulty metabolizing sugar.

Another predictor of increased risk is a high level of C-reactive protein (CRP), a chemical produced in the liver and released into the bloodstream in the presence of acute or chronic inflammation. Its presence can be measured by a simple, inexpensive blood test, performed twice two weeks apart with the two results averaged. A level of CRP of 1 to 3 milligrams per liter indicates moderate cardiovascular risk and calls for aggressive action to reduce it, via weight loss, smoking cessation, increased exercise, and possible use of cholesterol-lowering statins and the antidiabetic thiazolidinediones.

Preventive measures for atherosclerosis include periodic checks of blood pressure and, after middle age, of blood levels of cholesterol and triglycerides, followed by appropriate treatment if any of these levels rise beyond safe limits. Regular and vigorous physical exercise, stopping smoking, careful control of diabetes and weight control also help. Precautionary dietary measures also are recommended—some clinicians advise them for everyone, regardless of history—particularly reducing salt intake to avoid high blood pressure, reducing intake of foods that raise serum cholesterol, and replacing foods high in saturated fats, such as butter and pork products, with polyunsaturated fats, found in corn and other vegetable oils. A diet very low in fat (10 to 15% of a day's total calories from fat) also may provide protection. The American Heart Association recommends eating fish rich in omega-3 fats such as salmon and sardines at least twice a week, cutting sodium intake to 1,500 mg a day for people over 50 and, for women over 65, taking a daily low-dose aspirin (81 mg). Individuals with a high waist-to-hip ratio should be especially careful about diet and exercise, as well as about lowering other risk factors.

A diagnosis of coronary heart disease usually begins with an electrocardiogram and often includes a stress test, in which the patient exercises on a treadmill or stationary bicycle while hooked up to an electrocardiograph that measures the heart's electric activity at close to maximum capacity. A supplementary test is an image of the heart taken with echocardiography (in which sound waves construct a three-dimensional image) and/or a thallium scan (injecting a radioactive isotope that shows up on X-ray). A third test is a scan for calcium buildup in the arteries. Called *electron beam computed tomography* (EBCT), it uses a burst of X-rays to show how much calcium has been

RISK FACTORS FOR HEART DISEASE

Condition	Effects	Preventive Measures
High blood pressure	Stress on arteries paves way for arterial plaque deposits	Lose weight, exercise, restrict salt, medication
Diabetes	May damage arteries, raises blood pressure, worsens cholesterol levels	Lose weight, exercise, don't smoke; consider aspirin use
Poor lipid Profile	Low HDL (lower than 35; some say 45), high LDL, high triglyceride level (over 400)	Aerobic exercise; low-fat diet; consider estrogen replacement
Smoking	Increases risk in women 5 times or more	Quit smoking
Obesity and central-body obesity	Body mass index of 27 or more, waist-to-hip ratio of .9 or more	Lose weight, exercise
Sedentary lifestyle	Heart muscle, like other muscles, needs exercise	At least 30 minutes of moderate exercise a day

deposited in the coronary arteries, a good measure of how much plaque has accumulated there. High calcium scores suggest significant hardening of the arteries. In 2004 a government panel on preventive medicine concluded that for individuals who have no known risk factors, the risks posed by these procedures clearly outweigh the benefits, missing a significant number of disorders and producing an even larger number of false alarms. In patients who do need them, if any of these tests indicate abnormality, coronary angiography (also called cardiac catheterization) is performed. Dye is injected through a thin tube that has been inserted into the heart via an artery in the thigh or arm. An X-ray then reveals a kind of road map of all the blood vessels supplying the heart; those that are narrowed or blocked show up readily because they admit little or no dye.

Differences between men and women seem to exist at each stage of heart disease. Both are at

WOMEN'S EARLY WARNING SYMPTOMS OF HEART ATTACK*

Experienced more than one month before attack
- Unusual fatigue
- Sleep disturbances
- Shortness of breath

Acute symptoms
- Shortness of breath
- Dizziness
- Nausea
- Sweatiness
- Weakness
- Fatigue

*Unlike in men, chest discomfort and acute chest pain are largely absent.

risk if cholesterol levels are high, but in women high levels of another lipoprotein, triglycerides, seem to put them at higher risk even if cholesterol levels are low. Women are more likely to show abnormalities on their electrocardiograms (EKGs), which may lead a physician to ignore a slight EKG abnormality that would get more attention in a male patient. (Part of the problem may lie in the fact that a woman's breasts make it hard to place electrodes correctly on her chest; they also get in the way of a thallium scan.) Women also may have atypical symptoms of a heart attack, including shortness of breath, unusual fatigue or weakness, a cold sweat and dizziness. Women often have chest pain for a long time before a heart attack occurs; in men such pain usually signals that a heart attack has already begun. Because women heart patients often are elderly, they may not be able to tolerate an adequate stress test. Cigarette smoking sharply increases a woman's chance of having a heart attack; one study shows that it doubles the risk for women who smoke as few as one cigarette a day and increases it 11 times among heavy smokers (45 or more cigarettes a day). Finally, women are twice as likely as men to die within 60 days of a heart attack. The higher mortality rate probably is influenced by difficulties in diagnosis, more advanced age and a seeming reluctance by many physicians to treat women heart patients as aggressively as men. In any event, women do not do as well as

men after balloon angioplasty (inflating a balloon inside a narrowed diseased coronary artery so as to widen it)—one study showed they were 10 times as likely to die following this procedure—or after bypass surgery.

Findings from a federally funded Women's Ischemia Syndrome Evaluation study—*ischemia* means inadequate blood flow—indicate that in many women blockages occur not in large coronary arteries but in a network of smaller vessels that also nourish the heart. This condition, which may affect as many as 3 million American women, has been called *coronary microvascular dysfunction,* or *microvessel disease,* and *Syndrome X.* It is thought to account for the gender difference in symptoms of a heart attack (see table at left), why coronary angiography fails to identify the problem and why women who undergo angioplasty and bypass surgery do not recover as well as men. Stress tests and functional vascular imaging may diagnose the condition. The causes are unknown, but inflammation is a major suspect, and three proteins associated with inflammation—C-reactive protein, interleukin-6 and serum amyloid—may help assess the extent of the condition. Other cardiovascular risk factors (see accompanying table) also are implicated. Still other possible factors are premenopausal high blood pressure, anemia, and polycystic ovarian syndrome.

The later onset of heart disease in women gave rise to the idea that before menopause higher levels of estrogen protect against it. ESTROGEN REPLACEMENT THERAPY, long thought to reduce the risk of heart disease, has been found to be ineffective, but recent findings indicate that ORAL CONTRACEPTIVES may do so. Protective measures sometimes recommended include regular use of low-dose aspirin (75 to 100 mg daily) and moderate use of alcohol, especially red wine (4 ounces a day). Women who have already had a heart attack can cut their risk of a subsequent attack, stroke, and death by taking a cholesterol-lowering drug, even if their cholesterol levels are normal. Such medication also reduces the risk of a woman's need for bypass surgery (in which detours are built around clogged arteries) and angioplasty (which uses a balloon to widen arteries narrowed by plaque).

Anyone experiencing chest pain is advised to call 911 immediately for an ambulance and to take an aspirin. Even if it does not turn out to be a heart attack, it is better to err on the side of caution. An ambulance is preferable to other transportation because personnel are trained and equipped to deal with arrhythmias, start an intravenous line, give oxygen, and sometimes even administer an electrocardiogram. They also can radio information ahead to the hospital emergency room to enable faster treatment.

See also ANGINA PECTORIS.

artery One of a system of thick-walled, elastic muscular tubes that carry blood away from the heart. The major arteries lead to all structures of the body, branching and rebranching into smaller and smaller arteries, and finally *arterioles* and *capillaries* as they reach the organs they serve. Every contraction of the heart's ventricles forces a quantity of blood into the arteries, whose muscular walls stretch to accommodate these sudden surges. Each surge is followed by a contraction of the artery wall, which serves to push the blood along and so supplements the pumping work of the ventricles. Blood thus flows through the arteries in regular spurts rather than in a steady stream.

The distention of the arteries as blood surges through them can be detected in those vessels close to the surface of the body, such as the radial artery in the wrist, and is called the *pulse*. The rate of the heart's pumping thus can be determined by the pulse rate. The adult resting pulse is, on the average, somewhere between 50 and 90 beats per minute, but the normal range is wider still. A rapid heart rate—anywhere from 100 beats per minute or more (except in an unborn baby, where 140 beats per minute is not at all abnormal)—is called *tachycardia* and may be symptomatic of numerous disorders. However, the heart rate normally increases with vigorous exercise, sexual excitement, fear and under numerous other circumstances. The principal disease of the arteries is ARTERIOSCLEROSIS.

See also VEIN.

arthritis Also *rheumatism* (pop.). General name for a number of inflammatory diseases characterized by swelling, redness and/or tenderness of one or more joints. Not all joint aches, pains or stiffness constitute arthritis, a term usually reserved for conditions that are more or less chronic. A notable exception, however, is arthritis caused by infection, which generally can be totally cured by appropriate antibiotic treatment, although if it is not treated in time the affected joints can be permanently damaged. Among the infectious agents that can cause such arthritis are streptococci, staphylococci, pneumococci (which cause pneumonia), gonococci (which cause GONORRHEA) and the organisms that cause influenza, hepatitis, bacterial endocarditis and rubella. Another arthritic disease is *rheumatic fever*, which begins as an infection, usually by streptococci, and develops into an AUTOIMMUNE DISEASE. Both RHEUMATOID ARTHRITIS and SYSTEMIC LUPUS ERYTHEMATOSUS afflict women far more often than men; OSTEOARTHRITIS, the most common kind of arthritis, is more common in women than men when it strikes after the age of 45, as is usually the case.

artificial insemination Also *AI, alternative insemination, donor insemination, DI*. Inserting sperm into a woman's vagina by means other than sexual intercourse, in order for her to become pregnant. It is generally used by a heterosexual couple when the woman is fertile but the man's sperm is of poor quality (low count, low mobility, etc.), or he risks passing on a hereditary disease, or there are other barriers to sexual intercourse. For example, it may be used when the man is fertile but the woman has a disorder preventing the passage of sperm through her cervix; her own partner's sperm then is directly introduced into the uterus (*intrauterine insemination*). It also is used occasionally when a woman wishes to avoid heterosexual intercourse but wants to bear a child.

In *homologous* artificial insemination, the sperm is the husband's or regular partner's, and in *heterologous* artificial insemination, it is that of an unrelated donor. Some clinicians consider the latter a form of adoption—it has been called "semiadoption"—and many may insist that a couple considering donor insemination undergo interviews over a period to time in order to assess their emotional stability both individually and as a couple. Further, most insist that the woman be demonstrably fertile (based on a basal temperature chart to show she is ovulating as well as some other test to show that her tubes are not blocked, and sometimes also an endometrial biopsy) and that the man undergo extensive medical investigation for the cause of his infertility and any available treatment for it. Another criterion is that the man really wants the procedure performed—especially if it is heterologous—and is not just being pressed to agree by the woman.

Homologous artificial insemination sometimes is successful when a man has healthy sperm but in insufficient numbers (see OLIGOSPERMIA) or if there is an Rh factor or coital problem. Heterologous insemination is indicated when there are either no sperm (azoospermia) or no live sperm (necrospermia) or when the male partner has a hereditary disease carrying too great a risk for natural offspring. The choice of donor is, of course, very important. The main criteria are that he is fertile, as shown by semen analysis (see SPERM); that he is free of any illness, transmittable disease and history of hereditary diseases; that his intelligence is equal to that of the couple and that he is emotionally stable; that his physical proportions are similar to those of the husband or male partner; and that his blood group and type are compatible with those of the woman. For extra safety, some clinicians prefer to use only married donors with two or more healthy children of their own.

Some clinicians use *multiple donors*, that is, semen is inserted two or more times during a single ovulatory period with a different donor's used each time. Others prefer not to mix sperm. The time of ovulation is determined, and insertion, at the doctor's office or at a clinic, is by syringe into the vagina; generally a speculum is inserted first in order to expose the cervix. The woman is asked to remain prone for 20 minutes after insertion, with her pelvis somewhat higher than her head and shoulders, and before rising may insert a tampon or a cervical cap over the cervix to help retain the semen longer and enhance the chances of conception. Artificial insemination is usually performed twice a month (on the 12th and 14th days of a 28-day menstrual cycle, or at comparable times for longer or shorter cycles) for about four months. If the woman does not conceive, there may be further testing of her fertility. If no abnormality is discovered, the process is repeated for another six months. Statistics indicate that more than half of all women conceive during the first six months. Women with endometriosis, a history of pelvic disorders or ovulatory problems do not respond as well as others. Also, women over the age of 30 have a 30% lower pregnancy rate than younger women.

Although donor insemination may be performed by a woman herself, for heterologous insemination the American Society for Reproductive Medicine strongly recommends using only frozen semen (not fresh) because of the risk of contracting sexually transmitted diseases (including HIV). Therefore if she chooses a particular donor other than her partner, she must bring her donor's semen to a sperm bank or a physician with the appropriate facilities, where it is tested for HIV and other infectious agents and then frozen for at least three and up to nine months. The semen then is retested and only then can be used. It is not screened for genetic abnormalities, although donors are asked for their histories. This procedure is expensive and obviously slows down the process. Also, the thawed sperm has decreased motility, a shorter life span and reduced ability to penetrate cervical mucus. Using frozen sperm from an anonymous donor that has already been tested may represent a quicker and simpler solution.

To use fresh sperm from her partner, within 30 minutes of ejaculation the woman draws semen into a syringe (eye dropper, needleless hypodermic or even a kitchen baster), lies down on her back with a pillow under the buttocks and inserts the syringe into her vagina, depositing the semen near the cervix. She should remain in this position for 10 minutes or so, so as to prevent the sperm from leaking out. It is wise to repeat the procedure with a fresh sample every other day over the five-day period just before, during and following estimated ovulation. The same procedure can be followed at a women's health center or clinic. Reportedly most women succeed in conceiving after trying the procedure in three to five menstrual cycles.

At this writing the legal status of donor insemination varies from state to state, but there are no laws forbidding it. However, it is wise to check the laws in one's own state and to consult an attorney concerning the donor's paternity rights and the child's inheritance rights in case of death or divorce.

Human artificial insemination dates from the mid-19th century. In the United States it was first performed successfully by Dr. James Marion Sims in 1866; the first insemination using a donor's sperm was performed in the 1890s by Dr. Robert L. Dickinson.

See also EMBRYO TRANSFER; IN VITRO FERTILIZATION; SPERM BANK; SURROGATE MOTHER.

Ascheim-Zondeck test See PREGNANCY TEST.

Asherman's syndrome The presence of scar tissue (see ADHESION) in the uterine wall in amounts sufficient to prevent regular menstruation and cause infertility. Such scar tissue can result from repeated infection, as in chronic PELVIC INFLAMMATORY DISEASE, from repeated or overstrenuous curettage (see D AND C) or from an abnormally adherent placenta in a previous pregnancy. Although rare, Asherman's syndrome can cause AMENORRHEA (see def. 3) and lead to permanent infertility. Most often, however, periods are regular but scanty. Therefore, if a D and C must be performed in the presence of infection (as, for example, when infected placental tissue must be removed after a miscarriage or abortion), the curettage (scraping) of the endometrium must be done exceptionally gently and cautiously to avoid this condition.

Diagnosis is confirmed by X-ray. For women who wish to become pregnant, the usual treatment for Asherman's syndrome is to break up the scar tissue surgically, which may be possible using a hysteroscope and small scissors (when not by abdominal incision). An INTRAUTERINE DEVICE (IUD) is then inserted for a few months to keep the uterine walls open and to prevent adhesions from reforming while the endometrial tissue grows back. Also, a short-term (60-day) estrogen supplement is given to restore the endometrium. After normal menstrual periods have been reestablished, the IUD is removed.

aspermatogenesis See STERILITY.

aspiration See VACUUM ASPIRATION. For needle aspiration, see BIOPSY, def. 3.

asthma A lung disease characterized by attacks in which the bronchi become inflamed and narrowed by spasm, resulting in shortness of breath and wheezing. In severe cases an attack can be fatal. Asthma is most common in children and young adults. Before age 10 twice as many boys as girls have asthma, but by the age of 20 the disease afflicts nearly three times as many women as men. This difference may, studies indicate, be due to hormones, particularly to high levels of estradiol, progesterone or cortisol, which is consistent with the post-adolescent surge of asthmatic women. Obesity also appears to be a risk factor. Allergy is another contributing factor, particularly to agents that are inhaled and then bring on an attack. However, certain foods and drugs, especially aspirin and ibuprofen, can have a similar effect, as can respiratory infections, exercise or simply inhaling cold air. Birth control pills can exacerbate asthma.

It is important to end an asthmatic attack as quickly as one can. Treatment consists of medication, given orally and/or inhaled. The most common drugs are bronchodilators such as albuterol, theophylline or beta-2 agonists, which relax the involuntary muscles controlling the airways. Often they can be inhaled via an aerosol dispenser (they also come in the form of pills and injections). Once the attack is controlled, the clinician may prescribe preventive medications such as cromolyn, zafirlukast or zileuton to keep the airways open and help prevent attacks brought on by exercise or exposure to a specific allergen. In resistant cases anti-inflammatory agents, mainly corticosteroids, are needed. Oral corticosteroids (in pill form) are effective for suppressing symptoms, but their long-term use is associated with weight gain, high blood pressure, osteoporosis and cataracts. These complications occur far less with inhaled steroids.

Since most patients have normal lung function except during attacks, preventive measures are extremely important. They include avoiding smoke (including secondhand cigarette smoke) and other pollutants, and avoiding allergens, especially inhaled ones such as house dust, cat dander, pollen, plant molds (on house plants) and the like. Exercise-induced attacks may be avoided by inhaling a bronchodilator before running and breathing warm humid air during exercise (as in a heated indoor pool or gym). Also to be avoided are walking outdoors in cold weather or at least wearing a face mask when doing so. Holistic methods appear to help some asthma sufferers. Massage, yoga, acupuncture, biofeedback and meditation all have their advocates for this purpose, used in conjunction with bronchial dilators and the preventive measures already outlined.

In pregnancy about one-third of women who have asthma remain free from attacks; in another third the frequency of asthmatic attacks remains the same; and in the rest, asthma develops for the first time during pregnancy. A new study indicates that asthma in pregnancy can cause complications for both mother and fetus. Pregnant women with asthma are more likely to have high blood pressure, prebirth bleeding, amniotic membrane-related disorders, gestational diabetes and Cesarean sections than women without asthma. Also, infants born to women with asthma have lower birth weights and are smaller in size for their gestational age. Of the women in the study, 77% did not use daily asthma controller medications; 66% instead relied on quick-relief medications and 26% used them excessively. However, most asthma drugs are considered safe during pregnancy, although corticosteroids in pill form (rather than inhaled) should be avoided if at all possible. Treatment then must be adjusted and monitored so as to avoid compromising the pregnancy or harming the fetus.

asymptomatic Without symptoms, that is, without signs of a particular disorder or disease. For example, a man may have a *Trichomonas* infection without knowing it because he experiences no itching, discharge or other symptoms. He then may unwittingly transmit it to his partner.

atherosclerosis See ARTERIOSCLEROSIS.

athletic ability, women's The strength, coordination, speed of reflexes and other qualities and skills required in various sports as found in women, compared to those of men. Until the age of about 10, boys and girls are much the same in physical strength. The amount of oxygen a boy or girl can deliver to the muscles, known as *maximal oxygen uptake,* is identical, as are strength and endurance. By the age of 15, however, when sex hormones affect the body's development, there is considerable difference between the two sexes. Although female and male hormones are present in both, the comparative amounts are vastly different. The longer-term growth spurt and increased testosterone (male hormone) levels in boys make for a great increase in upper-body (arm and shoulder) strength, and the entire body becomes taller and heavier. After PUBERTY the female, in contrast, has a much larger percentage of fat to total body weight (25% compared to 14% in males) and less potential for developing muscle mass. In adulthood the average American man is 4 inches taller than the average woman and 30 to 40 pounds heavier. Women have smaller bones, smaller lungs and less muscle mass than men. In sports in which strength, height and speed are called for, therefore, as in basketball, the best women athletes are necessarily inferior to the best men. The same is true for sports requiring largely upper-body strength, such as the racket sports (tennis, squash, etc.). Where other qualities are required, however, such as flexibility for gymnastics, women excel. In some activities, moreover, women have been closing the gap between their performance and that of men, notably in swimming (both speed and long-distance) and in long-distance running.

One problem for women athletes who train very hard is that they may stop menstruating (see AMENORRHEA, def. 3). Preliminary results of studies currently under way suggest that when the ratio of a woman's body fat to lean weight drops below a certain threshold, as it does with vigorous training, a signal is sent to the pituitary gland to stop ovulation, causing menstrual periods to stop; when these women regain weight, their periods usually resume. What still is not known is the effect of training and exercise on hormones, raising questions such as whether, with heavy exercise, a woman's adrenal glands will, like her muscles, become larger, like those of men, and might then produce more androgens (male hormones), which in turn are linked with more aggressive behavior, higher bone density and increased muscle-protein synthesis.

See also ANABOLIC STEROIDS.

atrial fibrillation   A condition in which the heartbeat is quite irregular and usually quite rapid so that the heart pumps blood less effectively. It occurs when the heart's muscle fibers in the atrium (upper heart chamber) contract erratically (quiver, or fibrillate) instead of regularly. This kind of heart arrhythmia sometimes occurs in the absence of heart disease. In other cases it is caused by an overactive thyroid gland (hyperthyroidism), excessive alcohol or caffeine, or certain forms of heart disease. Some individuals with atrial fibrillation experience no symptoms, whereas others may feel palpitations or be acutely aware of their heartbeat. Formerly, atrial fibrillation was considered relatively benign because its most common symptoms (palpitations, dizziness, shortness of breath) were often short-lived. Now, however, it is recognized that atrial fibrillation allows blood to pool in the atria and form clots, which in turn may lead to strokes and heart attacks. Moreover, about one-third of strokes in patients aged 80 or older are attributable to atrial fibrillation and are more likely to be fatal than other types. Also, chronic atrial fibrillation may cause congestive heart failure. It is important to distinguish atrial fibrillation, which usually is not immediately life-threatening, from *ventricular fibrillation,* a rhythmic dysfunction of the ventricles that may be fatal if not treated within minutes.

Atrial fibrillation is usually treated with oral medication or cardioversion (defibrillation, delivery of an electric shock to the heart); however, even if the heart rhythm returns to normal, it may be necessary to continue drug treatment indefinitely. Because atrial fibrillation can lead to blood clots that can cause a stroke if they reach the brain, the first consideration for managing the condition is assessing the risk factors for stroke. With no risk factors, daily aspirin may be sufficient to prevent blood clots. With a single moderate risk factor, such as hypertension or diabetes, either aspirin or an oral anticoagulant (blood thinner) such as warfarin (Coumadin) may be required, whereas the latter is recommended for those at high risk for stroke. For those with persistent atrial fibrillation, other drugs used include Toprol or digoxin to control a rapid heart rate and amiadarone to regulate heart rhythm. A newer therapy for some patients is a minimally invasive procedure called *catheter ablation.* It involves inserting a tiny catheter through a leg vein and threading it up to the atria. The sources of abnormal electrical activity in the atria are located and destroyed either by radio-frequency energy or by freezing. Full-scale clinical trials have not yet shown the long-term benefits of catheter ablation. Occasionally patients will need subsequent ablation and also may have to continue with their former drug regimen or, in some cases, have a pacemaker implanted. Occasionally, in stubborn cases, surgery may be indicated. A form of open-heart surgery, it involves a series of small incisions in the atria that interrupt and channel the erratic electrical signals, as well as removal of the left atrial appendage, a prime source of blood clot formation. In a somewhat less invasive version of this procedure, slender instruments are inserted through small incisions in the chest so as to partition off the tissue causing fibrillation by means of radio waves, ultrasound, cryosurgery and similar techniques.

Atrial fibrillation can usually be well controlled and managed to allow patients to lead a normal life, so the condition warrants seeing a clinician to determine the cause and possible treatment.

augment anesthesia   See ANESTHESIA.

autoimmune disease   Any disorder in which the body in effect attacks itself by producing antibodies against its own normal tissues. There are at least 80 autoimmune diseases, and they affect an estimated 5 to 8% of the American population.

Examples include: Graves' disease and Hashimoto's thyroiditis (see THYROID), hemolytic anemia, MULTIPLE SCLEROSIS, MYOSITIS, MYASTHENIA GRAVIS, RHEUMATOID ARTHRITIS, SCLERODERMA, SJÖGREN'S SYNDROME and SYSTEMIC LUPUS ERYTHEMATOSUS. Also, CHRONIC FATIGUE SYNDROME, FIBROMYALGIA, INFLAMMATORY BOWEL DISEASE and psoriasis may be autoimmune disorders. Women are more likely to develop autoimmune diseases than men and at the same time have more immunologic protection against severe bacterial and viral infections. The reason, it is conjectured, is that during pregnancy women must support the growth of foreign tissue (the fetus) inside their bodies. This tissue is not rejected, as other foreign tissue usually is, presumably because certain substances produced during pregnancy suppress immunologic responses somewhat, though not so much as to risk death from dangerous infections. These same superior immunologic defenses may make women more susceptible to autoimmune disease.

Many autoimmune diseases are treated by suppressing the immune system, but that approach leaves a person vulnerable to infection. One such drug, Tysabri (natalizumab), used for multiple sclerosis, had to be taken off the market in 2005 after it was linked to a rare and often fatal viral brain infection. It has since returned on a limited basis (see under MULTIPLE SCLEROSIS). The most successful treatments so far have been drugs that block tumor necrosis factor, a protein in the body that spurs inflammation. Research is also being directed at ways to detect the diseases' symptoms by finding telltale antibodies or genetic markers.

See also IMMUNITY.

automanipulation   See MASTURBATION.

axillary   Of or in the armpit. Breast cancer that has begun to metastasize (spread) often involves the axillary lymph nodes, which usually are examined very carefully whenever the disease is suspected. The growth of axillary hair is one of the early signs of puberty.

Ayurveda   Also *Ayurvedic medicine.* A traditional medicine from India that incorporates medicinal, psychologic, religious and philosophic components. The name means "knowledge of life," and it has eight main branches of medicine: pediatrics, gynecology, obstetrics, ophthalmology, geriatrics, otorhinolaryngology (ear-nose-throat specialty), surgery and general medicine. Each type is addressed in terms of three doshas, or life forces, and the patient's constitutional type. Like traditional Chinese medicine, Ayurveda uses energy points, pulse diagnosis and herbal remedies as well as yoga and meditation. Good health, considered a state of balance where body, mind, spirit and environment are in harmony, is achieved through proper diet, exercise and lifestyle habits, through meditation and through psychological well-being. The Ayurvedic practitioner rarely treats symptoms but concentrates on removing the causes of a disorder. Following diagnosis, which involves pulse analysis and evaluation of one's constitutional makeup, treatment involves counseling concerning diet and lifestyle, and instituting a routine of massage, cleansing, meditation and exercise. It also may involve AROMATHERAPY, visualization and music therapy. Ayurveda is said to relieve such diverse complaints as insomnia, constipation, allergies and colds, back pain, arthritis, hypertension, tension headache, skin problems, nausea, obesity, anxiety, bronchitis, digestive disorders and various emotional problems. Although not recognized as a medicine in the United States (it is considered ALTERNATIVE MEDICINE), it may be used in conjunction with more conventional treatment.

azoospermia   A total absence of sperm in the seminal fluid, rendering a man sterile.

See also STERILITY.

B

back labor During childbirth, discomfort from uterine contractions that is felt principally in the lower back. It often occurs with a POSTERIOR PRE-SENTATION, presumably because the back of the baby's head is pressing against the mother's back. It may be eased by leaning forward or crouching on the hands and knees and by having the birth attendant apply firm hand pressure against the lower back. Lying across a BIRTH BALL also may afford relief.

bacterial vaginosis See VAGINOSIS.

balloon ablation Also *uterine balloon therapy.* A method of relieving hypermenorrhea (very heavy menstrual flow) that is not caused by fibroids, cancer or endometriosis. An outpatient procedure, it destroys the endometrium (uterine lining) but leaves the uterus intact and avoids the need for hysterectomy; however, it precludes a success-ful pregnancy and therefore can be used only for women who do not intend to have children.

Balloon ablation, inspired by the balloon angio-plasty that is used to open blocked coronary arter-ies, involves inserting a balloon-tipped catheter through the vagina and cervix into the uterus. The balloon is then filled with a sterile solution until it conforms to the shape of the uterus. A heat-ing element heats the fluid to about 189 degrees Fahrenheit (87 degrees Celsius), and the balloon remains in place for 8 minutes, during which the heat destroys the endometrial tissue. The balloon is then deflated and the fluid drained through the catheter, which is removed.

Balloon ablation is performed in a doctor's office or clinic with local anesthesia, a sedative and medi-cation to prevent cramping. Most patients return home after a few hours in the recovery room. Mild cramping, lasting about a day, and watery or spot-ted discharge, lasting about 10 days, are the most common aftermath. Performed on women whose heavy flows had not been controlled by oral con-traceptives or dilatation and curettage (D and C), the procedure is effective in about 90% of patients, who then have either significantly reduced men-strual flow or no menstrual periods.

ballottement See QUICKENING.

Band-Aid surgery See LAPAROSCOPY.

bariatric surgery Surgery to correct gross obesity. It is generally considered a last resort for persons who are morbidly obese, exceeding their ideal weight by at least 100 pounds and with a body mass index (BMI) of more than 40. (See OBESITY for an explanation.) The number of such surgeries for patients between the ages of 55 and 64 in the United States has soared from 772 procedures in 1998 to 177,600 in 2006, a 2,000% increase. There has been a similar increase in surgeries among patients aged 18 to 54. Women undergo bariatric surgery more than men, accounting for about 80% of the total in the years mentioned.

In the past, obesity surgery consisted of an *intestinal bypass,* bypassing a portion of the small intestine from the normal flow, reducing its length, and diminishing the surface for absorbing nutri-ents. However, the side effects were so severe that this procedure was abandoned. Today several other techniques are used. By far the most common is *gastric bypass surgery,* which closes off a portion of the stomach. The gold standard of these procedures, because of its high degree of effectiveness and durability, is the Roux-en-Y gastric bypass, whereby the upper part of the stomach is sectioned off by a line of staples converting it into a small pouch, the small intestine is cut and one end is connected to the stomach pouch and the other end reattached to the small intestine (this creates a Y-shape, hence the name). It allows food to bypass most of the stomach and upper small intestine, although both still secrete the juices and enzymes required for digestion. Patients lose weight rapidly for about two years following surgery and many maintain most of the weight loss as long as they do not resume overeating. Gastric bypass is performed either as open surgery or laparoscopically, with only tiny incisions, which is more difficult to perform and has a relatively high complication rate.

In another technique, called *gastric banding* or *lap-band surgery,* and always performed laparoscopically, silicon bands are tied around the stomach to reduce its size. Bypass surgery costs about twice as much as lap-band surgery. Two other techniques are *vertical sleeve gastrectomy,* which removes up to 95% of the stomach and leaves behind a thin, tubelike stomach roughly 2 ounces in volume, and *duodenal switch,* whereby a large portion of the stomach is removed and the small intestine rearranged. Insurance coverage for all bariatric surgeries is highly variable.

Bariatric surgery has some marked benefits. Most weight loss—anywhere from 40 to 85% of excess weight, depending on the type of surgery—occurs within 18 to 24 months following surgery. Even sooner, about four-fifths of patients with Type II diabetes and seven-tenths of those with hypertension achieve normal blood sugar and normal blood pressure without medication. Moreover, more than four-fifths with high cholesterol bring down their levels to normal. Other benefits include relief from joint and back pain, asthma, sleep apnea, gastric reflux and gallbladder disease.

However, bariatric surgery often leads to complications and occasionally to death. Studies have found that 10 to 20% of patients suffer complications while still in the hospital, and about 40% within 180 days of surgery. The most common complications included vomiting, diarrhea, abdominal hernia, infection, pneumonia and respiratory failure, as well as leaking of gastric juices owing to imperfect surgical connections between the stomach and intestines. About 1% of patients die from complications, mainly infections and blood clots. Long-term complications include an increased risk of bone loss and osteoporosis, owing to postoperative malnutrition, which produces deficiencies in fat-soluble vitamins A, E, K and D, and anemia, due to low vitamin B_{12}. Consequently, many patients are advised to take a daily multivitamin, B_{12} and calcium supplement.

Anyone considering bariatric surgery should find a highly qualified surgeon, preferably a member of the American Society of Bariatric Surgery, and if possible have it performed in a hospital bariatric center that has quality certification supplied by the American College of Surgeons or the Surgical Review Corporation (the latter is a nonprofit set up by groups interested in improving surgery outcomes). By early 2007 about 225 U.S. hospitals and 400 surgeons were approved, and many more have applied for approval.

barrier methods Contraceptive methods or devices that depend largely or entirely on blocking the passage of live sperm through the cervix. Among them are the CERVICAL CAP, CONDOM, CONTRACEPTIVE SPONGE, DIAPHRAGM and various kinds of SPERMICIDE.

Bartholin cyst See CYST, def. 3.

Bartholin's glands Also *vestibular glands, vulvovaginal glands.* A pair of pea-size glands on each side of the introitus (vaginal entrance) that open into the vagina. They are believed to secrete minute quantities of mucus to lubricate the vagina during sexual intercourse. Normally small and inconspicuous, these glands can become greatly enlarged when they are infected, a not infrequent occurrence. The infecting organism often is the gonococcus, which causes gonorrhea, but other bacteria also may be responsible. The first sign of infection usually is a hot, extremely tender lump near the introitus. It can become as large as a lemon. With severe infection an abscess forms, which must be opened surgically and drained. Antibiotic therapy alone is not likely to work quickly enough because the abscess is circumscribed and its blood supply reduced, so antibiotics cannot reach it in sufficient amounts. Following surgery, which generally is an office procedure performed under local anesthesia, a small drain is left in place for several days.

Sometimes the glands become chronically inflamed without a known cause (viral infection has been suspected but not confirmed). This painful condition sometimes responds to interferon, and sometimes to calcium citrate (found in over-the-counter calcium supplements).

Repeated infections of the glands can cause the formation of scar tissue that blocks the ducts, leading to accumulation of the secretions in a large cyst (see also CYST, def. 3). This too requires drainage to avoid repeated infection. Sometimes *marsupialization*—surgery that in effect converts the gland into a pouch—may prevent repeated infection, but if the condition continues to recur the gland may have to be removed. Both marsupialization and gland removal usually require general anesthesia and therefore should be performed in a hospital or surgical clinic. Recovery from these procedures tends to be rapid, although local tenderness and swelling may persist for several weeks afterward.

basal body temperature   Also *BBT, temperature method.* The lowest temperature of a normal healthy person during waking hours, which can be used as a means of determining whether a woman ovulates, and when. During the MENSTRUAL CYCLE the hormone progesterone, released after ovulation, causes a measurable increase in basal body temperature. A slight drop in temperature usually (but not always) occurs 12 to 24 hours before ovulation, and a sustained rise follows for at least three days, and sometimes until the beginning of the next cycle. In order to use this phenomenon for either birth control or conception, a specially marked thermometer (marked in tenths of degrees) is used to take a woman's temperature every morning immediately upon waking (before rising, eating, etc.). It remains inserted for a full four minutes, orally, vaginally or rectally, but always in the same way. The temperature is noted on a graph (another model involves a hand-held computer, with colored lights indicating safe and unsafe times). When it rises more than 0.1 degree Celsius (or 0.4 to 0.8 degrees Fahrenheit) and remains elevated for three days, ovulation presumably has occurred and the fertile period is over. If the temperature remains higher for 17 days (and the woman does not have fever), her pregnancy is confirmed. (See chart opposite.)

Records made over a period of six to eight months usually give a good indication of the pattern of ovulation, which can be used either to prevent or time a pregnancy. For birth control the temperature method is more accurate than the calendar method but still is far from totally reliable (see NATURAL FAMILY PLANNING). When combined with the CERVICAL MUCUS METHOD (and then called *sympto-thermic method*), it is somewhat more dependable. However, results may be made inaccurate by a cold or other infection, fatigue, emotional stress and other factors. Further, some women have no clear identifiable pattern of basal body temperature, even when they ovulate regularly.

basal metabolism   See METABOLISM.

beauty parlor stroke syndrome   The occurrence of cerebral vascular accident (stroke) symptoms following a shampoo in a beauty salon or a session in a dentist's chair. The symptoms, usually transient, include dizziness, difficulty speaking, poor coordination, blurred vision or nausea. It is believed that the condition is caused by compression of one of the two vertebral arteries that supply blood to the brain when a woman leans back with her neck extended and head hanging over the sink. Normally when one cerebral artery is compressed, there is sufficient blood flow through the other to supply the brain; however, when arteries are narrowed owing to atherosclerosis (see ARTERIOSCLEROSIS), blood flow can be impaired. Consequently women who have cerebrovascular disease are advised to avoid prolonging this position and should they experience any symptoms, to change position at once.

Basal Body Temperature Chart

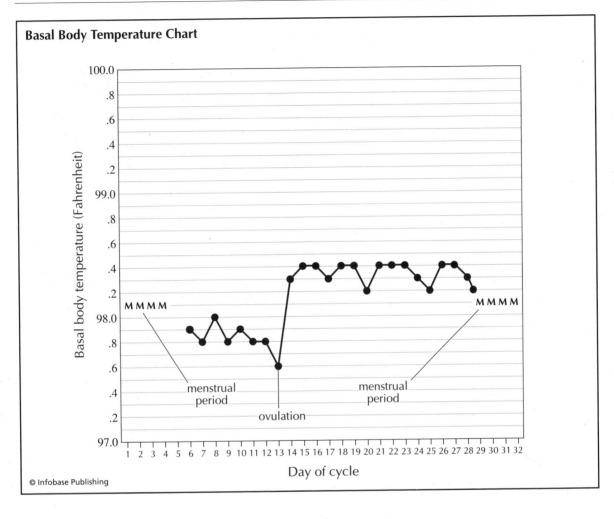

© Infobase Publishing

benign Describing a growth or tumor that is not cancerous. Although its presence means that a group of cells have multiplied more rapidly than normal, so that a mass of extra tissue has formed, a benign tumor differs in three ways from a malignant (cancerous) tumor: it cannot metastasize (spread) to a different part of the body; it cannot invade and destroy surrounding normal tissue; and it cannot recur (although a new benign tumor can develop). Benign tumors usually can be removed completely if they are not too close to vital organs (brain tumors can be a major exception), and the outlook for total cure is very favorable.

See also CANCER.

bilateral Affecting both sides. A bilateral oophorectomy, for example, means surgical removal of both ovaries.

bilirubin See NEONATAL JAUNDICE.

Billings method See CERVICAL MUCUS METHOD.

bimanual examination See GYNECOLOGIC EXAMINATION.

binge eating See BULIMIA.

biofeedback A technique for teaching individuals to become aware of their heart rate, blood pressure, temperature or other involuntary body functions in order to control them by a conscious mental effort. Often this technique involves learning to achieve complete relaxation, a physical state of deep rest. Biofeedback has proved particularly useful for helping patients lower their high blood pressure, and also for alleviating the side effect of nausea during chemotherapy. It has also been effective, in some cases, for disorders as diverse as Raynaud's phenomenon, epilepsy, chronic pain and severe eczema.

biopsy 1. Also, *incisional biopsy, surgical biopsy*. The surgical removal of tissue from a living person for evaluation and diagnosis by a pathologist. It is the primary diagnostic technique for many kinds of palpable solid tumor. Surgical biopsy can be performed under local anesthetic in a doctor's office or clinic, or under general anesthesia in a hospital or surgical clinic on either an inpatient or an outpatient basis. The excised tissue specimen can be examined in two ways: either quickly by a *frozen section*, while the patient is still anesthetized, or by a *permanent section*, a 48-hour process in which the tissue is fixed in formalin, embedded in paraffin blocks, and then sliced, stained and studied microscopically. A frozen section permits biopsy and surgical treatment to be combined in one operation; a permanent section allows for a more definitive analysis and time for both patient and physician to consider alternative treatments.

See also def. 5, 6, 7 and 8 below.

2. excisional biopsy. The removal of an entire growth, rather than a portion of it, for evaluation (see def. 1 above). In breast cancer, it is *not* the same as lumpectomy (removal of a tumor known to be malignant). It may require general anesthesia.

3. needle biopsy. The removal of tissue or fluid from a growth (tumor or cyst) by means of a hollow needle to determine whether it is cancerous. Technically, if only fluid is removed, the procedure is called "aspiration"; if tissue is removed it is a "biopsy." In practice the terms are used interchangeably. Needle biopsy frequently is performed in a clinician's office (rather than a

hospital) and requires either local or no anesthesia. After applying a small amount of local anesthesia to the breast, the clinician inserts a fine needle with a hypodermic syringe into the growth (this is called *fine needle aspiration*). If fluid can be withdrawn, it is analyzed for benign and malignant (cancerous) cells. If it is a benign cyst, it may be drained of fluid, surgically removed or simply observed. Fine needle aspiration has largely replaced the earlier procedure of *core needle biopsy* (also called *Tro-car* or *Tru-cut biopsy*), using a wider-bore needle, which yields a larger sample (easier for the pathologist to analyze) but also causes greater discomfort to the patient. However, if no fluid can be withdrawn, core needle biopsy may be tried. A positive biopsy (indicating cancer cells in the sample) is always conclusive, but a negative one may not be, because the needle may have missed the malignant portion of a growth. Thus, while needle biopsy is easier and less expensive than surgical biopsy, it is open to a wider margin of error. Nevertheless, it may be preferable to surgical biopsy when a patient cannot undergo even minor surgery owing to poor health or because the recuperation period would interfere with other necessary treatment. Other tests involving the removal of fluid for diagnostic purposes but not related to cancer tests are AMNIOCENTESIS, CULDOCENTESIS and various kinds of BLOOD TEST.

4. punch biopsy. The removal of a small wedge of suspicious tissue with a special instrument that, in effect, punches rather than cuts it out. *Multiple punch biopsy* (involving several punches) is almost always used to diagnose possible cancer of the cervix based on an abnormal PAP SMEAR and COLPOSCOPY, as well as a suspected cancer of the vulva.

5. breast biopsy. For palpable breast lesions, the simplest type of biopsy used is needle aspiration (see def. 3 above). If the lump is a fluid-filled cyst, the liquid will be extracted; if the fluid is bloody, it will be retained for analysis. Otherwise the cyst is assumed to be benign. If the lump is solid, the clinician will work the needle in and out several times to collect cells on the shaft and transfer them to a slide for analysis. This test can, however, miss cancerous cells, so more extensive biopsy—either incisional or excisional (def. 1 and 2 above)—may be called for. For excisional biopsy, the clinician makes an incision 3 to 4 centimeters (1 to 1½ inches) long over the nodule if the tumor or lump is near the surface. If the lump is deeply embedded, the incision may be made under the breast and the breast lifted up to expose the growth. The growth is then excised, together with surrounding tissue, and the small blood vessels in the area are closed off so that little or no blood is lost. In the case of a large or deep mass, a drain may be inserted and removable sutures (stitches) used to close the incision. Excisional breast biopsy often is performed as an outpatient procedure under local anesthesia in order to avoid delay, psychological distress, and unnecessary diagnostic studies for metastasis if the lump is found to be benign. MAMMOGRAPHY is indicated before any such biopsy (except in women under the age of 30) because there may well be other hidden lesions in the same breast or in the other breast. A less invasive form of biopsy, called *precision biopsy,* inserts a small device into the breast through a quarter-inch incision and vacuums tissue into position. The same device then cuts the tissue, taking several samples during one insertion; samples are drawn through a tube for collection and the incision is bandaged.

A special kind of biopsy called *wire-localization biopsy* is performed when mammography indicates a lesion that cannot be felt. Under direct X-ray or ultrasound observation and with local anesthesia, a very thin, hollow needle is inserted toward the mass and a thin hooked wire is passed through it. The needle is removed and a second mammogram is taken, to indicate if the wire is properly placed to guide the surgeon, who will then make an incision to remove tissue at the wire's tip for examination by the pathologist. A new ultra-fast staining technique makes it possible to obtain results within an hour or less.

Another newer technique is *stereotactic biopsy.* The woman lies face down on a table containing an opening for the breast, and, while a device compresses the breast, a mammogram is taken. The location of the lesion is then plotted by computer. With a device called a Mammotome, a probe guided by a computer or ultrasound is positioned in the breast and rotated to draw out tissue from the abnormal area's core. It provides a larger sample than needle biopsy but is still too new for a complete assessment of reliability. Because the results of biopsy are so important in determining treatment, it is now recommended that all women get a second opinion, or pathology review, on the biopsy tissue.

See also CANCER, BREAST; SENTINEL NODE BIOPSY.

6. vulvar biopsy. The removal and analysis of a small patch of skin from the vulva in order to test for skin cancer. It usually requires only local anesthesia, and if the incision is small or a punch biopsy (def. 4 above) is performed, sutures may not even required.

7. cervical biopsy. The removal and examination of a small amount of tissue from the cervix, usually performed if a PAP SMEAR has indicated abnormality. Examination by COLPOSCOPY may pinpoint the area from which tissue should be taken. Cervical biopsy often is an office procedure and requires no anesthesia; usually only a mild cramp or two can be felt when the specimen is taken. If the suspicious area extends up into the cervical canal (see CERVIX), the clinician may recommend an *endocervical curettage,* an office or outpatient procedure in which tissue from the cervical lining is scraped off and evaluated. In CONIZATION, a cone-shape piece of tissue is cut from the cervix.

8. endometrial biopsy. Also *uterine biopsy.* The removal and analysis of tissue from the uterine lining, or endometrium. There are two ways of obtaining the tissue. The first is *curettage,* in which a small scraper, called a curette or curet, is inserted through the cervical canal into the uterus and is scraped downward along the endometrium to remove shallow strands of tissue. A local anesthetic in the cervix may be used to minimize the pain, which ranges from moderate to strong cramping. An outpatient procedure, endometrial curettage often is used to evaluate abnormal bleeding, especially in women over 35 or in those who have a family history of endometrial cancer, and to evaluate fertility problems (the lining gives evidence of ovulation and of normal endocrine activity). The second principal method, rapidly becoming more common than curettage, is by VACUUM ASPIRATION (suction) and resembles the procedure used for an early vacuum abortion. A narrow, flexible tube is inserted into the uterus through the cervix and the application of suction removes a portion of the endometrial tissue. The procedure, also called an *office D and C,* is performed in the doctor's office and takes only a few minutes. There may be some mild cramping, but local anesthesia is rarely necessary. Vacuum scraping, like curettage, is used to make sure there is no abnormal thickening of the lining (endometrial hyperplasia) or cancerous tissue. It is quite accurate in identifying endometrial hyperplasia, and when used in conjunction with ultrasound it is close to 100% accurate. Consequently it has largely replaced the use of a salt solution to wash cells from the uterine cavity for examination in the laboratory.

bipolar disorder   See MANIC-DEPRESSIVE ILLNESS.

birth attendant   A person who assists a woman during labor and delivery. Most often the term is used for a person trained to do this work, such as a midwife, obstetrical nurse, nurse-practitioner or obstetrician. However, as health care costs have risen and an increasing number of Americans decide to have babies outside the traditional hospital setting, the birth attendant is sometimes a person without professional obstetric training—a husband or other relative, a friend or a practical nurse.

See also DOULA; MIDWIFE; PREPARED CHILDBIRTH.

birth ball   A large, colorful rubber ball, about 36 inches in diameter, that helps achieve a comfortable position in childbirth. Sitting on the ball helps dilate the cervix and relaxes the pelvis. Lying over it, face down, eases BACK LABOR.

birth canal   The corridor, or passage, through which a baby passes during childbirth, from the uterus down and out through the vagina. Some confine the use of the term to the vagina itself; others apply it more broadly to the entire bony pelvis, the cervix and the vagina, since constriction at any point in this area can prevent the passage of the baby.

birth center   Also *birthing center, childbearing center, maternity home.* A freestanding childbirth facility for labor and delivery. It is not a hospital but usually is staffed by certified nurse-midwives who provide prenatal and birth services. They generally work under the supervision of physicians, and there is an ambulance available to transport women who need hospital care. The center is equipped to handle normal labor and delivery, and generally screens women prenatally to make sure they do not represent a HIGH-RISK PREGNANCY or indicate in any way that they may have a complicated birth. Long popular in Europe, birth centers began to be used increasingly in the United States and Canada from the 1970s on. They are less expensive and less formal than hospitals, generally allow the husband and other family members to remain with a woman during much of the labor and use the same room for both labor and delivery. Childbirth education classes for both parents usually are held at the center prior to delivery and may be mandatory. Further, after a normal delivery the mother and child often are able to go home after 12 hours, rather than being required to remain for several days. A pediatrician usually examines the infant before discharge, and often a nurse from the center visits mother and baby at home several times during the first week or two. Advocates of birth centers regard them as an excellent compromise between hospital and HOME BIRTH.

With the proliferation of managed care, many free-standing birth centers have been taken over by local hospitals. They then must follow hospital rules, which may differ from their natural approach to childbirth. However, their value in terms of cost savings and low Cesarean rate has been acknowledged, and health care insurance generally covers their services. Today some birth centers are owned by hospitals, and others have contracts with HMOs. A good birthing center is licensed by the state and/or accredited by the Commission for Accreditation of Freestanding Birth Centers. (Also see resources in the Appendix.)

See also BIRTHING ROOM.

birth control   A term invented by Margaret Sanger (1879–1966), a pioneer in the early 20th-century movement to help women prevent unwanted pregnancies, for the means and methods so used. Until

1873 the kinds of CONTRACEPTIVE available—principally condoms and diaphragms—were not subject to legal restriction in the United States. In that year the Comstock Law was enacted that forbade information about contraception to be sent through the United States mails. It was not overturned until the 1930s, but during the intervening 60 years activists like Sanger pressed for its repeal. The first birth control clinic, devoted to teaching women how to prevent pregnancy, had been opened in Amsterdam in 1878 by Dr. Aletta Jacobs. Sanger, an American public health nurse, felt strongly that the poor especially should be able to limit the size of their families. In 1916 she opened a clinic in Brooklyn, New York, which was closed by the police, who also arrested her. A National Birth Control League had been formed the year before; in 1921 it became the American Birth Control League, with Sanger as president, and in 1923 it opened a permanent clinic in New York. Other state laws against birth control (22 in all) were eventually repealed, although the last of them was overturned only by a Supreme Court decision in the 1960s.

Though the term *birth control* is relatively new, various modes of birth control have been practiced since ancient times, despite the fact that understanding of the human reproductive system was very limited until the late 19th century. Over the years animal dung, serpent fat, honey, lemon juice, silk, paper and many other substances have been placed inside the vagina to prevent conception. Today a variety of tested contraceptives and methods are available. Most of them involve only the woman's body, although there are a few MALE CONTRACEPTIVES. All have advantages and disadvantages, and none is entirely risk-free, although methods of NATURAL FAMILY PLANNING carry only the risk of pregnancy. Moreover, even today birth control, which implicitly acknowledges that sexual activity without intent of reproduction is healthy and normal, is frowned on by certain groups, notably the Roman Catholic Church and other religious bodies, and some forms of it are expressly forbidden by them. The availability of birth control also implies a changing attitude toward female sexuality, acknowledging that—contrary to Victorian and other earlier ideas—women as well as men may enjoy the pleasure of sex and may have a sanctioned role other than that of motherhood.

Ideally, choosing a method of birth control should precede any heterosexual activity, except when pregnancy is desired. A woman's first birth control checkup, which can be performed at a birth control clinic or community clinic or by a private physician, should involve a breast and pelvic examination, blood pressure, urine and blood tests and a PAP SMEAR. If ORAL CONTRACEPTIVES are being considered, further tests may be needed. An important part of the checkup is the interview, during which the clinician tries to identify any relevant diseases and habits (for example, liver problems, high blood pressure, smoking) and educates the woman concerning the kinds of birth control available (see the discussion under CONTRACEPTIVE) and which of them might best suit her way of life. The interview should include a history of her reproductive life, including menstrual cycle, pregnancies and their outcome, sexual experiences and frequency, and previous contraceptive experience, and for oral contraceptives, family history concerning certain diseases. A follow-up visit should be scheduled for three months later to make sure that the method chosen is satisfactory.

See also PREGNANCY COUNSELING.

birth defects   Also *congenital abnormalities (defects).* Physical abnormalities in babies that are present from birth, which may or may not be hereditary. Some of them, such as phenylketonuria (PKU), can be detected and treated immediately, with a high chance of complete recovery. Others, such as Tay-Sachs disease and sickle cell disease, may not be detected for months or years and may be not only untreatable but fatal. Still others, such as mental retardation, occur in widely varying degrees, from very slight to very severe.

There are two principal sources of birth defects. One is outside influences during pregnancy and delivery, which include the mother's exposure to radiation, drugs (including alcohol and nicotine), virus infections, malnutrition, various chronic diseases, and damage during labor and delivery. The other is abnormalities of the baby's genes or chromosomes, which are sometimes called *genetic disorders.* Some genetic disorders, such as Gaucher's

IF YOU ARE PREGNANT, PROTECT YOUR UNBORN CHILD BY AVOIDING

- All nonessential medication (including antacids, laxatives, over-the-counter painkillers) unless prescribed by physician who knows you are (or might be) pregnant
- Alcoholic beverages (keep to minimum or abstain entirely)
- Excessive caffeine (reduce or stop consumption of coffee, tea, cola drinks, etc.)
- Immunization with any live virus vaccine, including flu vaccines
- Infection, especially with rubella, measles, mumps, herpes simplex, syphilis, gonorrhea, viral hepatitis, cytomegalovirus, influenza and toxoplasmosis
- Tobacco (reduce or, preferably, quit smoking)
- X-rays unless essential (in that case be sure to shield pelvic area with lead apron)

disease, are hereditary; others, such as Down syndrome, are not.

The number of known *teratogens*—agents with injurious effects on the development of a fetus—is large and growing quickly (as more is learned about various chemicals and their effects). Among them are methyl mercury (found in contaminated fish), which can cause CEREBRAL PALSY; the hormones estrogen and progesterone, which when administered during pregnancy can produce cardiovascular defects; the antibiotic tetracycline, which can produce hypoplasia (underdevelopment) of the teeth and stained dental enamel; the RUBELLA (German measles) virus, which can lead to early fetal death as well as serious abnormalities; the tranquilizer THALIDOMIDE, which prevents normal development of arms and legs; and various kinds of radiation, including high-dosage X-rays, which can produce an assortment of disorders. Rubella is by no means the only common infectious disease that causes damage. Other viruses also are dangerous, among them those causing chicken pox, herpes simplex, hepatitis, influenza, syphilis, smallpox and some kinds of encephalitis. (See also CONGENITAL INFECTION.) For this reason, it is highly recommended that women who are pregnant (or who could be pregnant) avoid all live vaccines (made with attenuated live organisms), anesthesia, chemicals, exposure to X-ray and other kinds of radiation, and drugs—not only prescription drugs but over-the-counter remedies such

as aspirin. They also should greatly restrict (if possible, stop) smoking and limit (or eliminate) intake of alcohol. The accompanying table summarizes these precautions. (See also ALCOHOL USE; DRUG USE AND PREGNANCY; SMOKING, TOBACCO.)

There are three basic kinds of genetic disorder: chromosome defects, single-gene disorders, and multifactorial or polygenic disorders. *Chromosome defects* involve either an excess or lack of chromosomal DNA (see NUCLEIC ACID), resulting in structural defects or in deviations from the normal number. Unlike the other genetic defects, they are seldom familial—that is, they usually constitute an isolated instance in a family. The most common chromosomal disorder is DOWN SYNDROME, usually caused by the presence of three copies of a chromosome, instead of two. It is also called *trisomy 21*, for the number given the chromosome. Two others are *trisomy 13*, which is usually fatal within days of birth, and *trisomy 18*, characterized by severe retardation and death during infancy. Like other chromosomal defects, Down syndrome often is associated with maternal age, that is, the older the mother, the greater the risk of this birth defect. Another chromosomal disorder is *hemochromatosis*, or *iron overload*. It causes the bowels to absorb too much iron, which is then stored in other organs that can later be damaged. It thus puts individuals at increased risk for diabetes, cirrhosis, chronic fatigue and heart disease. Symptoms often do not appear until middle age, by which time one or more of these diseases have occurred. Some researchers have recommended a routine blood test for excess iron. Another such disorder is *mitochondrial disease*, caused by abnormal genes on the chromosome inside a mitochondrion (every cell has mitochondria, structures responsible for energy production). When an egg is fertilized, only mitochondria from the egg become part of the fetus, those from the sperm being discarded. Hence mitochondrial disease is transmitted only by the mother, and it affects both men and women equally. The disorder causes damage to the brain, heart, liver, skeletal muscles and endocrine and respiratory systems, and at this writing it is incurable.

A special category of chromosomal defects are those affecting only the sex chromosomes, which produce ambiguities of sex differentiation in the child. Among these are TURNER'S SYNDROME and KLINEFELTER SYNDROME. The latter is associated with paternal age; the older the father, the greater the risk. Chromosomal defects in prospective parents are readily detected by examining the nuclei of white blood cells scraped from the lining of the mouth (a *buccal smear*) since they are present in every body cell. (See also CHROMOSOME; GENETICS.)

Single-gene defects occur when there is one or a pair of *mutant* genes. If the gene is *dominant*, its presence in either father or mother gives each of their children a 50% chance of contracting the disorder. (The terms *gene*, *mutant*, *dominant* and *recessive* are explained under GENETICS.) More than 1,200 dominant-gene disorders have been identified, among them Huntington's chorea, a progressive and fatal neurologic disorder, and primary hyperlipidemia, a predisposition to premature arteriosclerosis. (For Huntington's, which does not affect a person until mid-adulthood, there is now a blood test to detect the genetic marker that predicts its development.) If the gene is *recessive*, the presence in both parents gives each of their offspring a 25% chance of having it. Among the 950 or so such disorders known are TAY-SACHS DISEASE, SICKLE-CELL DISEASE, PHENYLKETONURIA and beta-thalassemia, an iron-storage disorder that affects mainly individuals of Mediterranean ancestry. If the gene is recessive and *X-linked* (present on the X chromosome only), it is transmitted only by mothers principally to their sons (their sons carry a 50% risk). Among the 150 disorders of this kind that have been identified are HEMOPHILIA A, which is characterized by lack of the clotting factor in blood; Duchenne MUSCULAR DYSTROPHY, a progressive weakening and degeneration of the muscle fibers; and a form of mental retardation associated with a fragile X chromosome, in which the X chromosomes are marred by constrictions that make them fragile, or easily broken. (See FRAGILE X SYNDROME.)

Multifactorial or *polygenic disorders* come from the interaction of pairs of genes with each other and with environmental factors. This kind of birth defect includes many congenital malformations, among them cleft lip and cleft palate, club foot and SPINA BIFIDA. Some of these, too, seem to be associated with older parents. In addition, it is believed that genetic factors are partly responsible for the development of arthritis, gout, stomach ulcers, multiple sclerosis,

high blood pressure, schizophrenia, diabetes, manic-depressive illness and some kinds of cancer.

Women, especially older mothers, have long been blamed as the main source of birth defects and genetic disorders. However, growing evidence suggests that men rather than women may be the source of most new genetic mutations, and the older the man, the more likely that his sperm carries such mutations. The sex cells that give rise to sperm continue to divide throughout his life, increasing the risk of mutation. Older men therefore have a greater risk of fathering children with such birth defects as, for example, Marfan syndrome, achondroplastic dwarfism and myositis ossificans (a bony tissue disorder).

Since 1968 AMNIOCENTESIS has been used to diagnose chromosomal abnormalities in the fetus, as well as a few biochemical disorders and some brain and spinal-cord defects. More recently developed tests include CHORIONIC VILLUS SAMPLING, ALPHA-FETO-PROTEIN TEST and NUCHAL TRANSLUCENCY-BIOCHEMI-CAL BLOOD TEST (see also GENETIC TESTING; PRENATAL TESTS). Also, GENETIC COUNSELING can be valuable for suggesting tests to determine the presence of a disease and assessing the risk of its transmission to children. In 1994 a baby was born who had been tested and found free of Tay-Sachs disease when she was only an eight-cell embryo. Other new methods include screening the unfertilized eggs of the mother before fertilization and screening the mother's blood for fetal cells showing chromosomal defects. Prenatal treatment also has evolved. In 1981 a baby who might have died because of its inability to use the vitamin biotin (a genetic defect) was diagnosed early, before birth, and was treated successfully by giving the mother large daily doses of the substance during the final three months of pregnancy. Also, a technique for monitoring a fetus directly through the umbilical cord, from which fetal blood can be withdrawn and through which drugs or blood transfusions can be administered, has been successful in treating fetuses with severe Rh disease, toxoplasmosis (a parasitic disease) and other severely damaging or potentially fatal conditions.

birthing room A hospital room for labor, delivery and recovery that is designed to be homelike and comfortable, with enough room for the father and close friends, easy chairs as well as a bed, and often a television set and magazines. Such rooms began to be used in American hospitals about 1970 in order to accommodate couples reluctant to use a hospital because of what they considered its sterile, dehumanized atmosphere and because hospital personnel tend to regard and treat childbirth as an illness rather than a normal process. To provide such couples with an alternative to HOME BIRTH, some hospitals began to offer more homelike facilities where childbirth could be treated as a family event; in fact, some even permit children and friends to be with a woman during labor and delivery (if she wants them).

Hospital policies vary with regard to the use of intravenous infusions and fetal monitoring in a birthing room, and equipment for emergency oxygen and suctioning may or may not be available in such a room. Critics of the birthing room say it contains too many objects that cannot be sterilized and therefore is not safe; it does not have adequate facilities for emergency situations; and it is a source of disappointment to women who must be moved to a traditional delivery room because of complications. Supporters say it offers family-centered maternity care to low-risk patients (high-risk patients are usually not permitted to use it) in a facility that can, if necessary, provide intensive care should either mother or baby require it.

See also BIRTH CENTER.

birth stool   A backless seat used by a birthing mother to help shorten and widen the pelvis and assist in pushing the baby through the birth canal. It looks like a footstool and is said to be particularly useful during the second (expulsion) stage of LABOR.

See also BIRTH BALL.

birth weight   The weight of a newborn baby, which often is directly related to its relative maturity and chances for survival. The average weight for a full-term white baby in America currently is 7 pounds (3,200 grams). Most PREMATURE babies, that is, babies born before 37 weeks of gestation,

weigh less than 2,500 grams (5½ pounds) and often are not well enough developed to survive without special care (sometimes not even then). Therefore, the birth weight of 2,500 grams long was considered a mark of adequate maturity, and any baby weighing less was considered a high risk. However, weight alone is not the only indicator of maturity, and some full-term or even postmature (past-term) infants weigh less than 2,500 grams and are in no special danger. Today, therefore, babies tend to be evaluated in terms of both weight and gestational age, and their care is based on these criteria as well as the APGAR SCORE and other factors. (Also see GESTATION.) However, very low birth weight, currently defined as 3 pounds, 4 ounces or less, remains closely associated with infant mortality, and also with CEREBRAL PALSY.

The cause of low birth weight may be genetic (parents who are of short stature themselves or transmitting a genetic disorder associated with short stature) or, more often, malnutrition. Malnutrition of the baby in turn may be caused by a disease of the mother, such as hypertension, kidney disease or severe diabetes, that prevents the passage of sufficient nutrients through the placenta. Cigarette smoking and drug addiction in the mother also appear to be associated with low birth weight, as is inadequate diet. Some researchers maintain that efforts to keep a pregnant woman from gaining too much weight—a popular strategy of obstetricians for many years—result in inadequate protein intake, which contributes to low birth weight (and other problems).

See DIET; WEIGHT GAIN, def. 2.

bisexual   The desire and/or practice of having sexual relationships with a person of either sex, that is, engaging in both HOMOSEXUAL and HETEROSEXUAL activities.

bladder   Also *urinary bladder*. A sac in the front of the pelvis that serves as a reservoir for urine, which it receives through the ureters from the kidneys and discharges through the urethra. Roughly triangular in shape when empty, the bladder is capable of considerable distention as it is filled, taking on an ovoid form. The inside of the bladder is lined with mucous membrane covering layers of involuntary muscle fibers, which are kept in a state of relaxation at the same time that the urinary SPHINCTER is contracted. The kidneys deposit urine in the bladder at the rate of about 30 drops a minute. When the bladder is full, there is a sensation of pressure, perceived as the need to void. The female bladder is very prone to inflammation and infection, usually caused by bacteria transported upward from the urethra (see CYSTITIS, def. 1). Relaxation of the muscles following pregnancy and childbirth occasionally causes loss of support, so that the bladder projects down, sometimes all the way into the vagina; see CYSTOCELE.

See also CANCER, BLADDER; FREQUENCY, URINARY; URINARY INCONTINENCE.

bladder infection   See CYSTITIS, def. 1.

bleeding, vaginal   After menarche and before menopause, bleeding that usually represents either normal MENSTRUAL FLOW or some disturbance of the menstrual cycle, called BREAKTHROUGH BLEEDING. Strictly speaking, the blood usually only passes through the vagina and exits from it, having originated in the uterus. Before menarche (the first menstrual period) and after menopause (defined as one year after the last period), any vaginal bleeding should be considered abnormal and, because it can be a symptom of cancer or some other serious disease, should be investigated promptly. Vaginal bleeding during pregnancy also is not normal and should be checked without delay. Some vaginal infections give rise to a blood-tinged discharge (see VAGINITIS). For other causes and kinds of vaginal bleeding, see ANOVULATORY BLEEDING; DYSFUNCTIONAL BLEEDING, VAGINAL; ENDOMETRIAL HYPERPLASIA; HEMORRHAGE, VAGINAL; POSTMENOPAUSAL BLEEDING, POSTPARTUM HEMORRHAGE.

See also withdrawal bleeding under ESTROGEN REPLACEMENT THERAPY.

blepharoplasty   See COSMETIC SURGERY.

bloating   See EDEMA.

blood clot   See THROMBUS.

blood count   See BLOOD TEST.

blood pressure   See HYPERTENSION.

blood test   Test of a sample of blood to detect disease or some abnormality. There are blood tests for syphilis, rubella and its antibodies, HIV antibodies (for the virus causing AIDS), thyroid function, liver damage and hundreds of other conditions. The most common kind of blood test is a *blood count* to detect ANEMIA, which can be performed by taking a small amount of blood from the finger or earlobe. (For most other blood tests a larger specimen must be drawn from a vein, in the arm or elsewhere.) Two techniques for a blood count are in common use. The *hemoglobin method* measures the concentration of hemoglobin (red pigment) in the blood; any hemoglobin value below 12 grams per 100 milliliters of blood indicates anemia. The *hematocrit method* measures the percentage of red blood cells in total blood volume; anything below 35% is considered anemia. Many authorities believe a blood count should be part of every standard medical checkup.

A more extensive test used for routine screening of all hospitalized patients is the *complete blood count,* or *CBC,* which measures the number, size and oxygen-carrying capacity of the components that make up blood. In adults the number of mature red and white cells remains fairly constant, with old cells being replaced by new ones created in the bone marrow. The CBC determines whether this process is functioning smoothly. Hemoglobin, which

COMPLETE BLOOD COUNT (CBC)	
Test	Normal values
hemoglobin	13.8–17.2 grams per deciliter (men) 12.0–15.6 grams per deciliter (women)
hematocrit	41–50% (men) 35–36% (women)
white blood cell count	3,800–10,800 per microliter
platelet count	130,000–400,000 per microliter

BLOOD CHEMISTRY PROFILE

Glucose (sugar) acts as the major fuel for bodily processes. Determining the amount of glucose in one's blood may be useful in diagnosing diabetes (high blood sugar) or hypoglycemia (low blood sugar).

BUN (Blood Urea Nitrogen) is the end point of protein breakdown in the body. One's BUN level varies with the amount of protein intake. Determining the amount of BUN in the blood may be useful in discovering diseases related to the kidneys or the urinary tract.

Creatinine is the waste material from the breakdown of creating phosphate, which interacts with other substances to produce energy used by the body. The level of creatinine in the blood remains fairly constant and is a good indicator of kidney function. An elevated level of creatinine may suggest that the kidney's ability to filter and remove waste from the bloodstream is damaged or that there is reduced blood flow to the kidneys due to blockage.

Enzymes are different proteins that function as biochemical catalysts aiding the processes of the body. Enzyme levels are checked to determine if the heart muscle and the liver are functioning properly.

Bilirubin is the waste product from the breakdown of hemoglobin. The substance exists in a non-soluble (indirect) and a soluble (direct) form. The levels of bilirubin may be assessed to discover disorders of the liver, bile ducts (ducts through which a digestive juice secreted by the liver is poured into the small intestine) or red blood cells. An elevated level of direct bilirubin may indicate that red blood cells are breaking down at an excessive rate. An elevated level of indirect bilirubin may indicate that the substance is backing up because the liver can't do its job effectively.

Calcium/Phosphorous By weight, calcium is the most plentiful mineral in the body; it is stored in the blood and bones. Phosphorous unites with calcium to form an insoluble combination that gives the skeleton its shape and structure. Proportions of calcium and phosphorous are delicately balanced, and testing the levels of these minerals may determine problems in muscle contraction, carbohydrate metabolism, kidney malfunction or the presence of kidney stones.

Uric acid is the endpoint of the breakdown of nucleic acids, which store genetic information needed to encode individual characteristics of each cell. Elevated levels of uric acid can be seen in a variety of conditions, one of which is gout—a condition in which a large amount of uric acid is being deposited in the vicinity of cartilage tissues such as joints.

Cholesterol is the basis for the synthesis of compounds that regulate many important bodily processes. The body manufactures cholesterol, mainly through the liver. Cholesterol is also available in foods such as fatty cuts of meat, dairy products and egg yolks. Two types of cholesterol exist: high-density lipoprotein (HDL) and low-density lipoprotein (LDL). A high reading of HDL is considered "good"; a low reading of HDL may indicate that plaque is being deposited in arteries, which may clog them. A high level of LDL is also undesirable.

Proteins are the major solid portions dissolved in the liquid portion of blood (serum). Various amounts of proteins may indicate how well the body's metabolic processes are functioning, how well the blood is transporting nutrients to various parts of the body and how well the body can defend itself against infection. Generally, tests for protein include specific tests for albumin and globulin, two types of protein vital for effective transportation of chemicals through the bloodstream.

---

transports oxygen from the lungs to other body cells, is checked for its efficient functioning. The number of white blood cells per sample is counted; an elevated number may indicate the presence of infection. The blood's smallest particles, the platelets, which aid in clotting, also are counted, and a description is presented of all the blood cells found (especially the structure of red blood cells).

A *serologic test* involves testing the serum, the portion of blood that remains after blood has clotted and the clot is removed; serum thus consists of all soluble materials in the blood, especially protein antibodies, and a serologic test is usually performed to detect and identify antibodies.

Serum cholesterol counts provide a measure of certain fatty substances in the blood. An elevated level may indicate potential problems, such as certain metabolic diseases or increased risk for heart disease or arteriosclerosis. The interpretation and significance of the serum cholesterol count vary with sex, age and level of activity. Generally, a count above 200 milligrams per deciliter is considered elevated and calls for reduction by diet changes, while 120 to 200 is considered normal. *Serum triglycerides* are a measure of one form of fat being carried in the serum. The normal values vary with age; marked increases appear to indicate a risk for atherosclerosis and other artery and heart disorders. (See also CHOLESTEROL.)

Serum glucose, also called *blood sugar,* is a measure of the number of milligrams of glucose per 100 milliliters of serum. Elevated serum glucose can be caused by DIABETES, but physical and emotional stress also can cause a rise, as can such conditions as pancreatitis and vitamin B_1 deficiency; a low reading, on the other hand, can reflect disorders in the pancreas or in the adrenal or other glands.

Serum potassium values of 3.5 to 5 are considered normal. Abnormal readings, either high or low, can indicate kidney disease. Low readings also may point to a number of gastrointestinal disorders.

Sedimentation rate measures the speed with which red blood cells settle out of a specially treated blood sample. The high end of the normal rate for men is 10 to 13 in one hour and that for women is from 15 to 20. Sedimentation rate sometimes is used as a measure of inflammation or for screening when there is some question about the presence of inflammation. It also can help differentiate between two disorders that cause similar symptoms, such as tension headache and temporal arteritis.

bloody show   Also *show.*
See also MUCUS PLUG.

board-certified   Certification by an official medical specialty board, awarded after passing a dif-

OFFICIAL MEDICAL BOARD SPECIALTIES	
American Board of . . .	
Allergy & Immunology	Orthopedic Surgery
Anesthesiology	Otolaryngology
Colon & Rectal Surgery	Pathology
Dermatology	Pediatrics
Emergency Medicine	Physical Medicine & Rehabilitation
Family Practice	Plastic Surgery
Internal Medicine	Preventive Medicine
Medical Genetics	Psychiatry & Neurology
Neurological Surgery	Radiology
Nuclear Medicine	Surgery
Obstetrics & Gynecology	Thoracic Surgery
Ophthalmology	Urology

ficult examination. Unlike a medical license, board certification is entirely voluntary, but it is often required by hospitals and managed-care companies. Owing to the prestige of such certification, doctors sometimes announce that they are board-certified, but by a self-designated board rather than an official one. Some of these have rigorous standards, but others are no more than clubs. The American Board of Medical Specialties (ABMS) recognizes 24 specialty boards (see the accompanying table), most of which also award certificates in subspecialties. To determine if such a specialty is recognized, check with the ABMS (see Appendix)

Board certification does not guarantee outstanding quality of care, but it does verify that a doctor who claims to be a surgeon, for example, actually is a surgeon. Lack of board certification may in some instances reflect a problem with a physician's training, competence or character.

body mass index   Also *BMI.*
See also OBESITY.

bonding   Also *maternal bonding, parental bonding.* Establishing a close emotional relationship between a baby and its parents, which should begin, according to current thinking, as soon as possible after birth. Proponents of this idea hold that the bond formed at the beginning of life has a lasting effect on subsequent relations between parents and their child. To encourage early bonding, the older practice of removing a newborn baby from the delivery room to the hospital nursery almost immediately is being replaced by letting the mother—and the father, when present—hold and cuddle the baby for a time after delivery and, if the mother intends to breast-feed, putting it to the breast at once. The practice of ROOMING-IN is encouraged, as is increased (in some hospitals, unlimited) contact between the father and baby.

Major obstacles to early bonding are the special equipment and care needed by a baby who is premature or has a serious physical problem. The parents then may have to make a considerable effort to make contact through an isolette, respirator, monitoring equipment, tubes and the like, which make it impossible to pick up and hold the baby in ordinary fashion. Parents determined to establish an early warm relationship with a baby who must remain hospitalized for some time after birth then must rely on frequent visits, touching and stroking their child through the appropriate openings in equipment, administering feedings themselves and similar measures.

bone density scan   A method of measuring bone mass, which decreases with age.

See also OSTEOPOROSIS.

bone loss   Also *bone resorption.*

See also OSTEOPOROSIS.

bone marrow transplant   A treatment for some forms of blood cancer (leukemia, lymphoma) in which healthy bone marrow from a carefully matched donor is transferred to the patient, where it grows healthy new blood cells, in effect giving the patient a new immune system. Since finding an immunologically compatible donor is difficult, ways of using the patient's own marrow for such transplants have been developed. In recent years this treatment has been used for patients with

advanced breast cancer, not because their marrow is cancerous but because it is damaged by the highly toxic chemotherapy required to treat the tumor. A portion of either the patient's bone marrow or of her blood-producing STEM CELLS are removed, she undergoes very aggressive chemotherapy, and the marrow or stem cells then are returned to her bloodstream to produce healthy blood cells. This treatment is also called *high-dose chemotherapy* combined with *autologous bone marrow transplant,* or *HDC/ABMT.* Still considered experimental, it is used only in women with metastatic cancer (spread to other organs) and newly diagnosed patients at high risk for recurrence. The best success rates are found in young women with limited metastasis who have had minimal doses of chemotherapy.

A still newer technique is using blood from the placenta and umbilical cord of a newborn infant, which has been stored in a *cord bank.* Like bone marrow, cord blood is rich in stem cells, which can help rebuild a blood supply and immune system compromised by high doses of radiation and chemotherapy. Cord blood also must be matched to the recipient, but it does not require as close a match as bone marrow does. Increasingly women are being urged to bank their own cord blood after childbirth, in the event that they will need it. Commercial cord banks charge an initial fee for collecting a sample and freezing it, and an annual fee to keep it stored in liquid nitrogen. Some medical centers with transplant programs perform the service without charge, as do some private companies.

bone scan   See RADIONUCLIDE IMAGING.

Botox   Botulism toxin used to erase wrinkles in COSMETIC SURGERY. Although not yet officially approved for these uses, the drug is also under study for treating chronic headache, especially tension headache and migraine; rectal fissures; hyperhidrosis (excessive sweating); spastic leg and arm movements related to central nervous system disorders; and a number of other conditions involving abnormal muscle contraction. It is approved for treating certain muscle spasms and two eye conditions, strabismus and blepharospasm (in which eyelid spasms squeeze the eye shut), and cosmetic surgery.

brachytherapy Also *interstitial radiation therapy*. Radiation applied to the site of a cancer by inserting catheters or other implants into the precise affected area. In men it has been used to treat prostate cancer. In women it is used after lumpectomy (removal of a breast tumor) as follow-up radiation.

See also RADIATION THERAPY.

Bradley method Also *husband-coached birth*. A method of PREPARED CHILDBIRTH devised in the 1940s by an American obstetrician, Robert A. Bradley. It differs from other methods in that it emphasizes the use of a trained, prepared husband to coach his wife in achieving a spontaneous delivery without medication. Bradley later conceded that another person might serve as the coach equally well—a mother, sister or friend—although he personally felt the husband was the ideal person. In this role the husband helps the wife learn and use relaxation and breathing techniques to facilitate the birth, helps her move into whatever position she finds comfortable and reassures her as to the progress of labor. Classes for both husband and wife—usually a series of eight—begin with one class held early in pregnancy (during the third or fourth month), followed by the remaining classes during the last trimester. The techniques taught include relaxation of all body muscle groups, normal diaphragmatic breathing (somewhat like that of the DICK-READ METHOD, which it most closely resembles), use of different positions during labor and pushing techniques. Although Bradley believed that birth should take place in a hospital, many later followers of his method believe that alternative settings, such as a birth center or the home, are equally safe.

Braxton-Hicks contractions Irregular contractions of the muscles of the uterus that occur during pregnancy. During the last weeks a woman becomes aware of the fact that her abdomen periodically becomes tense and firm (not painful). Actually, these contractions begin to occur early in pregnancy but are not noticeable until a few weeks before term, when they contribute to the EFFACEMENT and dilatation of the cervix. They are named for the physician who first observed them. Occasionally they are strong enough to be mistaken for true labor (see FALSE LABOR).

breakthrough bleeding Also *spotting, metrorrhagia*. Bleeding from the vagina between regular menstrual periods. One common form of breakthrough bleeding is *midcycle spotting*, light staining that occurs in about 10% of women for about two days halfway through the menstrual cycle, at the time of ovulation. It is harmless and requires no treatment. Persistent irregular bleeding can be caused by a disruption in the normal hormone balance and consequent failure to ovulate (see ENDOMETRIAL HYPERPLASIA). Such imbalances often occur at menarche and near menopause (see ANOVULATORY BLEEDING) but are not usual during the reproductive years (18 to 40). More often the cause is a condition such as cervicitis or another infection, or lesions such as a cervical or endometrial POLYP, adenomyosis, cervical eversion, the cysts of polycystic ovary syndrome, or cancer of the ovaries, uterus or cervix. Because of their potential seriousness, these conditions should be ruled out before beginning treatment. An ectopic pregnancy, the use of oral contraceptives or an intrauterine device (IUD) also can cause irregular bleeding. Breakthrough bleeding that is triggered by sexual intercourse often indicates cervical problems, such as cervicitis, a polyp or cervical eversion, but it also may be caused by an endometrial infection, an IUD or cervical cancer.

In women of reproductive age who are not ovulating, the principal means of dealing with irregular bleeding are the administration of hormones (usually progesterone alone or combined with estrogen) or a curettage—either a surgical D AND C or VACUUM ASPIRATION. In women who are ovulating, removing part of the endometrium (uterine lining) by curettage often stops heavy bleeding, at least for a time, and in the case of endometrial polyps serves to remove the cause as well. In either instance the tissue removed should be examined by a pathologist to rule out other, more serious conditions. Bleeding in girls before puberty and in women after menopause is definitely indicative of a possible serious disorder and should be investigated without delay.

See also BALLOON ABLATION; POSTMENOPAUSAL BLEEDING.

breast   One of a pair of modified sweat glands located in the superficial tissue of the chest wall, which in men have no function but in women are able to secrete milk. In women the breast usually extends from the second or third rib to the fifth or sixth rib; underlying it are the pectoral muscles. Each breast contains about 20 separate lobes, arranged like the spokes of a wheel. Each lobe consists of many smaller lobules and ends in tiny milk-producing glands called ACINI. The lobes, lobules and acini are connected to the NIPPLE by a complex network of ducts. There also is a network of blood vessels and lymphatic channels carrying blood and lymph that supply vital nutrients and remove wastes. The remainder of the breast is composed of fat and fibrous tissue.

Two kinds of fibrous structure support the breast and maintain its form. One is a layer of connective tissue that runs immediately under the skin of the breast. The second is made up of multiple fibrous bands, called *Cooper's ligaments,* which begin at the layer of connective tissue and run through the breast to attach loosely to the fascia (fibrous tissues) over the muscles of the chest wall. Many women also have crescent-shaped areas of thickened tissue at the lower border of each breast; these are called *inframammary ridges* or *folds* and have no known significance. The bulk of each breast's gland tissue is in the upper outer quadrant (closest to the armpit), and this also is the most common site for breast tumors. In fact, often a little breast tissue projects from this quadrant into the armpit, or axilla; it is called the *axillary tail* or *tail of Spence.*

The growth and development of the breast are regulated by hormones. Chief among them are estrogen and progesterone, from the ovaries, and prolactin, from the pituitary. Estrogen promotes growth of the milk duct system, stimulates the growth of glandular buds at the ends of the ducts, causes the deposit of fat and proliferation of fibrous

tissues within the breast and increases the pigmentation (coloring) of the nipple and AREOLA. Progesterone stimulates the growth and maturation of the gland tissues of the breast and causes the gland buds to develop into acini, but it can exert this effect only when the breast tissue first has been prepared by estrogen. Prolactin acts directly on the breast to stimulate gland growth and is responsible for the production of milk. Two other hormones, growth hormone (somatotropin or somatomammatropin) and adrenocorticotropin, are necessary for breast tissue to respond to estrogen, progesterone and prolactin, but the mechanism whereby this operates is not understood.

Breast development in girls usually begins around the age of 10 or 11. If it occurs much before the age of nine or if none has occurred by the age of 16, it is advisable to check for possible abnormalities. At first only the nipple begins to protrude from the chest, and then gland tissue begins to grow under it; this is sometimes called a *breast bud* and may occur on one side much sooner than on the other. A woman's breasts rarely are identical in size, but if the difference is very great one should check for abnormality caused by a tumor or other problem.

The size of the breasts depends on heredity, the influence of estrogen and progesterone, and nutrition (weight gain or loss often affects breast size). Almost any size is considered normal. Some women who are very unhappy about the appearance of their breasts undergo surgery to enlarge or reduce them (see MAMMAPLASTY). Massive breast growth may occur during puberty or pregnancy as the result of abnormal sensitivity of one or both breasts to increased estrogen levels; some women find that oral contraceptives have a similar effect, although usually to a lesser extent. The shape of the breasts depends on heredity, fat deposits and the strength of the Cooper's ligaments; changes in shape occur primarily as a result of stretched ligaments, which sooner or later occurs with age. The use of a brassiere for heavy breasts may delay such stretching, but the main purpose of wearing brassieres is for comfort and appearance.

The breast is subject to a number of disorders, ranging in seriousness from an occasional cyst or minor infection to cancer. The three most common lesions are FIBROADENOMA, FIBROCYSTIC BREAST SYN-DROME and cancer (see CANCER, BREAST).

See also BREAST-FEEDING, BREAST SELF-EXAMINA-TION; CALCIFICATIONS, BREAST; CYSTOSARCOMA PHYL-LODES; DUCTAL PAPILLOMA; INFLAMMATORY BREAST CANCER; LACTATION; LIPOMA; MAMMALGIA; MAMMARY DUCT ECTASIA; MAMMARY DUCT FISTULA; MASTITIS; PAGET'S DISEASE, def. 1.

breast augmentation, reduction, reconstruction See MAMMAPLASTY.

breast cancer   See CANCER, BREAST.

breast-feeding   Also *nursing*. Suckling an infant, the oldest form of feeding human babies and a method shared by all mammals. (See LACTATION for an explanation of milk production.) In Western civilization breast-feeding has from time to time fallen into disrepute. Wealthy women who did not wish to be tied down to regular feedings of an infant would employ a *wet nurse*, a woman lactating after having given birth herself, who was willing and able to breast-feed another woman's child. Wet nurses were indispensable when a mother died during or soon after childbirth, a frequent occurrence until sterile methods of childbirth were introduced in the 19th century. In the 20th century, with the development of a special baby-food industry that also manufactured milk formulas to be fed to newborn babies, an alternative to the wet nurse became available in grocery stores and pharmacies. Various means were employed to stop lactation in mothers not planning to breast-feed, such as breast binding and ice packs. These actually do not stop lactation (only lack of suckling does), and one method, the administration of hormones (particularly DIETHYLSTILBESTROL, or DES), is dangerous to the mother. Other drugs used to suppress lactation include bromocriptine (Parlodel), estrogen and estrogen-testosterone combinations. All are of doubtful efficacy and may be dangerous. With bromocriptine lactation resumes when the drug is discontinued (in about 40% of cases). Also, it has been associated with such dangerous side

effects as stroke, hypertension and seizures, as well as such milder ones as nausea, vomiting, dizziness and headache. When one wishes to discontinue nursing, therefore, it is advisable to treat breast engorgement by wearing a tight bra, applying cold compresses or ice packs and using a mild pain reliever. In most cases discomfort will subside and lactation will cease in a few days. The woman who stops breast-feeding at eight months usually suffers few or no such symptoms, since by then the rate of milk production has decreased considerably.

In the 1950s a counterrevolution was begun among American women who wished to breast-feed and found themselves thwarted by lack of help from—and sometimes even active interference by—hospital personnel. In 1956 a group of nursing mothers in Franklin Park, Illinois, founded an organization called La Leche League (*la leche* means "the milk" in Spanish), which today has chapters all over the United States and Canada. The national organization will send information about breast-feeding on request, and local chapters, often listed in the telephone book, have an experienced nursing mother on call 24 hours a day to advise women on any problems they might encounter.

Most authorities agree that breast-feeding is the ideal form of nourishing an infant, and since 1997 the American Academy of Pediatrics has been recommending that mothers breast-feed for at least one year (twice as long as its previous recommendation). Breast milk is highly digestible and transmits an arsenal of immunologic weapons (both antibodies and antiallergens) to an infant's still immature body, immobilizing otherwise harmful infectious organisms and allergens. It is thought to decrease the incidence of infant ear infections, allergies, diarrhea and bacterial meningitis, and may also protect against childhood lymphoma, sudden infant death syndrome and diabetes. Breast-feeding is regulated by the infant. The amount of milk produced is directly proportionate to the amount the baby suckles, and hence overfeeding and early obesity are prevented. Breast milk is always warm, fresh, sterile and conveniently available.

Breast-feeding has advantages for the mother as well. Suckling after childbirth stimulates the pituitary to release oxytocin, the hormone that makes the uterus contract during labor and afterward helps it return to its normal state. Extra weight gained during pregnancy is lost more easily; breast-feeding uses up about 500 calories a day. The nursing mother need not follow any special diet other than making sure she drinks enough liquids—almost any liquid. Breast-feeding usually delays the resumption of ovulation and menstruation, but birth control still must be used to avoid pregnancy since one is never sure when ovulation resumes until after the fact. The principal disadvantage of breast-feeding is that it ties down the mother. Usually, however, substitute bottles can be given as often as once a day—more often if they are made with her breast milk, expressed manually or with the aid of a breast pump, and refrigerated—and of course she can discontinue breast-feeding whenever she wishes. However, it is recommended that babies be fed breast milk exclusively until the age of six months, when solids are usually introduced.

There are a few contraindications to breast-feeding. Among them are active tuberculosis and chicken pox in the mother, both of which can be transmitted to an infant through her milk. The AIDS virus also can be transmitted through breast milk, so that any woman at risk for AIDS infection should be tested before she nurses her baby. Also, women taking anticancer drugs, radioactive medications of any kind or hormones are advised not to breast-feed. Drugs such as PCP, cocaine, heroin, barbiturates, some antibiotics and tranquilizers, and alcohol should be avoided. (Even one alcoholic drink a day may pass on enough through the milk to retard the baby's motor development, one study showed, so the most one can safely drink is two glasses of wine per week.) Smoking also should be avoided, since nicotine hampers milk production. On the other hand, most antibiotics are safe, as are over-the-counter cold medications and drugs for heart conditions and high blood pressure, and caffeine (up to six cups of coffee a day). Acetaminophen (sold under Tylenol and other brand names) is a safer pain-reliever than aspirin. Antidepressants are not considered risky since only very small amounts enter the breast milk.

Women who have had breast reconstruction surgery with silicone implants may be able to breast-feed, as can women who have had breast reduction surgery (unless very large amounts of secretory tissue have been removed or several mammary ducts have been cut). Women who have had a mastectomy usually can nurse with the remaining breast. Breast engorgement and local infections—even a breast abscess—need not interfere with nursing; indeed, the pain of these conditions may be relieved by nursing, which reduces the pressure of fluids on the affected parts. A woman can continue to nurse while pregnant with another child; although nursing does trigger the release of oxytocin, it does not induce miscarriage. However, some authorities warn that since dietary calcium tends to go to the breast milk first, the fetus may thus be deprived of it, thereby risking a low birth weight and impaired development. Following the birth of another child a woman can continue to nurse both the new baby and a toddler. Many women have successfully nursed twins and triplets. A premature infant who must be placed in an incubator can be fed milk expressed from the mother's breasts by hand or with an electric breast pump, thus maintaining her milk supply and giving the child the benefits of breast milk until it can nurse.

There is no evidence that breast-feeding has any permanent effect on the size and shape of the breasts (see BREAST). Although for a time it was believed that women who breast-fed had a lower risk of developing breast cancer, there is no clear-cut evidence that breast-feeding affords such protection.

Breast-feeding may be begun immediately after delivery (even before the umbilical cord is cut), although many hospitals delay the initial feeding for eight hours or longer. Some also offer one or two feedings of water first to help the infant regurgitate any mucus or other secretions swallowed during delivery. Those who strongly favor breast-feeding oppose this practice, believing a baby should be put to the breast as soon as possible after delivery. *Colostrum,* a protein-rich yellow fluid that precedes milk secretion (see LACTATION), is the chief source of nourishment for the first three or four days, but suckling stimulates earlier milk production. To breast-feed effectively, the infant must place the NIPPLE well back in the mouth, close the lips tightly around the AREOLA and squeeze the nipple against the palate with the tongue. This procedure compresses the lactiferous sinuses behind the areola and draws milk into the mouth. (Complicated as this may sound, most infants accomplish it almost immediately.) For the first few weeks, until the milk supply is well established and the baby is growing at a normal rate, most authorities recommend letting the baby nurse whenever it wants to, approximately every three or four hours or even more often, a method called *demand feeding.* After this initial period of adjustment, the mother can to some extent regulate the feeding schedule according to her convenience.

A number of HERBAL REMEDIES have been used to help women with the problem of sore nipples. One is rubbing the nipples with resin of balsam fir or with sweet almond oil; another is simmering three tablespoons of common spurge or milk purslane (*Euphorbia maculata*) in a cup of olive oil or glycerine for 15 minutes and then rubbing on the nipples. The herb milkwort (*Polygala vulgaris*), eaten raw or made into a tea, has been used to increase the milk supply but may be toxic.

Today some communities in the United States have human *milk banks,* which store the breast milk of human donors for distribution to infants who cannot tolerate any other nourishment or formulas but for whom no milk from their own mothers is available. Human milk can be kept frozen for up to two years, but in practice hospital milk banks usually limit storage time to a month or two.

In recent years there has been some return to wet-nursing, that is, hiring a woman to breast-feed one's baby. Another new trend is cross-nursing, in which mothers breast-feed one another's babies. These trends are fueled by the fact that more American babies are again being breast-fed and, since more than 50% of women work outside the home and more young women undergo breast surgery, there is a shortage of breast-feeding mothers.

breast implant See MAMMAPLASTY.

breast reconstruction See MAMMAPLASTY.

breast self-examination A systematic examination by a woman of her own breasts in order to detect any abnormalities. Ideally it is carried out every month, but if one forgets it is better to do it occasionally than not at all. Breast cancer is the most common malignancy in women (current statistics estimate that 1 of every 8 women in America will develop it over a life span of 85 years) and has the second highest fatality rate of cancer in women. Since early detection makes it much easier to treat breast cancer successfully, breast self-examination, along with MAMMOGRAPHY, is one of the first and best lines of defense. Approximately four out of every five breast lumps so detected turn out to be a cyst or other benign (noncancerous) lesion. If a lump is found, however, it is essential to determine as quickly as possible if it is cancerous or not.

Self-examination long was recommended for all women from age 20 on. However, three cancer organizations—the American Cancer Society, the National Cancer Institute, and the U.S. Preventive Services Task Force—now consider it optional, since it has not been demonstrated to save lives. See the illustration on page 68.

breech presentation Also *breech birth.* In childbirth, the position of the baby in which its buttocks (breech) are the presenting or leading part (that is, leading its descent into the birth canal). Breech presentation occurs in 3 to 4% of all deliveries. In a *frank breech* presentation, the baby's hips are flexed but the knees extended. In a *complete breech* the baby is virtually in sitting position, with both hips and knees flexed. Occasionally the breech is *incomplete,* with one or both feet or knees presenting (sometimes called a *single* or *double footling breech*). Unlike the far more common CEPHALIC PRESENTATION (head first), where, after the baby's largest part—the head—passes through the birth canal, the rest of the body follows with little difficulty, in a breech birth successively larger portions of the baby are born: first the buttocks, then shoulders and last the head. Moreover, in cephalic presentation the head, which is still very malleable, is molded by the forces of the contractions pushing it through the birth canal, as a result of which it may decrease as much as half an inch in diameter. In breech presentation there is no such opportunity, so that a larger pelvic diameter is needed to accommodate the passage of the head.

Breast Self-examination (BSE)

Breast self-examination should be done once a month so you become familiar with the usual appearance and feel of your breasts. Familiarity makes it easier to notice any changes in the breast from one month to another. Early discovery of a change from what is "normal" is the main idea behind BSE.

If you menstruate, the best time to do BSE is 2 or 3 days after your period ends, when your breasts are least likely to be tender or swollen. If you no longer menstruate, pick a day, such as the first day of the month, to remind yourself it is time to do BSE.

Here is how to do BSE:

1　Stand before a mirror. Inspect both breasts for anything unusual, such as any discharge from the nipples, puckering, dimpling, or scaling of the skin.

2　Watching closely in the mirror, clasp hands behind your head and press hands forward.

3　Next, press hands firmly on hips and bow slightly toward your mirror as you pull your shoulders and elbows forward.

　　Some women do the next part of the exam in the shower. Fingers glide over soapy skin, making it easy to concentrate on the texture underneath.

4　Raise your left arm. Use three or four fingers of your right hand to explore your left breast firmly, carefully, and thoroughly. Beginning at the outer edge, press the flat part of your fingers in small circles, moving the circles slowly around the breast. Gradually work toward the nipple. Be sure to cover the entire breast. Pay special attention to the area between the breast and the armpit, including the armpit itself. Feel for any unusual lump or mass under the skin.

5　Gently squeeze the nipple and look for a discharge. Repeat the exam on your right breast.

6　Steps 4 and 5 should be repeated lying down. Lie flat on your back, left arm over your head and a pillow or folded towel under your left shoulder. This position flattens the breast and makes it easier to examine. Use the same circular motion described earlier. Repeat on your right breast.

© Infobase Publishing

Opinion differs as to whether breech labors are more prolonged than cephalic ones—many clinicians believe they are—but all agree that their risk to the baby is almost four times greater. Part of the reason for this is that breech babies often are premature; indeed, this may be the main cause of breech presentation, the smaller (premature) fetus having room to turn upside down inside the uterus. Another risk is the danger to the baby's head; intracranial hemorrhage, pressures on the head, the clinician's attempts to pull the head through the cervix, which has closed somewhat before the head can emerge—all contribute to this danger. Also, there is danger of compressing the umbilical cord, thus cutting off the baby's oxygen supply. In view of these risks, most clinicians try to prevent breech presentation. If it is recognized in the last few weeks of pregnancy (from palpating the mother's abdomen), attempts may be made at *external version,* that is, gently but firmly maneuvering the baby's position from the outside of the abdomen. Unfortunately, even when such version (turning) can be accomplished readily, the baby often will turn back to breech position.

In spontaneous breech delivery there usually is no problem until the baby's umbilicus is reached. From that point on, the clinician must be extremely watchful. If the head is larger than the pelvic girdle, a CESAREAN SECTION must be performed. While dangerous in itself, Cesarean section is safer than a difficult extraction and should be used if the baby is premature, the mother's pelvis is small and the baby is very large, or if contractions are weak. An X-ray before or during labor may show whether a baby's head is too large for the pelvis and help in weighing the risks and benefits of vaginal versus surgical delivery. In the United States by far the majority of breech babies are delivered surgically, because physicians now prefer to avoid rotating such babies manually or with instruments during labor, lest they injure the brain or other organs. If the baby is full term and in the most common, frank breech position and the clinician is experienced with breech births, vaginal breech delivery has the backing of the American College of Obstetricians and Gynecologists.

brow presentation In childbirth, the position of the baby when its brow (forehead) is the presenting or leading part (the part that leads the baby's descent into the birth canal). Often a brow presentation will convert itself into either a vertex or a face presentation as the baby moves down the birth canal, forcing the baby to flex its chin into its chest (see CEPHALIC PRESENTATION). If brow presentation persists, with a very small baby vaginal delivery may be possible, but with a full-term baby of average size it usually is not, and a CESAREAN SECTION will have to be performed. Brow presentation is, however, the least common form of abnormal presentation.

bruising Also *easy bruising, purpura simplex.* A benign condition in which bruises develop upon slight impact or no impact, especially on the arms, hands, thighs and buttocks. Occurring more in women than in men, it results from aging skin, when the dermis (the layer just below the surface) thins and collagen fibers decrease, lessening support for the blood vessels. Although such bruising does not indicate blood-clotting failure, it should be evaluated by the health care practitioner to rule out other signs of abnormal bleeding, such as VON WILLEBRAND DISEASE. There is no effective treatment. Smoking and taking aspirin and oral corticosteroids (often used by the elderly for arthritis) aggravate the condition. Younger women who use sunscreen regularly can slow collagen loss. Older women can try to protect themselves by wearing gloves, long sleeves and long pants, and by removing or padding sharp-edged pieces of furniture. Skin tears should be washed with mild soap (not iodine or alcohol), treated with antibiotic ointment and covered with a dressing that holds moisture but lets air through.

bubo A painful inflammation or swelling of a lymph gland, usually in the groin, developing especially in the course of a venereal infection.

See also CHANCROID; LYMPHOGRANULOMA VENEREUM.

bulimia Also *bulimarexia.* A cycle of alternate gorging and self-starvation that continues over a period of time. The term *bulimarexia* was coined by an American psychologist, Marlene Boskind-White, in the 1970s, but today it is usually shortened to bulimia. An eating disorder, the condition occurs chiefly in young women who have abnormally low self-esteem and become obsessed with attaining an ideal figure, which they perceive as an extremely thin body. They tend to view themselves as fat when in fact their weight is generally normal. The cycle frequently begins with an eating binge, in which the woman eats anything and everything available—1,000 to 60,000 calories in a short time, usually in secret—until she literally feels ill. It is followed by feelings of self-disgust and shame, which she deals with by extreme dieting or complete fasting and sometimes also by purging (self-induced vomiting, laxative abuse, use of amphetamines, overstrenuous exercise). This aberrant behavior then becomes a regular routine. Unlike ANOREXIA NERVOSA, bulimia rarely prohibits functioning in day-to-day life or requires hospitalization, although the bizarre eating pattern takes up considerable time and energy. Women who abuse laxatives may have chronic diarrhea and develop RECTOCELE. In extreme cases bulimics may be dehydrated, have gastric bleeding and suffer from life-threatening electrolyte imbalance. In most cases, however, hospitalization is not required.

It is not known how widespread the condition is, partly because it was recognized only recently and partly because one of its characteristic features is that the binging and purging take place secretly. Attempts to cure the condition usually involve some form of psychotherapy. Group therapy in particular appears to show promise, since it forces patients to acknowledge that neither their behavior nor the feelings prompting it are unique. Therapy is directed largely at building up self-esteem. Antidepressant medication, especially fluoxetine (Prozac), has helped some bulimics, reducing the number of binge-eating episodes by two-thirds and vomiting sessions by half.

Like anorexics, the overwhelming majority of bulimics are women (90 to 95%). The weight fluctuations and poor nutrition engendered by the disorder can alter their menstrual and reproductive cycles, resulting in irregular or no menses. Also, frequent vomiting and/or high doses of laxatives may alter the effectiveness of oral contraceptives, putting some patients at risk for an unwanted pregnancy.

A related eating disorder is *binge eating*, whose symptoms are similar to bulimia except that binge eaters do not purge and usually are significantly overweight. Binge eating disorder is characterized by eating an excessively large amount of food in a two-hour period at least twice a week for six months, feeling a lack of control over the episodes and experiencing marked distress concerning the practice. Far more common than anorexia and bulimia, it is estimated to affect one in 35 adults. It is prevalent among obese individuals. Treatment may consist of cognitive-behavioral therapy and some form of weight control.

bunion A foot deformity, a painful protuberance at the base of the big toe. Nine times more common in women than in men, it results from *hallux valgus,* a condition in which the joint at the base of the toe bulges outward and the toe points inward. The tendency to bunions is hereditary, but ill-fitting shoes, especially those that crowd the toes, exacerbate it. Continued friction with the shoe irritates the bunion and leads to increased bone growth and further swelling and, in time, arthritic changes in the joint. Treatment ranges from wearing pads to shield the bunion and wearing wider shoes to injecting the bunion with a corticosteroid mixed with a local anesthetic. Severe cases may require surgical correction of the toe's position, which usually affords considerable pain relief but does not guarantee a total cure. Called *bunionectomy* and usually performed on an outpatient basis, it aims to remove the protuberance and, often, involves *osteotomy*, that is, cutting and repositioning the bones to align them properly. Depending on the severity of the bunion, which affects the precise techniques required, recovery takes anywhere from 3 to 12 weeks.

A bunion may also form on the joint of the little toe. It is called a *bunionette* and involves the same kinds of treatment.

burning mouth syndrome Burning sensations on the tongue, lips or in the whole mouth. Affecting women seven times more often than men and usually occurring after the age of 60, it is not evident on examination of the mouth. Causes include chronic infection, gastric reflux (see GASTROESOPH-AGEAL REFLUX DISORDER), blood diseases, vitamin deficiency, hormone imbalance, allergy or the side effect of an antibiotic or other medication. In some women an oral yeast infection is responsible, which is treated with anti-yeast lozenges dissolved in the mouth four times a day. If this helps, treatment is continued for 8 to 12 weeks. Easy to diagnose but difficult to treat, the burning sensation may be accompanied by a dry mouth, increased thirst and altered taste. If simple measures such as frequent drinks of water and chewing gum do not help, an antidepressant such as nortriptyline or an antianxiety drug such as clonazepam may be tried.

Caesarean section   See CESAREAN SECTION.

calcifications, breast   Tiny deposits of calcium that accumulate in breast tissue. They cannot be felt on manual examination but show up as a white sprinkling on a mammogram. Although they most often are not associated with any malignancy, a cluster of small calcifications—so-called *microcalcifications* (larger ones are called *macrocalcifications*)—may signal a cancerous or precancerous condition. In questionable cases, therefore, a biopsy is indicated to rule out malignancy (see BIOPSY, def. 5). Even then about three-fourths turn out to be benign. Calcifications are caused by a variety of benign factors, including fibrocystic changes, fibroadenomas or fat necrosis. They do *not* result from too much calcium in the diet.

calcium   A vital dietary mineral, needed for building bones and teeth, for blood clotting and for regulating nerve and muscle activity. In addition to its primary role in forming and maintaining strong bones and teeth, calcium has been found to reduce the risk of colon cancer in men at high risk for the disease and reduce life-disrupting premenstrual symptoms in women who suffer from congestive dysmenorrhea (see DYSMENORRHEA, def. 5). It also helps contribute to normal blood pressure, especially when consumed in dairy products.

The best dietary sources of calcium are milk and milk products, broccoli, canned fish containing bones, and leafy green vegetables (except that the oxalic acid also contained in spinach, beet greens and Swiss chard interferes with the body's ability to absorb the calcium in these foods). Calcium supplements vary markedly in effectiveness. Among the many kinds available, calcium-citrate-malate (CCM) is most readily absorbed, and calcium oxalate most poorly. Calcium carbonate, the most widely marketed variety (it is found in antacids such as Tums) lies between these two. (It is also found in oyster shell supplements, which should be avoided since they may contain harmful contaminants; the same is true of bone meal and dolomite.) Also, some pills have a coating that resists digestive enzymes so that they pass through the system unabsorbed. Consequently one should test a pill by dropping it into a glass containing six ounces of vinegar and stirring every few minutes; if it has not completely dissolved in 30 minutes, it probably will not dissolve inside the body. Supplements are most effective when taken in doses of 500 milligrams or less. Further, vitamin D is essential for calcium absorption, and 800 International Units of it a day are recommended. Fortified milk is the most common source of vitamin D, but many other products, such as calcium-fortified orange juice, also include some vitamin D.

In addition to the oxalic acid in spinach, a number of important medications not only interfere with the body's absorption of dietary calcium but undermine its bone-building processes. Among them are glucocorticoids (including cortisone, hydrocortisone, prednisone and prednisolone), especially if taken by mouth over a long term; thyroid hormone; phenytoin and barbiturate anticonvulsants such as Dilantin, used to control epilepsy; large amounts of over-the-counter aluminum-containing antacids such as Maalox, Rolaids and Gelusil. When such drugs are necessary to control serious or chronic conditions, their calcium-inhibiting side effect should be counteracted with such measures as increasing calcium intake, exercising with weights and strength training, avoiding smoking and limiting alcohol and caffeine consumption.

The recommended amounts of daily calcium intake are 1,200 to 1,500 mg (milligrams) for ages 11 to 24 and for pregnant and lactating women, 1,000 mg for ages 25 to 50, and 1,500 mg from age 51 on (earlier if postmenopausal). If those are difficult to obtain in the daily diet, as they may be by older women, calcium supplements in some form probably are advisable. It is possible, however, to consume too much calcium, usually by taking a few extra supplements a day. It can result in constipation, increase the risk of kidney stones in those susceptible to them, increase blood calcium (which can lead to calcification in the kidneys and arteries) and impair absorption of iron, zinc or magnesium. The upper limit, according to the National Research Council, is 2,500 milligrams from the age of 19 upward. Similarly, too much vitamin D—more than 2,000 International Units per day—can lead to high blood calcium.

See also DIET; OSTEOPOROSIS.

calendar method   See NATURAL FAMILY PLANNING.

Canavan disease   An inherited neurological disorder that usually results in death before the age of 10. Symptoms, which tend to appear between the ages of three and six months, include delays in development, poor head control and an enlarged head. Eventually seizures, severe feeding problems, significant motor delays and possibly blindness occur. There is no treatment. Canavan disease is most prevalent among Ashkenazi Jews (Jews of central and eastern European descent), among whom about 1 in 40 is a carrier. When both parents of a child are carriers, their child has a risk of Canavan of about 1 in 6,400. Despite this relatively low risk, the fact that the disorder is invariably fatal has made the American College of Obstetricians and Gynecologists recommend screening by means of a blood test for all individuals who may be carriers, ideally before conceiving a child. When both parents are carriers, prenatal testing through CHORIONIC VILLUS SAMPLING or AMNIOCENTESIS can reveal if the fetus has the disease.

cancer   Also *carcinoma, malignancy, malignant tumor, neoplasm.* A general name for what is thought to be some 200 different diseases that have certain traits in common. First, all of them are characterized by *abnormal cell division;* instead of normal cells reproducing in an orderly fashion to carry on the process of tissue growth and repair, cancer cells begin an uncontrolled process of dividing, creating a mass of extra cells or tissue that, when it takes a solid form, is called a TUMOR. The process begins with one damaged cell, which divides and multiplies unchecked—a capacity that all of its copies share. There are several different kinds of cancer cell, each with a different rate of growth and spreading ability, but virtually all of them behave in this way. Moreover, cancer cells look much like healthy cells; they are simply somewhat less organized and somewhat misshapen. Second, cancer is usually *invasive;* that is, it infiltrates and actively destroys surrounding healthy tissue (but see also CANCER IN SITU). Third, cancer can metastasize—it can spread to other parts of the body, forming new growths called *metastases.* It was long thought that metastasis takes place by means of cancer cells spreading through the blood or lymph (the clear fluid that bathes body cells). Today most cancers are regarded as a systemic disease, one that affects the entire body in the same way as a generalized infection; almost from the time it is formed, a tumor sheds malignant cells into the circulatory system. Finally, cancer tends to *recur.* After a period of improvement or seeming cure, called *remission,* it may strike again, in the same part of the body or elsewhere. Untreated, cancer usually is fatal, displacing healthy tissue and causing organs to cease functioning until the patient dies. Occasionally, however, the disease will go into spontaneous remission, with the symptoms decreasing or disappearing altogether.

Cancer can attack just about any of the body's organs—the respiratory system, digestive system, reproductive system, bones, brain, skin, blood, lymph. Indeed, cancers often are named for the organ where they originated (lung cancer, breast cancer, etc.). Cancers also may be classified according to the kind of tissue in which they arise. ADENOCARCINOMAS involve glandular tissue; SARCOMAS involve connective tissue; adenosarcomas involve both connective and gland tissue; leukemias involve the blood cells; lymphomas involve the lymph nodes. Approximately 85% of all cancers consist of solid tumors, that is, adenocarcinomas and sarcomas.

In women, nearly half of all cases of cancer affect the reproductive system. Breast cancer accounts for about half of those, and the rest attack the pelvic area (vulva, vagina, cervix, endometrium, fallopian tubes, ovaries). Of the latter, endometrial cancer is the second most common malignancy in women, followed by ovarian cancer. Cervical cancer tends to strike women in their mid-40s, while endometrial and ovarian cancers are more common after menopause. Tubal cancers are very rare. The leading cause of cancer deaths in women, however, is lung cancer, followed by breast cancer.

Ultimately cancer is caused by damaged genes. Since each gene is the stored blueprint for a protein, the chemical that does most of the work (including growth) of cells, anything that damages genes can cause cancer. Some factors are environmental *carcinogens* (cancer-causing agents), among them high doses of ultraviolet or ionizing radiation; the use of tobacco (implicated in an estimated 80% or more of all cases of lung cancer); exposure to asbestos, coal dust and numerous toxic industrial substances; and infection with viruses, such as HTLV-I (human T-lymphotropic virus), which causes a form of adult leukemia (blood cancer), and Epstein-Barr virus, linked with Burkitt's lymphoma and other cancers. These substances appear to cause changes in the genes of a normal cell that prime it for uncontrolled growth. Before a cell can reproduce it must copy out its genes, written on DNA (see GENETICS for further explanation). Some cancers are caused by errors that creep in when DNA is being copied or the disruption of DNA by a virus. The changed genes are called *oncogenes* (cancer genes). Another kind of change cripples a gene that normally makes a protein that checks cell growth. It is called a *suppressor gene*. Suppressor genes are missing in almost all lung and bone cancers, many bladder cancers and some breast cancers. Several other cancers appear to have missing genes on particular chromosomes, the cell structures on which DNA is arranged, and these may well be suppressor genes. Moreover, in a process as complex as cell growth, it may take more than one genetic error

to cause cancer, which may explain why cancer is more likely to occur with advancing age (which allows time for more genetic changes to occur). Another promising avenue of research is into *cancer stem cells*, cells that in effect function as a tumor's master print and therefore enable it to recur and spread. Harvesting stem cells from a tumor and identifying the stem-defining proteins might, it is hoped, be used for targeted drug therapy that would be more effective.

Genetic research also indicates that, for many kinds of cancer, there is an inherited predisposition. Although the specific genes for only very few such cancers have been identified so far, family history may reveal individuals who are at risk. Recent research indicates that every individual is born with various genetic susceptibilities, a finding that explains why some heavy smokers never get lung cancer and others who have never smoked do. Apparently some individuals have genes enabling their bodies to detoxify harmful chemicals rapidly, whereas others have slow-acting forms of these genes. Locating markers for these genetic traits, it is hoped, will enable more accurate prediction of who is at risk for what kind of cancer. Among genetic mutations so far implicated in cancer risk are the P53 gene, which constitutes a 50% risk for developing cancer by age 30 and 90% by age 60 (breast cancer, leukemia, sarcomas, brain cancer or adrenal gland cancer); BRCA1 or BRCA2, up to 85% risk for breast cancer and up to 60% for ovarian cancer; CDKN2A, up to 76% risk for melanoma; and any of five genes for 80% risk of colon cancer. (See also separate entries for various cancers.)

To minimize one's risk, it may be wise to change one's diet. Based on worldwide studies of cancer incidence, animal studies and laboratory findings, the American Cancer Society has concluded that diet is a primary factor in one-third of all deaths from cancer. While there are no guarantees that a better diet will prevent cancer, it is plausible that one's risk may be reduced by means of a diet rich in whole grains, fruits and vegetables, moderate in animal protein (especially red meat) and low in fat, simple sugars and alcohol.

Treatment of cancer consists of surgery (excision of malignant tumors) and chemotherapy, hormone therapy and radiation (to kill malignant cells). While causing serious side effects because they also kill healthy cells, radiation and anticancer drugs work mostly on the oncogenes—that is, they attempt to block growth, usually by blocking cell division. A particularly promising avenue is the use of so-called *targeted drugs* and *smart drugs,* which precisely block the abnormal genetic pathways or mutations that cause and maintain cancer. Among them are *angiogenesis inhibitors,* which inhibit the formation of new blood vessels around cancer cells and thus starve them of nourishment; *growth-factor inhibitors,* which block a cancer cells's link to critical proteins that help it divide and grow; *chemoprevention* therapies, such as the hormone blocker tamoxifen, which keeps cells from dividing by binding to estrogen receptors; *gene therapies* that replace defective suppressor genes with healthy ones; and *monoclonal antibodies,* such as trastuzumab (Herceptin) for advanced breast cancer, proteins that bind to and attack a particular target (usually another protein called an antigen, such as those displayed by tumor cells) and can carry radioactive and chemical toxins that directly destroy malignant tissue. Another approach is IMMUNOTHERAPY, that is, strengthening the body's immune system so that it can better fight cancerous growths, either using such drugs as alpha-interferon and interleukin-12 or by developing vaccines (dozens are being tested) or proteins to stimulate the immune system. One such approach, still experimental, is a vaccine enhancing the ability of dendritic cells, which mobilize the immune system, to target cancer cells and enable the body's killer T cells to recognize and destroy them. Therapies that also are still experimental at this writing include *antimetastatic factors,* to keep cancer cells confined to a single spot; and *anti-oncogenic factors,* combating a tumor's ability to activate oncogenes. Still another approach being investigated is *virotherapy,* the use of genetically engineered viruses to target and kill diseased cells without affecting healthy cells. A promising new approach is to target only the molecular problems (the mutated genes) that drive a tumor's growth. Often these drugs must be used in conjunction with more traditional agents or combined with other targeted agents. To find

DIET TO REDUCE CANCER RISK

Food	Benefits
Soy, dried beans	Contain plant estrogens that may reduce risk of breast and pelvic cancers
Tomatoes, carrots, carotenoids, red peppers	Rich in vitamin C; may reduce risk of prostate cancer
Cruciferous vegetables (broccoli, cabbage, brussels, sprouts, bok choy, cauliflower, kale, other greens)	May reduce risk of lung, colon, rectum, stomach and esophageal cancers; also possibly breast, bladder, pancreas and larynx cancers
Garlic, onions, leeks	Contain allium compounds; may reduce risk of breast cancer
Olive oil	May reduce risk of breast cancer
Milk and milk products	Rich in calcium and vitamin D; may reduce risk of breast and colon cancers
Salmon and other oily fish	May reduce cancer risk

the correct target, identifying mutations in particular genes, is a DNA microarray or *gene chip.* Gene chips can show which genes in a tumor are more active than they should be.

Many cancers detected at an early stage are potentially curable. For this reason and because many cancers are not associated with warning symptoms such as pain until they are far advanced—often too far for any treatment to be effective—early cancer detection is of prime importance. Thus all women are advised to have regular tests of their cervical cells, to examine their own breasts monthly for lumps or other irregularities and, after age 40, to have regular mammograms (see BREAST SELF-EXAMINATION; MAMMOGRAPHY; PAP SMEAR). With early detection, before a cancer has had time to destroy much surrounding tissue or to spread to other parts of the body, the chances for a complete cure (using surgery, radiation, drugs or some combination of these treatments) are thought to be much greater. Newer diagnostic techniques, such as RADIONUCLIDE IMAGING, also assist early detection. Moreover, researchers currently are developing simpler blood and urine tests that may not only track the course of early cancers and monitor cancer treatment but may detect the first signs of malignancy. One newer test for high-risk women is *ductal lavage,* which washes cells from milk ducts, where 95% of breast cancers start. It can be done in a doctor's office or outpatient clinic. After a local anesthetic is applied to the nipple area, a suction device draws tiny amounts of fluid from the milk duct to the surface, indicating the duct's opening. A slender catheter is inserted into the duct, releasing anesthetic fluid, and saline is delivered through it to rinse the duct and collect cells, which are sent to a laboratory. However, a study of women about to undergo mastectomy who were given ductal lavage before surgery indicated that the procedure detected cancer in only five of the 38 known to have cancer, and it was concluded that ductal lavage is unacceptable as a screening test.

Preliminary findings announced in 2004 indicate that a simple urine test may detect breast cancer early and accurately track tumor growth. Researchers continued to investigate urine tests for other cancers. If successful, these would be more convenient and less expensive than the scans, blood tests and biopsies commonly used to screen for and diagnose cancers.

A new noninvasive test for breast cancer, the Halo Breast Pap Test System, is said to diagnose early breast cancer before a lesion has developed (see also CANCER, BREAST). Another new test under development aims at making sure that, following surgery, cancer has not spread. It employs a molecular "paint," a blend of chlorotoxin and a fluorescent molecule that emits near infrared light. The chlorotoxin binds to cancer cells. After tumor removal, a special camera is used to capture near infrared photons in the body and see if any cancer cells have been missed.

Another avenue being explored is developing DNA tests to determine the possibilities of recurrence and the best treatment. Such a test profiles a tumor's genes and tailors treatment accordingly. Several have already been introduced for certain lung and breast cancers, and more are under development for prostate, kidney, and colon cancers, chronic leukemia and other malignancies.

Some patients reject surgical, radiation and chemical treatment in favor of nutritional, manipulative or psychological therapies, or choose to combine these with conventional medical treatment. The nutritional approaches, which regard cancer as a systemic disease, include fasting, said to eliminate poisons from the body and deprive developing cancer cells of nourishment; raw foods (after fasting), to encourage the body's elimination of toxins and to starve the cancer cells; eliminating or limiting salt, refined sugar and caffeine from the diet; vitamin therapy, with large doses of vitamin A (to build immunity, fight infection, keep cells from aging), the B vitamins (to cope with stress and facilitate estrogen metabolism), laetrile (B_{17}), found in apricot pits, which allegedly kills cancer cells without harming normal cells, vitamin C in massive doses, vitamin E and such minerals as potassium, magnesium, selenium and zinc; and various herbal combinations. Manipulative techniques include acupressure, acupuncture and shiatsu (a Japanese massage technique involving acupressure). None of these has been recognized as an effective treatment by any reputable medical organization or shown to be effective in careful controlled studies, but many are being studied by the National Institutes of Health's Office of Alternative and Complementary Medicine. Those who do choose an alternative therapy along with more conventional treatment are urged to inform their physicians, since some of these therapies may interfere with standard treatment.

See also CHEMOTHERAPY; HORMONE THERAPY; RADIATION THERAPY.

One kind of psychological therapy used in conjunction with traditional (surgical, chemical, radiation) therapies and/or nutritional treatment is VISUALIZATION.

The National Cancer Institute has a computerized database, Physician Data Query (PDQ), that tells where new treatments are being tried for a particular cancer and what treatments currently are considered best. See the Appendix for the phone number and Web site of the PDQ. A number of other Web sites give more information: treatment guidelines at http://www.nccn.org and www.facs.org/cancer/qualitymeasures.html; approved cancer programs at www.facs.org/cancerprogram.

AMERICAN CANCER SOCIETY SCREENING GUIDELINES FOR EARLY DETECTION OF CANCER IN ASYMPTOMATIC PERSONS

Test or procedure	Sex	Age	Frequency
Sigmoidoscopy, preferably flexible	M&F	Over 50	Every 3–5 years
Fecal occult blood test (for bowel cancel)	M&F	Over 50	Every year
Digital rectal examination	M&F	Over 40	Every year
Pap test (for cervical cancer)	F	All women who are or have been sexually active or have reached age 18 should have annual Pap test and pelvic exam. After three or more consecutive satisfactory normal annual exams, Pap test may be done less often at physician's discretion.	
Pelvic examination	F	18–40 Over 40	Every 1–3 years Every year
Endometrial tissue sample	F	At menopause	At menopause and thereafter at physician's discretion if at high risk*
Breast self-examination	F	Over 20	Every month
Breast clinical examination	F	20–40 Over 40	Every 3 years Every year
Mammography†	F	40–49 50 and over	Every 1–2 years Every year
Health counseling and cancer checkup‡	M&F M&F	Over 20 Over 40	Every 3 years Every year

*History of infertility, obesity, failure to ovulate, abnormal uterine bleeding, or unopposed estrogen or tamoxifen therapy.
†Screening mammography should begin by age 40.
‡To include examination for cancers of the thyroid, ovaries, lymph nodes, oral region and skin.

With more successful treatments for cancer, there are more and more *cancer survivors.* Consequently, there is a growing need for a survivorship care plan, providing information about proper long-term care; a detailed list of treatments received and their potential consequences; a monitoring plan to check for delayed effects of treatment, such as heart or bone damage; a plan to check for recurrence or a new cancer, with indication of symptoms that might indicate these; advice about diet and exercise; information about a CANCER SUPPORT GROUP.

The aftereffects of radiation and chemotherapy have long been known, especially for survivors of childhood cancers, but only in recent years has there been increased awareness of and support for these individuals. Although many do not suffer from toxic side effects, a large study indicated that more than 62% had at least one chronic health condition, and women were at greater risk than men. Survivors of bone tumors, central nervous system tumors and Hodgkin's disease had the highest risk of a serious chronic disease. Often they find that their ability to engage in and/or enjoy sexual relationships has been impaired—by the disease, the treatment, or both. In men, radical surgery may lead to lasting impotence and temporary or permanent loss of fertility. In women, chemotherapy or radiation in the pelvic area can cause vaginal changes that makes intercourse painful, and other treatment may cause infertility and induce early menopause. Even when treatment does not result in physical problems, the effects of cancer on one's image, to oneself or one's partner, can inhibit sexual relationships. It is prudent, therefore, to discuss with one's surgeon or oncologist how fertility and sexual functioning may be affected by various treatment options. A man may want to bank his sperm. A woman may want to harvest eggs for later fertilization. After treatment, various devices may counter a man's impotence or a women's vaginal discomfort, and SEX THERAPY may help with the attendant emotional problems. The American Cancer Society publishes two booklets called "Sexuality and Cancer," one for women and one for men, and their partners, available from their local divisions (see the Appendix for address).

The question of whether or not a cancer patient or cancer survivor can or should undergo childbirth has no simple answer. For example, in cases where surgery removed a non-estrogen-sensitive breast tumor, pregnancy would not affect risk of recurrence. Radiation for Hodgkin's disease can be so performed that the ovaries and uterus are out of the radiation field, and other cancer treatments to reduce their effect on fertility and pregnancy are increasingly being used. Even women diagnosed with breast cancer while they are pregnant are not necessarily advised to terminate the pregnancy; the estrogen produced in pregnancy is weaker and less likely to stimulate breast cancer growth, even if the tumor is estrogen-sensitive. Further, fear that potent anticancer drugs will damage a woman's eggs or man's sperm and result in birth defects has proved unfounded. Even women operated on for cervical cancer may preserve their fertility if only part of the cervix is removed. And women whose ovaries are destroyed by cancer treatment may still sustain a pregnancy achieved through in vitro fertilization with a donor egg. In 2004 a 32-year-old woman became the first to give birth to a healthy baby after having ovarian tissue removed, frozen and then reimplanted in her body. The tissue had been removed seven years earlier because she had to be treated for cancer with drugs likely to damage her ovaries and cause infertility. However, it is still considered unwise to become pregnant during cancer treatment because the chances of survival are not known, and radiation therapy (as opposed to chemotherapy) definitely can harm the fetus.

Researchers have formulated seven warning signs of cancer and advise anyone who observes any of these symptoms to seek medical advice as quickly as possible:

1. A change in bowel or bladder habits
2. A sore that does not heal
3. Unusual bleeding or discharge
4. A thickening or lump in the breast or elsewhere
5. Persistent indigestion or difficulty in swallowing
6. Changes in a wart or a mole
7. A nagging cough or unusually hoarse voice

Most often these symptoms indicate some condition other than cancer but it is safer to make sure. See also the following entries on specific cancers affecting women; also PRECANCEROUS LESIONS.

cancer, bladder A CANCER of the urinary bladder, three times as common in men as in women. However, the symptoms of bladder cancer resemble those of cystitis and other common urinary disorders; they include blood in the urine, pain on voiding, burning and frequency. Since early diagnosis enables some 90% of bladder cancers to be treated successfully (and advanced cases rarely respond to treatment), such symptoms or any other changes in bladder function should be investigated promptly. On manual examination a palpable mass may be felt, and urinalysis may reveal cancer cells. Diagnosis first must rule out other possible causes of blood in the urine, mainly through testing a urine sample, and then identify a bladder tumor by means of cystoscopy (visual examination by inserting a tube and dye through the urethra into the bladder) or by surgical biopsy. Treatment depends on how widespread and aggressive the cancer is. Many bladder cancers have not invaded adjacent muscle and usually are removed by cystoscopic resection. It may be followed by immunotherapy with *bacillus Calmette-Guerin*, a bacterium placed inside the bladder through a catheter; it triggers the body's immune response. Superficial bladder cancer often recurs, so cystoscopy needs to be repeated every few months. For more advanced cancers, treatment consists of surgical removal of the entire bladder and, sometimes, also ovaries, ureters, urethra, and part of the vaginal wall. Traditionally it was followed by a UROSTOMY, but newer methods, which permit more normal urination through an artificial bladder, are replacing it. Chemotherapy and/or radiation therapy may follow surgery.

The single greatest risk factor for bladder cancer is cigarette smoking; the cancer-causing agents in tobacco smoke concentrate in urine, which touches the bladder lining. Another risk factor is diabetes, but since this disease requires frequent monitoring of urine, early detection may have skewed study results.

cancer, breast   The second most common kind of CANCER in women (after skin cancer) between the ages of 25 and 75 and the second leading cause of cancer deaths among women (after lung cancer). Younger black women who get breast cancer are more likely to get a particularly aggressive and lethal form of the disease; hence theirs is a higher death rate from cancer than white women in the same age group. However, incidence of breast cancer in the United States decreased markedly in 2003, most likely because the results of a large study on its link with estrogen replacement therapy (ERT) had been widely disseminated.

Like other cancers, breast cancer develops when changes in the DNA alter the proteins produced, transforming a normal cell into a malignant one. Such genetic mutations can be present at birth, predisposing a woman to getting breast cancer earlier in life, or be caused by exposure to hormones and carcinogens (cancer-causing agents). Women whose mothers contracted breast cancer before the age of 40 are likely to have inherited mutant genes, and their risk is thought to be about twice as great as the average. However, recent findings show that family history of the disease is linked with only about 6% of all cases. Further, researchers have discovered two genes, called BRCA1 and BRCA2, in which mutations are thought to be implicated in 10% of all breast cancers, as well as in ovarian cancers, and by 2002 six more were identified. Women found to have such a mutant gene have an 85% chance of developing breast cancer by the age of 70, and about 60% develop ovarian cancer. Such a finding may lead a woman to have more frequent testing (mammograms and clinical breast exams), and some may even consider preventive surgery to remove their breasts and ovaries. Unfortunately, the test for BRCA1 and BRCA2 genes missed them in about 12% of women from families with multiple cases of breast or ovarian cancer. Consequently, it cannot be wholly relied upon to discover early cancers.

Exposure to estrogen also is thought to be a factor. Thus women who began to menstruate fairly early (before the age of 12) and who stopped menstruating late (after 55) are at higher risk, as are those who had their first child after age 30 or have never given birth. Taking estrogen, in the form of the Pill for birth control or estrogen replacement after menopause, appears to increase risk. Some authorities cite cigarette smoking as another risk factor, holding that some women are particularly sensitive to the carcinogens found in tobacco (because they have a slow-acting form of a liver enzyme that detoxifies carcinogens).

About 15% of women with cancer in one breast are likely to develop it in the other breast, and recurrence in the same breast also may occur. An injury or blow to the breast is not related to the development of breast cancer, nor is breast-feeding.

The presence of FIBROCYSTIC BREAST SYNDROME, long thought to be unequivocally precancerous, is no longer considered indicative of a definitely increased risk. The ordinary lumpiness experienced by many women does not increase risk. However, a history of benign breast cysts, confirmed by biopsy or aspiration, is still thought by some to increase the risk of breast cancer. Atypical hyperplasia, a change in which breast cells are abnormally shaped and more numerous than average, also can be a precancerous condition; it is seen on a mammogram but must be confirmed by biopsy.

Environmental carcinogens also appear to be causative factors. Exposure to ionizing radiation increases the risk. Other prime suspects are the pesticide DDT (banned in 1972 but widely used until then), another kind of pesticide called PBBs (polybrominated biphenyls), and insulating fluids called PCBs (polychorinated biphenyls). Other toxins are being investigated as well. Several studies have implicated heavy use of antibiotics with increased risk. Some studies indicate that a diet high in fats, especially animal fats, and alcohol consumption increase the risk of breast cancer, but these findings are not yet conclusive.

Breast cancer is not a single disease. There probably are at least 15 different kinds, each with a different rate of growth and different tendency to metastasize (spread to other parts of the body). It is local only briefly and can develop in many parts of the breast: in the milk ducts, between ducts, in fat, in lymph or blood vessels, in the nipple, in the lobes where milk is manufactured (see PAGET'S DISEASE, def. 1). The most common type is invasive ductal carcinoma, accounting for about 70 to 80% of all breast cancers. It starts in a milk duct, breaks through the duct wall and invades the breast's fatty tissue. Another 10 to 15% of breast cancers are invasive lobular carcinomas, which begin in the milk-producing glands and can spread elsewhere. Still other, rarer kinds of breast cancer tend to have a better prognosis than these two most common types. Men also can get breast cancer, but they account for only 1% of all cases.

Estimates vary, but 80 to 95% of breast cancers are first detected by women themselves, making regular self-examination one of the principal means of early detection (see BREAST SELF-EXAMINATION). Besides lumps (80% of which turn out to be benign growths or cysts), other early symptoms are thickened areas, irregularities of shape, nipple retraction, nipple discharge, redness, flaking, puckering, enlarged pores or other skin changes. Pain is rarely a symptom until the cancer is quite far advanced. The principal means of diagnosis—and many believe the only definitive one—is BIOPSY (see def. 5), although such means as MAMMOGRAPHY and ULTRASOUND (see def. 1) also are employed, mainly as screening devices. Of these, the most reliable screening method by far is mammography (see the box on screening guidelines under CANCER). However, in women with very dense breast tissue, both ultrasound and mammograms may miss tumors, which, however, can be detected by a MAGNETIC RESONANCE IMAGER (MRI). MRI is also more accurate for detecting cancer in women who carry the breast cancer genes BRCA1 and BRCA2. Breast cancers may or may not be hormone-dependent, so any positive biopsy should be combined with an ESTROGEN-RECEPTOR ASSAY.

A new test for breast cancer, an experimental ultrasound technique that measures how readily breast lumps compress and bounce back, may help determine whether a biopsy needs to be performed. Called *elastography* or *elasticity imaging,* it is noninvasive and expected to cost far less than a biopsy. A cancerous tumor shows up larger on an elastogram than on a traditional ultrasound image. Larger trials are needed before the technique is considered conclusive. Still another new test, the Halo Breast

IF YOU HAVE BREAST CANCER, DOES YOUR PHYSICIAN/SURGEON:

- Treat many breast cancer patients? How many a year? (A specialist averages 10 a week, a general surgeon 10 a year.)
- Object to presurgery counseling and support given to his/her patients by other health care professionals?
- Perform only surgical biopsy?
- Perform a one-step procedure (both biopsy and surgery while the patient is under general anesthesia)?
- Use local anesthesia for biopsy if a woman requests it?
- Send cancerous tissue out for estrogen-receptor assay?
- Consider doing different surgical procedures, such as lumpectomy, simple mastectomy or modified radical mastectomy?
- Encourage patients to get a second opinion about alternative procedures?
- Encourage consultation with a plastic surgeon before surgery?
- Perform surgery so as to enable breast reconstruction afterward?
- Recommend radiation to the armpit after any kind of mastectomy?
- Advocate radiation or chemotherapy after surgery if lymph nodes in armpit all are negative? One node positive? Two nodes?
- Administer further treatment (drugs, radiation, hormone, etc.) after surgery or refer patient to cancer specialist?
- Arrange psychological counseling for women who have difficulty adjusting to diagnosis and/or treatment or refer them to self-help or professional counseling and support organizations?
- Encourage patients to become involved in National Cancer Institute clinical trials to compare different treatments?
- Refer patients to a comprehensive cancer center?

Pap Test System, combines a test for collecting nipple aspirate fluid with a laboratory analysis of ductal cells in that fluid. Using cups similar to those in a breast-milk pump, it applies heat and suction to collect aspirate. A five-minute procedure that can be performed in a doctor's office, it detects risk of cancer before a tumor has developed.

See also BIOPSY, def. 5.

Treatment generally involves surgery of various degrees, ranging from removal of a tumor alone to removal of the entire breast, underlying muscle and axillary lymph nodes (see MASTECTOMY for the various kinds of surgery). Formerly, it was

ASSESSING RISK FOR BREAST CANCER

Highest risk	*Familial:* One or more close relatives (mother, daughter, sister) have had breast cancer. *Genetic:* Inherited alteration in BRCA1 and BRCA2 genes.
Other risks	*Age:* Risk at age 45, 1 in 93; at age 55, 1 in 33; at age 65, 1 in 17; at age 85, 1 in 8. *Menarche/menopause:* Menstruation before age 14, menopause later than age 55 (increased exposure to estrogen). *Childbearing:* First child at age 30 or later, or no children. *Breast density:* Masks tumors in mammograms.

believed that a cancerous tumor remains local at the site of origin, spreads to nearby LYMPH NODES and then continues spreading through the body via the lymphatic system. If adjacent lymph nodes are removed with the tumor, it was reasoned, the route of spread is cut off. The current view holds that cancer is a systemic disease involving a complex spectrum of host-tumor relationships, with cancer cells spread via the bloodstream, and therefore variations in local or regional therapy are unlikely to affect a patient's survival. Rather, the cancer must be attacked systemically, through the use of RADIATION THERAPY, CHEMOTHERAPY (anticancer drugs), HORMONE THERAPY (changing the body's hormone levels and balance) and IMMUNOTHERAPY. The American Cancer Society recommends that before any therapy is directed at a primary breast tumor and regional lymph nodes, the patient be checked to make sure metastasis (cancer spread) to other parts of the body has not begun. The most frequent sites of metastasis for breast cancer are the lungs, pleurae, bones and liver. A bone scan is recommended for all Stage III and IV patients and for Stage II patients with evidence of lymph node involvement (see STAGING for an explanation of how cancer progresses), and routine laboratory tests should include liver function tests.

In mid-2007 the FDA approved the first molecular-based laboratory test that can tell surgeons, within minutes, if the breast cancer has spread and requires more extensive surgery. The test, called GeneSearch Breast Lymph Node Assay, focuses on the SENTINEL NODE removed. If that lymph node contains cancer cells, surgeons normally remove additional nodes. The new test quickly measures the presence and concentration of genes that should not normally be present and are correlated with breast cancer. Results appear in 40 minutes while the patient is anesthetized, so if they are positive the surgery can continue immediately. If they are negative the woman is spared unneeded further surgery and possible side effects such as LYMPHEDEMA.

Treatment is most effective in the early stages of the disease (some 60% of women found to have axillary lymph node involvement when first treated eventually die of cancer), and the spread of the disease is not always detectable. Therefore, a focus of current research is to pin down distant metastases that are microscopic in size, or *micromestastases*, which, it is believed, often are overlooked entirely in preliminary diagnoses.

A new approach to very large tumors is preoperative chemotherapy. Called *neoadjuvant therapy*, it allows determining if a specific chemotherapy works and thus spares using postsurgical therapy that is ineffective. And it sometimes eliminates the need for mastectomy. Two kinds of tumor benefit most from this approach—one too big to excise but with no cancerous tissue around it or one large tumor that might be shrunk in this way, then requiring only lumpectomy instead of mastectomy.

Because 30% of breast cancers recur, the National Cancer Institute urges all women with breast cancer to have chemotherapy or hormone (endocrine) therapy following surgery, even if there is no evidence that the cancer has spread. Such *systemic adjuvant therapy*, as it is called, can prevent or delay about one-third of recurrences. Many clinicians now advocate radiation therapy following excision of a small

BREAST CANCER SCREENING GUIDELINES*

Annual mammogram every one to two years from age 40 on

Clinical breast exam every two to three years for women aged 20 to 40, annually from age 40 on

Annual breast MRI for women whose lifetime risk of breast cancer is greater than 20%; women whose risk is 15 to 20% should discuss risk-benefit with their physicians

*Source: American Cancer Society

tumor with no lymph node involvement, and chemotherapy if lymph nodes have become involved.

Not everyone agrees that all patients need such aggressive treatment, and those who oppose it urge assessing the risk of recurrence by means of various tests. The most important of these tests are *tumor size* (the larger it is, the more likely it has spread); *estrogen and progestin receptor status,* that is, cancer cells that respond to these hormones suggest a less aggressive cancer and lower risk; *histological type,* grading the cell according to appearance (the higher the grade, the higher the risk); *DNA flow cytometry,* assessing the number of chromosomes and rate of DNA synthesis (the higher the number and faster the rate, the greater the risk); *HER2/oncogene,* in which extra copies of this gene signal aggressive cancer; and *cathepsin D,* with high levels suggesting high risk. Also, for women over the age of 70 who have small breast tumors, recent studies show they need not routinely undergo radiation therapy; for them surgery and estrogen-blocking tamoxifen (see below) may suffice. However, for women whose tumors are ER negative (do not require estrogen to grow), chemotherapy is usually advisable.

Studies are now underway for using genetic information to plan therapy for early-stage breast cancer. A test called Oncotype DX will be studied to determine the presence of a set of 21 genes known to be linked to higher risk of recurrence in patients with estrogen-receptor positive, lymph-node negative cancers. It is hoped to identify those who may have surgery alone and those who need chemotherapy. A similar test, MammaPrint, was approved by the FDA early in 2007; it examines the pattern of activity of 70 specific genes in a breast tumor that has been excised. The test is not totally accurate.

Several drugs are now available to treat or prevent breast cancer. They include two estrogen-blocking drugs. One, *tamoxifen,* first approved for advanced breast cancer, is now used for estrogen-receptive cancer patients and also for high-risk individuals who are still menstruating and producing considerable estrogen. Given by mouth, it may increase the risk of endometrial cancer and also may worsen vaginal dryness and hot flashes. Its use is not recommended for more than five years. However, after five years, postmenopausal women may take *letrozole* (Femara), which cuts

the risk of recurrence by 50%. The second kind, *aromatase inhibitors,* block aromatase, an enzyme that converts androgens produced by the adrenal gland into estrogens, and are used in postmenopausal women in whom androgens are the only source of estrogen. The aromatase inhibitors, such as anastrozole (Arimidex), fetrozole (Femara) and exemestane (Aromasin), seem to work as well or better than tamoxifen in postmenopausal women with advanced disease. They can cause bone loss, and they are not used in premenopausal patients because they do not effectively inhibit estrogen production in the ovaries. Many authorities suggest that an aromatase inhibitor be the initial treatment for early-stage, hormone-sensitive breast cancer in postmenopausal women, and that women who have taken tamoxifen for five years follow up with five or more years of Femara. One recent study indicated that this regimen reduced the risk of cancer spreading to other areas by 61% and the risk that a tumor would develop in the unaffected breast by more than 80%. A 2004 study reported that women taking tamoxifen for two and a half years and then switching to exmestane had much lower rates of cancer recurrence. Still another drug for treating advanced breast cancer is *fulvestrant,* which not only blocks cells from estrogen but breaks down and degrades the estrogen receptor. Like aromatase inhibitors, it suppresses new tumors but also keeps the disease at bay longer. Both kinds, however, are linked to gastrointestinal disturbances and hot flashes. In addition, progestins sometimes are used for advanced cancers.

A recent study showed that a drug used to prevent bone loss during cancer treatment also substantially cut the risk of cancer recurrence. The study tested Zometa, a bisphosphonate now used for cancer that has already spread to the bone. In the study of 1,800 premenopausal women taking hormone-blocking treatment for early-stage breast cancer, Zometa cut the risk of recurrence—in bones or other organs—by one-third.

Two other drugs are derived from compounds in the yew tree and act by disrupting the internal structure of forming cancer cells. A newer form of paclitaxel, Abraxane, is delivered more efficiently and helps shrink tumors more effectively. The other, Taxotere (docetaxel), improved long-term survival in patients with early-stage breast cancer. Both are used in advanced cases but have serious side effects. Herceptin (trastuzumab), a genetically engineered monoclonal antibody, is used to treat those breast tumors that have spread to other organs and overproduce a protein called HER2. Although only about 30% of malignant breast tumors are so involved, they are a particularly aggressive kind, and Herceptin, approved in 1998, slowed their progress by three to five months. Two tests to identify the presence of the HER2 gene are available. One looks at the amount of protein on the surface of a sample of tumor cells. The other looks for extra copies of the gene that governs HER2 production. Herceptin, if used after surgical removal of a tumor, cuts the risk of recurrence by 50%. However, a recent investigation showed that women who actually tested negative for HER2 still benefited from Herceptin, either indicating that the tests are imperfect or Herceptin has greater benefits than anticipated. A newer targeted drug, lapatinib (Tykerb), has been approved for patients with advanced metastatic HER-positive cancer who have tried other therapies and for whom Herceptin no longer works. It is administered orally along with another chemotherapy drug, capecitabine (Xeloda). Researchers are also investigating a promising vaccine that targets HER2/neu receptors, but more studies are needed.

Until the 1970s surgeons most often combined biopsy and mastectomy into one operation (the *one-stage approach*). When research began to indicate that less radical surgery or nonsurgical treatment sometimes was just as effective, women began to campaign for a *two-step procedure*. After biopsy (step 1) they would determine which of the available treatments was best for them. In 1979 Massachusetts passed the first state law requiring physicians to tell breast cancer patients about all the alternatives available to them and not to proceed until the patient reached a decision. This practice has become increasingly widespread but is not universal.

Older women who take hormone pills that combine estrogen and testosterone, sold under the brand names Estratest and Estratest H.S., more than double their risk of breast cancer. Similarly, medications combining estrogen and progestin greatly increase the risk (see also ESTROGEN REPLACEMENT THERAPY).

Recent years have seen a spate of studies that link low incidence of breast cancer with various environment factors, especially diet. For example, a study of Greek women seemed to show that their high consumption of fruits, vegetables and olive oil affords protection; another showed that as Japanese women ate more saturated fats, incidence of breast cancer rose. Another food touted to be a cancer preventive is soy (in such foods as tofu, tempeh, soy milk and vegetarian meat substitutes), but there is no clear evidence for this supposition. While it is clear that consuming more fruits and vegetables, eating less red meat (perhaps substituting soy protein) and avoiding cholesterol (olive oil has none) have health benefits, their relationship to preventing breast cancer has not been clearly established. A chemical found in broccoli, cabbage and other cruciferous vegetables may help prevent estrogen-related cancers. Called indole-3-carbinol or I-3-C, it changes how estrogen is metabolized; it is now available as a diet supplement, but more study is needed before it can be definitively considered a preventative. Another possible preventive measure is regular use of anti-inflammatory drugs. Several studies have shown that women who used standard doses of such drugs as ibuprofen and aspirin two or more times a week over a five- to nine-year period lowered their risk for breast cancer by 21%. The 10-year risk reduction was even higher, nearly 50% for ibuprofen and 22% for aspirin. Acetaminophen and low-dose aspirin, less than 100 mg, had no effect on breast cancer risk.

IF YOU HAVE CANCER, ASK YOUR CLINICIAN:

1. What is the stage of my cancer? (See STAGING)
2. How many tumors do I have? How large are they?
3. What is my tumor's grade (how abnormal the cells appear) and histology (type and arrangement of cells) as seen under a microscope?
4. Do I have any positive (cancerous) lymph nodes: If so, how many?
5. Is my cancer estrogen receptor-positive or progesterone receptor-positive?
6. How does my status as having (or not having) reached menopause affect my treatment?

National Comprehensive Cancer Network and American Cancer Society

A recent study showed that exercise helps prolong life for breast cancer survivors. Walking three or more hours a week or exercising more strenuously for shorter periods lowered the rate of recurrence. The precise mechanism is not known, but it is suspected that physical activity lowers hormone levels, decreases insulin resistance and reduces weight gain, all factors in breast cancer.

See also CANCER, INFLAMMATORY BREAST; CANCER IN SITU.

cancer, cervical A CANCER of the cervix, that is, the neck of the uterus. The second most common kind of pelvic cancer in women (after endometrial), it is almost 100% curable if it is caught in its early stages and treated surgically by hysterectomy and/or radiation therapy. However, because it typically gives no warning whatever, it may be present for as long as 4 to 10 years before it invades the deeper cervical tissues and gives rise to symptoms. Even then it is curable in 80% of cases. Thereafter, however, it spreads to the vagina, uterus, bladder and even the rectum, usually quite rapidly, and the outlook for cure is much less hopeful. Because its presence as a rule is unannounced, it is extremely important that all women, from the age of 18 on or when they become sexually active (whichever is first), undergo regular screening for cervical cancer, which is done by a very simple procedure called a PAP SMEAR.

Cervical cancer attacks about 2 to 3% of all American women, mostly between the ages of 35 and 55. But the disease is not unheard of in older women; of all new cases of cervical cancer, 25% develop in women 65 and older. If it is diagnosed very early, as a severe DYSPLASIA, it often responds to treatment, the method chosen depending on the location. Inside the cervical canal it is treated surgically with CONIZATION, which removes only part of the cervix and preserves the patient's ability to bear children; on the outside (ectocervix) it may be treated with CRYOSURGERY, the LOOP ELECTRO-SURGICAL EXCISION PROCEDURE, electrocoagulation (destroying tissue by heat) or laser surgery. In the next stage, when it is confined to the surface of the cervix (sometimes called CANCER IN SITU), treatment usually consists of surgical removal of both cervix and uterus (a hysterectomy); the ovaries can be left intact, since cervical cancer does not spread to the ovaries and is not affected by the production of estrogen. In young women who want to bear children, a new surgical technique, called *radical trachelectomy*, spares the uterus, but whether the cancer will return is not yet known. If the cancer has advanced to the deeper tissues of the cervix, it usually is treated with radiation, although sometimes extensive surgery may be undertaken. At this stage there still is a 75 to 85% chance of cure. With more advanced cancers, radiation was long the treatment of choice, but several major studies indicate that radiation combined with chemotherapy greatly improves the outlook.

There is overwhelming evidence that cervical cancer is caused by sexually transmitted viruses belonging to a group called human papilloma viruses, or HPV. Very common and hard to avoid, they are spread by skin contact and inhabit more territory than a condom can cover. One type, HPV-16, is found in 50% of cervical cancers; another, HPV-18, causes 20%, and others cause the rest. The vaccine Gardasil was approved by the FDA in 2006 and was widely recommended for all women, beginning at age 11 or 12. It will immunize against HPV 16 and HPV 18, and also HPV 6 and HPV 11. It is administered intravenously in three doses, the second following the first by one month and the last after six months. It also protects against genital warts, genital HERPES, and other HPV-associated disorders. (See also under HUMAN PAPILLOMA VIRUS.)

A new HPV test added to the conventional Pap smear diagnoses suspicious tissue samples for HPV infection. A recent study of more than 10,000 women showed that the test correctly spotted 95% of cervical cancers, opposed to only 55% found with a Pap test. Like the Pap, it uses cells scraped from the cervix. Currently the HPV test can be given only along with a Pap test. Investigations are underway to determine if the HPV test can be used alone and in place of a Pap test. Herpes simplex II might be involved in at least some cancers, since women with genital HERPES INFECTION develop cervical cancer far more often than women never so infected. Further, women who smoke are about three times as likely to develop cervical cancer as nonsmokers, and women exposed to heavy smokers for three or more hours a day are at the same risk as active smokers. Other risk factors are use of oral contraceptives and infection with other sexually transmitted diseases.

See also ADENOCARCINOMA, def. 2.

cancer, colorectal   Also *colon cancer, rectal cancer.* A CANCER of the colon and rectum, which is the third leading cause of cancer deaths in American women (after lung and breast cancers). Colon cancer is more common in women; rectal cancer, in men. It is a relatively silent killer, growing slowly for years before it is large enough to produce symptoms.

In rectal cancer the most common symptom is bleeding with a bowel movement. Therefore, whenever rectal bleeding occurs, even in the presence of known hemorrhoids, cancer needs to be ruled out. In colon cancers the symptoms depend on the lesion's location, type and extent. A tumor in the right colon may be symptomless, with fatigue and weakness the only complaints. In the left colon, it may cause alternating constipation and diarrhea, colicky abdominal pain and blood-streaked or black stools.

Experts maintain that most colorectal cancers could be stopped even before they become a threat by means of early detection tests. These tests find not only early, symptomless cancers but even precancerous conditions, permitting their removal and cure. A digital rectal examination, in which the physician inserts a finger into the rectum and feels for abnormalities, is recommended as part of the annual physical from age 40 on. Another such test is the fecal occult blood test, which involves smearing samples of one's stool on a card for three consecutive bowel movements. The smears are then tested with a chemical revealing the presence of hidden blood. Although this test has shortcomings—retrieval is imperfect (can be contaminated) and it can show blood from sources other than cancer (consuming aspirin, hemorrhoids, ulcers, etc.), the American Cancer Society recommends that everyone have a fecal occult blood test annually from age 50 on. (The risk of these cancers begins to rise at age 40.) Kits for it can be bought at a drugstore, but in most cases the cards are issued by and returned to the physician. A more effective but also costlier examination is flexible sigmoidoscopy, using an 18-inch flexible instrument to look into the lower third of the bowel. It also permits the removal of premalignant polyps, and should be done, it is recommended, every three to five years after age 50. Another test consists of administering a barium enema, which gives an X-ray image of the colon. If suspicious areas appear, the most effective procedure, COLONOSCOPY, is indicated. It uses a longer flexible instrument to examine the entire 5-foot length of the large bowel. It is generally performed when an occult blood test is positive, when growths are found with sigmoidoscopy or when family history suggests a high risk. For the latter, colonoscopy is recommended, starting at age 35 or 40, every five years. For the general population colonoscopy is recommended every 10 years. Still another test is a CEA assay, a blood test used to measure a protein (carcinoembryonic antigen) that is sometimes higher in individuals with colorectal cancer. Another way of screening for very early colon cancer is looking for traces of a gene called APC, which regulates faulty cell growth in 90% of early colon cancers. APC is sloughed off in colon cells contained in stool, but the test is still experimental and requires further study. Another test currently being studied is a noninvasive fecal DNA test, using an entire bowel movement that is packaged and sent to the lab. While research indicated it has a high degree of sensitivity, it also may mistakenly indicate cancer where there is none.

Individuals at high risk include those who have had previous malignant or precancerous polyps removed, those with a parent, sibling or child who developed colorectal cancer before age 56, and those who have had endometrial or ovarian cancer before age 50. In recent years researchers have discovered the defective genes that are responsible for 95% of all hereditary colon cancers (constituting about 20% of all colon cancers diagnosed in the United States each year). Having mutations in any of five particular genes constitutes an 80% risk for developing colon cancer, and their presence makes the development of colorectal cancer by one's forties a virtual certainty. Genetic tests can reveal their presence, which, if verified, calls for having frequent colonoscopies beginning in adolescence.

Colon cancer usually develops from benign tumors. These adenomatous polyps are either flat spreading growths (adenomas) or tubular growths (polyps) protruding from the bowel wall. The larger growths, wider than 1 inch, are more likely to become cancerous, but even so only a small percentage do so, and over a period of time. Their presence, however, puts a person at fairly high risk. Another risk factor, besides the genetic one, is inflammatory bowel disease (Crohn's disease, ulcerative colitis).

Treatment depends on how much the cancer has progressed (see the accompanying table on staging). Generally it consists of complete excision of the tumor, sometimes followed up with radiation or chemotherapy. (Also see COLOSTOMY.) Immunotherapy may also be effective. A less invasive technique for removing colon cancers uses LAPAROSCOPY, which shortens the hospital stay and results in fewer postoperative complications among patients whose cancer has not spread. It is still considered experimental and more study is needed. Another technique applies radiation therapy during surgery, but it is effective only if the cancer is confined to the colon. It is currently available. In 2004 a new drug, Avastin, was approved for advanced colon cancer. It blocks the development of blood vessels that feed tumors and, administered with other chemotherapy, lengthens the patient's survival.

Colon cancer appears to be a disease of highly industrialized nations, suggesting that preventive measures may consist of changing one's lifestyle. Associated with reduced risk are a diet rich in vegetables, fruits and cereals (400 mcg. of the B vitamin folate may also be helpful); adequate intake of calcium; use of NSAIDs (non-steroidal anti-inflammatory drugs) such as ibuprofen, aspirin, celexoxib (Celebrex) or sulindac (Clinoril); not smoking; and use of postmenopausal estrogen. A recent study showed that taking one baby aspirin (81 mg) a day reduced both the number and size of colorectal polyps.

cancer, endometrial　A CANCER of the lining of the uterus, the most common pelvic cancer in women. It appears most often between the ages of 50 and 70 and is often associated with previous menstrual irregularity (irregular periods), sporadic ovulation, infertility or prolonged estrogen therapy. It also is found more often in obese women, in women with high blood pressure and in women with diabetes. These conditions and other evidence suggest that endometrial cancer is associated with a chronic excess of estrogen relative to progesterone.

The most common symptom of endometrial cancer is irregular bleeding, with or without abdominal discomfort. For this reason women past menopause—defined as no menstrual periods for one year—who experience any bleeding or spotting, even just a pink stain, should be checked immediately. They may require a suction curettage and biopsy, or, if the condition is strongly suspicious, surgical D and C followed by examination of the tissue scrapings by a pathologist. (See BIOPSY, def. 8.) A Pap smear is not reliable for detecting endometrial cancer because the abnormal cells shed by the endometrium usually degenerate before reaching the vagina. In women still menstruating, grossly irregular periods and/or bleeding or staining between periods are cause for suspicion and, since about one-fourth of all endometrial cancers occur before menopause, should be promptly investigated.

Endometrial cancer in its early stages, when the tumor is confined to the uterus, is very curable if treated with a total hysterectomy and bilateral salpingo-oophorectomy (surgical removal of the uterus, both fallopian tubes and both ovaries), with or without radiation treatment. Further, following surgery ESTROGEN REPLACEMENT THERAPY probably

STAGING COLON CANCER	
Stage	Treatment
I: Tumor confined to colon wall	Bowel resection
II: Tumor protrudes through colon wall	Bowel resection; sometimes also radiation
III: Colon tumor and malignant lymph nodes	Bowel resection; also radiation and/or chemotherapy; possible immunotherapy
IV: Colon tumor and spread to other organs	Bowel resection; radiation, chemotherapy; possible surgery to remove liver metastases; immunotherapy

should be avoided (even for women suffering unpleasant menopausal symptoms) because most endometrial cancers are estrogen-dependent (see ESTROGEN-RECEPTOR ASSAY).

See also ADENOCARCINOMA, def. 3; ENDOMETRIAL HYPERPLASIA; STAGING.

cancer, inflammatory breast An uncommon type of breast cancer that usually grows rapidly and often spreads to other parts of the body. It occurs when cancer cells block the lymph vessels in the skin of the breast, causing the breast to become red, swollen and warm. The skin may appear bruised and may have ridges or appear pitted, and the nipple may be retracted. Sometimes lymph nodes under the arm and/or above the collarbone are swollen. Usually a tumor cannot be felt or seen on a mammogram. Diagnosis is based on the doctor's clinical judgment and results of a biopsy. Treatment usually consists of chemotherapy prior to mastectomy (breast removal), which is often followed by radiation. African Americans have a higher incidence of inflammatory breast cancer than Caucasians or other ethnic groups. Researchers currently are investigating the effectiveness of hormonal therapy and immunotherapy, sometimes combined with chemotherapy.

cancer, liver A cancer that originates in the liver (rather than spreading to the liver from another cancer, such as breast or colon cancer). Prevalent in Southeast Asia and sub-Saharan Africa, primary liver cancer is relatively rare in the United States, but the incidence is rising rapidly. Liver cancer often causes no symptoms until it is far advanced, not curable by surgery and/or having spread to other organs. Moreover, it grows rapidly, doubling in size every four months. Symptoms include pain in the upper right abdomen, a swollen abdomen, weight loss, loss of appetite and feeling of fullness, fever, and jaundice (yellowing of the skin and eyes).

Blood tests and screening for liver cancer are not completely accurate, biopsy yielding the only certain finding. When diagnosis is confirmed, the outlook is not good and death may occur within a few months. Most treatments are unsatisfactory.

The only possible cure for an early liver cancer is a transplant with a healthy liver from a cadaver or a lobe from a living donor. Because the liver regenerates, both donor and recipient soon have a full-size liver.

Liver cancer most often results from chronic infection by the viruses for hepatitis B and C (see HEPATITIS), which damage the liver and can lead to cancer many years after an infection begins. These infections also can cause cirrhosis, a scarring of the liver, and about 5% of patients with cirrhosis from any cause (alcohol abuse, infection) eventually develop liver cancer.

cancer, lung Also, *pulmonary cancer.* A CANCER affecting the respiratory system. Long the leading cause of cancer death in men, in the mid-1980s it passed breast cancer to become the leading cancer killer in women. Lung cancer is very difficult to detect early, hence its high fatality rate. Symptoms often do not appear until the disease has advanced considerably. Warning signs are a persistent cough, sputum streaked with blood, chest pain and recurring attacks of bronchitis or pneumonia. The single most important risk factor is cigarette smoking, especially for 20 or more years; it is estimated that 85% of lung cancer cases are caused by smoking. Moreover, recent studies show that women who smoke are twice as likely to get lung cancer as their male counterparts; the reason is not known. Inhaling secondary smoke—that is, being exposed to smoke without smoking oneself—is also an important factor. Other contributing agents include industrial materials such as asbestos, uranium, radon, nickel, arsenic and chromates. They are even more dangerous for smokers than for non-smokers. Recent studies indicate that nonsmoking women are more vulnerable to lung cancer than nonsmoking men; one study indicated they are twice as vulnerable. The reasons are not known, but secondhand smoke or the fact that they absorb more cancer-causing chemicals from smoke may be major factors. Moreover, nonsmokers' tumors respond differently to drugs than those of smokers. Research is underway to clarify gender differences in lung cancer, the hormone estrogen being a leading suspect.

Diagnosis involves such procedures as a sputum cytology test and fiberoptic bronchoscopy, but the single most reliable procedure is a chest X-ray. However, standard X-rays often do not spot a tumor until it is 1 centimeter in size, and by then the disease is often in a late stage. A low-dose CAT SCAN can pick up much smaller cancers, so individuals at risk (because of long-time smoking or exposure to smoke) might consider CAT-scan screening. Screening with a low-dose, spiral-computed CAT scan is still more accurate and may eventually be recommended for all high-risk patients. For this procedure the patient lies on a narrow table and passes through a donut-shaped X-ray machine. The machine rotates around the patient, producing images at different angles that can reveal tiny growths long before they produce symptoms. At this writing the procedure is not covered by insurance, and a study is underway to compare it to X-rays and normal CAT scans. If the scan detects a nodule larger than 1 centimeter, irregular in shape or otherwise suspicious, a biopsy may be indicated. Treatment depends on the type of lung cancer and its stage of advancement.

Approximately 15 to 20% of all lung cancers are small-cell lung cancer. The remainder, non-small-cell lung cancers, include adenocarcinoma, the most common type in women and nonsmokers, which spreads early on to other organs; squamous cell carcinoma, the most common in men and smokers; and large-cell carcinoma, the least common, but which spreads quickly.

For many localized tumors, surgery is the treatment of choice. Since most patients with lung cancer show metastases (spread), radiation therapy and chemotherapy often are combined with surgery. In small-cell cancer of the lung, chemotherapy alone or combined with radiation has largely replaced surgery. This treatment leads to remission in a large percentage of cases—sometimes even long-lasting remission. A new genetic test identifies those patients who are at greatest risk for recurrence by identifying patterns of active genes present in a tumor. Initially it was to be used to identify patients with stage 1 non-small-cell lung cancer who would benefit from chemotherapy. It was also expected to identify those with later stages of the disease who were unlikely to benefit from chemotherapy.

Other treatments include directed radiation or intensity-modulated radiation therapy, for which a CAT scan and computer map organs and direct radiation to the desired spot; this enables giving higher doses of radiation with less chance of damaging healthy cells but has severe side effects. Less invasive surgery called video-assisted thoracic surgery removes only the tumor but does not remove lymph nodes; cryotherapy freezes early-stage tumors; and photodynamic therapy uses laser light to destroy tumors. However, the survival rate of lung cancer patients is poor. The five-year survival rate for lung cancer patients is only 15%, but it is 50% in those whose cancers have not spread to other organs. In addition to primary lung cancer, there is secondary lung cancer, that is, metastasizing from malignancies in the breast or elsewhere, and the outlook for these is even less hopeful.

cancer, ovarian   A CANCER of the ovaries, third in incidence of pelvic cancers but currently the most common cause of death from gynecologic cancer in the United States. The most asymptomatic of the pelvic cancers and the most difficult to diagnose, ovarian cancer is too far advanced for successful treatment by the time there are symptoms, and three-fourths of all cases are not diagnosed until the cancer has spread beyond the ovarian capsule. Once it has so advanced, there is a less than 10% chance of cure. There usually are no early signs, it tends to spread rapidly and it generally involves both ovaries simultaneously. It can occur at any age; under 5 and over 80 are not uncommon, but the highest rates of occurrence are between the ages of 40 and 70. The first warning signs are persistent indigestion and abdominal discomfort, particularly a sense of pelvic fullness, because the cancer produces fluid in the abdominal cavity.

Other early symptoms are nausea, loss of appetite and frequent urination. One study indicated that 43% of patients had a combination of bloating, increased abdominal size and urinary symptoms at least four months before diagnosis. (See accompanying table.) Women with this pattern of symptoms are advised to see their primary care physician or gynecologist for an evaluation that

EARLY WARNING SIGNS OF OVARIAN CANCER

Experiencing any of these symptoms more than a dozen times a month warrants contacting a physician.

- Pelvic pain
- Abdominal pain
- Increased abdominal size
- Bloating
- Difficulty eating
- Feeling full
- Frequent need to urinate

could include a pelvic exam, ultrasound, and a blood test for CA-125, a protein that is elevated in most ovarian cancer cells.

Some 90% of ovarian cancers are epithelial carcinomas; that is, they start in the epithelial cells on the outer layer of the ovaries. Germ cell tumors begin in the cells that form eggs; stromal cell cancers arise in the connective tissue of the ovaries.

Although ovarian cancer strikes only one woman in 70, it is deadly in its late stages. However, 90% of patients survive if it is caught early, so researchers are seeking new and better ways to screen women for early signs. Annual pelvic examination, recommended for all women of childbearing age, is not sensitive enough to detect small ovarian tumors. Ultrasound is more sensitive but cannot distinguish a tumor from an ovarian cyst (see CYST, def. 6). A newer refinement is *transvaginal sonography,* which will pick up many early tumors but also cannot always distinguish between malignant and benign lesions and is expensive (and rarely covered by insurance). Therefore, if a mass is detected, a biopsy must determine whether it is cancerous. Biopsy may be done via LAPAROSCOPY, or if initial tests strongly suggest cancer, exploratory surgery for viewing the entire abdominal cavity and ovaries. There also are blood tests to detect proteins produced by a cancer. The most common one, for CA-125, often yields false positive results and also misses half of early ovarian cancers. A promising newer blood test that investigates patterns of small proteins in the blood of cancer patients has so far been able to identify ovarian cancer at even very early stages. Until it becomes widely available, for women at high risk, annual or semiannual screening with transvaginal

ultrasound and CA-125, beginning at age 25, is recommended by many authorities.

The single biggest risk factor is heredity. If a close relative (mother, sister or daughter) has had ovarian cancer, the risk is five times the average, or a lifetime risk of 9.4%; if two such relatives are affected, it jumps to 50%. Another risk factor is how many times a woman has ovulated. Beginning menstruation before age 12, never giving birth to children and starting menopause after age 50 all increase risk. Mutations in two genes also linked to breast cancer, BRCA1 and to a lesser degree, BRCA2, raise the lifetime risk to 15 to 60%, and some authorities advise women with these genetic mutations to undergo prophylactic oophorectomy (removal of ovaries) and sometimes also mastectomy. Moreover, some studies show that genetic transmission also may occur through a woman's father. Other factors seem to serve as protection. Among them are infrequent ovulation owing to multiple pregnancies, use of oral contraceptives, breast-feeding, hysterectomy or tubal sterilization. Further, a diet high in vegetables and low in fat appears to reduce the risk.

If an ovary is found to be cancerous, the uterus, both tubes and both ovaries generally are removed immediately, along with any growths on the diaphragm or bowel, and some lymph nodes (for examination). However, if the cancer is quite small and localized and the woman is quite young, only the diseased ovary and fallopian tube are removed (see OOPHORECTOMY). Surgery is usually followed by chemotherapy with such agents as paclitaxel (Taxol) or platinum, administered intravenously, and occasionally also radiation. Other drugs also are available. In some cases chemotherapy is delivered directly into the abdomen, where ovarian cancers typically spread, and at least one study showed that combined intravenous and intra-abdominal treatment prolonged life. Chemotherapy leads to complete remission in about 50% of cases; however, only about 15% of patients survive for five years after diagnosis.

Unlike endometrial cancer, ovarian cancer is rarely estrogen-dependent; therefore removal of the ovaries may be followed by estrogen replacement therapy to relieve severe menopausal symptoms, but that is not without other risks.

See also box under STAGING.

cancer, pelvic General name for any CANCER of the reproductive organs in the pelvis in women, particularly the uterus (cervix and endometrium) and ovaries, but also the fallopian tubes, vagina and vulva. Of these, cancer of the cervix is the most common, followed by cancer of the uterine lining, or endometrium. Cancer of the fallopian tubes and of the vagina is extremely rare.

See CANCER, CERVICAL; CANCER, ENDOMETRIAL; CANCER, OVARIAN; CANCER, VAGINAL; CANCER, VULVAR; CHORIOCARCINOMA.

cancer, skin The most common form of CANCER in human beings, with about a million new cases (not including melanoma) per year in the United States alone (more than all other kinds of cancer combined). Of these about 90% are cured, but perhaps as many as 50,000 cases recur. The most common forms are *basal cell carcinoma* and *squamous cell carcinoma,* usually caused by cumulative excessive exposure to the sun and other ultraviolet light. These cancers generally are highly curable. The most serious skin cancer is MELANOMA, which accounts for about 5% of all cases of skin cancer.

Basal cell carcinoma, which accounts for 75% of skin cancers, usually appears as a shiny, pearly gray nodule surrounded by swollen capillaries. It occurs most often on the face, neck and back of the hands. Removal by surgery, radiation, CAUTERIZATION or CRYOSURGERY easily cures such cancers; they rarely if ever metastasize (spread).

Squamous cell carcinoma usually appears as a scaly, slightly red lesion with a crusty surface,

---

SYMPTOMS OF BASAL CELL CARCINOMA

- An open, oozing or bleeding sore that persists for three weeks or longer.
- A reddish, irritated spot, often on chest, shoulders, arms or legs, that itches or is crusty and persists.
- A shiny bump, pearly or translucent, and often pink, red or white (in dark-haired people, tan, black or brown).
- A pink growth with raised rolled border and crusted center.
- A scarlike, waxy area with poorly defined borders in which skin is yellow or white and appears shiny and taut.

---

and it may become nodular, with a warty surface. Treatment is by surgical excision, radiation or some other special means. For basal cell and squamous cell carcinoma, which often spread beyond the visible margins on the skin, a special surgical technique, called Mohs micrographic surgery, is said to yield the best results. This technique removes the tumor in stages, layer by layer, examining each for cancer cells, until no cancer cells can be found. The patient must wait between the stages of excision, typically two or three. Once the cancer is removed, the surgeon may do reconstructive surgery to avoid unsightly scars. The principal advantage of Mohs surgery is that it appears to prevent recurrence more than other treatments.

A precursor of squamous cell cancer is *actinic keratosis,* a flat, well-defined, scaly lesion with a rough, crusty texture, pink, tan or multicolored. About 5 to 10% of keratoses will progress to skin cancer within a decade, so they should be removed promptly and biopsied if suspicious. The best protection against skin cancer is prevention, begun in childhood. Avoid peak exposure to the sun, from 10 A.M. to 3 P.M., use a strong sunscreen (with a skin protection factor, or SPF, of at least 17) and wear protective clothing. The SPF factor in sunscreens protects against only one type of harmful ray, the ultraviolet B (UVB) that causes sunburn. Also important is a block against ultraviolet A (UVA), which penetrates more deeply than UVB and also contributes to skin aging. Unfortunately there is no federal regulation concerning UVA blockers. In 2006 the FDA approved Anthelios SX, which contains Mexoryl SX (a UVA protecter) in an over-the-counter sunscreen made by L'Oreal. Another recommended product is Neutrogena's Ultra Sheer Dry-Touch sunblock. One study shows that using sunscreen actually may cause keratoses to disappear, but another more recent study has indicated it may not prevent cancer nearly as well as protective clothing does.

Early detection yields the best chances for cure. Consequently, women are advised to have their clinician examine their skin for irregular moles or skin color once every three years between the ages of 18 and 40 and annually thereafter and to see a dermatologist to examine any suspicious lesions.

See also CANCER, VULVAR; MELANOMA.

cancer, thyroid A cancer of the THYROID gland whose cause is not known. There are four general kinds of thyroid cancer, depending on which type of cell they affect. The most common and most curable kind is papillary, which accounts for 60 to 70% of cases and affects women two to three times more than men. It is more common in individuals who received radiation therapy in the head, neck or chest. The first sign usually is a painless lump in the neck, and diagnosis proceeds with a fine-needle biopsy. Treatment consists of surgical excision, either of the nodules (small growths) in the gland along with surrounding tissue, or of most or all of the thyroid gland. Radioactive iodine and thyroid hormone then are given to destroy any remaining thyroid tissue. Another 15% of cases are follicular cancer, more common in the elderly and also more common in women than men. It is apt to spread more quickly and widely and hence requires near total or total thyroidectomy followed by radioactive iodine and thyroid hormone therapy. It is curable, but less so than papillary cancer. Anaplastic cancer accounts for fewer than 5% of thyroid cancers and is more common among older women. It grows very fast, tends to produce a large growth in the neck, and has only a 20% survival rate after one year. The fourth kind, medullary cancer, gives rise to unusual symptoms and can also spread very fast. It often occurs together with other endocrine cancers, and then is relatively curable; when occurring alone the chances of survival are not as good.

cancer, uterine A CANCER of the uterus. The most common kinds are cervical cancer and endometrial cancer (see CANCER, CERVICAL; CANCER, ENDOMETRIAL). Much rarer is CHORIOCARCINOMA.

cancer, vaginal A CANCER of the vagina. Primary vaginal cancer (originating in the vagina) is quite rare except in daughters of women who were treated with DIETHYLSTILBESTROL during their pregnancy. (See also ADENOCARCINOMA, def. 2.) Cancer may spread to the vagina from the cervix but then is still regarded as cervical cancer. Treatment depends on the stage, location and cell type of the cancer. In the upper vagina it is similar to treatment of cervical cancer. In the lower vagina it is usually treated with radiation.

cancer, vulvar A CANCER of the VULVA, usually affecting the labia (lips) surrounding the vagina. This type of cancer is essentially a skin cancer and appears as a lump or sore on the vulva that can be readily seen and felt. However, women often tend to ignore such a lesion, which, if malignant, then can grow considerably. Another kind of vulvar cancer is MELANOMA, also a skin cancer; although it is rare, it is the second most common kind of vulvar malignancy.

The warning signs of vulvar cancer are a persistent sore or wartlike growth on the skin of the vulva, persistent itching, redness or thickening of the vulvar skin, or change in a mole. The lesions sometimes look very much like those of CONDYLOMA ACUMINATA (genital warts), and the only way to distinguish the two conditions is by biopsy (see BIOPSY, def. 6). A precancerous lesion or early-stage malignancy is called *vulvar intraepithelial neoplasia (VIN)*, which must be treated lest it spread to nearby tissues and become invasive.

Treatment of VIN, if the area is small, consists of a chemotherapy drug applied in cream form. For larger lesions or more advanced malignancy, treatment is surgical, consisting of local excision for precancerous lesions, and, if there is cancer, a simple vulvectomy (removal of skin from the labia, clitoris and surrounding area). The use of laser surgery for this procedure tends to reduce scarring and promote healing. Invasive cancer is treated with a more radical vulvectomy (removal of the labia, clitoris, underlying glands in the groin, about one-half of the vagina and several inches on each side of the vulva). If there is lymph node involvement, surgery is followed up by radiation. Despite such extensive excision, sexual intercourse is still possible afterward and can be satisfactory.

See also PAGET'S DISEASE, def. 2.

cancer in situ Also *carcinoma in situ*. Literally, cancer "in place." A growth disturbance in which normal cells are replaced by abnormal-appearing cells that do not yet have two fundamental characteristics of advanced cancers: invasiveness and metastasis (see CANCER). Instead, the lesion is confined to the site of origin and has not yet invaded neighboring tissues or spread elsewhere. Some authorities regard it as a very early and localized (hence "in place") cancer, also called Stage O (see STAGING), but believe that it can become invasive and then spread. Further, since there is no way to predict which lesions will remain localized and which will spread, they recommend immediate surgical removal. Two kinds of cancer in situ occur in the breast. One is *ductal cancer in situ (DCIS)*, which consists of abnormal cells confined to the lining of the milk ducts. If the abnormal cells break through the duct wall and invade the adjacent fat tissue, they are no longer cancer in situ but invasive cancer. Ductal cancer in situ forms a palpable mass and can be detected by a mammogram. Before mammography was widely used, the diagnosis of DCIS was rare. Now it makes up some 25 to 30% of the cases of breast cancer detected in the United States. Once suspected on a mammogram, it should be biopsied (see BIOPSY, def. 5) and treated, that is, surgically excised, with either the lesion and its margins removed (lumpectomy) or the entire breast removed (mastectomy). Untreated, one out of every three will develop into an invasive cancer. Even when excised, there is a chance of developing invasive cancer within 10 years, a risk reduced by following surgery with radiation therapy. However, since there are at present no markers to determine which DCIS will become invasive, the decision concerning follow-up radiation can be controversial.

The other kind of breast lesion is called *lobular cancer in situ (LCIS)* and involves the breast's lobules. Its cells do not seem to progress to invasive cancer, but their appearance is a sign that the breast tissue has a higher than average risk of becoming cancerous, that is, a 25 to 35% chance that cancer will develop, though perhaps not for 40 years. Since about 90% of all breast cancers are similar in cell structure to ductal and lobular tumors, it is important, following diagnosis, to rule out metastasis (spread), by means of physical examination for enlarged lymph nodes, skin lesions and liver enlargement, a chest X-ray, blood count and liver function studies. Because several lobules in both breasts often are involved, local treatments like lumpectomy or radiation are not appropriate. Consequently careful monitoring through clinical breast exams every few months and annual mammography are advisable. Occasionally a woman will opt for removal of one or both breasts.

Another option for both DCIS and LCIS is tamoxifen, the estrogen-blocking drug given in advanced breast cancer that also is used as a preventive agent.

See also DYSPLASIA; PRECANCEROUS LESIONS.

cancer support group   A group of cancer patients who meet to share their experiences in living with a serious disease, that is, coping with cancer and the effects of treatments. Usually such groups are led by a social worker, nurse or other health practitioner. Cancer patients may be concerned about holding their jobs, caring for their families, keeping up with daily activities or starting new relationships. Women in particular may be worried about the effects of pelvic and breast cancers and their treatments on their sexuality. Meeting with others who face similar problems can be helpful to those who want to talk about their feelings or discuss their concerns. Information about programs and local resources is available through the Cancer Information Service (see the Appendix).

Candida albicans   See YEAST INFECTION.

carcinogen   A physical or chemical agent that has the potential of producing cancer. The connection between a carcinogen and cancer is often hard to establish because the resulting tumors may not appear for as long as two or three decades, but most authorities believe that environmental or nutritional carcinogens account for as many as 90% of human cancers. Among them are exposure to sunlight, chemicals and drugs as well as certain lifestyle habits. Ultraviolet light is a causative factor in skin cancer, and overexposure to ionizing radiation (including X-rays) plays a role in leukemia, lymphomas and other cancers. Carcinogenic industrial chemicals include arsenic and asbestos (lung cancer), benzene (leukemia), nickel (lung and sinus cancer) and vinyl chloride (liver cancer). Tobacco smoke is involved in numerous cancers (lung, esophagus and bladder) as are alcohol (esophagus, pharynx) and betel nuts (mouth, pharynx). Some drugs also have carcinogenic potential, notably DES (see DIETHYLSTILBESTROL), alkylating agents (leukemia) and others. Finally, certain viruses, such as human papilloma virus (cervix), appear to cause malignancies.

See also CANCER.

carcinoma Strictly speaking, a malignant (cancerous) tumor of epithelial tissue, as opposed to one involving connective tissue (sarcoma) or lymph tissue (lymphoma). However, in general medical usage the term often is used interchangeably with CANCER.

carcinoma in situ See CANCER IN SITU.

carpal tunnel syndrome A kind of repetitive strain injury in which the median nerve in the hand is compressed or damaged as it passes through swollen tissue in the carpal tunnel of the wrist. Found more often in women than men and affecting either one or both hands, it is caused by forceful and repetitive hand and wrist motions, which give rise to sensations of burning, aching, numbness or tingling of the fingers. In time the thumb muscle weakens so it becomes hard to grip anything. The condition is diagnosed by tests of nerve conduction and muscle fiber activity. Treatment includes splinting the hand to hold it in a neutral position, painkillers such as nonsteroidal anti-inflammatory drugs (NSAIDs) and sometimes corticosteroid injections. If all else fails, surgery may be indicated to cut away the fibrous tissue bands that press on the nerve.

Although carpal tunnel syndrome also can occur during pregnancy or with rheumatoid arthritis, underactive thyroid, diabetes or gout, most often it results from repetitive stress, as in using a computer keyboard that is not positioned properly. To avoid the last, the keyboard should be adjusted so that forearms are parallel to the floor, wrists straight and in line with the forearms, and elbows relaxed.

castration Surgical removal or destruction by radiation of both gonads (sex glands)—that is, both ovaries in women or both testes in men. When those glands can no longer fulfill their function of hormone production, permanent sterility results.

See also OOPHORECTOMY; STERILIZATION.

cataract A clouding of the eye's lens that blocks the transmission of light enough so as to disturb vision. Some clouding of the lenses occurs by age 65 in 95% of the population, but cataracts occur 13% more frequently in women than in men. Provided they do not significantly impair vision, cataracts require no treatment. When they do, surgery can largely correct the condition.

Smoking, drinking alcoholic beverages, corticosteroid drugs and exposure to ultraviolet light and ionizing radiation can cause cataracts, but the principal cause is aging. Surgery, which is relatively risk-free and can be performed even on very old patients, generally involves replacing the lens with an artificial lens—a silicone or acrylic intraocular implant—but retaining the capsule that holds it in place, which also helps to protect the retina. Occasionally the artificial lens cannot be inserted during surgery; it then may be done in a second operation, or a contact lens may be fitted instead. Cataract surgery usually is done on an outpatient basis except for patients with serious medical conditions, who may require overnight hospitalization. Generally topical or local anesthesia is used. One can normally resume regular activities within a day or two but should avoid heavy lifting and strenuous exercise. Full recovery of vision takes four to six weeks, and thereafter new eyeglasses may be required to further correct vision. In up to 50% of cases a membrane from the cataract (left to anchor the new lens) thickens and causes blurred vision. This secondary cataract can readily be treated later, often by laser.

catheter, urinary A flexible tube inserted through the urethra into the bladder, either to obtain a urine specimen uncontaminated by bacteria on the skin or in the urethra, or to ensure the flow of urine when the usual sphincter muscles are not working owing to trauma or disease. Since the insertion of a catheter itself can transport bacteria into the bladder, it is extremely important that sterile procedures be followed. Catheterization often is used after operations in the genital-urinary area, including Cesarean section, to ensure emptying of the bladder; sometimes an indwelling catheter (commonly a *Foley catheter*) is allowed to remain inserted for several days until normal function returns.

Patients who catheterize themselves on a long-term basis—a procedure called *intermittent self-catheterization* that is used by some paraplegics and others—generally use only clean rather than sterile technique but develop surprisingly few urinary infections.

CAT scan Also *computerized axial tomography, CT scan*. A diagnostic tool used since the mid-1970s. In this sophisticated X-ray technique a picture is taken of a plane in the body, sometimes after the intravenous injection of dye. Cross-section pictures are constructed that may show, for example, the exact shape of a tumor or an aneurysm in the brain or aorta with great precision, enabling better treatment.

The use of CAT scans has increased enormously during the past decade and consequently has exposed patients to increased ionizing radiation, which can damage cells and lead to problems like cancer. Even though the total dose delivered by a scan is relatively low, repeated scans can lead to an unacceptable increase. Further, individuals who request a CAT scan to identify any possible problems that have presented no symptoms should probably be discouraged from doing so.

See also MAGNETIC RESONANCE IMAGER.

caudal anesthesia A kind of REGIONAL ANESTHESIA that is administered during childbirth into the caudal canal, a space below the last sacral vertebra. It is usually administered on a continuous basis; that is, a catheter is inserted into that area when the woman is almost through the first stage of active LABOR (when the cervix is dilated about 8 centimeters of the required 10) and a small quantity of anesthetic solution is injected repeatedly. It serves

to anesthetize the entire pelvis and legs so that no pain is felt from the uterine contractions or from the stretching of the perineum when the baby is expelled. It thus is effective through the transition and second stage of labor. However, this method impairs the frequency and strength of contractions, thereby prolonging labor, and requiring a larger amount of anesthetic. Therefore it has been largely replaced by EPIDURAL ANESTHESIA.

caul See AMNIOTIC SAC.

cauterization Also *cautery, electrocautery, electrodesiccation*. Destroying cells by applying chemicals or heat to them. Cauterization commonly is used to treat warts on the vulva (see CONDYLOMA ACUMINATA), inflammation of the cervix (see CERVICITIS) and precancerous lesions of the cervix (see DYSPLASIA). The heat that kills the cells is produced by a controlled high-frequency electric current at the tip of a cautery probe, which is touched to the desired area. The heat kills only the surface cells. The procedure is mildly to moderately painful, depending on the kind of tissue being treated, and creates an unpleasant odor of burning, but it takes only a few seconds. Before electrocautery was available, clinicians applied agents such as silver nitrate to the cervix, but these were far less effective. Cauterization may cause some swelling in the cervix, which might temporarily narrow the cervical canal (see also CERVICAL STENOSIS). It usually causes a profuse watery vaginal discharge that lasts several weeks and occasionally some staining or bleeding. Complications rarely occur. Newer treatment for similar disorders are freezing, or CRYOSURGERY, and laser surgery. Cauterization also is used to close the fallopian tubes in TUBAL LIGATION and the vas deferens in VASECTOMY.

celibacy The state of abstinence from any sexual relationship. The term long was associated almost exclusively with persons who abstain from sexual relations in order to fulfill a vow, such as those required by various religious orders. Today it often means choosing to have no sex for a time, either no sex with a partner or, sometimes, no masturbation as well.

cellulite Dimpling in areas of the body where fat deposits are greatest, especially on the buttocks and thighs but also on the abdomen and upper arms. The puckered, bumpy appearance, resembling orange peel, results from the pull of bands of connective tissue that connect the outer layer of skin, or dermis, to deeper tissues. It is common in women and rare in men, probably because women's dermis is thinner and the fat layer below it is thicker than in men. Cellulite is normal and harmless, but many women deplore it and try to correct it with products that claim to remove it. A recently approved hand-held massage device, called Endermologie, purportedly helps by drawing the skin into a fold between two motorized rollers and kneading it. Designed for operation by a trained technician, it is expensive and improves appearance only temporarily. A more effective measure is cosmetic surgery, specifically liposuction, which involves removing excess fat, breaking up the bands of connective tissue and inserting fat into the depressed areas. It is even more expensive and will not prevent recurrence.

cephalhematoma In a newborn baby, a blood clot under the scalp, between the bone and the membrane covering it (periosteum). Usually resulting from a difficult delivery, it may not appear for 12 to 24 hours after birth. It tends to enlarge more during the next few days, remains stable for a few weeks and then begins to disappear. No treatment of any kind is needed, nor does any permanent damage result from it.

cephalic presentation In childbirth, any position of the baby in which its head presents (that is, will emerge first). The ideal and most common presentation is *vertex,* that is, with the crown or top of the skull (called "occiput") the presenting part; it is by far the easiest position for delivery. All others are called "abnormal," including other cephalic presentations, each of which raises special problems; see BROW PRESENTATION; FACE PRESENTATION; POSTERIOR PRESENTATION.

cerebral palsy General name for a group of motor disorders that result from damage to the central nervous system occurring before, during or after birth (up to the age of six). The symptoms, all stemming from lack of motor muscle control by the brain, range from mild to severe and include awkward or involuntary movements, shaking of the limbs, lack of balance, irregular gait or inability to walk, and a delay in growth and development. Spasticity occurs in almost three-fourths of all cases. Cerebral palsy also is linked to learning disabilities and, sometimes, mental retardation. Intelligence may or may not be affected, depending on what part of the brain suffered injury. Therefore a cerebral palsy patient's difficulties in communicating and inability to control the voluntary muscles do not necessarily mean he or she is deficient in understanding or has impaired mental ability.

The ultimate cause of cerebral palsy is not known, but precipitating factors include a very difficult labor, birth trauma, neonatal asphyxiation, severe childhood illness (such as meningitis), exposure to lead or arsenic, and, especially, prematurity and low birth weight (it afflicts 1 of every 20 babies who weigh less than 3 pounds at birth). The risk of cerebral palsy has been found to be almost 12 times as great in twins as in single-birth babies, and if one twin died before birth the risk rises to 108 times. This factor should be taken into account if a woman is considering fertility treatments that increase her risk of multiple births. A recent study overturned the long-held belief that oxygen deprivation was the main cause in premature infants. Rather, it is bacterial infection, especially with staphylococcus but also other organisms.

Cerebral palsy is not progressive; on the contrary, the handicaps can be considerably lessened by physical therapy, speech therapy, bracing and/or orthopedic surgery, and anticonvulsants to control seizures. For women with cerebral palsy, menstruation and fertility are unaffected. Pregnancy is possible in the less severe forms of the disorder, although delivery may be complicated by muscle spasms and the woman's inability to bear down at will. Sexual stimulation and arousal may trigger spastic and other involuntary movements, which also may make sexual intercourse difficult in certain positions, and some women find they lack vaginal lubrication, which can be assisted by using a water-soluble lubricant. Sensation and orgasm, however, are not affected.

cerebral vascular accident   Also *cerebrovascular accident, CVA, stroke.* A sudden disturbance of the brain's blood supply, usually caused by an EMBOLISM, a blood clot (see THROMBUS) or a stenosis (severe narrowing) in a blood vessel supplying the brain. This happens in 80% of cases, termed *ischemic.* Hemorrhage (uncontrolled bleeding) accounts for the remaining 20%; it occurs when a blood vessel inside the brain erupts and bleeds, most often because of hypertension or an *aneurysm* (weak spot in the artery wall, believed to be hereditary). A CVA is potentially fatal and may be permanently disabling. Deprived of oxygen-filled blood, some brain cells are either paralyzed or destroyed and cease to control the body functions that normally are under their direction. An accident in one side of the brain may cause *hemiplegia* (paralysis and numbness) of the opposite side of the head and body (face, arm, leg). Other manifestations of CVA include loss of bladder control, emotional instability, speech and language problems, memory impairment and visual disturbances.

As the word *accident* implies, the onset of this condition usually is abrupt and constitutes a medical emergency. Early symptoms include weakness on one side of the body, numbness, visual disturbance such as double vision, and/or seizures.

Except in rare cases, a cerebral vascular accident usually is secondary to atherosclerosis (see ARTERIOSCLEROSIS) or high blood pressure (see HYPERTENSION) or both. Other conditions contributing to its occurrence are DIABETES and heart disease, especially a condition involving deformities of the heart valve. Obesity, high CHOLESTEROL, heavy smoking, physical inactivity and stress also seem to increase the risk, probably because they predispose a person to the circulatory disorders and heart disease so often associated with stroke. Women may have an increased risk of CVA at times of radical hormonal changes, especially pregnancy and childbirth. The risk may also increase at menopause.

An early warning sign of stroke is a kind of ministroke called a *transient ischemic attack,* or *TIA.* It, too, is caused by a temporary interruption of the brain's blood supply, but it lasts only a short time, from a few minutes to an hour, and symptoms disappear completely within 24 hours. Among the symptoms are weakness or numbness in an arm, leg or on the face, usually just on one side of the body; double vision or blurred vision in one or both eyes; deafness or ringing in the ears; dizziness or fainting; difficulty in performing a familiar task or inability to control one's movements; difficulty swallowing; difficulty speaking or understanding spoken language; sudden headache; and abrupt personality changes, impaired judgment or forgetfulness. It is believed that 80% of all stroke victims have a history of TIAs. Treatment of these attacks to help prevent a future stroke includes the use of aspirin or anticoagulants to prevent clot formation and in some cases surgery to improve circulation to those parts of the brain supplied by damaged arteries. Carotid endoarterectomy, whereby plaque is removed from the carotid arteries, can reduce the risk of stroke in cases where TIAs result from arterial blockages, and aneurysms also may be surgically repaired.

Cerebral vascular accident accounts for approximately one-third of all causes of paralysis in women between the ages of 17 and 44 and is the most common cause of neurologic disability among men and women of all ages. The risk for stroke rises with age, since contributing factors such as atherosclerosis and hypertension also occur more often after the age of 50. Stroke is the third leading cause of death among American women. Women have a greater risk of stroke during their lifetimes than men and account for about 60% of all stroke deaths. Women are likely to be older than men when they experience their first stroke, and it will probably be more severe and disabling. But younger women may also be stricken. The outcome of a stroke is highly variable. About one-fifth of all hospitalized patients die. Of those who survive, about half recover enough to walk and take care of their basic needs, and the remainder remain more or less partly handicapped (and some remain severely handicapped for life).

The key to optimum recovery is quick treatment, with immediate transfer to a hospital and preferably to a hospital's specialized stroke center. In 1996 the U.S. Food and Drug Administration approved a tissue plasminogen activator (TPA), long used for heart attacks, as the first treatment for ischemic CVAs. It works by dissolving the causative blood clot and restoring blood flow before there is brain damage and has been found to reverse the effects of stroke completely in 30% of cases. A successful outcome depends on quick treatment, preferably within three hours of onset. It should be given as soon as a CAT scan has determined the stroke is caused by a clot. If the clot does not respond to TPA, two other treatments might be considered. One is delivering a clot-dissolving drug directly to the site of the clot through a catheter. Another is to remove the clot by means of a device called the Merci retriever. This procedure involves an incision in the groin, threading a catheter up to the carotid artery that feeds the brain and having the retriever snare and remove the clot. It is still considered experimental, and long-term results are unknown. In hemorrhagic stroke, treatment involves breathing aids and medications to control seizures, reduce brain swelling, maintain normal blood pressure and ease pain. Surgery also may be required, either to clip off an aneurysm or insert a glue-like substance near the aneurysm to control bleeding. Currently researchers are investigating drugs that promote clotting in hemorrhagic stroke.

In general, the extent of neurologic recovery from stroke depends on a person's age and general health, the location and dimensions of brain damage, and rehabilitation therapy that is begun early and pursued aggressively. The sooner improvement begins, the better the outlook. About half of those with moderate or severe hemiplegia and most of those with minor hemiplegia recover partially by the time they leave the hospital. Rehabilitation therapy should begin almost immediately and be pursued even when it seemingly exhausts the patient. Physical and speech therapy both can be of great benefit. The extent of recovery usually is established by the end of six to nine months, but some patients continue to show steady improvement over a longer time.

However, survivors are at high risk for a second stroke (about 13% have one within the

WARNING SIGNS OF A STROKE

1. Sudden weakness, numbness or paralysis of an arm, leg or the face*
2. Sudden dimness or loss of vision
3. Loss of speech; trouble talking or understanding language
4. Sudden severe headache with no apparent cause
5. Unexplained dizziness, unsteadiness or sudden falls

*Especially if affecting one side of the body.

next 12 months). Preventive measures include changes in lifestyle, medication and sometimes surgery. Stroke survivors are urged to cut down on dietary fat and salt, exercise regularly, abstain from smoking and limit alcohol intake (especially if the stroke was caused by hemorrhage). A recent study indicates that a diet high in potassium (found in bananas, tomatoes, spinach and other fruits and vegetables) reduces the risk of stroke, especially in those with high blood pressure. A potassium supplement of 1 gram a day was also beneficial. In addition, antihypertensive agents may be needed to control high blood pressure, and cholesterol-lowering drugs may be needed if LDL levels are high, as well as anticoagulants to reduce clot formation. For ischemic stroke caused by an embolism or thrombus in the carotid artery, surgery to reopen the artery may be considered, but usually only if the artery is severely narrowed. Occasionally surgery is considered for hemorrhagic stroke if tests show a slowly leaking aneurysm, in which case the weakened vessel is tied off to stop the bleeding.

Women who have had a cerebral vascular accident may experience lack of interest in sex for several months. Nearly all stroke victims experience extreme fatigue, sometimes persisting for as long as a year, and it frequently affects sexual responses. Spasms of the affected leg (in those with hemiplegia) and urinary incontinence (loss of bladder control) may hamper sexual intercourse, and orgasm may be more difficult to achieve. Menstruation and fertility are not affected at all. Pregnancy may lessen bladder control even more. If an intrauterine device (IUD) is used, one should be alert to any associated increases in menstrual bleeding.

cervical cancer vaccine See under HUMAN PAPILLOMA VIRUS.

cervical cap A flexible rubber or plastic cap that fits tightly over the cervix, holding spermicide against it, and prevents sperm from entering the cervical opening. It is about 1½ inches (3¾ centimeters) long, is widest at the opening and has a thick, semirigid rim. The cervical cap is held in place by suction. Used together with a SPERMICIDE (preferably cream, but jelly is also effective), it works much as a DIAPHRAGM (see def. 2) does and like it must be fitted to an individual woman. However, it may be left in place considerably longer (authorities differ on this point; see below) and therefore is more convenient to use. The cap should not be relied on as a contraceptive during menstrual periods, because the menstrual flow breaks the suction holding it in place (although it can be used to collect the menstrual flow).

Women who cannot use a diaphragm because of a very short anterior (front) vaginal wall, extreme cystocele (fallen bladder) or other anatomical problems often can be fitted for a cervical cap, provided the cervix protrudes at least ¼ inch (7 millimeters) from the vaginal wall. The cap also requires less refitting than a diaphragm, since in most women the CERVIX changes less in size (with pregnancy, weight gain or loss) than the vagina. There are, however, some contraindications for its use, among them severe cervical laceration, an unusually long or short or irregularly shaped cervix, and inflammation of the vagina (vaginitis), cervix (cervicitis) or ovaries and fallopian tubes (pelvic inflammatory disease). The last three conditions are temporary contraindications; once the inflammation is cleared up there is no reason to avoid using a cervical cap. Other contraindications for its use are the same as those for the DIAPHRAGM.

Used correctly, the cervical cap is believed to have nearly the same effectiveness as the diaphragm, with a theoretical success rate of about 91% (in practice, 88%). However, these figures apply only to women who have never borne a child. For those who have, the success rate drops to 74% (theoretical) and 68% (practical).

The cervical cap does have some drawbacks. It requires careful fitting, it is a little more difficult to insert than a diaphragm and the number of sizes is limited. Long available in Great Britain, it was approved in the United States in 1988, although American women had been obtaining imported caps at women's health centers for some years. Some women cannot be fitted for the cap. Also, it has been associated with some incidence of abnormal PAP SMEAR results. Consequently, the U.S. Food and Drug Administration (FDA) recommends that only women with a normal Pap smear use it and that they obtain another Pap smear after using the cap for three months, to make sure no cervical changes have taken place.

The cap appears to have no side effects except possible irritation from the spermicide; when that occurs, a different brand may solve the problem. Occasionally the cap is dislodged during intercourse; if it happens more than once or twice, the fit should be rechecked. Because of this possibility, use of a condom during the first eight times of intercourse with a cap is recommended. Also, some women do have marked cervical changes during their menstrual cycle and have therefore found it necessary to use two sizes of cap to accommodate these changes.

The cervical cap was invented in the early 1800s in Europe and by the end of the 19th century was used there fairly widely. It was originally used without spermicide, but the use of spermicidal

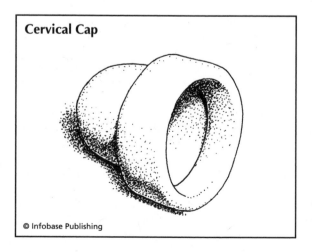

Cervical Cap

© Infobase Publishing

cream or jelly is definitely recommended; some say that cream adheres better and longer than jelly. The cap is filled one-third full with cream or jelly and carefully inserted so as to cover the cervix. It may be inserted up to 40 hours before intercourse but should not be removed for at least 6 to 8 hours after the last intercourse. It may then be left in place but authorities differ as to how long; some say a maximum of 72 hours, but the FDA suggests a maximum of 48 hours. After removal, which is accomplished by lifting the rim away from the cervix to break the suction, the cap should be washed with soap and water. Should it retain some odor, it can be soaked in rubbing alcohol for 24 hours, or in 1 cup of water with 1 tablespoon cider vinegar or lemon juice for 20 minutes; odor also can be avoided by inserting one drop of liquid chlorophyll on top of the spermicide before next inserting the cap. There is some difference of opinion concerning wear. Some recommend that the cap be replaced after one year, while others say it lasts two to five years.

A newer kind of cervical barrier is Lea's Shield, approved by the FDA in 2002. It comes in one size that fits nearly all women and does not need a clinician to fit it. Made of silicone rubber, it is shaped like an elliptical bowl with a loop at one end to facilitate removal. Unlike the cap, it has a valve that allows the passage of cervical secretions and creates a better fit over the cervix. It may be used without spermicide, but is more effective with it. The Lea's Shield should be replaced after one year. A still newer intravaginal barrier recently approved is the FemCap. Obtainable by prescription, it comes in three sizes (one's size is determined by obstetrical history—no childbirth, miscarriage, childbirth) and is so designed that it protects both cervix and upper vagina. It is used together with spermicide, which must be reapplied (without removing the cap) before each repeated intercourse within 48 hours. It is removed six hours after the last intercourse, and then cleaned and dried. The FemCap can be reused for two years.

cervical cyst See CYST, def. 4.

cervical erosion See CERVICITIS.

cervical eversion Also *ectropion*. The replacement of normal tissue on the surface of the CERVIX with tissue that is usually found farther up inside the cervical canal. The surface of the cervix normally consists of several layers of flat, shiny cells called *squamous epithelium;* the lining of the cervical canal consists of tall, red, velvety cells richly supplied with mucous glands and called *columnar epithelium.* The junction of the squamous and columnar tissue usually is located near the opening of the cervical canal. In cervical eversion, the columnar cells have spread beyond that normal junction and over the surface of the cervix, making it look red and bumpy, although smooth to the touch. Many women have no symptoms at all. When they do, the most common is a heavy mucus discharge (caused by the increased number of mucous glands). Cervical eversion most often occurs when estrogen levels in the body are high, as at puberty, during pregnancy or while oral contraceptives are being used. Most clinicians believe cervical eversion requires no treatment at all. Some say the moist environment provided by the extra gland secretions increases the risk of infection, and the abnormal tissue therefore should be destroyed by freezing (see CRYOSURGERY). Opponents point out that the treatment represents a higher risk than any such infection. If the discharge is troublesome, douching with vinegar and water or vitamin C and water, or any of the herbal remedies for cervicitis, may afford relief.

See also CERVICITIS.

cervical intraepithelial neoplasia Also *CIN, squamous intraepithelial lesions, SIL.* A condition characterized by abnormal tissue on the CERVIX. More common names for this condition are cervical DYSPLASIA for mild to moderate CIN, and CANCER IN SITU for severe CIN.

cervical mucus method Also *ovulation method.* A method of determining the time of OVULATION based on the fact that the cervical mucus secreted by most women changes in volume and consistency during the course of each menstrual cycle. After menstruation the mucus is scarcely noticeable in amount. It gradually increases in quantity and becomes thick, sticky and opaque. Just before ovulation occurs the amount of mucus increases and it becomes clear and slippery, similar in consistency to raw egg white. It has a quality called *Spinnbarkeit* (a German word meaning "ability to be spun"), meaning it is stringy and stretchable. Soon after it reaches a peak of stretchability, in a day or two, ovulation takes place. After ovulation the mucus again becomes thicker and stickier, though not as much as before, until menstruation, when the cycle begins again. The regular checking of cervical mucus consistency for purposes of preventing conception (birth control) is also called the *Billings method,* after two Australian doctors (husband and wife) who recommend it.

The cervical mucus method in its simplest form consists of having a woman check her mucus manually every day. If she becomes familiar with her own pattern and that pattern proves to be quite regular, it is a fairly reliable method of birth control. Combined with taking BASAL BODY TEMPERATURE, it becomes even more reliable (see also NATURAL FAMILY PLANNING). However, the presence of seminal fluid (after intercourse), spermicides (creams, jellies, foam), douching, or any vaginal or cervical infection can obscure or remove natural mucus, making the method useless.

Also, a woman can perform simple tests on her own cervical mucus to determine what stage of the cycle she is in. At ovulation the mucus contains an abundant amount of glucose (sugar); by using chemically treated paper (special fertility kits for this purpose are sold over the counter in many drugstores) and applying a small sample (fingertip) of mucus to the paper, she can determine by the color of the paper how much glucose the mucus contains. Another test, the *fern test,* requires the use of a microscope. At ovulation the cervical mucus, placed on a slide under the microscope, shows a distinctive branching pattern resembling that of a fern. Before ovulation the mucus looks unfernlike or has at most only a few branches. After ovulation the fernlike appearance disappears within two or three days. The fern test, however, does not work in women who bleed slightly at ovulation or who have an inflammation of the cervix (cervicitis).

See also MENSTRUAL CYCLE; MITTELSCHMERZ; OVULATION.

cervical os   See CERVIX.

cervical polyp   See POLYP, def. 2.

cervical stenosis   Narrowing of the cervical canal, a complication of CAUTERIZATION caused by the formation of scar tissue. It usually occurs only after repeated cauterization and is a principal reason why CRYOSURGERY, which substitutes freezing for burning abnormal tissue, is a preferable procedure. However, stenosis also occasionally results from cryosurgery or from any other instrumentation of the cervix, such as dilation for a D and C or abortion.

cervicitis   Also *cervical erosion.* Inflammation of the CERVIX, often caused by infection but sometimes by chemicals or a foreign body (tampon, IUD string, penis). Mild cervicitis has no symptoms at all. A more severe case will cause a heavy vaginal discharge, sometimes with a foul odor. It may be thin or thick in consistency, ranges from grayish white to yellow in color and occasionally is tinged with blood. Pain may be felt during vaginal intercourse or when the cervix is touched with a fingertip or tampon, and sometimes there is spotting or bleeding after intercourse. It is advisable to identify the cause of the infection, which may be yeast, trichomonas, gonococcus (which causes gonorrhea) or some other organism, and do a PAP SMEAR as well to make sure no precancerous condition exists. Once the cause is identified, specific treatment may be begun. If the cervicitis is caused by bacteria normally residing in the vagina, sulfa cream or suppositories may be tried and, if ineffective, followed by antibiotic treatment, usually in the form of vaginal creams or suppositories. In the case of trichomonal or gonorrheal infection, the woman's partner also must be treated. In instances where the condition persists and is bothersome, CAUTERIZATION or CRYOSURGERY, which destroys the abnormal tissue on the surface and helps induce healing and growth of new tissue, may be considered. Apart from the unpleasantness of chronic discharge, women who wish to become pregnant may not be able to conceive because a thick secretion is blocking the passage of sperm. In women using an intrauterine device (IUD) to prevent conception, treatment of cervicitis usually can proceed without removing the device, but in severe and recurrent cervicitis many clinicians believe it should be removed and another mode of birth control used. Also, avoid using tampons for menstrual flow until the inflammation has healed.

Among women who prefer more conservative therapy, a number of kinds have been tried. They include the use of birth control jellies and creams (see SPERMICIDE); vitamin E capsules inserted as a vaginal suppository at bedtime; an acidic douche, made from crushed vitamin C tablets or vinegar or lemon juice diluted with water; and HERBAL REMEDIES, specifically an infusion made from rosemary (*Rosmarinus officinalis*), sanicle (*Sanicle europaea* or *mariandica*), comfrey (*Symphytum officinalis*) and heal-all or self-heal (*Prunella vulgaris*) used either as a douche or to soak a tampon that is then inserted into the vagina; or a douche made from goldenseal (*Hydrastis canadensis*), one-quarter teaspoon dried herb in one quart of water, used twice a day for two to three weeks.

See also CERVICAL EVERSION.

cervix A cylindrical structure that is part of the UTERUS, specifically the narrow lower end, most of which protrudes into the vagina. It often is called the *neck* of the uterus, the rest being called the *corpus* or *body*. The bulk of its 2.5-centimeter (1-inch) length is the *cervical canal*, or *endocervix*. At the lower end, inside the vagina, is a small opening called the *external os*. Before childbearing the external os is a small regular opening, about 5 millimeters (⅕ inch) in diameter. During labor it dilates to a diameter of 10 centimeters (4 inches), and thereafter it never returns to its former shape, instead resembling a transverse slit 6 millimeters (about ¼ inch) long. At the upper end of the cervical canal is another small opening into the body of the uterus, which is called the *internal os*. In nonpregnant women the cervix is pink; in pregnancy it assumes a bluish color, a result of increased blood supply. This color change is one of the earliest presumptive signs of pregnancy.

The cervix is lined with numerous small glands, which furnish constant thick secretions. Occasionally some become blocked, forming a Nabothian cyst (see CYST, def. 14). The secretions change in response to stimulation by different hormones during the menstrual cycle, making it possible sometimes to determine when ovulation is taking place (see CERVICAL MUCUS METHOD). The cervix is subject to a number of disorders, the most serious of which is cancer, largely symptomless but detectable by a PAP SMEAR (see CANCER, CERVICAL). Less serious but often very annoying are CERVICAL EVERSION, POLYPS (see def. 2), CERVICITIS and DYSPLASIA.

See also INCOMPETENT CERVIX.

Cesarean section Also *Caesarean section, C section, abdominal delivery, surgical delivery.* Delivery of a baby through a surgical incision in the uterus. Although this kind of surgery dates from ancient times, until recently it was performed only to save the life of the child because it almost invariably caused the death of the mother (unless she was already dead; Cesareans were and still are performed to extract live infants from dead mothers). Today the use of blood transfusions and antibiotics has enormously reduced the maternal death toll from hemorrhage and infection. By 1980 it also had become, at least in the United States, one of the procedures performed so frequently that many began to consider it unnecessary surgery. It currently is the most common major operation performed on American women.

In 1957 the American College of Surgeons judged that the normal rate for Cesareans was approximately 3% of all births, but between 1968 and 1975 the rate of Cesarean sections performed in the United States tripled from 5 to 15% and by 1988 it was 25% (it had dropped to 21% by 1998). By 2005, however, it had again risen, to more than 30%. Part of the earlier increase was due to the widespread use of FETAL MONITORING, which picks up more sounds that may be interpreted as fetal distress, part was due to the insistence of most American physicians that a previous surgical delivery made vaginal delivery impossible and part was due to the delivery of nearly all breech births by Cesarean. Other factors are medical insurance policies that pay more for surgical than vaginal delivery; the increase in hospital deliveries by obstetricians trained in surgery; the older age of mothers with first babies, who are more likely to experience complications; the trend toward multiple, high-risk births as a result of fertility treatments; a 1999 study that found vaginal delivery after a previous Cesarean section can be dangerous (although a later study said risk of uterine rupture was less than 1%); and the increase in malpractice suits when babies suffer damage during delivery. Vaginal breech deliveries are no longer recommended and have been largely abandoned. Better data about the complications associated with the use of forceps or vacuum extractors—chiefly birth injury to the baby, perineal injury and incontinence for the mother—have led to a decrease in operative vaginal deliveries. Also, an increase in the induction of labor has led to increased Cesareans. Finally, in the late 1990s the number of women requesting elective Cesarean delivery (with no medical reason given) for sheer convenience was beginning to rise. However, in at least one group of hospitals, a concerted effort to reduce the Cesarean rate succeeded in cutting it by 25% over a four-year period. Measures to do so included admitting a woman only when her contractions were strong and the cervix was thinning; replacing the traditional "due date" with a two-week interval when birth might take place (to allay anxiety about "lateness"); deferring regional anesthesia (epidural) until later in labor (allowing the woman to move freely about for a longer time); and delaying or avoiding use of a fetal monitor.

The principal indication for a Cesarean section is dystocia, that is, abnormal or too-slow progress of labor, which accounts for 28.9% of Cesareans. Dystocia covers a wide range of problems, including too small a pelvis, too large a baby (especially if the head is too large for safe delivery), too weak contractions or a combination of these factors. Another 35.6% of Cesareans are so-called *repeat Cesareans,* to avoid the alleged risk of rupturing the scar of a previous Cesarean delivery and thereby rupturing the uterus. In 1916, when this policy was first promulgated, most Cesareans involved a long vertical uterine cut (the classical incision described below), which sometimes ruptured during a subse-

quent labor. Since that time, however, horizontal incisions have largely replaced it, and in 1982 the American College of Obstetricians and Gynecologists announced that vaginal deliveries following a Cesarean were safe under many circumstances. In 1988 it further recommended that in the absence of medical complications of pregnancy, *all* women with previous Cesareans be encouraged to attempt *VBAC,* or *vaginal birth after Cesarean.* This is principally advisable in women whose Cesarean was performed with a low transverse incision (see below), and a 1999 study advised much more caution. (The group currently advises against vaginal delivery for women who have had a classical section; see below for explanation.) Abnormal presentation of the baby, especially BREECH PRESENTATION, accounts for another 12.3% of surgical deliveries, and fetal distress, principally asphyxia, for only 9.9%. Other indications for a Cesarean are hemorrhage caused by either ABRUPTIO PLACENTAE or PLACENTA PREVIA, the presence of PREECLAMPSIA or ECLAMPSIA, RH FACTOR incompatibility, serious infection (including HIV, hepatitis B or C and human papilloma virus), and other serious maternal disease, such as heart disease or diabetes.

To prevent the risk of an unnecessary Cesarean section, pregnant women are advised to ask their clinician what percentage of his or her patients is delivered surgically; if that figure exceeds 15% they might consider looking for another clinician. Other questions to ask are whether he/she offers "trial of labor" (attempted vaginal delivery) to women who have had a previous Cesarean, and if so, what percentage of them deliver vaginally; how is labor monitored (electronic fetal monitoring? fetal blood sampling to confirm fetal distress?); does he/she attempt external version after 37 weeks for breech presentation? However, ultimately, a woman needs to be flexible about her birth decisions, striving for a vaginal delivery but not insisting on it if the attending clinician strongly recommends against it.

A Cesarean section is much safer than it used to be, but it still constitutes major surgery. The risk of death to the mother is 2 to 4 times greater than with vaginal delivery (about 1 in 2,500), and recovery from it is much slower than from a vaginal delivery. Two main kinds of operation are in current use, differentiated by the location of the uterine incision. A *cervical incision,* which may be either transverse (crosswise) or vertical (longitudinal), is made in the lower segment of the uterus, above the cervix and behind the bladder. The second, a low transverse incision (*Kerr incision*), is used whenever possible because it involves less blood loss during surgery, less risk of rupture in subsequent pregnancies and subsequent vaginal deliveries, less postoperative infection and easier repair. Sometimes, because of fetal size (very large or very small) or position, lack of space or other problems, a low vertical incision (*Kronig-Selheim incision*) is performed. It is generally thought to be associated with more morbidity than the low transverse technique but is still considered preferable to the classical Cesarean.

The older *classical section,* a vertical incision, is made in the body of the uterus (rather than its lower portion). It allows a greater length for the surgical opening and more room for delivery of the fetus. It is used when there are problems with the mother (as when the placenta covers the lower uterine segment) or, more often, problems relating to the fetus's size and position (such as a crosswise, or transverse, lie). This incision is associated with more bleeding at the time of surgery and more intraabdominal infection postoperatively. It continues to be used, especially in emergency cases when time is of the essence, because it is quicker and easier to perform, but only in about 1% of all Cesarean deliveries.

The incisions just described are into the uterus, not the abdomen, and therefore do not affect the visible scar. There are also two kinds of abdominal incision: a vertical one that extends from the umbilicus almost to the pubis and a transverse, or PFANNENSTIEL INCISION, just above the pubic mound. If the Cesarean delivery is an emergency, the baby is very large or in abnormal position, or the mother is obese, the vertical incision may be necessary. With either kind of abdominal incision, the uterine incision may be either vertical or transverse. Either general or regional anesthesia may be used.

The principal complication from Cesarean section is infection of the uterus, urinary tract or surgical wound, which occurs in up to 40% of cases. Most such infections respond to antibiotic treatment but many require additional time spent in the hospital. One study of elective Cesareans showed that hospital stays are 77% longer and cost 76% more than normal deliveries. Further, mothers who had an optional Cesarean were 2.3 times more likely to return to the hospital within 30 days, usually because of wound complications or major systemic infection. Another, less frequent complication is excessive blood loss that requires transfusion. Blood clots may form in the legs and travel to the lungs, a potentially life-threatening complication, and paralytic ileus, in which the bowels stop functioning temporarily, may cause abdominal cramps and nausea. Even without these complications, the pain and fatigue that normally follow major surgery make it hard for the mother to care for her baby. Another complication is the development of a keloid or other abnormal scar from the incision. Medically harmless but unsightly, it is thicker, wider and less even in appearance than a normal scar and tends to pucker. A subsequent Cesarean will not eliminate it, nor is there any effective means of prevention. A Cesarean delivery also can affect the mother's future reproductive health. Subsequent pregnancies are associated with increased risk of miscarriage, ectopic presentation, placenta previa and placenta accreta. These risks have been well documented but tend to be overlooked when an elective Cesarean is being considered.

A Cesarean also can harm the baby. If delivered too soon, it may be unexpectedly premature and at risk for respiratory distress (although tests to determine fetal maturity can prevent too early a delivery). Further, it is thought that the contractions of a vaginal delivery help the baby absorb fetal lung fluid in preparation for breathing air. While consequent lung problems may be transient and respond well to supplemental oxygen, this difficulty tends to be avoided in vaginal delivery.

For women who looked forward to a vaginal delivery and planned to use one or another method of PREPARED CHILDBIRTH, a Cesarean can be a very upsetting experience. A few hospitals now provide Cesarean birth counselors to assist such women, and some classes for prepared childbirth include educational material to prepare a woman for surgical delivery if it should become necessary.

See also POSTPARTUM.

CFS   See CHRONIC FATIGUE SYNDROME.

Chadwick's sign   A change of color in the tissues around the entrance to the vagina and the cervix that helps in the presumptive early diagnosis of pregnancy. Normally these tissues are pink, but in pregnancy they take on a purplish, dusky color. The color deepens in the course of the pregnancy, and it is most apparent in second and subsequent pregnancies.

chancre   A sore that is the first visible sign of SYPHILIS.

chancroid   Also *soft chancre, ulcus molle.* A SEXUALLY TRANSMITTED DISEASE caused by a rod-shaped bacterium, *Hemophilus ducreyi,* that is most common in the tropics; in North America it occurs largely in the southeast United States but has, like many sexually transmitted disorders, been found more often in recent years. It is transmitted by vaginal, anal or oral-genital intercourse and is most apt to invade the genitals through an existing lesion, such as a small cut or scratch. In most women chancroid gives rise to no symptoms, so they may be unknowing carriers of the disease. In men one or, more often, several small sores appear on the penis or in the urethra one to five days after the infecting contact. The sore is a raised bump surrounded by a narrow red border. It soon becomes pimplelike, filled with pus, and then ruptures to form a painful open sore with ragged edges. Chancroid sores bleed easily when touched and sometimes spread along a line to form a single long, narrow sore. In women the sores appear on the vulva, thighs, vagina, cervix or inside the urethra and may be centered at the base of pubic hairs. Sometimes the chancroid sores disappear by themselves within a few days. In half of untreated cases, however, the bacteria infect the lymph glands in the groin. Within five to eight days after the first sore appears, the glands on one or both sides of the groin become enlarged, hard and painful. They fuse together to form a single rounded painful swelling called a *bubo.* The overlying skin is red. If untreated the bubo may push to the surface and rupture, oozing pus. A large open sore results, which is highly susceptible to infection by other organisms as well.

Diagnosis of chancroid often is confused with other venereal diseases, especially SYPHILIS and LYMPHOGRANULOMA VENEREUM (the latter also characterized by buboes). A culture of pus from an open sore will reveal the causative organism. Treatment is antibiotics, either ceftriaxone injected intramuscularly or erythromycin, azithromycin or ciprofloxacin taken orally for 7 to 10 days. Buboes about to burst should be aspirated and drained. Occasionally plastic surgery may be needed if they have disfigured the genital area. After treatment, there should be follow-up tests every three months for a year to make sure the disease has been eradicated. Unfortunately, the bacterium has a tendency to develop resistance to antibiotics, so that tetracycline and sulfa drugs, once effective, no longer work very well.

change of life   See MENOPAUSE.

chastity   Sexual purity, referring either to abstinence from unlawful sexual intercourse (that is, outside of marriage) or to total abstinence (CELIBACY).

See also VIRGINITY.

chelation therapy   An alternative treatment that has been approved only for lead poisoning but that some proponents believe can rid the body of arterial blockages and thus cure arteriosclerosis. It involves intravenous infusions of a chemical, ethylenediaminetetraacetic acid (EDTA), along with vitamins, iron supplements and trace elements. Each treatment, given 3 times a week, lasts from 1½ to 3 hours, and 30 to 50 treatments are typical. In the bloodstream EDTA works like a magnet, attracting metals and minerals (such as calcium in atherosclerotic plaques), which are then excreted through the urine. To date there have been no well-documented studies attesting to the effectiveness of the treatment, which is also very expensive.

chemotherapy Also *anticancer drugs.* Strictly speaking, any treatment with chemical substances, or drugs, but generally the term is reserved for drugs used to treat CANCER. Anticancer drugs are very powerful agents that kill cancer cells shed into the bloodstream and lymph system by the original tumor as well as the tumor itself, especially when injected directly into it. They also affect healthy cells. The drugs presently in use are most effective against tumors whose cells are actively growing (making DNA and dividing). For this reason they also destroy certain normal tissues that have a high proportion of actively growing cells, such as white blood cells, hair roots and various gastrointestinal tissues, especially mucous membranes. They also may increase susceptibility to infection, create blood-clotting problems and disrupt the menstrual cycle. The number and severity of these side effects varies widely, and new drugs often are able to counterbalance the effects.

Because they are so toxic, it is especially important (but difficult) to establish dosages for these drugs sufficient to kill a tumor but not to damage too much normal tissue. Although many cancer experts feel that the more of a drug they can give, the better the chance of cure, recent studies show that higher dosages are not necessarily more effective. However, chemotherapy doses that would have depleted red and white blood cells in the mid-1980s can now be used, because other drugs that stimulate bone marrow to step up blood-cell production have since been developed. Other considerations in planning chemotherapy include timing, so as to attack cells while they are dividing, and monitoring toxicity.

Newer, more selective and less toxic drugs are constantly being developed (for example, the U.S. Food and Drug Administration approved two dozen between 1994 and 1996 alone), and oral and wafer forms of anticancer drugs have made chemotherapy more convenient. Since cancer is caused by defective genes that in turn give rise to defective proteins, the newer cancer drugs take direct aim at these proteins, disrupting them in various ways. Unlike the earlier drugs, they do not poison the tumor, which consequently damaged healthy cells, but instead aim at the process that makes a cancer cell function. More and more of these so-called *targeted therapies,* which attack molecular mechanisms that spur tumor growth, are the focus of current research, and a number of them, although still considered experimental, are being successfully used in cancer patients. The newest class of cancer drugs are *radioimmunotherapies.* They deliver radioactive particles directly to cancerous cells to kill them. They tend to be very expensive, costing about $25,000 per treatment, but one dose is usually sufficient. Because they are radioactive, they are almost always administered in hospitals rather than doctors' office. Consequently doctors are not paid by insurers for prescribing them and hence tend to give patients more common types of chemotherapy.

Chemotherapy is used in four principal ways: (1) as a primary treatment for certain cancers; (2) as an attempt to cure a cancer when metastasis (spread) is openly present; (3) as a follow-up to surgery when there is no obvious metastasis, to help prevent spread or recurrence; (4) to reduce symptoms and prolong survival when cure is not possible. Recent research indicates also that sometimes chemotherapy administered before surgery can lengthen survival time considerably over surgery alone.

Different cancer drugs work in different ways. Some inhibit cell growth, much as radiation does, and others prevent cell division altogether. Others block cell division by interfering with enzymes needed for synthesis of RNA and DNA building blocks (see NUCLEIC ACID for an explanation of RNA and DNA), and still others adhere to DNA and therefore interfere with cell reproduction. Certain kinds of cancer respond better to one drug than another. For example, CHORIOCARCINOMA is one cancer that responds very well to drugs that block cell division. In some cancers combinations of several drugs work more effectively than any one drug; each attacks a different stage of the cancer's growth. Among these are certain cancers of the blood and lymph, notably acute lymphocytic leukemia and Hodgkin's disease. In breast cancers with lymph node involvement, surgical removal of the affected breast and all the lymph nodes plus radiation treatment does not yield as high a rate of recurrence-free survival as the same treatment combined with drug therapy, most often a combination of two or three drugs. Because chemotherapy is most effective against cancers whose cells are actively dividing, many authorities feel it should be used much earlier for solid tumors, such as breast cancers, while they are actively growing. One such drug, Taxol (paclitaxel), produced from the bark of the Pacific yew tree, has a 50% success rate in significantly reducing breast cancer tumors, but only in patients previously treated with other anticancer drugs. Unlike other agents, Taxol interferes with the skeleton-like system of structural supports inside malignant cells, making it effective against some tumors that do not respond to other drugs. However, its side effects include damage to bone marrow cells, causing anemia and immune system impairment, nerve damage and gastrointestinal problems. Moreover, a recent study indicated that Taxol does not work for the most common form of breast cancer, that is, women whose tumors are HER-2 negative (and are being helped to grow by estrogen; see under CANCER, BREAST for more information).

Chemotherapy is administered orally or by injection into a muscle or vein, weekly or monthly, occasionally daily, or in special cycles. For advanced cancers some physicians prefer to use a continuous infusion, that is, intravenous administration of one or more drugs in an uninterrupted flow for about five days. In most cases a combination of drugs is used. A newer approach, called CHRONOTHERAPY, tries to synchronize treatment with the body's own circadian cycles through a 24-hour day, which appears to make the drugs more effective. Rather than being administered in single injections or steady infusions that remain constant day and night, some drugs have been found to work better when given at gradually increasing and decreasing doses through the night, whereas others are more potent during the day. Side effects also seem less severe with this approach, which is based on the fluctuating cycle in which the body releases hormones, produces new blood cells and so on.

The most common side effects of chemotherapy are nausea and vomiting, ulcers in the mouth, skin rashes and the loss of hair, the last usually a temporary problem. Often nausea and vomiting can be controlled by administering corticosteroids or other antinausea drugs. Nutritional changes,

relaxation and behavior-modification techniques may also be helpful. Recommended measures include eating frequent small meals, eating at least one hour before treatment, avoiding fried and fatty foods, restricting fluids with meals, eating foods cold or at room temperature, limiting exposure to sounds, sights and smells that cause nausea and wearing loose-fitting clothes. Menstrual periods may become irregular or cease. In men the sperm count may be reduced, either temporarily or permanently; therefore some oncologists (cancer specialists) advise men to deposit some sperm in a SPERM BANK before undergoing chemotherapy; there it can be stored for 10 years or longer. Sometimes intravenous administration will cause a burning sensation at the site of the injection for several days. More serious possible toxic effects, not apparent for some time, include bone marrow depression (a reduction in the bone marrow's production of white blood cells), which reduces resistance against other diseases; damage to the heart muscle; a decrease in blood platelets (thrombocytopenia); cystitis; hepatic fibrosis (death of liver tissue); and, after long-term use, the development of acute leukemia. Indeed, one of the major problems of chemotherapy—and all other cancer treatment—is that agents potent enough to treat a cancer sometimes cause another cancer elsewhere in the body. However, since most cancers have a very long latency period (take long to develop), the risk of carcinogenic drugs is considered worthwhile for many patients. Another effect experienced by women after chemotherapy for breast cancer, in possibly 20% to 30% of cases, is a lessening of cognitive function that has been called *chemo brain*. Sometimes lasting as long as a decade, it is generally described as increased distractibility and inattentiveness. At this writing the condition is still insufficiently documented, but studies of causes, incidence and treatment are underway. One recent study indicated that cancer drugs can cause a temporary shrinkage in brain structures involved in cognition and awareness, which tended to subside after three years. Another study showed that three specific drugs used for a range of cancers tend to be more toxic to healthy brain cells than to cancer cells. These results are preliminary and should not deter necessary treatment.

In addition to these effects, chemotherapy can erode the quality of life. Anticancer drugs may decrease a patient's libido, indirectly by causing fatigue, nausea, constipation or muscle pain, and more directly by causing vaginal atrophy (shrinkage), dryness or bleeding. In men they may impair erection maintenance, limit semen production or lessen control over ejaculation. Because many such drugs suppress the immune system, they also make patients more susceptible to genital infections such as herpes and yeast infections. Further, changes in appearance, such as weight loss and hair loss, may damage self-esteem. Most courses of chemotherapy last from six months to two years and often are coupled with surgery and radiation therapy (which also can affect sexuality). To maintain sexual intimacy, open communication between partners is necessary, and, if needed, professional counseling may be advisable. Vaginal dryness can be eased with the use of water-based lubricant. In some men and women, treatment with testosterone may restore desire temporarily. Medication through a port (implanted tube) need not limit physical contact, provided one avoids rubbing against the dressing. Abstinence generally is advised only if there is bleeding in the genital area or intercourse provokes pain. And if drugs have significantly lowered the white blood count, it is important for one's partner to be free of any infection.

See also HORMONE THERAPY; IMMUNOTHERAPY; RADIATION THERAPY.

childbearing, age for   See AGE, CHILDBEARING.

childbearing center   See BIRTH CENTER.

childbed fever   See PUERPERAL FEVER.

childbirth education   See PREPARED CHILDBIRTH.

chiropractic   A treatment method that involves manipulating the muscles and spine, usually by hand, based on the idea that adjustment of the spinal column will restore normal function to the nervous system and the body's own natural healing ability. Although manipulative massage is an ancient practice and is still used in many non-Western cultures, chiropractic as known today was founded by Daniel David Palmer in 1895. Despite the opposition of conventional medicine, chiropractic thrived, and today it is the third most widely practiced form of treatment in the United States (after medicine and dentistry) and is licensed in every state.

Most patients go to a chiropractor to relieve pain, especially back pain, but also neck and joint pain. Chiropractors typically look for subluxations, partially misaligned or biochemically dysfunctional vertebrae and other off-center joints that may be impinging on normal neurological function. They also look for trauma to muscles and bones from falls and accidents, for postural distortions that may cause joints or muscles to function abnormally, and inquire about physical and mental stress. The treatment appears to work best for mechanical dysfunction, such as injured muscles and joints, and has become very popular with individuals who experience low back pain, slipped disks and sports injuries. Some chiropractors limit their practice to musculoskeletal problems, but others claim to offer effective treatment for a huge variety of ailments, from irritable bowel syndrome to gallbladder problems, asthma and angina (heart pain). Critics point out that few if any chiropractors have sufficient training to function as family doctors and therefore such claims should be viewed skeptically, at best.

Chiropractic treatment is not without risk. Complications of manipulation can range from increased pain to ruptured disks, paralysis and even death, but these are rare. Another risk is that some chiropractic patients delay seeking more appropriate medical care. Finally, the older widespread chiropractic practice of subjecting patients to repeated full-spine X-rays, overexposing them to radiation, fortunately has abated, but some practitioners still follow it. To avoid risk, it is recommended that one first see a physician to rule out back pain caused by cancer as well as conditions that are made worse by manipulation (fractures, rheumatoid arthritis, severe osteoporosis, bleeding disorders, spinal inflammation). Then select a chiropractor recommended by the American Chiropractic Association and who is licensed by your state. First discuss your condition with him or her carefully. Watch out for chiropractors who take repeated or full-spine X-rays, fail to take a history or do a clinical examination, offer vitamin or other nutritional remedies, or claim to improve immune function or organ systems unrelated to the presenting problem. When pain has been relieved or if there has been no improvement within four to six weeks, it is reasonable to stop treatment after discussing expected outcomes with the chiropractor.

chlamydia infection A sexually transmitted (venereal) disease named for the bacterium that causes it, *Chlamydia trachomatis,* which in the 1980s surpassed gonorrhea as the leading venereal disease in the United States. In 2006 more than 1 million new cases were reported, the most ever for a sexually transmitted disease. However, the number of infected individuals was probably much greater, since the disease often is overlooked or misdiagnosed. Peak incidence occurs in sexually active adolescent and young adult women, and, despite recommendations to use a simple urine test to screen young women, screening rates remain low. A recent study indicated that 25% of American teenage women had at least one sexually transmitted disease, and the number was twice as large in black women as in white.

In women, chlamydia may first affect the urethra and cervix, often without any symptoms at all. If there are symptoms, they usually appear slowly, within three weeks after contact with an infected person, and include a discharge from the cervix and/or urethritis, marked by itching inside the urethra and burning on urination. If the infection is not treated, it may progress to become pelvic inflammatory disease, which can lead to infertility. Although most women with chlamydia are symptom-free, men with the disease nearly always have symptoms, such as a discharge from the penis and local discomfort. It also can cause prostate gland infection as well as infect the epididymis, the canal that carries sperm. Untreated chlamydia may cause infertility. Further, in both men and women

it can cause conjunctivitis (eye inflammation), and in individuals with an impaired immune system, pneumonia. Chlamydia can cause postpartum fever, a potentially serious infection in the mother following delivery, and can be transmitted to her infant as it passes through the birth canal. It also has been linked to miscarriage, ectopic pregnancy and premature delivery. The U.S. Preventive Task Force recommends testing for all pregnant women. Moreover, since 1993 it has recommended screening for all sexually active nonpregnant women aged 24 or younger and those older nonpregnant women who are at increased risk. Women also can transmit chlamydia to their female sexual partners by way of the fingers or artificial stimulators.

Chlamydial infections are diagnosed in several ways. One consists of taking a cell sample from the sexual organs and adding monoclonal antibodies; if chlamydial organisms are present, they combine with the antibodies, producing a radioactive signal visible in an ultraviolet microscope. However, it is not entirely reliable. Newer, simpler and more accurate urine tests make possible much easier screening in sexually active men, in whom it is more difficult to obtain tissue samples (by inserting a swab into the urethra). When such screening becomes more widespread, the older advice of giving treatment for anyone at high risk on statistical grounds—those with gonorrhea or pelvic inflammatory disease, women with cervical discharge unaccounted for by other tests and individuals in sexual contact with those whose symptoms suggest chlamydia—will become unnecessary. Treatment consists of a seven-day course of oral doxycycline, which cannot be taken during pregnancy, or a single dose of azithromycin, not to be taken if allergic to erythromycin. Erythromycin, often prescribed instead of doxycycline, is safe during pregnancy. Chlamydial eye infection is treated with local antibiotic agents.

chloasma Also *mask of pregnancy, melasma.* Irregular brownish patches of varying size that appear on the face during pregnancy, often in a winglike pattern over the cheeks, forehead and upper lip, giving rise to the name "mask of pregnancy." They usually disappear, or at least fade considerably, after delivery. Similarly, ordinary freckles tend to become darker during pregnancy. Women who experience such pigment changes in pregnancy also may experience them when they use oral contraceptives or estrogen replacement therapy, supporting the theory that they result from increased melanin production triggered by higher levels either of estrogen and/or progesterone or of melanocyte-stimulating hormone. Women with chloasma of pregnancy should avoid or minimize their exposure to the sun and always use a sunscreen outdoors, since sunlight tends to aggravate the pigmentation and may make it less likely to fade.

chocolate cyst   See ENDOMETRIOSIS.

cholesterol   One of several lipids (blood fats) that combine with proteins, forming *lipoproteins,* and transport fat in the bloodstream. High-density lipoproteins (HDL) carry fat away from body cells, thereby preventing its accumulation in the artery walls. Low-density lipoproteins (LDL), which contain a high proportion of cholesterol, appear to promote the buildup of fatty materials in artery walls and therefore are associated with an increased risk of coronary heart disease and stroke (CEREBRAL VASCULAR ACCIDENT). These two diseases together account for nearly half of all deaths in U.S. women. It seems likely that their risk can be reduced by lowering LDL levels through dietary changes, particularly by reducing the consumption of foods rich in cholesterol and saturated fatty acids (intake of these foods is comparatively high in the United States). Further, weight loss and exercise often raise HDL levels. Dietary recommendations include eating skinless poultry and fish instead of red meat and pork, limiting red meat to lean cuts, replacing butter and shortening with unhydrogenated, monounsaturated and polyunsaturated vegetable oils (canola, safflower, sunflower, corn and olive oils), reducing egg yolk consumption to no more than three per week and using low-fat dairy products (low-fat milk, low-fat cheeses, yogurt, etc.), and increasing intake of soluble fiber (oat bran, etc.). Since just which fats are present in a particular food is sometimes unclear, it is safest to limit dietary fat to 30% of total calorie intake (and preferably even less) and saturated fat

GUIDELINES FOR DIETARY CHANGES TO LOWER CHOLESTEROL*

	Maximum total calories
• Total fat	Reduce to no more than 30%
• Saturated fat (found in meat, dairy products, coconut and palm oils)	Reduce to less than 10%
• Polyunsaturated fat (found in fat of plant foods, especially safflower, sunflower, corn and cottonseed oils)	Increase, up to 10%
• Monounsaturated fat (found in olive and peanut oils, some margarines and shortening)	Reduce to 10–15%
• Cholesterol (found in all foods of animal origin, mostly meat and dairy products)	Less than 300 mg a day
• Carbohydrates	Increase to 50–60%

HOW MUCH FAT SHOULD YOU EAT?

Total daily calories**	Maximum amount of fat in grams
1,500	50
2,000	67
2,500	83
3,000	100

*From *Eating to Lower Your High Blood Cholesterol,* National Institutes of Health publication
**Average woman aged 23–50 needs 2,000 calories a day; aged 51–75 needs 1,600 calories a day

to one-third of those (10% or less of total calories). An exception to the warnings about dietary fat relates to the *omega-3 fatty acid* (alpha-linolenic acid) and *omega-6 fatty acid* (linolenic acid), found in fish, especially sardines, salmon and mackerel; soybean, safflower and corn oils; and nuts and seeds. They are polyunsaturated fats, are essential to a number of body processes, and must be consumed since the body cannot manufacture them. Studies show they appear to decrease triglyceride levels and slow the growth of atherosclerotic plaque (leading to heart disease), so eating 3 ounces of fatty fish (mackerel, herring, whitefish, lake trout, salmon, tuna, bluefish) twice a week is highly recommended.

Current federal labeling rules require manufacturers to list only saturated and total fat. Some nutritionists feel that *trans fat*, found in hard margarine and other products that have been treated with a process called partial hydrogenation, are as harmful as saturated fat and therefore should also be listed on labels. In 2003 the Food and Drug Administration ruled that products containing trans fats be so labeled, and manufacturers had until January 1, 2006, to comply (see TRANS FAT).

Cholesterol levels can be revealed by a blood test, but authorities differ as to what constitutes a desirable level. Most agree, however, that 200 milligrams per deciliter or less is acceptable, although some maintain 160 is a far more desirable goal. There is fairly general agreement that 240 or higher puts an individual at much greater risk, and 200 to 240 is considered borderline. Preliminary results of a recent study show that high cholesterol levels (and low HDL levels) seem to have little bearing on heart disease and mortality after the age of 70, particularly in women. Nevertheless, the American Heart Association recommends limiting dietary cholesterol intake to 300 milligrams per day.

Cholesterol measurements are not always reliable, and a high value usually should be confirmed with a second measurement. If cholesterol still appears to be high, a lipoprotein analysis is recommended in order to determine LDL and HDL values. To perform this test, blood is drawn the morning after an overnight fast. Three substances are measured: total cholesterol, HDL-cholesterol and triglycerides. (Triglycerides are ordinary fat molecules stored in body fat, and some circulate in the blood.) The amount of LDL-cholesterol is calculated according to a formula: LDL = total cholesterol - HDL - (triglycerides ÷ 5). For example, if total cholesterol is 200, HDL is 45, and triglyceride is 150, the LDL level works out to 125 (200 - 45 - 30). Values for LDL ideally are below 100; 100 to 129 is close to ideal, 130 to 159 is borderline high, 160–189 is high, and over 190 is very high. The average HDL level for men is 40 to 50 mg/dl, and for women 50 to 60. (These figures are provided by the American Heart Association.) Incidentally, this formula works only if the triglyceride level is below 400; at higher levels, a more accurate but costlier method must be used to determine LDL.

GUIDELINES FOR CHOLESTEROL LEVELS*

- Total cholesterol below 200 milligrams per deciliter (mg/dL)
- HDL cholesterol above 50 mg/dL
- LDL cholesterol below 100 mg/dL
- Triglycerides below 150 mg/dL

*American Heart Association

An even more refined test calculates not only the number but the size of the lipoproteins that carry cholesterol in the blood. Small and dense LDL particles penetrate artery walls more easily than large ones and so are considered riskier. A test using nuclear magnetic resonance spectroscopy, which places lipoproteins into a high field magnet, reveals not only standard information (total cholesterol, LDL, HDL, triglycerides) but also the size and number of lipoproteins, including small, dense LDL and very-low-density lipoproteins (VLDL), which carry triglycerides in the blood. Not everyone needs such an advanced test. It should be used mainly for patients with normal or slightly elevated cholesterol who are at risk due to other factors.

Until recently it was believed that high HDL offset high LDL, but new findings indicate that LDL may play a more important role in elevating risk. Thus, even if total cholesterol is within the normal range, high LDL may require more aggressive means for lowering it. New guidelines say the highest-risk individuals need to aim for an LDL of 70, and the American Heart Association recommended that those who have had a heart attack, diabetes, chest pain, or surgery to clear blocked blood vessels and have an LDL over 100 should be medicated. Those considered at moderate risk should take medication if their LDL is 130 or higher. Moreover, proper diet and exercise also must be followed, in addition to medication. (High risk applies to the following for women: smoking; postmenopausal; high blood pressure; diabetes; a relative who had a heart attack before age 55.) If LDL is over 100, begin dietary treatment, and if ineffective, consider drug therapy as well. Similarly, triglyceride levels of 200 to 400 milligrams call for dietary changes, and drug treatment if other risk factors are high; over 400 calls for drug treatment. (Also see TRI-

GLYCERIDES.) Occasionally high cholesterol is caused by an underactive thyroid; when that is the case, administering thyroid hormone generally brings cholesterol down to a normal range.

Treatment recommendations also vary, and some clinicians believe that all "borderline" cases should be treated. Further, recent studies have shown that female heart attack survivors can cut their risk of another heart attack, stroke and death by taking a cholesterol-lowering drug, even if their cholesterol levels are normal. Numerous cholesterol-lowering drugs are available; all require a lifetime commitment, and none is free of side effects. The principal kinds of cholesterol-lowering drugs are the statins (see STATIN), niacin, and fibrate drugs such as gemfibrozil (Lopid) or fenofibrate (Tricor). The statins lower LDL. Fibrates and niacin are particularly effective in patients with high numbers of small, dense LDL particles, and niacin raises HDL, but only slightly. Both cholesterol levels and liver function should be checked within two months of beginning any of these medications. Thereafter they should be monitored every 6 to 12 months. Medications and a vaccine to raise HDL are currently being tested.

Nonprescription treatments to lower cholesterol include taking a psyllium fiber supplement (1 tablespoon twice a day) to lower cholesterol by 10 to 15 percent; red yeast, which contains some lovastatin; fish oil capsules to lower triglycerides; plant sterols found in Benecol and Take Control spreads used three times a day on bread or crackers. Regular exercise and weight loss also are recommended.

Cholesterol tests generally are conducted in a doctor's office. At this writing, however, several companies have developed home cholesterol tests, which went on the market in 1994. The Advance Cholesterol Home Test measures the sum of LDL, HDL and VLDL (another type of cholesterol). Taking it involves sitting quite still for five minutes (to allow cholesterol levels in the blood to stabilize), pricking one's finger with a lancet, and squeezing a few drops of blood into a plastic container holding a specially treated strip. Within 15 minutes a color change in the strip indicates how much cholesterol is present in the sample. To determine the level, one compares the strip with an enclosed chart. Although a high finding generally indicates a problem, a low finding is not necessarily accurate because it can be caused by too little HDL. False results also may be due to not sitting still long enough before testing, "milking" too much blood from the finger and thereby diluting the sample, or taking either acetaminophen (Tylenol) or vitamin C pills within four hours of testing.

The first available figures for cholesterol all were based on studies of *men*. Recent work indicates that the link between cholesterol and heart disease is different for women, especially elderly women, and different for black and white women.

choriocarcinoma   A kind of cancer resulting from a HYDATIDIFORM MOLE (after it has been expelled through the vagina) or, more rarely, following normal delivery, when it develops from tissues of the baby. The chief symptom is bleeding, often very heavy and sometimes so profuse that the hemorrhage is fatal. This kind of cancer spreads very fast, to the lung, brain, bone and even skin, so that prompt treatment is essential. Fortunately choriocarcinoma has been found to respond very well to anticancer drugs, which have largely replaced the surgical treatment (hysterectomy) formerly necessary.

chorion   The outermost membrane covering the fertilized egg, part of which—the chorionic villi—will develop into the PLACENTA. The chorionic villi become embedded in the uterine lining and are bathed in a pool of maternal blood where the exchange of nutrients and waste products takes place.

chorionic gonadotropin   See HUMAN CHORIONIC GONADOTROPIN.

chorionic villus sampling   Also *CVS*. A prenatal test that can identify numerous common birth defects after 9½ to 12 weeks of pregnancy. To perform it, the clinician, guided by ultrasound, inserts a catheter into the uterus through the vagina and removes small amounts of the villi, tiny projections surrounding the CHORION, whose composition is similar to the embryo's. Analysis of the villi can reveal the presence of Down syndrome and other chromosomal defects, and most cases of cystic fibrosis, Tay-Sachs, Gaucher disease and sickle-cell disease but not neural tube defects. In some cases it is preferable to use a fine needle placed through the abdominal skin and uterus into the villi.

Like other prenatal tests, CVS is not without risk. It is approximately twice the risk of AMNIO-CENTESIS, and if it is done too early it may lead to limb abnormalities in the baby, mainly in the form of missing fingers and toes. It is also technically harder to perform than amniocentesis, and fewer doctors are trained to do it. Consequently it is recommended only for women with an extremely high risk of carrying a genetically abnormal fetus.

chromosome A microscopic body in the nucleus of almost every living cell containing coded instructions that tell the cell what it can produce and do during its life and that are transmitted to its offspring. A chromosome can be regarded as a strand of *genes* (see GENETICS). Human beings normally have 46 chromosomes in each and every cell, 23 coming from each parent. Significant abnormalities in chromosomes occur in approximately one of every 250 live human births, and an estimated three-fourths of these genetic "errors" are considered undesirable. In addition, about one-third of all miscarriages are believed to be caused by chromosomal abnormalities.

See also BIRTH DEFECTS.

chromosome test A test sometimes administered to women athletes to determine whether or not they are in fact biologically female. The test consists of taking a buccal smear (a tiny scraping from inside the mouth) and examining the cells for their chromosomes. The chromosomes of particular interest are the so-called *sex chromosomes*, two X chromosomes in every female and one X and one Y chromosome in every male (see GENETICS). The use of the test allegedly was made necessary by the growing use of ANABOLIC STEROIDS to increase

athletic strength as well as by the performance of TRANSSEXUAL surgery.

chronic Developing over a period of time and having a long duration. The opposite of chronic is ACUTE.

chronic fatigue syndrome Also *CFS, chronic fatigue dysfunction syndrome, CFIDS*. A condition of extreme fatigue that limits one's daily activity to less than half of its previous level and persists for at least six months. It generally is accompanied by any or all of the following symptoms: mild fever, sore throat, painful lymph nodes in neck or armpits, generalized muscle weakness and/or discomfort or pain, headache, intermittent joint pains, visual or other disturbances suggesting central nervous system involvement, sleep disturbances, disabling fatigue lasting more than 24 hours after vigorous exercise that is normally tolerated, and the onset of symptoms within hours or a day or two (many patients can pinpoint the exact time). On physical examination, a low-grade fever, throat inflammation and/or tender lymph nodes often are found.

The syndrome, which affects mostly young adults, and women twice as often as men, resembles a persistent case of flu, with fatigue being the main problem. At this writing the cause of chronic fatigue is not known, but a virus or some other immune system defect is strongly suspected. There is no certain diagnosis by blood test. Since many of the symptoms are common to numerous ailments, a key factor in diagnosis is whether a person is suddenly experiencing them for the first time or to a markedly different degree. More specifically, according to a revised definition issued by an international committee of experts in 1994, the patient must be suffering from unexplained, persistent or relapsing chronic fatigue that is new or of definite onset, does not result from increased physical activity, is not much relieved by rest, and has caused significantly diminished levels of activity (compared to previously). Also, at least four of the following symptoms must have appeared since the start of the illness: short-term memory or concentration problems severe enough to interfere with work, school, or social activities; sore throat or tender lymph nodes in the neck or underarm area; muscle and joint pain; severe headache; sleep that fails to refresh, and malaise that persists for a day or more following physical exertion.

There is no specific treatment. Although the condition may be quite disabling and lasts for months, it is not progressive (does not get worse). Those who are severely affected must learn to rearrange their lives so as to minimize fatigue, maintain good nutrition, get ample rest and exercise insofar as possible and take advantage of those times when they have more energy. Low doses of tricyclic antidepressants—lower than those used for depression—sometimes improve sleep and assuage muscle pain. Eventually the disease seems to run its course.

chronic obstructive pulmonary disease Also *COPD, chronic bronchitis, emphysema.* A lung disease in which the airways are partly obstructed, making it hard to get air in and out. The airways lose their elasticity, their walls become thick and inflamed, and cells in the airways produce more sputum than usual, which also clogs. A major cause of death and illness, COPD develops slowly and cannot be cured. The major cause of COPD is smoking; inhaling other irritants, such as pollution, dust or chemicals, over long periods also may cause or contribute to the disorder. The principal symptoms are shortness of breath, a chronic cough, excess sputum production and wheezing. A diagnosis is confirmed with a breathing test called *spirometry,* which measures the amount of and speed of air a person exhales. Based on this test, your clinician can determine if you have COPD and its severity, ranging from at risk (chronic cough, increased sputum), mild (mild airflow limitation), moderate (more airflow limitation, shortness of breath during brisk activity) and severe (severe shortness of breath, risk of respiratory failure and heart failure). Treatment, based on the severity of the disease, includes inhaled bronchodilators, inhaled glucocorticosteroids, annual flu shots (important for COPD patients), pneumococcal vaccine, oxygen for severe cases and sometimes surgery.

chronic pain Pain that last six months or more and does not respond to any conventional treatment. It may be the result of serious injury, surgery or diseases such as ENDOMETRIOSIS, FIBROMYALGIA or IRRITABLE BOWEL SYNDROME, or nerve damage as an aftermath of shingles. It often comes to dominate the sufferer's life. Medications used to treat acute pain become less and less effective against chronic pain; indeed, prolonged daily use of narcotics or tranquilizers often worsens pain, in addition to making the patient drug-dependent. Consequently, managing chronic pain requires a different approach, including treatment for specific physical symptoms and behavioral counseling to alter the patient's perception of pain. The best place to obtain such care is a pain center or pain clinic where anesthesiologists, physical therapists, neurologists, psychiatrists, acupuncturists, biofeedback technicians and other specialists work together. The underlying principles of chronic pain management are to encourage the patient to take an active role in dealing with her pain, change her response to pain, and understand the relationship between physical pain and stress, which she can be taught to minimize by means of muscle relaxation and other techniques. The therapies used may include ACUPUNCTURE, biofeedback, hypnosis, electrical stimulation, neural blockade, steroid therapy, diet counseling, physical and occupational therapy, psychological counseling, behavior modification and stress management training. Skin patches containing various analgesics often help relieve pain and avoid the side effects of oral medication (see also ANALGESIC). Other topical treatments include wraps, creams and ointments that produce cooling or heat, thereby interfering with pain signal transmission. Other nondrug therapies include massage and physical therapy for musculoskeletal pain. Another option is transcutaneous electric nerve stimulation (TENS), which delivers a mild electrical current to a painful area to interfere with pain signals. There also are implantable spinal cord stimulators to block nerve signals, and implantable pumps that release small amounts of strong medication. These last treatments are largely reserved for extreme cases, such as pain secondary to failed back surgery or a vascular condition, interstitial cystitis (see CYSTITIS, def. 2) or other kinds of neuropathic pain. Exercise, which stimulates the release of endorphins (natural pain suppressants), can be very beneficial. For a particular syndrome of chronic pain, see REFLEX SYMPATHETIC DYSTROPHY SYNDROME. To find a good pain clinic, consult your physician, county medical association, hospital or medical school, or contact the American Chronic Pain Association (see the Appendix).

chronotherapy Timing treatment on the basis of the body's own circadian rhythms (regular cycles that run their course in about 24 hours). Chronotherapy is especially useful when symptoms vary predictably over a 24-hour period, when treatment aims at supplementing or replacing hormones or when drugs are metabolized at different rates or side effects are worse at certain times of day. The last is especially true for chemotherapy. Rather than administering cancer-fighting drugs in single injections or steady infusions that remain constant day and night, some drugs have been found to work better when given at gradually increasing and decreasing doses through the night, whereas others were more potent during the day. Side effects also seemed less severe with this approach, which is based on the fluctuating cycle in which the body releases hormones, produces new blood cells, etc.

Another approach is timing treatment according to a woman's menstrual cycle. At this writing a large study of premenopausal women is investigating whether breast cancer surgery—lumpectomy or mastectomy—is best performed during the first or second half (follicular or luteal phase) of the menstrual cycle so as to reduce the risk of cancer recurrence. Earlier studies yielded conflicting results, although most suggested that the second half (luteal phase) is more beneficial. The opposite appears to be true for menstrual timing of mammography, probably because breast density appears to be lower during the first half (follicular phase).

Sudden heart attack, sudden death from heart arrhythmias, and stroke occur three times more often in the morning as at other times of day. Traditionally drugs to lower blood pressure, lower cholesterol or prevent angina (chest pain) are prescribed to be taken in the morning. If they are not very effective, a sustained-release pill taken in the evening might be more effective. Similarly, severe asthma attacks tend to occur in the very early morning (some 80% of breathing failures and two-thirds of asthma deaths take place between midnight and 8 A.M.). Therefore medication for this condition might best be taken in the late afternoon or early evening. Pain from rheumatoid arthritis is worst in the morning, whereas pain from osteoarthritis peaks in the evening. Both kinds benefit from nonsteroidal anti-inflammatory drugs, but one may call for evening medication and the other for morning. Estrogen therapy for hot flashes may work best when taken late in the day.

Coordinating over-the-counter pain relievers, antihistamines or decongestants with body rhythms may be a helpful strategy. With prescription drugs, however, it is not advisable to change one's schedule without consulting one's physician. Further, it should be noted that taking a drug at a different time may increase side effects rather than its effectiveness.

CIN Abbreviation for *cervical intraepithelial neoplasia:* see DYSPLASIA.

circumcision Surgical removal of the foreskin, or PREPUCE, of the penis in men and of the clitoris in women. This operation sometimes was performed on women until the late 1930s in the United States, in order to curb masturbation (to some extent it replaced clitoridectomy; see under CLITORIS), and is still performed in some non-Western cultures. There is no valid medical reason for ever performing it on women. For a good part of the 20th century circumcision was performed in American hospitals almost routinely on male babies, usually a few days after birth, for purposes of hygiene and, as some experts believed, to prevent penile cancer. Both purposes then began to be questioned. Recent studies suggest it may afford some protection against AIDS and other infections. In 2007 the World Health Organization officially recommended circumcision as a way to prevent heterosexual transmission of the AIDS virus. Circumcised men still can contract and transmit the virus, but they have a much lower risk of doing so. Opponents to circumcision hold that good hygiene can prevent problems. So long as the foreskin can be retracted easily, cleaning it and the area under it reduce the risk of penile cancer and infection. In recent years the rate of circumcision has fallen; one agency reports it was performed for only 57% of births in the United States in 2005. Much of the decline is attributed to immigration from Latin America and Asia, where the procedure is rare. Also, Medicaid no longer covers the surgery routinely, so many low-income families cannot afford it. Circumcision also is a ceremonial ritual in certain religions, mandatory for all males in Judaism and Islam, and used for women and/or men among other groups.

climacteric See MENOPAUSE.

climax See ORGASM.

clinic A health care facility that deals principally or entirely with outpatients and sometimes is devoted to a specific area of health care (family planning, alcoholism, chronic pain or sexually transmitted diseases only). In North America four principal kinds of clinic provide routine women's health care: the outpatient gynecological clinic of a teaching hospital (a hospital associated with a medical school); a gynecological clinic within a public or community hospital, which may provide only limited outpatient services; a freestanding clinic (not associated with a hospital), which includes such facilities as neighborhood or community health centers and family planning clinics as well as SELF-HELP clinics; and a prepaid group practice health plan (health maintenance organization, or HMO), which provides a range of services from outpatient care to hospitalization.

The practices followed by clinics vary greatly. In some a patient is seen by whatever health care provider is available at the time; in others one may see a particular clinician by appointment. Originally, clinics were designed for patients of low income who could not afford a private physician. Today this distinction has been largely eliminated, and many persons who can afford private care prefer to use a clinic that has the advantage of providing a variety of specialists within one center.

clitoris A small cylindrical structure at the upper front of the VULVA, between the *labia minoris* (see LABIA), which form its prepuce (hood), or foreskin. Lying just above and in front of the urethral opening, it resembles the male penis in that it contains many nerve endings and erectile tissue (capable of stiffening). Like the penis, it is extremely sensitive, especially at the glans (tip), and becomes engorged with blood during sexual stimulation. However, it is much smaller, usually less than 1 inch (2½ centimeters) long, even when it is erect. Highly responsive to touch, so much so that many women find its direct stimulation painful, the clitoris is the primary focus of ORGASM in women; indeed, its only known function is for sexual pleasure.

The importance of the clitoris in sexual response was long overlooked. Even as late as the 1950s, some physicians and alleged experts on sex differentiated between what they called a "clitoral" and "vaginal" orgasm, maintaining that the former was an "immature" response and the latter the only one appropriate for adult women. This differentiation was based on where the source of stimulation was located—vaginal penetration, not manual stimulation—rather than on a genuine difference in response, and has been largely discounted as a misconception.

In 19th-century Europe (and in other parts of the world even today) the clitoris was sometimes surgically removed—an operation called *clitoridectomy*—for a variety of purposes. In 1885 this surgery was first performed in England to check female "mental disorders," a practice that soon spread to America. Later it was performed to check MASTURBATION. Today the operation is considered, in most advanced countries, to be cruel and unnecessary mutilation, except in those rare cases where cancer has spread to the external genitals (see CANCER, VULVAR). In 2006 a large medical study of female genital cutting showed that the procedure has deadly consequences when a woman gives birth, raising by more than 50% the likelihood that she or her baby will die.

clomiphene citrate   See FERTILITY DRUG.

coitus   Also *copulation, sexual intercourse.* Vaginal intercourse, with the man's penis placed inside the woman's vagina.

See also ANUS; ORAL SEX; SEXUAL RESPONSE.

coitus interruptus   Also *French method, pulling out, withdrawal method.* A Latin term meaning "interrupted intercourse" and referring to a method of BIRTH CONTROL in which the male pulls his penis out of his partner's vagina before he ejaculates ("comes"). It is one of the oldest and simplest methods of preventing conception, requiring no equipment of any kind, but it also has the highest failure rate. Some seminal fluid may leak from the penis before ejaculation, and even a drop or two can contain thousands of sperm. Further, many men are unable to withdraw completely in time, and spilling of even a little seminal fluid on the outer female genitals may deposit sperm that migrate up inside the vagina. In any event, this method requires great self-control and is considered, at best, 81% effective, and often far less so. Many couples also find it unsatisfactory, the man because he must constantly monitor his level of excitement in order to withdraw in time, the woman because she may not trust his ability to withdraw and also may not be ready for orgasm at the same time and consequently have to rely on other means of stimulation for gratification.

colonoscopy   A diagnostic test that examines the large intestine using a flexible viewing tube. It is used in cases of inflammatory bowel disease and in screening for COLORECTAL CANCER. It is considered far more accurate than sigmoidoscopy, which views only the bottom third of the intestine. Performed in a clinic or hospital, colonoscopy requires clearing the digestive system of stool, accomplished by taking a strong laxative and/or one or more enemas. Sometimes fasting is recommended as well. If the tube detects intestinal polyps, which may be precancerous, they can be removed during the procedure, simply being snipped off. Because many individuals dislike or fear this unpleasant and invasive procedure, researchers have developed a substitute called *virtual colonoscopy,* which uses digital data generated by multiple computer scans to create a three-dimensional image of the intestine displayed on a computer screen. After a 48-hour low-fiber diet and complete bowel cleansing, the bowel is filled with air and serial X-rays are taken. Much less expensive than the conventional procedure, it cannot, however, remove any polyps it locates. In a new 2008 study, it identified nine out of 10 individuals with cancers and large growths seen by regular colonoscopies. While superior at detecting large knobby polyps, it is not as good in detecting flat growths on the colon. Recommended to be performed every five years, it is also called CTcolonography.

For individuals with no family history of colorectal cancer, traditional colonoscopy is recommended at age 60 and every 10 years thereafter. For those with a family history or who are otherwise considered at high risk, the test is recommended at age 35 or 40 and repeated every five years. In 2008, the U.S. Preventive Services Task Force decided not to support virtual colonoscopy and held that while everyone between the ages of 50 and 75 should be screened once every 10 years, most people over 75 should stop getting routine cancer tests because the benefits decline and the risks rise.

colostomy   A surgical opening of the colon (large intestine) through the abdomen for discharge of solid waste (feces), which is made when a diseased or injured colon and/or rectum cannot be treated medically. The principal cause of such disease is cancer of the colon and/rectum; other causes are inflammatory bowel disease (ulcerative colitis and Crohn's disease), diverticulitis, familial polyposis, birth defects and severe injury. Occasionally a *temporary colostomy* is performed in order to allow the lower part of the colon and/or rectum to heal; in such cases there are usually two stomas (openings), one to discharge waste and the other only mucus, and when the injured parts have healed the openings are closed. In a *permanent colostomy,* usually part of the colon and all of the rectum are removed, and the end portion of the remaining colon is brought through the abdominal wall to form a single stoma. A newer technique for this major surgery involves, when possible, fashioning an internal reservoir or pouch in the remaining portion of bowel, allowing the patient to defecate normally instead of through an artificial opening in the abdomen.

Colostomies are performed in different parts of the colon, depending on where it is diseased, and are generally named for the relevant portion. A *sigmoid colostomy* is an opening in the upper end of the sigmoid colon. In a *descending colostomy* the opening is somewhat higher, in the descending colon. Most colostomies are in the sigmoid or descending colon, and stomas for either type are on the left side of the abdomen. Sigmoid colostomies usually are permanent. Evacuation of fecal matter is often controlled by irrigation, that is, periodic enemas, so that no collection appliance is needed. A *transverse colostomy* is an opening in the transverse colon, and the stoma is located on the upper abdomen, in the middle of the right side. Evacuation sometimes can be controlled by irrigation, but more often an appliance (bag) is used to collect fecal matter. A transverse colostomy is usually a temporary procedure, with two stomas. Occasionally, however, it is an end colostomy with a single opening, with most or all of the colon beyond removed. For the operation's effect on a woman's reproductive and sexual functioning, see OSTOMY.

colostrum   See LACTATION.

colposcopy   A technique for examining the cervix and vagina with a *colposcope,* a low-power microscope that has a strong light source with a green filter. It is generally undertaken when a PAP SMEAR had indicated areas of abnormal cells in order to locate and identify the area of abnormal structure, but it also can be used to examine external sores or other abnormalities on the vulva or to help determine the reasons for pain or bleeding caused by intercourse. The colposcope magnifies the cervix 6 to 40 times, enabling a view of the area where squamous epithelial cells join columnar epithelial cells on the face of the cervix (see CERVICAL EVERSION for further explanation), called the *transformation zone,* and also showing the pattern of blood vessels and white patches. These areas—the transformation zone, white patches and blood vessels—can indicate precancerous changes and the

actual presence of cancer. If any area viewed looks suspicious, a biopsy (tissue sample) can be taken and examined in the laboratory with the assurance that the specimen actually comes from the most abnormal area. If abnormalities extend upward into the cervical canal where they cannot be seen, even when using a tiny speculum to dilate the cervix, the clinician may recommend further investigation, either endocervical curettage (scraping tissue from inside the cervical canal) or possibly CONIZATION. Colposcopy is quite painless (the instrument does not actually touch the body). The physician inserts a speculum into the vagina, washes the vagina with acetic acid to reveal any abnormal areas and positions the colposcope in front of the vagina. The entire process takes 15 to 20 minutes. Regular colposcopic exams are recommended for DES daughters (see DIETHYLSTILBESTROL).

colpotomy   See CULDOSCOPY.

compression fracture   Also CRUSH FRACTURE. A bone that is broken by compression, that is, simple pressure without severe injury of any kind. It most commonly occurs as a complication of OSTEOPOROSIS in the weight-bearing vertebrae of the spine. The pain is usually acute, as with any other fracture, and is aggravated by weight-bearing (any upright position). There may be local tenderness as well. Usually the pain subsides in a few days or weeks. Persons with numerous compression fractures of the vertebrae may develop exaggerated curvatures of the spine (see DOWAGER'S HUMP), may lose several inches of height and may experience chronic, dull, aching back pain. For acute severe back pain caused by a compression fracture, treatment includes use of an orthopedic support, analgesics and, if there is muscle spasm, heat and massage.

compulsive overeating   See OBESITY.

conception   See FERTILIZATION.

condom   Also PROPHYLACTIC, RUBBER, SAFE. A delicate sheath, usually made of rubber (latex), that is used to cover the penis during sexual intercourse, preventing the sperm that are ejaculated from entering the vagina. The oldest and most common form of barrier MALE CONTRACEPTIVE, it still is widely used for BIRTH CONTROL. It also reduces the spread of sexually transmitted diseases, such as gonorrhea, syphilis, herpes, and condyloma acuminata (genital warts; see also SEXUALLY TRANSMITTED DISEASE), and, used with spermicide, is considered an important form of protection against HIV infection (the cause of AIDS). A condom is placed on the penis while it is erect but before it comes in contact with even the woman's external genitals. In order to make sure the device does not break, about half an inch of empty air space should be left at the tip in order to allow enough room to hold the ejaculated seminal fluid. (Some condoms are made with nipple-shaped tips to hold the ejaculate.) After ejaculation the man or his partner must hold the condom rim firmly against the base of the penis as he slowly withdraws his still-erect penis, taking care not to spill any seminal fluid on the woman's external genitals. For lubrication, either water-soluble jelly or saliva can be used; petroleum jelly (Vaseline) should be avoided because it makes the rubber of the condom break down. Prelubricated condoms also are available. Condoms are readily obtainable in drugstores without prescription, as well as from vending machines. A condom can be stored in its package up to two years before use but should not be kept in a warm, moist place (such as a wallet or pocket), because heat makes it disintegrate.

A condom should be used for only a single act of intercourse. Should it tear or break while the man is withdrawing, the woman should immediately insert contraceptive foam or jelly in order to be protected (see SPERMICIDE). She should avoid douching, which might serve to spread the sperm. Used alone, a condom is in practice 86% effective in preventing pregnancy; if the woman also uses foam at the same time, it is slightly more effective. There are no side effects from using condoms for either man or woman. Their only disadvantage is that there is some interruption in lovemaking while the condom is put on, and some men believe they lessen penile sensation.

Most condoms are made of latex rubber and currently one brand of synthetic material is available for those allergic to latex. Early condoms were made from animal intestines (most often sheep cecum). Some condoms of this material are still available, but there is no advantage in using them. They are more expensive, and some authorities maintain that the manufacturing standards for them are less well defined than those for rubber condoms, so that they may be less reliable. All condoms carry an expiration date, mandated by the U.S. Food and Drug Administration. Most nonspermicide models are good for five years, and spermicide models for two to three years.

Today there is little difference in designs of condom. Most are 7½ inches (18¾ centimeters) long, and the open end has a wider ring of stronger latex to help keep it in place. Some brands come in different colors or with ribbing. Most condoms are prerolled and lubricated. When they are not, they should be rolled up just before use and then unrolled onto the erect penis up to its base. Air should be expelled from the tip before the condom is rolled on. Using two condoms at one time is *not* recommended, since the friction between them could cause them to tear.

The consistent use of condoms protects against transmitting the HUMAN PAPILLOMA VIRUS (HPV), a cause of genital warts, cervical cancers and other sexually transmitted infections. Indeed, the AIDS crisis is believed to have greatly increased the use of condoms, which are considered the best available protection against infection. It also led to the development of several kinds of *female condom,* devices that line the vagina and extend over the labia. The first kind to win approval from the U.S. Food and Drug Administration (1992), marketed as the Reality Vaginal Pouch, consists of a soft, loose-fitting polyurethane sheath mounted on two flexible rings; the inner ring at the closed end covers the cervix and the second ring remains outside the vagina. Because it covers a larger area—it is about 7 inches (17½ centimeters) long—this type of condom may provide better protection against sexually transmitted diseases than either the diaphragm or the cervical cap. It comes prelubricated and may be inserted up to eight hours before intercourse. The failure rate of the female condom is 21%, considerably higher than for the diaphragm or male condom, but this initial high finding may reflect relative inexperience. To insert the female condom, squeeze the inner ring and place inside the vagina past the pubic bone, so that the inner ring covers the cervix. If the sheath is not twisted (one can check with one's finger), it will create a completely covered passage for the man's penis. The female condom is sold over the counter, without a prescription, and can be used for only a single episode of intercourse. At least two potential female condoms are currently being tested. Made of latex and prelubricated, one kind is pushed into the vagina by the male partner at the time of intercourse. Possible disadvantages are the potential for latex allergy and for dislodgement.

conduction anesthesia   See REGIONAL ANESTHESIA.

condyloma acuminata   Also *genital human papilloma virus (HPV), genital warts, venereal warts.* A virus infection that causes small benign tumors to grow around the moist folds of the vulva and inside the vagina in women and on the shaft of the penis in men (sometimes also around the anus in both sexes). They are caused by several types of *human papilloma virus (HPV)*—they were the first tumor in human beings definitely known to be caused by a virus—that are usually transmitted by sexual contact. The virus is transmitted, it is believed, through sexual intercourse, whether heterosexual or homosexual, by direct skin-to-skin contact. Poor hygiene is also a contributing factor. The virus has a long incubation period, so the warts may not appear until one to six months after one has been exposed to them. Moreover, only an estimated 10% of those exposed ever developed the warts; the virus often remains asymptomatic.

The warts begin as tiny, discrete, pinkish or tan growths about the size of a rice grain, either singly or in clusters (looking somewhat like cauliflower), and they grow rapidly. They sometimes itch, and scratching helps spread them. Often, however, the warts are too small to be readily seen or are hidden too deeply in the genital tract to be noticed. The standard screening test for women is the PAP SMEAR. Sometimes the warts can be revealed by applying a vinegar solution, which turns them white and makes them visible through a magnifying instrument. Because the warts resemble a cancerous growth, and because they frequently have been found in women with cervical cancer, in which they are thought to play a contributing role, a biopsy (see BIOPSY, def. 6) may be taken to establish diagnosis.

Treatment for small warts consists of applying podophyllin or trichloroacetic acid to them two or three times at weekly intervals, taking extreme care to avoid touching the surrounding healthy tissue, and washing off the medication after six to eight hours. If the warts are large or the patient is pregnant, cryosurgery (freezing), cauterization (burning), laser surgery or surgical excision is preferable; the warts are limited to the superficial layers of the skin and can be removed readily in this way. (Pregnant women must avoid podophyllin because it can damage the fetus if applied inside the vagina.) In 1988 the U.S. Food and Drug Administration approved the use of alpha-interferon to treat genital warts. Injections into the warts three times a week for three weeks eliminate warts in about half of all patients and reduce symptoms in another 25%. The treatment is less painful than surgery, cryosurgery or cautery, and unlike those procedures it causes no scarring. However, alpha-interferon must be avoided by pregnant women, and it may give rise to side effects that consist of flulike symptoms. Intramuscular injection of interferon B also appears to be effective but has not yet been approved in the United States.

Even if treatment eliminates the warts, they tend to recur, and treatment then must be resumed. The sexual partner, too, should be examined to avoid a cycle of reinfection; use of a condom can help prevent their spread. Oral contraceptives and pregnancy both appear to stimulate the growth and spread of warts. No treatment currently available is known to eliminate the virus from the body. Because the virus is associated with cervical cancer (some say the virus is associated with 90% of all cervical cancers) and cancers of the vulva, vagina and anus, careful follow-up with lab tests of cervical tissue or colposcopy at yearly intervals may be necessary.

A vaccine against four types of HPV (HPV-6, HPV-11, HPV-16, HPV-18) was approved in 2006, including two that cause genital warts. For more information see under CANCER, CERVICAL; HERPES; HUMAN PAPILLOMA VIRUS. See also SEXUALLY TRANSMITTED DISEASE.

cone biopsy   See CONIZATION.

congenital abnormalities (defects)   See BIRTH DEFECTS.

congenital infection   An infection present in a baby at birth, having been acquired from the mother before or during delivery. It is caused by an organism transmitted to the fetus across the placenta or to the baby as it passed through the birth canal. Various infectious diseases, notably rubella and chicken pox, can be transmitted to a baby in this way, and even when they are mild in the mother they can be very serious—sometimes fatal—in the infant. Venereal diseases such as HERPES INFECTION and AIDS also can be transmitted to a baby as it passes through the birth canal. In addition to such infections, a baby can be born addicted to an opiate such as heroin or cocaine, or to alcohol, and suffer withdrawal symptoms when the source of supply—the mother's body—is removed.
    See ALCOHOL USE; BIRTH DEFECTS; DRUG USE AND PREGNANCY.

congestive   Referring to an abnormal accumulation of blood in the body's tissues. In *pelvic congestion syndrome*, a catchall term for a combination of symptoms including painful menstruation, lower abdominal and lower back pain and other pelvic discomfort, the term "congestion" refers to engorgement of the blood vessels of the pelvis.
    See also DYSMENORRHEA, def. 5.

congestive heart failure   A disorder in which the pumping action of the heart is inadequate, so that blood flow is reduced, leading to congestion of blood in the lungs and veins. Although it can occur at any age, it is most common after the age of 65, when such causes as hypertension (high blood pressure) and coronary artery disease are more common (see ARTERIOSCLEROSIS). There are two kinds of heart failure, *systolic,* when the heart doesn't pump adequately, and *diastolic,* when the heart does not relax adequately. More women than men have diastolic heart failure, although some have both kinds. In most cases, symptoms develop slowly over days or months. Symptoms include fluid accumulation and swelling in the feet, ankles, legs and abdomen or shortness of breath during exertion. Often all these symptoms are present. In addition, patients feel tired and weak during physical activity. Diagnosis often can be based on these symptoms, verified by chest X-ray, electrocardiogram and sometimes other procedures. Treatment, in addition to correcting physical heart problems such as a leaking valve or coronary artery blockage, involves various drugs, among them diuretics to eliminate excess fluid and, especially, angiotensin-converting enzyme (ACE) inhibitors, which cause blood vessels to dilate and decrease the amount of work the heart must do. Other drugs that may be used are beta-blockers, to help the heart's ability to relax and lower blood pressure, and digoxin, which strengthens heart contractions. An important dietary measure is lowering salt intake, to less than two grams of sodium (less than two teaspoons) a day.
    See also HYPERTENSION.

conization   Also *cone biopsy.* The surgical removal of a cone-shaped piece of tissue from the cylindrical cervix. Formerly used principally as a diagnostic tool to make sure abnormal tissue was not actually cancerous, conization today is used more cautiously, since COLPOSCOPY for a directed biopsy usually affords an adequate diagnosis. Conization requires regional or general anesthesia and therefore nearly always is performed in a hospital. The surgeon cuts a cone-shaped wedge out of the cervix, removing the upper portion of the cervical canal along with the entire outer surface of the cervix. After the center cone is removed, the cut edges of the cervix are sutured (stitched).
    Conization is a major surgical procedure, with the risk of several complications. Of these, the most common is heavy bleeding, during or immediately after surgery, or even a week or two later, when the stitches are absorbed. Hemorrhage may require further treatment (transfusion and/or other surgery). Less common complications are perforation of the uterus and infection. Long-term complications include cervical incompetence (see INCOMPETENT

CERVIX), leading to miscarriage in future pregnancies; infertility, owing to inadequate cervical mucus production (the portion of cervix removed contains a substantial number of mucus-producing glands); and narrowing or stenosis of the cervical canal by scar tissue, which can interfere with later delivery or even, in the case of blockage, trap menstrual flow. For these reasons colposcopy is now performed instead of conization whenever possible. The American Cancer Society recommends the following indications for performing a diagnostic conization: (1) persistent abnormal Pap smear and colposcopically directed biopsies that have not confirmed abnormal cell findings; (2) inability to view the entire transformation zone (where cells have changed from normal to suspicious) because it extends up into the endocervical canal; (3) positive findings on endocervical curettage; or (4) microinvasion (the beginnings of cancer cells). A newer technique, LOOP ELECTROSURGICAL EXCISION PROCEDURE, may be a less risky alternative.

See also BIOPSY, def. 7.

constipation Infrequent or difficult bowel movements (elimination of feces and/or hard stools), defined as needing to strain more than 25% of the time. Contrary to earlier thought, a daily bowel movement is not essential to good health. Although regular evacuation of feces is important, what is regular for one person is not for another; some individuals normally have three bowel movements a day while others have one every three or four days. Occasional constipation usually presents no great problem, nor does the occasional use of a mild laxative. It is only when constipation becomes chronic, so that a person becomes largely or wholly dependent on laxatives, that serious disease needs to be ruled out. Organic causes of constipation include an intestinal obstruction, a tumor, anal fissures, hemorrhoids, diabetes, diverticulitis or some other gastrointestinal disorder, or rectocele, and usually can be readily diagnosed. Most constipation, however, is functional, due to a mistaken belief that a daily movement is essential; to an inactive colon (especially in the elderly, the bedridden or a younger laxative-dependent person); or to social and emotional factors, such as irregular eating habits, inadequate exercise, overly demanding schedules or too little fiber or liquid in the diet.

Some women regularly have trouble with constipation during pregnancy, especially during the later months, when the enlarged uterus presses on the descending colon. Others experience it monthly during the few days preceding a menstrual period (see DYSMENORRHEA, def. 5), and still others are troubled with it during the menopausal years, suggesting that changing hormone levels may affect the muscle tone of the intestinal tract. For the most part, functional constipation is best treated with regular exercise, a diet high in fiber (whole grains, nuts, fresh fruit, raw vegetables) and drinking plenty of water. Some medications cause constipation, among them oral contraceptives, iron, diuretics, various heart drugs, some antacid preparations and narcotics such as codeine. Many experts believe that adding 15 to 20 grams (½ to ¾ ounce) of fiber to the daily diet (the amount in two servings of a high-fiber bran cereal) should maintain regularity. Some believe that rhubarb, although not a source of fiber, is a natural laxative (cook and puree three stalks of rhubarb, and add 1 cup of apple juice, a quarter of a peeled lemon, and 1 tablespoon of honey). If proper diet and adequate exercise do not relieve constipation, a bulk-forming laxative (usually a seed preparation with psyllium or cellulose that creates a softer, bulkier stool) or a stool softener such as docusate may help. There are numerous over-the-counter laxatives, some of them based on herbs such as cascara. Various HERBAL REMEDIES for constipation range from mild (licorice root, or *Glycyrrhiza lepidota*) to quite strong (senna pods, or *Cassis acutifolia*). Dependence on these, however, is no more desirable than dependence on an inorganic laxative, and they should definitely be avoided during pregnancy.

contact dermatitis An inflammation of the skin resulting from contact with irritating agents or substances. Any part of the skin may be involved. For contact dermatitis of the genital area, see under VULVITIS.

contraceptive Any device, substance or method used to prevent pregnancy. These include abstaining from intercourse, either entirely (celibacy) or during a woman's fertile period (after ovulation; see NATURAL FAMILY PLANNING); withdrawing the penis from the vagina before ejaculation (see COITUS INTERRUPTUS); breast-feeding a baby, which temporarily delays ovulation (but note that one never knows for how long until after menstruation has resumed, indicating ovulation did occur); destroying sperm or making them inactive (see SPERMICIDE; THERMATIC STERILIZATION; ULTRASOUND, def. 2); imposing a physical and/or chemical barrier to prevent the passage of sperm through the cervix (see CERVICAL CAP; CONDOM; CONTRACEPTIVE SPONGE; DIAPHRAGM); flushing sperm out of the vagina after intercourse (see DOUCHING); making the uterine lining unreceptive to a fertilized egg (see INTRAUTERINE DEVICE); suppressing ovulation and/or sperm production by means of hormone medications (see ORAL CONTRACEPTIVE; MALE CONTRACEPTIVE; PROGESTIN) or by STERILIZATION; preventing preparation of the uterus for an embryo (see CONTRAGESTIVE); and terminating pregnancy (ABORTION). Their effectiveness varies widely, from virtually 0% (douching) to nearly 100% (sterilization, abortion). See also the accompanying table.

Safety and freedom from side effects also vary. The diaphragm, cervical cap, contraceptive sponge and condom are considered freest of risk to the user (other than accidental pregnancy) and oral contraceptives, inserted implants (Implanon) and intrauterine devices (IUDs) carry the highest risk of side effects. For safety from unwanted pregnancy the ratings are exactly the reverse; oral contraceptives and implants have the lowest failure rate (2 and 1% respectively), followed by IUDs (4.2%) and then all other forms.

Two newer oral contraceptives limit the number of periods a woman experiences. Seasonique or Seasonale, prescribed in a three-month package, limits periods to four per year. For the first 84 days the pills contain both progestin and estrogen; for the last seven days they contain estrogen only. Side effects may include breakthrough bleeding and spotting, weight gain, and acne. The second kind, approved by the FDA in 2007, is Lybrel, which will stop periods for as long as it is taken.

One implant method uses capsules of long-acting progesterone, surgically implanted under the

ESTIMATED EFFECTIVENESS OF COMMON CONTRACEPTIVES

Method	Theoretical Effectiveness*	Practical Effectiveness*
Abortion	100%	100%
Cervical cap with spermicide		
women who have had children	74%	60%
women who have had no children	91%	80%
Coitus interruptus (withdrawal)	96%	81%
Condom		
male	97%	86%
female	95%	79%
Contraceptive sponge	91%	80%
Diaphragm with spermicide	94%	80%
Douche	?	50%?
Hysterectomy	100%	100%
Implant (Implanon)	99.5%	99.5%
Intrauterine device (IUD)		
copper	99%	99%
progesterone	98.5%	98.5%
NuvaRing	98%	98%
Oral contraceptive, combination-type pill	99.66%	99.66%
progesterone alone	99.5%	99.5%
Spermicide alone (foam, jelly, vaginal suppository)	93%	74%
Tubal ligation	99.5%	99.5%
Vaccine (Depo-Provera), every three months	99+%	99+%
Vasectomy	99.5%	99.5%

*Theocretical effectiveness is the effectiveness when the method is used without error and exactly according to instructions; practical effectiveness takes into consideration all the users of a method—those who use it correctly (and perfectly) and those who are careless.

skin, that slowly release a hormone blocking ovulation. The brand Norplant, approved in 1989, consists of six matchstick-size capsules containing the hormone levonorgestrel, which are placed under the skin of the woman's forearm. The contraceptive is released into the bloodstream for five years.

However, difficulties with removal and some suspicion as to effectiveness caused the discontinuance of Norplant in the United States in 2002, although women already using it were not told to remove it. A newer form of implant, Implanon, using only one rod and a custom-made, disposable inserter to ease insertion and removal, recently became available. It uses a slightly different form of progestin and is intended to be removed after three years. Another method is an injected vaccine. One kind, DEPO-PROVERA, injects synthetic progesterone every three months, preventing ovulation. Another was Lunelle, a monthly injectable combination of low-dosage estrogen and progestin that also was recalled in 2002. Newer contraceptives now being investigated are a contraceptive ring (NuvaRing), a clear plastic hoop inserted like a tampon, which slowly releases low levels of estrogen for three weeks and then is removed and discarded to permit menstruation (a new ring is inserted on or before day 5 of the menstrual period); a five-year intrauterine device, Mirena, that contains only progestin and limits or entirely eliminates menstrual bleeding; a hormone skin patch, Ortho Evra, applied weekly for three weeks and left off for a fourth week, which can be worn on the buttocks, abdomen, upper torso or upper outer arm (it stays on through swimming or bathing). However, a consumer advocacy group has urged the FDA to take Ortho Evra off the market because several studies have shown that women who used it have twice the risk of blood clots in the legs and lungs as women who take the pill. The reason is that up to 60% more estrogen is absorbed from the patch than from the pill, and, indeed, the patch's label bears warnings about clots. Most contraceptive devices are available only by prescription, the principal exception being some barrier methods (spermicidal cream, jelly, foam and condoms).

Like most medications, contraceptives are not without side effects. Depo-Provera has been associated with altered menstrual bleeding, bone loss, mood disorders and a delay in the return of fertility. The patch delivers more estrogen than a pill and is most effective in women weighing less than 200 pounds, but it may raise the risk of blood clots in the legs and lungs. Mirena can cause breakthrough bleeding during the first three months and

increased rates of acne, dizziness, headache, breast tenderness and weight gain, symptoms associated with most hormonal contraceptives.

Various plants and herbs have been used since ancient times as contraceptives, emmenagogues and abortifacients. Hippocrates wrote that the seeds of Queen Anne's lace or wild carrot (*Daucus carota*) are contraceptive and also induce abortion; modern studies indicate that they block progesterone production. Pennyroyal or squaw mint (*Mentha pulegium*) was also so used in ancient times and is still occasionally used today in Appalachia; it contains pulegone, a chemical that terminates pregnancy but also is toxic to the liver. All the cautions that apply to HERBAL REMEDIES must similarly be observed with contraceptive use.

See also BIRTH CONTROL; EMERGENCY CONTRACEPTION; MALE CONTRACEPTIVE.

contraceptive implant See CONTRACEPTIVE; PROGESTERONE.

contraceptive sponge   A soft, disposable polyurethane foam body, about 2 inches (5 centimeters) around, with a small depression in the center of one side to fit over the cervix and a loop of tape to grasp for removing. It comes presoaked with spermicide and, inserted into the vagina, acts as a contraceptive by killing sperm, trapping sperm and blocking the cervix. Introduced in the United States in 1983 as the Today brand, it was no longer available after 1995 owing to manufacturing problems but continued to be sold in Canada; it returned to the U.S. market in 2005. A newer sponge, called Protectaid, is available in Canada by prescription and is expected to become available in the United States within two or three years. It contains three different spermicides that may have antiviral properties as well.

The sponge is moistened with tap water and inserted. Unlike the DIAPHRAGM, the sponge may be left in place for 24 hours without reapplying more spermicide for additional acts of intercourse during that period. However, it should be left in place for at least six hours after intercourse. Critics of the sponge report a variety of problems: difficulty in removal; disintegration of the sponge, possibly with fragments being retained in the vagina; vaginal soreness; inflammation of the cervix; and a higher failure rate than is admitted. The contraceptive sponge occasionally gives rise to an allergic reaction, and it should not be used by women who have had toxic shock syndrome (see TAMPON), or during a menstrual period, when risk of infection is greater. Also, it affords no protection against sexually transmitted diseases or AIDS.

contraction, uterine   Also *labor pain, pain.* The temporary shortening of the muscle fibers of the UTERUS, which occurs involuntarily during labor and serves to push the baby down through the birth canal. The uterine muscles actually begin to contract periodically early in pregnancy, but these contractions usually are perceived only in the ninth month or so and are painless (see BRAXTON-HICKS CONTRACTIONS). When labor begins, the contractions become regular. During the first stage of LABOR they are short, mild and separated by intervals of 10 to 20 minutes. Often they are first felt as discomfort in the small of the back, but soon they begin to be felt in the lower abdomen as well. The contractions gradually recur at shorter intervals and become stronger and longer in duration. As the cervix dilates to about 4 to 7 centimeters (1.6 to 2.8 inches), they last approximately 60 seconds and occur every four to eight minutes. At the end of the first stage of labor, or with 7 to 10 centimeters' (2.8 to 4 inches') dilation, they may last as long as 1½ minutes, with intervals as short as 30 seconds between contractions. After the cervix is fully dilated, during the second stage of labor (the expulsion of the baby), contractions continue to last fairly long (50 to 100 seconds) and occur at intervals of 2 to 3 minutes. At this point the muscles of the abdomen are brought into play, and most women (if anesthesia does not prevent it) feel an urge to strain or bear down strenuously and thus assist the uterus in expelling the baby. Following delivery, there may be a few minutes' wait; then uterine contractions resume at regular intervals until the PLACENTA separates from the uterine wall and is expelled. After delivery of the placenta, the attending clinician usually massages

the woman's abdomen at regular intervals to make sure the uterus continues to contract. If it does not, there is danger of excessive bleeding (see POSTPARTUM HEMORRHAGE). Thereafter the uterus continues to contract periodically, the contractions sometimes giving rise to somewhat painful sensations called *afterpains.* In some women these are severe enough to require mild analgesics and may last for a number of days. They are particularly noticeable when the baby is put to the breast, probably because of the release of oxytocin (see LACTATION for further explanation). Usually, however, they decrease in intensity and become quite mild within 48 hours after delivery. The afterpains further reduce the uterus to its former prepregnant size and also help stop bleeding.

Uterine contractions are involuntary. They occur in laboring women who receive a regional anesthetic, such as CAUDAL or EPIDURAL ANESTHESIA, as well as in women who have no control over other muscles in their pelvis, such as paraplegics. They occur not only in labor but sometimes during menstruation (cramps; see DYSMENORRHEA, def. 4) and, in much milder form, during ORGASM. Why strong contractions hurt is not known; some authorities believe the pain comes from the stretching of the cervix and perineum, others that it comes from hypoxia (oxygen lack) in the contracted muscles and still others that it comes from the compression of nerves in the pelvis.

See also ANESTHESIA, def. 2.

contragestive   Also *contragestant, abortion pill.* A substance called *mifepristone,* or *RU-486,* which was developed by Dr. Etienne Baulieu and the Roussel-Uclaf company. The contragestive blocks progesterone receptors in the endometrium (uterine lining), preventing its buildup by progesterone; hence the uterus cannot sustain a pregnancy. It does not prevent fertilization or implantation, so technically it is an ABORTIFACIENT rather than a contraceptive. Administered orally, intravaginally or by injection, it prevents gestation, that is, the maintenance of a pregnancy.

RU-486 can induce abortion of an early known pregnancy or, taken every month close to the time of an expected menstrual period, it can be used as birth control. In early pregnancy (the first two months) it causes abortion in about 95% of cases, tending to be more effective if followed in 48 to 72 hours by a prostaglandin such as misoprostol given orally, by suppository or injected. The prostaglandin strengthens contractions. Expulsion occurs in about four hours. Potential side effects include dizziness, nausea, heavy or prolonged bleeding and severe cramps. It should not be used by women older than 35 or by heavy smokers. In any case, it is important to return to one's healthcare provider 14 days later to make sure the pregnancy was ended and there are no complications. When the procedure fails (as it does in about 2% of cases), a vacuum abortion or D and C should be performed.

In 1989 the Roussel-Uclaf company, which markets RU-486 under the name mifepristone, decided to distribute it only in France for about a year and later market it only in countries where abortion is legal, medical facilities are adequate and distribution can be tightly controlled to prevent a black market. It was widely used in France, China, Great Britain and Sweden, but owing to pressure from antiabortion groups, the only manufacturer, Hoechst AG of Germany, closed its plant in 1997. In that year a French company, Exelgyn, obtained rights to RU-486 and made it available in small quantities. They later signed American rights over to the Population Council. In the United States, opposition by antiabortion groups delayed its approval, even though the Food and Drug Administration had deemed it safe and effective in 1996. Final approval was vigorously sought not only by feminist groups but by those eager to use it to treat breast cancer (trials are still under way), meningioma (a brain tumor) and CUSHING'S DISEASE (where it has been effective), and possibly also endometriosis and fibroids. All these conditions appear to be aided by RU-486's progesterone-blocking action. It was finally approved in 2000. A large study published in 2007 showed that medical abortion (use of the contragestive) results in no more risk of subsequent miscarriage, ectopic pregnancy, premature births or low birth weight than surgical abortion (vacuum abortion or D and C).

Misoprostol, a drug approved for ulcer therapy, also can be used alone to induce abortion, though it is more effective in conjunction with methotrexate (a cancer drug). These are available in the United States but take longer to work than RU-486, up to two weeks.

contraindication Any condition that makes a particular treatment or procedure undesirable. An *absolute contraindication* means that the treatment is hazardous to the patient and should not be used; a *relative contraindication* means that the risks must be weighed carefully against the benefits before undertaking the treatment. For example, a history of cardiovascular disease (blood clots, heart attack, stroke) is an absolute contraindication for taking oral contraceptives; a history of diabetes or gallbladder disease is a relative contraindication to oral contraceptives. Similarly, pregnancy is an absolute contraindication to the insertion of an intrauterine device (IUD); a history of severe anemia is a relative contraindication, because the IUD makes many women bleed more heavily.

coronary artery disease Also CAD.
See ARTERIOSCLEROSIS.

corpus luteum The structure formed from a ruptured GRAAFIAN FOLLICLE after ovulation. The term is Latin for "yellow body," the "yellow" referring to a pigmented substance called *lutein* that accumulates inside the ruptured follicle, and "body" referring to the rearrangement of follicle cells into a cluster. In the course of the MENSTRUAL CYCLE, the follicle produces both estrogen and, under the influence of luteinizing hormone (LH), progesterone. If the released egg is not fertilized, the levels of estrogen and progesterone gradually drop, and in time the corpus luteum disintegrates into a tiny speck of scar tissue. Sometimes, however, the corpus luteum does not shrink but remains abnormally large. It then constitutes a cyst, called a *corpus luteum cyst,* which is especially common in the early weeks of pregnancy and which secretes progesterone (see also CYST, def. 6).

If the egg is fertilized and a pregnancy is established, the corpus luteum continues to be maintained, not by LH but by the hormone of pregnancy, human chorionic gonadotropin (HCG), which begins to be produced by the placenta soon after fertilization. Six to eight weeks later, when the placenta has developed sufficiently to produce high enough levels of progesterone and estrogen, luteal function gradually dwindles and the corpus luteum disintegrates.

cosmetics   Also *makeup*. General name for products that are designed to improve the appearance of the face, skin, eyes, hair and other features but are not absorbed in amounts significant enough to alter body functions. Lipstick, nail polish, mascara, eye shadow, perfume, hair dye, powders and lotions generally and harmless but occasionally can cause health problems. The most common is an allergic reaction (marked by itching, swelling, tearing of the eyes and/or rash), usually but not always caused by the perfume in the product. So-called *hypoallergenic cosmetics* are virtually odorless. Some face makeup aggravates acne, and some hair dyes and tints contain aniline, a common allergen; also, long-term use of black hair dye (more than 20 years) has been associated with the development of some cancers. Mascara that does not contain sufficient preservatives may contain bacteria that, if they come in contact with the eyes, can cause serious infection and even permanent eye damage.

Occasionally manufacturers have added estrogen to cosmetics on the theory that it prevents signs of aging, such as wrinkles. There is no evidence that it does; moreover, estrogen can be absorbed through the skin, possibly leading to side effects.

See also DEODORANT.

cosmetic surgery   General name for surgical procedures that are undertaken solely to improve one's appearance rather than to correct any disorder. Included are face lifts to minimize the appearance of wrinkles, changing the shape of the nose, removing acne or other scars by dermabrasion or laser resurfacing, reducing or increasing breast size (see MAMMAPLASTY), as well as *liposuction* and other procedures to slenderize the abdomen, thighs or buttocks. A popular procedure is *blepharoplasty*, a surgical eyelid lift that tightens the skin of drooping or hooded eyelids; it can be performed on the upper or lower eyelids, or both, usually on an outpatient basis, with full recovery taking two to eight weeks. A less invasive procedure is the endoscopic brow lift, which raises the brow, lessens wrinkles on the forehead and around the eyes, and eliminates sagging lids. Still another procedure is the cheek lift, which repositions the cheek's fat pad and reduces the appearance of deep smile lines between the nose and corners of the mouth. There is less experience with either procedure concerning how long it lasts and for whom it is most appropriate.

Unlike weight loss due to diet and exercise, fat reduction from liposuction does not reduce the risk of diabetes, high blood pressure or high cholesterol, and in fact has no health benefits whatever. However, it not only removes fat tissue from certain parts of the body but does so permanently, sucking it out through a cannula (narrow hollow tube) connected to a vacuum pump; once gone, fat cells will not be replaced. A newer technique, ultrasonic liposuction, uses a rapidly vibrating probe to liquefy the fat so that greater amounts can be removed. This technique is potentially harmful, since the probe also breaks up fibrous tissue and can liquefy the skin, causing both internal damage and scarring.

Cosmetic surgery is not without risk. The chances of death from complications from general anesthesia for a healthy woman are about 1 in 10,000, and postoperative infection is also possible. Other risks are permanent skin discoloration and scarring, severing of a facial nerve, hemorrhage, impaired vision and even blindness incurred during eyelid lifts, and blockage of a blood vessel in the heart or brain. Women who regularly take aspirin should stop a week before surgery, to avoid its interference with clotting. For women with a chronic illness such as diabetes, heart or kidney disease, or vascular disorder, the risk of complications increases, and recovery may be more difficult. Also, after face lifts heavy smokers may experience skin slough, the death of skin from inadequate blood supply.

If despite these risks one decides to undertake cosmetic surgery, which is generally considered elective and therefore not covered by insurance, it is best performed by a plastic surgeon, although any licensed physician (even one without surgical training) may perform it. It may be wise to determine if the surgeon is board certified, in plastic surgery or reconstructive surgery (by the American Society of Plastic and Reconstructive Surgeons) for liposuction, face lifts or repairing damages from accident or disease; in ophthalmology for eyelid surgery; in ear, nose and throat surgery for face lift or rhinoplasty (nose surgery); or in dermatology for wrinkle treatments such as collagen injections. Board certification means he or she has met certain requirements and standards for specialized training. (Note that the cosmetic surgery board is not a member of the American Board of Medical Specialties and therefore cannot be assumed to have the same standards.) Further, it may be wise to select a doctor with expertise in the particular procedure being considered.

Other questions to ask are how often the physician has performed the particular procedure and his or her complication rate; what risk there is of infection, and what is done to prevent it; and if any former patients are willing to talk about their experience. Since most such surgery is done on an outpatient basis, it also is wise to check on the facility where it is to be done. Is it accredited by the American Association for Accreditation of Ambulatory Surgery? Is there a certified nurse or anesthesiologist to provide monitoring throughout the procedure? Although most procedures do not require an overnight hospital stay, recovery may last a number of weeks. Furthermore, results are not guaranteed, and even in cases where the surgery is a technical success, the woman may not be pleased with the result.

A newer type of cosmetic surgery is the toxic facelift, which involves the injection of the botulin toxin or Botox (which causes botulism, a deadly food poisoning) into areas around the forehead and eyes as a means of temporarily smoothing frown lines, crow's-feet and furrowed brows. The toxin temporarily paralyzes facial muscles, preventing the contractions that help form lines and wrinkles. The skin smooths in two to three days and the effect lasts three to six months, after which the injections must be repeated. The procedure has side effects, ranging from pain, redness or bruising at the injection site, weakness of adjacent muscles, and loss of some facial expression. About 5% of patients treated on the upper face develop weakness and a drooping eyelid, eyebrow or brow. In the lower face, adverse effects include drooling, asymmetry, and repeatedly biting the inside of one's weakened cheek. Pregnant women should not receive Botox. Further, it is not useful for all patients, since not all wrinkles are caused by muscles; many result from lack of elasticity due to aging. As with all such surgery, one should seek out a dermatologist or plastic surgeon experienced with the technique.

Another technique for erasing wrinkles is injecting a wrinkle filler. Among them are hyaluronic acid gel and a collagen-based filler. They are injected into such sites as frown lines that run from nose to mouth. The effects are usually immediate and last three to six months for collagen and 6 to 12 months for hyaluronic acid gels. Side effects include pain, redness and swelling at the injection site, and occasional allergic reactions. Another option is laser surgery for erasing wrinkles, removing tattoos, eliminating birthmarks and spider veins and making similar dermatologic repairs. Different lasers are used, depending on the treatment, which is usually on an outpatient basis and is followed by some swelling and pain. Exposure to the sun must be avoided both before and after treatment. Recently the Food and Drug Administration approved a nonsurgical, noninvasive approach to tightening loose and sagging skin. Through radiofrequency technology, which heats the deeper layers of the skin and underlying tissue, collagen is contracted. No healing or downtime is required. Following the immediate procedure there is gradual collagen remodeling and visible tightening over two to six months. Called Thermage, it can be performed on all skin types except not in areas recently treated with fillers such as collagen. Also, the degree of improvement varies among patients and, because the procedure is still new, it is not predictable. With newer treatments it is especially important to select a doctor experienced with the procedure.

counseling See FEMINIST THERAPY; GENETIC COUNSELING; PREGNANCY COUNSELING; PSYCHOTHERAPY; SEX THERAPY.

crabs   See PUBIC LICE.

cramp   A sudden, painful contraction of a muscle or group of muscles. *Menstrual cramps* are uterine contractions like those of labor (labor pains) but both milder and less regular (see DYSMENORRHEA, def. 4). *Leg cramps* are common during pregnancy and childbirth. Often a pregnant woman will wake in the night to find the muscles of one calf or foot in painful spasm; it is best relieved by local massage, kneading the muscles until they relax, by lengthening the muscle by pointing the toes toward the head or by standing on the affected foot. Leg cramps also may occur during the second stage of labor, when the baby's head presses on the pelvic nerves; they can be relieved by massage.

C-reactive protein   See ARTERIOSCLEROSIS.

critical weight   The proportion of body fat tissue to lean tissue that appears to be necessary for both menarche (the first menstruation) and the maintenance of more or less regular menstrual cycles. Before the adolescent growth spurt that precedes menarche, most girls show a 5 to 1 ratio of lean to fat tissue; by menarche this ratio has changed to 3 to 1, or 24% fat and 76% lean, an increase in fat tissue of 125% in two to three years. The average critical weight at menarche in the United States currently is 103 pounds (47 kilograms); this may explain why plump girls tend to menstruate earlier than very slender ones.

The first year or two of menstrual cycles are usually ANOVULATORY (there is no ovulation). By the time OVULATION begins (at an average age of 15), fat tissue makes up 28% of the body composition. Many adolescent girls continue to gain weight during the two years following the growth spurt, for reasons not wholly understood.

Before the early 1970s many reasons were advanced for what triggers the onset of menstruation: climate, genes, education, height, weight, diet. An American physician, Rose Frisch, then suggested that critical weight was the necessary factor, but exactly how the higher proportion of fat tissue

stimulates hormone production is not completely understood. One theory is that metabolic changes signal the hypothalamus to begin producing the factors that trigger menstruation (see MENSTRUAL CYCLE). Whatever the mechanism, it also operates in girls with ANOREXIA NERVOSA (self-starvation) as well as in professional athletes and dancers, who, when their body makeup is less than about 15% fat (in some cases even below 22%), have either very irregular periods or none at all, but whose menses resume regularity when they gain weight.

cryosurgery   Also *cryotherapy*. Destroying abnormal cells by freezing. Cryosurgery is commonly used to treat various skin lesions, among them warts on the vulva (CONDYLOMA ACUMINATA), some precancerous lesions of the cervix (DYSPLASIA) and occasionally inflammation of the cervix (CERVICITIS). For these procedures many physicians prefer it to CAUTERIZATION (burning) because it is less painful, produces a more even level of tissue destruction and causes less scarring and narrowing of the cervical canal. It may also be used to remove benign breast tumors (see FIBROADENOMA).

Cryosurgery is performed with a hand-held metal-tipped instrument, a *cryoprobe,* connected to a tank of compressed nitrous oxide, carbon dioxide or Freon. When the compressed gas is released into the cryoprobe, it expands rapidly and produces intense cold, about 6 degrees Fahrenheit (−15 degrees Celsius). The metal tip of the instrument, cooled by conduction, is held to the affected area, such as the outer surface of the cervix, for two minutes or so, in order to freeze the tissue thoroughly. The procedure is virtually painless; the only sensations are a feeling of coldness and, sometimes, mild cramping. Like cauterization, cryosurgery can cause temporary swelling that narrows the cervical canal for a time as well as a profuse watery vaginal discharge that lasts for a few weeks. The flow at first is heavy enough to require using a pad (tampons should not be used). If the discharge smells, powdering the labia with cornstarch may eliminate odor. Cryosurgery should be performed soon after the end of a menstrual period so as to avoid contact with menstrual flow during the early stage of healing. Also, infection is more apt to occur near the time of ovulation or menstruation. Nothing should be placed inside the vagina for two weeks afterward, and tampons should not be used for six to eight weeks. An IUD usually need not be removed for cryosurgery on the cervix.

cryptomenorrhea See AMENORRHEA, def. 2.

cryptorchidism Also *undescended testes*. The incomplete or improper descent of one or both testes at birth, which occurs in approximately 8 of every 1,000 boys born. In some cases the testes descend spontaneously in the first year of life, so a diagnosis cannot be accurate before the age of one. In *total cryptorchidism* the testis remains within the abdominal cavity as a result of mechanical or hormonal abnormalities. In *incomplete descent* it lies within the inguinal canal but is obstructed by mechanical factors. In *hypermobile testes,* the most common such condition, the testes may lie within the scrotum sometimes (as during a hot bath) but then retract into the inguinal canal. In most cases of hypermobile testes descent will occur of its own accord before or during puberty. In the other kinds, however, surgical repair—preferably before the age of three or four—is indicated, with simultaneous repair of the inguinal hernia that often accompanies the condition. Delay beyond the age of five or six may impair sperm formation after puberty and be a cause of eventual infertility. If only one testicle is affected, fertility is not compromised, but it is still associated with a 20% increased risk of cancer developing in the normal testicle.

C section See CESAREAN SECTION.

cul-de-sac Also *Douglas cul-de-sac, rectouterine pouch*. A blind pouch that lies between the lower back portion of the vagina and the rectum. It is through the cul-de-sac that CULDOCENTESIS and CULDOSCOPY are performed.

culdocentesis Withdrawing fluid from the pelvic cavity by placing a needle through the vagina into the CUL-DE-SAC portion of the abdomen, behind the uterus, in order to determine the presence of blood. If nonclotting blood is withdrawn, there is a strong possibility of a ruptured ECTOPIC PREGNANCY, and further diagnostic procedures, such as CULDOSCOPY or LAPAROSCOPY, should follow. Culdocentesis can be performed in the office or in an outpatient clinic. Occasionally it is performed in cases of PELVIC INFLAMMATORY DISEASE in order to identify the infecting organism.

culdoscopy Also *colpotomy.* The insertion of a special instrument, a *culdoscope,* through a small incision in the vagina, just behind the cervix, into the CUL-DE-SAC, which enables visual examination of the pelvic organs and performance of TUBAL LIGATION. Through the culdoscope the fallopian tubes can be examined for any blockage that prevents conception or for the presence of a tubal pregnancy (see ECTOPIC PREGNANCY; also CULDOCENTESIS). By inserting instruments, each of the fallopian tubes can be pulled out through the incision, a portion of them removed and the cut ends ligated (tied), occluded or cauterized, rendering the woman sterile. This operation can be performed under local or general anesthesia and, because the incision is made through the vagina, leaves no visible scar. However, it is difficult to perform on women who have scarring or adhesions from previous surgery, pelvic infection or severe endometriosis. It carries a relatively high risk of postoperative infection and hemorrhage. Further, it is an awkward procedure because the patient must be placed on her knees, with her head down and her buttocks up toward the surgeon, a position difficult to maintain under either general or local anesthesia. Consequently, for purposes of sterilization culdoscopy has been largely replaced by other forms of tubal ligation, principally LAPAROSCOPY and MINILAPAROTOMY.

culture The growing of microorganisms, such as bacteria or living cells, in the laboratory, in a medium designed to encourage them to reproduce. Also, the product of such a procedure. Cultures are made from samples of sputum, urine, blood, spinal fluids, stools, and cells from the throat, vagina or other organs in order to determine what organism is causing an infection. Under favorable conditions the organism usually multiplies in a matter of hours or days and then can be readily identified, but cell cultures often take three to five weeks.

cunnilingus   Also *eating* (slang). A form of oral sexual intercourse in which a woman's partner uses his or her mouth (lips, tongue) to stimulate her genitals. Some authorities believe it should be avoided when a woman is in the advanced stage of pregnancy, at least in any form that might involve blowing air into her vagina, lest it cause an air embolism (potentially fatal).

See also FELLATIO; ORAL SEX.

curettage   Literally "scraping," referring to the removal of thin strands of tissue from the uterus or some other organ. The instrument used for this purpose is called a *curette* or *curet*.

See also BIOPSY, def. 8; D AND C; VACUUM ASPIRATION.

curvature of the spine   See SCOLIOSIS.

Cushing's syndrome   Also *Cushing syndrome*. A disorder of the adrenal glands that is characterized by overproduction of the hormone cortisol. Originally discovered in 1932 by Dr. Harvey Cushing, who believed it resulted from a pituitary tumor or other growth, it has been found to occur also in the absence of such a tumor but in the presence of an adrenal tumor or of malfunction of the hypothalamus. (When the cause lies in the pituitary, it is called *Cushing's disease*. This is a relatively rare condition affecting mostly young to middle-aged women.) Most often, however, it results from large doses of corticosteroid drugs taken over a long time to treat another illness, such as rheumatoid arthritis or asthma.

Cushing's syndrome occurs mostly in women of childbearing age. It is characterized by rapidly developing obesity affecting the face, neck and trunk. A moon face and a pad of fat between the shoulder blades producing a round-shouldered look are characteristic. Other symptoms are oligomenorrhea or amenorrhea (infrequent or no menstruation); hirsutism (excess body hair); acne; purplish striae (stretch marks) of the skin, especially on the abdomen; a tendency to bruise easily; hypertension (high blood pressure); fatigue; and weakness. Diagnosis is based on the presence of a large amount of corticoids in the urine. Treatment depends on whether the cause lies in the pituitary or the adrenals and usually involves radiation therapy to the pituitary, removal of tumors and/or removal of one or both adrenal glands (and subsequent cortisone replacement therapy for life). For those who develop Cushing's syndrome owing to excess steroid medication, dosages must be adjusted or an alternative remedy found. However, steroids should never be stopped abruptly but tapered off gradually to avoid sudden adrenal failure.

CVS   See CHORIONIC VILLUS SAMPLING.

cycle   See MENSTRUAL CYCLE; for the ovarian cycle, see OVULATION; for the cervical cycle, see CERVICAL MUCUS METHOD.

cyst   **1.** A small, fluid-filled sac of tissue that can develop in various parts of the body, including the breasts, ovaries and cervix as well as the skin. Some cysts contain semisolid material.

2. sebaceous cyst. A slow-growing tumor of the skin, frequently found on the scalp, ears, face, back, scrotum, vulva or breasts. It rarely causes discomfort unless it becomes infected, but then it may form an abscess. The treatment, if any is needed, consists of applying moist heat every few hours until it comes to a head and drains. It this is not effective, the cyst is drained, either through a small stabbing incision or, in the case of larger cysts, through surgical incision. An infected cyst generally requires the insertion of a drain for a week or so; thereafter the wall of the cyst must be removed if the cyst is not to recur.

3. Bartholin cyst. A cyst that develops when a duct of one of the BARTHOLIN'S GLANDS, located near the opening of the vagina, becomes blocked. If the cyst is small, no treatment is needed. However, if it is large or, as is often the case, it becomes infected, surgical treatment is indicated. Such infections can be extremely painful and the gland, normally tiny, can grow to the size of a lemon. Treatment usually involves oral antibiotics, applying hot compresses, and surgical incision and drainage. Among the organisms responsible for such infection is gonococcus, so a GONORRHEA culture also is necessary. Bartholin cysts tend to recur because scarring from one infection often creates new blockage of the gland's secretions. Then either the entire cyst has to be removed (*cystectomy*) or even the entire gland. Occasionally this can be avoided by *marsupialization*, in which, after the cyst is removed, the gland is so cut and stitched that a permanent opening (pouch) is created.

4. Nabothian cyst. Also *cervical cyst.* A cyst formed when one of the many mucus-producing glands that line the cervix becomes blocked. Nabothian cysts may occur singly or in groups and most often occur on the surface of the cervix. In size they usually grow no bigger than a small pea; they look like small, white pimplelike bumps on the surface of the cervix. Unless such cysts are associated with other irritation of the cervix, they usually cause no problem and require no treatment, but if they occur in conjunction with CERVICITIS they are treated in the same way, with cauterization or cryosurgery.

5. chocolate cyst. Also *endometrical cyst.* (See ENDOMETRIOSIS.)

6. ovarian cyst. A cyst that develops on the ovary. Ovarian cysts may occur at any age, singly or in numbers, on one or both ovaries. The cyst consists of a thin, transparent outer wall enclosing a center of clear fluids or jellylike material. Such cysts range in size from that of a raisin to that of a large orange. They may cause a feeling of fullness in the abdominal area or pain on vaginal intercourse. Often, however, there are no symptoms at all, and the cyst is discovered only during a gynecologic examination when the clinician finds one ovary is considerably enlarged. At that point it is important to rule out malignancy (see CANCER, OVARIAN), since ovarian cancers in their early stages also have no warning symptoms and can occur at any age.

Many ovarian cysts—some authorities say more than half—are *functional*, that is, they arise out of the normal functions of the ovary during the MENSTRUAL CYCLE. A cyst can form when a FOLLICLE has grown in preparation for ovulation but fails to rupture and release an egg; this type is called a *follicle cyst* or *follicular cyst*. Sometimes the structure formed from the follicle after ovulation, the CORPUS LUTEUM, fails to shrink and forms a cyst; this is called a *corpus luteum cyst*. If there is no severe pain or swelling, a clinician may decide to wait for one or two more menstrual cycles to be completed, during the course of which such functional cysts frequently disappear of their own accord. Sometimes this process is hastened by administering oral contraceptives for several months, which establishes a very regular menstrual cycle. (Women already taking oral contraceptives rarely develop ovarian cysts.)

A different kind of ovarian cyst found most often in younger women is a *dermoid cyst,* which contains particles of teeth, hair or calcium-containing tissue that are thought to be an embryologic remnant; such cysts usually do not cause menstrual irregularity. Ovarian cysts cause problems when they become very large, when they rupture and cause severe internal bleeding, or when their pedicle (a tail-like appendage) suddenly twists and cuts off their blood supply, creating severe pain. In these cases surgical treatment is indicated, preferably a *cystectomy,* which means removal of the cyst only and preservation of as much of the normal ovarian tissue as possible. Sometimes, with a very large cyst, the ovary cannot be saved and must be removed.

The diagnosis of an ovarian cyst is determined by the patient's age, medical and family history, symptoms and size of the enlarged ovary. In women under 30, clinicians usually will recommend waiting through one or two menstrual cycles to see if the ovary will return to its normal size. If it does not and pregnancy has been ruled out, an abdominal X-ray and/or sonograph (see ULTRASOUND, def. 1) can determine the exact size of the ovaries and distinguish between a cyst and a solid tumor. In older women (over 40) X-ray and sonograph may be done sooner and, if uncertainty still exists, the clinician may recommend LAPAROSCOPY to look at the ovaries through a small incision, or a larger incision and a biopsy.

See also POLYCYSTIC OVARY SYNDROME.

7. breast cyst. See FIBROCYSTIC BREAST SYNDROME.

cyst, breast   See FIBROCYSTIC BREAST SYNDROME.

cyst, cervical   See CYST, def. 4.

cyst, ovarian   See CYST, def. 6.

cystic disease, breast   See FIBROCYSTIC BREAST SYNDROME.

cystic fibrosis   A severe and chronic inherited disease of the exocrine (externally secreting) glands that affects principally the pancreas, respiratory system and sweat glands, causing them to overproduce normal secretions and/or produce abnormal secretions. It also may affect the intestines, causing malabsorption syndrome, that is, failure to absorb needed nutrients. It occurs primarily in persons of North European ancestry and is carried as a recessive trait (see GENETICS for explanation), so if both parents are carriers, any of their children (of either sex) has a 25% chance of inheriting the disease. If only one parent carries it, the disease is not passed on. Approximately 1 in 25 women and men are carriers, even though they themselves are completely healthy and often have no family history of affected children. Genetic tests can detect the majority of adults who carry the disease, which is the most common fatal disorder of young Americans. A simple blood test identifies a carrier, and either amniocentesis or chorionic villus sampling will identify a fetus who has the disease.

Cystic fibrosis usually is recognized in infancy or early childhood, but in some patients few or no symptoms appear until late adolescence. The principal symptoms are respiratory problems and failure to grow despite normal appetite and vigor. Male patients usually are infertile. No cure has yet been found, but life can be prolonged by close atten-

tion to respiratory difficulties—young children, for example, may need regular suctioning of mucus several times a day—and prompt treatment of any infections so as to avoid involvement of the lungs. Treatment includes administering pancreatin, to make up for inadequate pancreatic functions, and careful attention to adequate diet—more calories than normal, especially in the form of fats—as well as treatment of specific manifestations of the disease when they occur. The most recently developed treatment for the disease is gene therapy, transferring copies of the gene patients lack directly into their lungs; at this writing it is still experimental.

cystitis   **1.** Also *bladder infection, urinary tract infection, UTI.* Infection of the bladder, which usually is caused by bacteria and may be triggered by mechanical irritation. A common trigger in women is frequent sexual intercourse; in fact, cystitis of this origin is called *honeymoon cystitis* because so many women used to be affected in the early weeks of marriage, when engaging in intercourse for the first time and/or very frequently. Intercourse, especially in the conventional position with the woman on her back and the man lying on top of her, directs the penis along the roof of the vagina and against the floor of the urethra and bladder. The pumping action of the penis irritates those structures and pushes bacteria normally resident on the external vulva into the urethra. In recent years, use by men of the anti-impotence drug Viagra has seen an increase in honeymoon cystitis in their partners, especially women aged 55 to 75, in whom the vaginal dryness of aging also contributes to the condition. The best way of preventing such infection is to empty the bladder before intercourse and again immediately afterward and to drink considerably more water than usual, so as to dilute the urine and make it less hospitable to bacterial growth. A diaphragm also can irritate the urethra if the rim rubs against it during intercourse. Some clinicians believe diaphragms tend to be fitted too large; since they do not act as a seal but simply to hold spermicide against the cervix, a smaller size can be just as effective and less irritating. Bubble baths and swimming pools with chemically treated water occasionally are irritants.

Sexual intercourse is by no means the only way of contracting cystitis, for even young children can be afflicted. The causative bacteria often are such normal residents of the intestinal tract as *Escherichia coli*. They may move from the rectum into the vagina (as a result of wiping from back to front after a bowel movement, for example) and thence into the urinary tract; or they may be introduced by instruments used to withdraw urine (a catheter) or to examine the urinary tract (cystoscope). A CYSTOCELE (fallen bladder) also may contribute to infection by preventing the complete emptying of the bladder; the urine that remains is hospitable to bacteria. For a similar reason, cystitis is common during pregnancy, when the fetus is pressing on the bladder.

The symptoms of cystitis are urgency, frequency (needing to void much more often, but producing less urine at one time) and pain—usually a burning sensation—felt on urination. Some blood or pus may appear in the urine, and there may be a feeling of pressure just above the pubic bone. Diagnosis should include a urine culture and sensitivity test to determine what organisms are responsible and which drugs will be most effective against them. Treatment involves drinking six to eight glasses of water per day (in addition to other beverages) and taking appropriate medication—sulfonamides (sulfa drugs) or antibiotics to kill the bacteria and perhaps also phenazopyridine hydrochloride (Pyridium) to soothe the mucous membranes in the area and to relieve urinary frequency. (This drug tends to turn the urine a bright orange and stains underwear.) Drinking cranberry juice helps make the urine more acid and therefore inhospitable to bacteria, and also enhances the effect of some drugs used against the infection (especially tetracycline but not the sulfa drugs); cranberry juice contains benzoic acid, a natural preservative used to prevent the growth of molds, yeasts and bacteria in foods. (If cranberry juice increases the burning sensation, drink lots of water with a teaspoon of sodium bicarbonate, or baking soda, per glass; however, omit the baking soda if you have high blood pressure or heart disease.) A follow-up urine test should be done after medication relieves the symptoms to make sure the infection has been eliminated completely.

Women who prefer HERBAL REMEDIES report that relief from pain is provided by a tea made from cornsilk (*Zea mays*), buchu leaf (*Barosma betulina*) or pipsissewa (*Chimaphila umbellata*). For infections with bleeding they use a tea made from a combination of shepherd's purse (*Capsella bursa pastoris*), burdock root (*Arctium lappa*), bearberry (*Arctostaphylos uvaursi*) and echinacea root (*Echinacea augustifolia*). Some women use the herbal extract *Coleus forskolin*, which is said to flush out bacteria from the bladder lining that are not reached by antibiotics.

Cystitis is one of the most common ailments affecting women; nearly every woman contracts it at some time during her life. (A woman's bladder is only about 1 inch [2.5 centimeters] from her urethra; in a man the distance is 6 or more inches [15+ centimeters], and therefore cystitis is much less common in men.) Although distressing, it usually is not serious. However, cystitis should be treated, for it tends to recur, and chronic bladder infection over a period of years can result in permanent kidney damage. Recurrent urinary tract infections are not unusual in postmenopausal women, in whom urinary incontinence also increases the risk. If urologic evaluation rules out an underlying cause, such as a kidney stone or anatomic abnormality, a prophylactic antibiotic may be prescribed. It is safe to take such an antibiotic for up to several years. Among those used for this purpose, Bactrim 400/80 is one that has been widely studied (the numbers mean each dose contains 400 mg of sulfamethoxazole and 80 mg of trimethoprim). The most common side effects are diarrhea, nausea and yeast infection.

See also URETHRITIS.

2. interstitial cystitis. A painful condition of the bladder with many of the same symptoms as bacterial cystitis (see def. 1 above), including pain and urinary frequency. It affects mainly middle-aged women. A urine culture will reveal no causative organism. The condition is thought to be due to a chronic inflammation of the bladder wall, which produces symptoms that come and go, or to an oversensitive bladder, or to pain originating from nerves and muscles around the bladder. The underlying reason for the inflammation is not known, but among the suspected causes are previous urinary infections, defects in the cells of the bladder wall, disorders of nerve functions, an allergic process or a combination of these factors. The affected bladder wall is hypersensitive to stimulation, so that even a small amount of urine causes it to contract, in turn creating almost constant discomfort that is relieved only briefly by voiding. In severe cases bladder capacity can be drastically reduced and the bladder walls become ulcerated. The use of antibiotics to treat cystitis when bacteria are not the cause actually may give rise to interstitial cystitis, destroying the inner protective layer of bladder tissue. This exposes the delicate underlying layers to acid urine, so that they become irritated, leading to pain, frequency and a burning sensation on urination.

For diagnosis, based on the principal symptoms of urinary frequency (up to as much as every 15 minutes), urgency, and bladder pain, anatomic defects, infection and cancer are first ruled out. Then either a cystometrogram or cystoscopy is performed under local or general anesthesia. With the former, a catheter is inserted into the urethra and a tiny electronic sensor threaded into the bladder, which is then infused with fluid. As the bladder fills, the sensor measures changing pressures that indicate contractions of the muscular wall; most patients with interstitial cystitis experience contractions well before the bladder reaches normal capacity. With CYSTOSCOPY, the bladder is distended, enabling the clinician to see the multiple pinpoint hemorrhages that characterize the disease. Another sign is Hunner's ulcer, a wedge-shaped erosion that extends into several layers of the bladder wall. A newer diagnostic aid, a potassium-sensitivity test, which also uses a catheter, may be still more accurate; it is based on the idea that cystitis involves an abnormality in the bladder lining that allows potassium to be absorbed and cause discomfort.

Treatment includes "stretching" the bladder by filling it with fluid under anesthesia, or using a bladder instillation of dimethyl sulfoxide (DMSO), which coats the bladder wall, and other medications, but none has proved to be consistently effective. Other bladder instillation drugs are currently being tested. Another option is *transcutaneous electrical nerve stimulation (TENS)*, a procedure in which pain pathways are modified by a device worn on

PREVENTING URINARY TRACT INFECTION

- Urinate frequently to prevent urine pooling in bladder
- Urinate before and after sexual intercourse, and wash genital area
- Avoid feminine hygiene sprays and douches
- Avoid spermicide nonosynol-9, which can irritate urethra
- Drink lots of water
- Wipe from front to back after bowel movement

the body. It produces electrical impulses through electrodes, which reduce pain in about 25% of patients who have tried it. An implantable device called InterStim, which stimulates the sacral nerve in the lower back, is also being investigated.

An oral medication, *pentosan polysulfate sodium,* marketed as Elmiron, may help by forming a protective coating on the bladder lining. Another drug is the antihistamine *hydroxyzine hydrochloride* (Atarax, Vistaril), because histamine can cause bladder inflammation. Other medications include drugs for nerve pain and alkalyzing agents to reduce irritation. Laser treatment may be used to vaporize the lesions of Hunner's ulcers.

Bladder surgery is considered a treatment of last resort for those who are not helped in any other way and find their symptoms unbearable. It generally involves removing nearly all of the bladder and replacing it with either an internal pouch or an external appliance to collect urine. Often, however, pelvic pain persists long after the surgery. Simpler measures such as eliminating bladder-stimulating foods, especially alcohol, caffeine, chocolate, lemons, limes, tomatoes, artificial sweeteners and brewer's yeast, may change the composition of urine enough to ease symptoms. Patients urinate at least eight times a day and three times during the night. Bladder training to increase the interval between voiding by a given amount (such as 15 minutes) each week many help reduce symptoms; holding urine seems to increase bladder capacity significantly.

cystocele Also *dropped bladder, fallen bladder.* A bulging of the bladder into the vaginal canal, owing to pelvic relaxation, that is, impairment of the muscles that normally hold the bladder in place. It may occur alone or in conjunction with a PROLAPSED UTERUS and usually is, like the latter, a result of childbirth (a long, difficult labor, very large babies or many pregnancies). Cystocele usually gives rise to some symptoms, the most common of which is leaking of urine, especially when coughing, laughing or sneezing (see stress incontinence under URINARY INCONTINENCE). However, symptoms may not appear until after menopause, when reduced estrogen production causes further muscle relaxation. It often leads to repeated urinary infections, marked by frequency of urination, a burning sensation when voiding and a feeling of incomplete voiding (see also CYSTITIS). The condition is readily diagnosed with a pelvic examination. Treatment for minor cystocele may consist merely of KEGEL EXERCISES to strengthen the pelvic muscles. For more severe cases surgery is indicated, after other causes for chronic incontinence have been ruled out. In the standard repair procedure, the surgeon makes an incision along the front wall of the vagina, pushes the bladder upward and sews it into normal position. This may be combined with repairing the back wall of the vagina (near the rectum) for better support (see also RECTOCELE). About four out of five patients find relief in this way. For the remaining 20% more complicated surgery, called a *Marshall-Marchetti procedure,* may be needed to eliminate incontinence. In this procedure the surgeon makes an incision in the abdomen and changes the angle of the bladder opening. For other techniques see URINARY INCONTINENCE. Some clinicians recommend hysterectomy, but others view it as a last resort.

See also URETHROCELE.

cystosarcoma phyllodes A rapidly growing but relatively uncommon tumor of the breast. It usually is benign (noncancerous) but occasionally is malignant; moreover, it is not easy to distinguish the benign form from the malignant, and therefore evaluation of the tumor tissue by at least two pathologists is recommended. Treatment consists of surgical removal; because this kind of tumor grows so fast, sometimes the entire breast must be removed to eliminate the whole tumor, even when it is benign.

cystoscopy Examination of the urethra and bladder with a cystoscope, a slender metal tube with a lens and light source, inserted through the urethra into the bladder. Samples of urine and bits of tissue can be removed through the cystoscope for further examination. Performed by a urologist under local anesthesia, cystoscopy is used to diagnose interstitial cystitis (see CYSTITIS, def. 2) or other abnormalities.

cytology The study of cells, including their structure, function, origin and pathology (diseases and other abnormalities). A PAP SMEAR is one of the most common cytologic studies.

danazol A synthetic male hormone used to treat ENDOMETRIOSIS, and sometimes also premenstrual syndrome (see DYSMENORRHEA, def. 5) and fibroids, and for EMERGENCY CONTRACEPTION. It suppresses production of LH (luteinizing hormone) and FSH (follicle-stimulating hormone) by the pituitary, causing amenorrhea, during which the endometrial implants waste away. Danazol appears to work best in women with mild or moderate endometriosis. In severe cases it may be combined with surgery. Menstruation resumes four to six weeks after stopping the drug, and the best chances for becoming pregnant occur about two months later. Danazol, however, has side effects severe enough so that some women must stop using it. They include depression and other mood changes, unexplained muscle cramps, decreased breast size, flushing, sweating, fatigue, oily skin, acne, abnormal hair growth and water retention. The drug also is associated with unfavorable blood cholesterol changes. It should not be used by women with undiagnosed abnormal genital bleeding, women who are pregnant or breast-feeding or those who have serious liver, kidney or heart disease. Further, the drug is quite expensive, with a month's treatment costing several hundred dollars. Usually three to nine months of treatment are required before it is effective.

D and C Abbreviation for *dilatation and curettage,* or scraping of the uterine lining, for years the single most frequently performed surgical procedure in the United States. It involves dilating (stretching) the cervix, or neck of the uterus, sufficiently to allow the insertion of a curet (curette), a small instrument that is used to scrape away part of the endometrium (uterine lining). Among the principal reasons for performing a D and C are to determine the cause of abnormal bleeding or staining; to stop heavy bleeding (see ENDOMETRIAL HYPERPLASIA); to remove bits of placental or other tissue remaining after childbirth, miscarriage or abortion; to determine if ovulation has occurred in cases of infertility; to detect early uterine cancer or a FIBROID; and to remove endometrial POLYPS (see def. 3). Even when the principal purpose of a D and C is not diagnosis, the tissue removed always should be examined in the laboratory to make sure no cancer cells are present.

Until about 1960 a D and C was the principal method of performing an early abortion (during the first trimester of pregnancy), but since then VACUUM ASPIRATION has largely replaced it. Further, for purposes of biopsy as well as to stop heavy bleeding, many clinicians prefer to use the simpler vacuum procedure first, following it up with a surgical D and C only if necessary (see BIOPSY, def. 8).

Most often an outpatient procedure, a D and C requires general, regional (epidural, spinal or caudal) or local anesthesia. The last, usually a paracervical block, is generally accompanied by a sedative and/or painkiller, to ease cramps felt during the procedure. The patient is placed in the same position as for a pelvic examination. Next the surgeon inserts a speculum, holds the cervix steady with a special clamp (a *tenaculum*) and determines the angle of the cervical canal and depth of the uterus by inserting a narrow metal rod called a *sound* through the cervix to the top (fundus) of the uterus. The cervix then is gradually dilated by inserting a series of ever larger rods; the largest is about ½ inch (12 millimeters) in diameter. Sometimes LAMINARIA are used for this purpose, but they take about 24 hours to dilate the cervix and generally are reserved for procedures where considerable dilatation is needed, more than for a diagnostic D and C. If there are polyps, they are located and removed, and a spoon-shaped curet is used to scrape shreds of tissue from all around the endometrium. The entire procedure takes 15 to 20 minutes. The instruments then are removed and the procedure is finished; no sutures (stitches) are required.

Women usually go home as soon as the anesthetic has worn off. Recovery from a D and C takes anywhere from a few hours to a couple of days. There may be some bleeding and staining for about two weeks and mild cramps or backache for the first day or so. Fever, severe cramps or abdominal pain, heavy bleeding or foul-smelling discharge all are signs of infection and should be reported to the clinician promptly. Such infections, which are the most common complication of a D and C, usually respond to antibiotic treatment but should never be ignored, because they can become serious. Most clinicians advise patients to avoid vaginal intercourse, douching and the use of tampons for two weeks, because the cervix takes time to return to its normal closed position and any of these activities is a potential source of infection. If a woman does wish to engage in vaginal intercourse, her partner should use a condom (to prevent entry of bacteria). After two weeks most clinicians see patients for a postoperative checkup.

Complications after a D and C are rare. It is possible for the uterus to be punctured (perforated) by a surgical instrument, but even then no treatment may be needed, the injured tissue simply healing by itself. There also can be damage to bladder or bowel, both of which are adjacent to the uterus, but this rarely happens. Relatively safe as a D and C is, it still constitutes surgery and should be undertaken only if there is a genuine need for it. For irregular bleeding in young women, for example, many clinicians prefer first to try hormone therapy for several months (see BREAKTHROUGH BLEEDING). Further, not only is it essential that pregnancy be ruled out before performing a D and C—provided that the woman wishes to continue the pregnancy—but if there is any infection or inflammation of the uterus, tubes or cervix, these conditions should, if possible, be cleared up before surgery.

In recent years the D and C often has been avoided through less invasive techniques. Highly sensitive ultrasound can help pinpoint physical causes for abnormal bleeding before menopause and noncancerous bleeding after menopause. To enhance the image, a small amount of saline can be instilled into the uterus, a procedure called *sonohysterography.* Also, *transvaginal ultrasound* can show if a woman has ovulated or if the uterine lining (endometrium) is normally thickened before menstruation and thinned afterward. However, if there is a high suspicion of cancer, or if there are polyps or fibroids that can be removed, a D and C is still indicated.

See also ASHERMAN'S SYNDROME.

D and E   See DILATATION AND EVACUATION.

deafness   Hearing loss, most often associated with aging. Age-related hearing loss, called *presbycusis,* affects about one-third of all adults by the age of 65. Often such loss is caused by damage to the sensory nerves or hair cells that line the cochlea of the inner ear, a condition called *sensorineural hearing loss.* The hair cells are tuned to sounds from high to low frequencies; men tend to be affected in the high frequency range, women more in lower frequencies. Another kind, conductive hearing loss, involves the tiny vibrating bones or ossicles in the middle ear. This may be due to *otosclerosis,* in which the bone in the ear canal grows across the ligament so that the bone does not vibrate. Otosclerosis affects women four times more often than men. Hearing loss also can be caused by a tumor that grows on the auditory nerve, infections, wax buildup, head injuries and some medications.

Hearing loss tends to come on slowly over time. Hearing is tested by an audiologist, who can determine the extent of loss and the frequencies affected and can fit one with a hearing aid. An ear, nose and throat specialist can decide if there is a medical cause for the hearing loss. Individuals with mild to moderate conductive hearing loss can benefit from analog hearing aids, which amplify sound over all frequencies. Sensorineural hearing loss benefits more from digital hearing aids, which can be tuned specifically to a given problem.

defloration Literally, "deflowering," meaning a woman's first vaginal intercourse, when penile penetration breaks the HYMEN.

See also VIRGINITY.

delayed puberty See AMENORRHEA, def. 2; PUBERTY.

delivery The birth of a baby; childbirth.

See also LABOR.

demand feeding A schedule of BREAST-FEEDING based on the infant's wish to nurse rather than on specific times.

Demerol Brand name for meperidine, a synthetic narcotic widely used for the relief of pain in childbirth as well as other severe pain. Formerly it was regularly used in labor together with SCOPOLAMINE (it replaced an even stronger narcotic, morphine) to induce a relatively pain-free "twilight sleep." It is very effective as a pain reliever, but its principal disadvantage is that it has a depressant effect on the baby's respiratory center if it is in the baby's bloodstream at delivery. Demerol also makes a newborn baby sleepy for a day or more. Further, some women cannot tolerate the drug because of such side effects as nausea and vomiting.

See also ANALGESIC.

deodorant A class of COSMETICS that helps eliminate the odor of perspiration by killing some of the bacteria that cause it, or by adding a fragrance to mask it, or both. Deodorants generally are harmless when used on the armpits but should not be used in the pubic area. Occasionally they give rise to an allergic reaction, most often caused by their perfume component. Switching to another brand may solve the problem. A deodorant does not stop perspiration; if it does, it is classed as an *antiperspirant*, which contains a substance—usually aluminum salts—that temporarily closes the openings of the sweat glands and thus blocks their secretions.

Depo-Provera Also *DMPA*. A synthetic progesterone (medroxyprogesterone acetate) that was the first injectable hormonal contraceptive approved by the U.S. Food and Drug Administration for use in the United States. (Several other injectable products exist but are not yet marketed in the United States.) Approved earlier for treatment of terminal endometrial cancer, Depo-Provera was not approved for contraception until 1992. It works by preventing ovulation. A single intramuscular injection every three months affords 99% protection against pregnancy (for up to 14 weeks). However, it should be administered only during the first five days of a normal menstrual period to make sure a woman is not already pregnant. It may be administered within five days of childbirth or, if the woman is breast-feeding, within six weeks of delivery. After that it is safest to perform a pregnancy test before injecting it.

Side effects include irregular menstrual cycles—bleeding between periods or no periods at all—and fertility can be delayed six months to a year after stopping injections; however, it is restored in 90% of women within two years. Among other side effects are weight gain, dizziness, headache, depression and moodiness, and decreased libido. Also, it provides no protection against sexually transmitted diseases, including HIV, and some authorities believe it may be linked to an increased risk of breast cancer. In 2004 the FDA warned that long-term use could permanently weaken bones. Depo-Provera should be avoided by women with liver disease or hepatitis, gallbladder disease, a history of or current breast cancer, severe high blood pressure, heart disease and diabetes. However, its high degree of effectiveness and convenient administration will for some women offset possible concerns about its long-term health effects.

depression **1.** Also *melancholia*. An emotional disorder that ranges in severity from unusually intense or long-lasting feelings of sadness, disappointment and frustration to chronic insomnia, inability to concentrate or perform ordinary tasks and attempts at suicide. Depression is one of the most common afflictions of American adults, affecting an estimated 8 to 20% of the entire population.

SYMPTOMS OF DEPRESSION*

blues

anhedonia (inability to feel pleasure)

marked change in appetite, with weight loss or gain

constipation

sleep disturbances, sleeping too much or insomnia
   (especially waking during night or early morning)

diminished energy, fatigue, lethargy

restlessness, agitation

slowed-down speech, movement, thought

stooped posture, sad facial expression

decreased sex drive

loss of interest in work

feelings of worthlessness, self-reproach, guilt

diminished ability to think and concentrate

forgetfulness

indecisiveness

low self-esteem

feelings of helplessness, anxiety

pessimism, feelings of hopelessness

thoughts of death, suicide attempts

self-absorption, bodily complaints

*None alone is symptomatic of a clinical depression, but the persistent presence of six or more simultaneously may be suspicious.

It is at least twice as prevalent in women as in men; estimates range from a ratio of 4 to 5 depressed women to every man down to only 1½ or 2 to 1 in the form known as MANIC-DEPRESSIVE ILLNESS, or bipolar depression. The symptoms of depression are very numerous indeed (see the accompanying chart), and some of them are experienced by practically every man, woman or child at some time or another. They constitute an illness called *clinical depression* only when they are long-lasting or severe enough to interfere with normal functioning for a number of months or years.

Depression afflicts people of all ages; in older individuals, one person in seven over the age of 65 suffers from it, but relatively few seek treatment. Another group who may be neglected are pregnant women, among whom 10 to 20% suffer from moderate to severe depression during pregnancy. Depression is often overlooked in pregnant women, and they are reluctant to take antidepressants even if prescribed. Untreated depression has been linked to higher rates of miscarriage, stillbirths, premature deliveries and low birth weight babies. On the other hand, some antidepressants expose the newborn baby to other risks, some of them serious. Thus, the decision to treat or not must involve careful assessment of the known risks and benefits. (See also def. 2 below.)

Clinicians frequently distinguish between a *reactive depression* (also called *exogenous depression*), which begins as a natural reaction to a particular situation or event (such as death of a parent) but persists for more than a normal amount of time and seems more extreme than the situation that provoked it, and *endogenous depression,* which has no discoverable cause. They also distinguish between very severe or *major depression* and less severe depression, sometimes called *dysthymia.*

The more severe depressions respond better to drugs and electroshock therapy than do milder ones (see ANTIDEPRESSANTS), which supports the general view that they are caused by biochemical factors. Some studies suggest that certain individuals may have a genetic predisposition for such illness. Others maintain that some persons lack or have an excess of some chemical that affects the activity of neurotransmitters in the brain or some other objective physical factor. Depression is known to be associated with certain physical illnesses; for example, mononucleosis and infectious hepatitis both are linked with mild depression, and arteriosclerosis with more severe depression. Further, some researchers have linked clinical depression to the use of oral contraceptives.

There is no conclusive evidence yet concerning these hypotheses, but certain social and emotional aspects of depression have been long observed. Consequently therapists continue to treat depression with psychotherapy, ranging from psychoanalysis to various behavior therapies, as well as with drugs and electroshock treatment, with varying degrees of success. Many feminists maintain that depression often is, at least in part, a normal response of women to a repressive sexist society. They therefore tend to endorse treatment that teaches women (in particular) to cope more effectively, principally by changing their behavior so as to receive more positive reinforcement of their self-esteem. Such treatment may involve keeping records to discover the relationship between one's mood and one's expectation of reinforcement, consciousness-raising contacts with other women, assertiveness training to learn to express appropriate anger and to take independent action, and similar measures.

See also FEMINIST THERAPY.

2. postpartum depression. Also *after-baby blues.* A form of depression experienced by many—perhaps most—women three to four days after giving birth. Typically it is characterized by feelings of fear or apprehension about being able to take care of the baby as well as a general letdown following the exhilaration of giving birth. Because it is so common, many authorities believe postpartum depression may be caused by physical changes, especially the marked drop in estrogen levels following delivery (back to normal within 24 hours) and the drastic reduction in total blood volume (30%). The feelings generally last anywhere from a day or two to 10 days. For about 15% of new mothers, however, symptoms may last for several months. If depression persists or is severe enough for a woman to withdraw from her family, professional help may be indicated. However, contact with a support group of other new parents often is sufficient.

A few women—an estimated 1 in 600—suffer from more severe (but also temporary) mental illness following childbirth. This condition comes on suddenly, within two weeks of delivery, and ends in about three months, with the woman fully recovering. Symptoms here are more marked than a mood of sadness or withdrawal, and may include confusion and rambling speech, hallucinations and occasionally severe psychotic episodes. Some women become euphoric and hyperactive, unable to sleep; others are incapable of caring for their babies and ask for help or supervision in even the simplest tasks. Most women with this condition, one study indicates, have particularly high levels of estrogen and low levels of progesterone, as well as abnormal levels of other hormones, suggesting an endocrine imbalance. Counseling, antidepressant medication, electroconvulsive therapy and/or hospitalization may be indicated, depending on the nature and severity of the condition. Some practitioners use a two-month estrogen/proges-

terone regimen that gradually reduces the mother's hormone output rather than letting it drop abruptly. One study found that an estrogen skin patch hastened recovery from severe postpartum depression.

Occasionally postpartum depression is combined with or takes the form of panic disorder (see ANXIETY), which also may require professional help (counseling, medication).

Note that some of the drugs used for postpartum emotional disorders may pass into breast milk, an issue requiring evaluation if the mother is breast-feeding.

3. seasonal affective disorder. Also *SAD, winter blues.* A form of depression that occurs during the winter months, when days are shorter and sunlight scarcer, and that also seems to affect women more than men. (One study says 80% of patients are women, most of whom first developed symptoms while in their 20s.) Unlike other forms of depression, which have been linked to the neurotransmitter (brain chemical) serotonin, SAD is linked with melatonin, a hormone that responds to differing amounts of light, and possibly also the neurotransmitter dopamine. Estrogen also may be involved, accounting for the fact that women afflicted with SAD frequently find it subsides after menopause. SAD often responds to *phototherapy,* exposure to high-intensity light, that is, sitting less than 3 feet (1 meter) away from a bank of fluorescent lights emitting about 10,000 lux (20 times brighter than ordinary light) for 20 minutes to 2 hours a day, depending on the severity of the condition. Symptoms subside within a few days and may disappear entirely in a week or two. It should not be used by anyone whose eyes or skin are sensitive to light. For these patients aerobic exercise in sunlight or a well-lighted area, stress management techniques, psychotherapy and antidepressant medication are other measures to try.

DeQuervain's tendinitis   Also *DeQuervain's tenosynovitis.* A painful condition caused by inflammation of the tendons of the thumb. It causes pain on the thumb side of the wrist during grasping or wrist movements. It is so common among women who have given birth recently that it is sometimes called *new mom's syndrome*. Such women are susceptible because the fluid gain of pregnancy causes the tendons to swell and chafe against surrounding encasement. Also, tendons and joints become lax in late pregnancy. Afflicted women then tend to pick up their baby with their hands angled downward, aggravating the condition. The tendinitis may be treated in a number of ways: with rest, ice, and a nonsteroidal anti-inflammatory drug (NSAID); a cortisone shot to reduce inflammation; ultrasound treatment; a brace to immobilize the wrist; physical therapy to strengthen the area and teach new ways of picking up the baby. Left untreated, the inflammation may progress to fibrosis, or scarring, which limits thumb movement.

DES   See DIETHYLSTILBESTROL.

designer estrogen   See SELECTIVE ESTROGEN-RECEPTOR MODULATOR.

detoxification   See ADDICTION; ALCOHOL USE.

diabetes   Also *diabetes mellitus, sugar diabetes.* A disorder characterized by failure of the pancreas to provide enough effective insulin, a hormone that removes excess sugar from the blood and stores it in the liver, or the inability of body cells to receive insulin. Its prevailing sign is the presence of increased quantities of glucose (sugar) in the blood (*hyperglycemia*) and urine (*glycosuria*). Symptoms include urinary frequency, increased hunger and thirst, and weight loss. In women frequent vaginal yeast infections and vaginal itching also occur. The ultimate cause is not known, although diabetes does appear to be connected with age, overweight, hereditary factors and virus infection. In the case of Type I diabetes (see below), the cause is clearly an autoimmune response (see AUTOIMMUNE DISEASE), the body's immune system attacking the pancreas and destroying its ability to make insulin. The condition cannot be cured, but it usually can be controlled, by diet alone or by oral medica-

tion or by administering insulin in various forms. Uncontrolled, diabetes may have serious complications, especially in the circulatory system, where in extreme cases it causes impairment leading to gangrene and the loss of limbs, and in the eye, where blindness may result. It also is associated with dangerously high blood pressure and accelerates atherosclerosis, increasing the risk of heart attack or stroke; destroys the kidney's filtration system; slows the healing of wounds; and in women who bear children, may increase the incidence of birth defects.

Type I diabetes tends to begin in childhood and appears to be due to a defect in the pancreas itself, rendering it unable to produce insulin. Also called *insulin-dependent* or *juvenile-onset diabetes,* it afflicts about 10% of all diabetics. An autoimmune response (see AUTOIMMUNE DISEASE), in which the body's immune system attacks the pancreas and destroys its ability to make insulin, it is more apt to develop serious complications and usually requires insulin therapy for life. Insulin-dependent diabetics can monitor their blood glucose with small handheld meters; usually they must check it before each meal and at bedtime. A promising new approach to treating Type I diabetes is targeting T cells, which destroy the cells of the pancreas. Work with cloned antibodies known to target T cells appears to halt the disease's progress, although patients must still take insulin because of the damage already done.

Type II diabetes, also called *non-insulin-dependent* or *adult-onset diabetes,* usually (but not always) attacks after the age of 30, with incidence peaking between 45 and 65, and is slightly more common in women than in men. It occurs when organs become resistant to the insulin produced by the body and is progressive; in the final stages the body stops producing insulin. Far more common than Type I, it afflicts about 10% of all adults in the United States; 90% of them are obese. Because it does not always give rise to overt symptoms, many patients—some authorities believe as many as half—are not even aware of the disease. Individuals who develop Type II diabetes have usually been *prediabetic* for years, that is, their blood-sugar levels have been elevated but not high enough to qualify as diabetic. Type II diabetes, which tends to run in families more than Type I does, is often

WARNING SIGNS OF DIABETES

- Increased thirst
- Frequent urination, especially at night
- Constant hunger
- Blurred vision
- Unusual fatigue
- Sores that do not heal
- Unexplained weight loss
- Menstrual irregularity and chronic yeast infections

controlled simply by following a strict diet (high in carbohydrates and fiber) and exercising for weight control; it may or may not require the administration of insulin. Type II diabetics also can use the self-monitoring glucose meters; used faithfully, especially before and after meals and physical exercise, they have made it easier to control the disease. The main ways to reduce the risk of developing Type II diabetes are regular exercise and avoiding obesity.

A number of oral medications can help control Type II diabetes. At this writing a number of drugs are approved for treating the condition, but a government study published in 2007 analyzed 10 of them and found some differences among them. They are metformin (Glucophage, Riomet, Fortamet), acarbose (Precose), glimepiride (Amaryl), glipizide (Glucotrol), glyburide (Micronase, DiaBeta, Glynase Pres Tab), miglitol (Glyset), nateglinide (Starlix), pioglitazone (Actos), repaglinide (Prandin) and rosiglitazone (Avandia). All of them are similarly effective for reducing blood glucose, but metformin and acarbose do not increase weight, whereas the others do by two to 12 pounds. These two drugs cause more gastrointestinal problems, such as diarrhea, but this may be mitigated by using a lower dose of metformin and combining it with one of the other drugs. Metformin also tends to decrease LDL ("bad cholesterol"), which tends to increase with pioglitazone and rosiglitazone. However, the latter two tend to raise HDL ("good cholesterol") as well. Glimepiride, glipizide and repaglinide are associated with hypoglycemia (when blood glucose levels go too low) more than the other drugs. Pioglitazone and rosiglitazone (Avandia) are also linked with greater

risk of congestive heart failure, and patients who have underlying heart disease or are at high risk of heart attack should consult their clinicians to evaluate this treatment, especially with Avandia. Still another drug developed for Type II diabetes is Byetta, injected twice a day, which causes significant weight loss (unlike most other such drugs). All of these medications have side effects and should only be taken under the direction of a watchful clinician.

Because unrecognized Type II diabetes may be so widespread, the American Diabetes Association has recommended wider screening and a change in diagnostic criteria. It recommends a fasting plasma glucose test (FPG) for all adults at age 45 and every 3 years thereafter. It is performed at least eight hours after eating and measures the amount of glucose in the blood. Some clinicians use the oral glucose tolerance test, in which blood samples are taken after the patient drinks a special glucose solution. The traditional glucose tests merely measure blood-sugar levels. A newer recommended test is the A1C test. It measures blood levels of hemoglobin A1C, which indicates how well glucose levels have been controlled for the previous three months. Home tests for A1C are available; the ideal number is less than 7% A1C. Formerly an FPG of 140 milligrams per deciliter indicated diabetes, a measurement that might be altered to 110 for normal levels and 110–126 for high risk. These guidelines are particularly applicable for persons at high risk for the disease (see table).

In addition to monitoring blood sugar levels, diabetic patients, being at increased risk for heart attack and stroke, are urged to monitor their blood pressure and cholesterol levels. Blood pressure should be less than 130 over 80, and LDL cholesterol under 100 mg, preferably 70 to 80 mg.

In 2007 the FDA approved a new kind of medication for Type II diabetes. The drug, sitagliptin phosphate (Januva), increases a hormone that triggers the pancreas to produce more insulin to turn glucose into energy and at the same time blocks an enzyme that makes the liver stop producing glucose. It appears to have lower side effects than older drugs. When oral medications fail, patients typically moved to insulin injections. In 2007 the

FDA approved an inhaled form of insulin, a relief for patients who struggle with daily injections. The brand Exubera is a powdered form taken just before meals; it is released into the mouth and lungs through an inhaler similar to those used by asthma patients and can be used for either Type I or Type II diabetes. However, the product was withdrawn from the market in 2008 because a small number of patients developed lung cancer, and FDA approval was deemed premature.

A third form of diabetes is found to occur during pregnancy and sometimes (but not always) disappears after delivery. Some authorities believe that in such cases pregnancy may "unmask" an already existing disease, but others regard it as a separate form called *gestational* or *Type III diabetes*. Women who develop gestational diabetes are at 20 to 50% more risk of developing Type II diabetes within 5 to 10 years.

Gestational diabetes affects 4 to 8% of pregnant women, or about 135,000 in the United States. However, recent studies have shown that the higher a pregnant woman's level of blood sugar, the greater risk to her newborn, whether or not she has diabetes. These findings may lead to more women being diagnosed with diabetes and given stricter diet advice or medication to lower blood sugar. Currently the goal for a pregnant woman's fasting blood sugar (the measure of blood glucose after she has had no food for eight hours) is below 95 mg by deciliter during the last few months of pregnancy. It is now suggested that 90 mg be a better goal, although new guidelines for this have not yet been publicized. Also, a recent study indicated that the children born of a woman with untreated gestational diabetes are almost twice as likely to be obese or overweight by the ages of 5 to 7, underlining the importance of treatment during pregnancy. Studies show that treatment with metformin, alone or with supplemental insulin, does not result in complications in the fetus or baby.

Diabetes poses a considerable problem in pregnancy, so a pregnant woman with diabetes is usually classed as a HIGH-RISK PREGNANCY. Too much insulin or too little food cause a diabetic to go into shock (*hypoglycemia*); too little insulin causes another dangerous condition, ketoacidosis. The balance of insulin is a delicate one, and whenever

RISK FACTORS FOR DIABETES*

More than 20% above ideal weight

Blood pressure at or above 140/90

HDL cholesterol of 35 or less and/or triglycerides of 250 or more

Have parent or sibling with diabetes

Are African American, Hispanic American, Native American or Asian American (high-risk ethnicities)

Have borne a baby weighing more than 9 pounds or had gestational diabetes

*Indicating that testing for the disease should begin before age 45.

the body goes through a major metabolic or hormonal change, as during the adolescent growth spurt (see PUBERTY) or during pregnancy, that balance is upset. Babies of diabetic mothers, for reasons that are not understood, tend to be very large, with oversize organs, but not well developed (mature) for their size. They also tend to be born prematurely and consequently are more likely to develop hypoglycemia and respiratory distress syndrome. The babies also seem to run a higher risk of becoming obese and developing Type II diabetes later in life. The diabetic mother has a much greater risk of developing hypertension (high blood pressure), preeclampsia and eclampsia (four times that of the nondiabetic) as well as infections of various kinds during pregnancy. The larger size of the baby often makes for difficult delivery. The incidence of still-birth is high, HYDRAMNIOS is common and postpartum hemorrhage frequently is a threat.

Because of these risks, it is important to determine at the outset of pregnancy if and what type of diabetes is involved. Further, since women developing gestational diabetes have no prior history of the disease, all pregnant women should be screened for it routinely; it occurs in 4% of all women (higher in some ethnic groups), and the incidence has been rising considerably. One factor is the increased incidence of obesity, which predisposes to it. Both preconception counseling and diabetic control throughout the pregnancy are vital. Type II diabetics, even though they may not require insulin normally, almost always seem to need it during pregnancy. For Type III diabetics insulin is not routinely recommended but should be given when needed.

Although fastidious prenatal care of the diabetic mother usually will safeguard her during the pregnancy, the outlook for her baby is less optimistic: Perinatal mortality (before, during or just after delivery) is estimated to be 10 to 15%, and those babies who survive often have one or more disabling birth defects. Since the main cause of infant death is congenital malformations of major vital organs, many clinicians recommend a maternal blood test or ALPHA-FETOPROTEIN TEST at 16 to 18 weeks and ultrasound at 18 to 22 weeks to uncover such defects.

Especially vigilant monitoring is essential during the third trimester. Formerly many clinicians insisted that all their diabetic patients be delivered by Cesarean section by the 38th week. Today a more conservative approach prevails. Women with Type III diabetes usually can be delivered at term and vaginally. INDUCTION OF LABOR may be used to make sure they do not go beyond term (42 weeks), since the fetus then is greatly endangered. If labor does not progress well or the baby is too big for the birth canal, a Cesarean may be performed. In Types I and II, close monitoring for the baby's well-being begins at about 35 weeks, and many clinicians recommend ultrasound examination and amniocentesis at 37 to 38 weeks. If these reveal that the baby's lungs are sufficiently mature, labor may be induced and vaginal delivery effected unless some problem develops.

After delivery the mother's insulin dosage must be lowered drastically to meet her body's new needs and must continue to be monitored carefully and the baby's health carefully assessed. Some clinicians feel that diabetic women who already have several children and who have circulatory or kidney impairment of any kind should seriously consider sterilization to avoid the hazards of another pregnancy.

diagnosis Determining the presence and nature of a disease. Diagnosis is based on a variety of measures, ranging from simple observation by a trained eye to detect, for example, chicken pox or poison ivy, to elaborate studies and tests involving sophis-

ticated machinery. A careful history is important. Diagnosis may require laboratory analysis of the blood, urine, semen, cerebrospinal fluid, sputum or stool; the use of electrical machinery to trace heart and brain activity (electrocardiograph and electroencephalograph); special kinds of photography ranging from X-rays to mammography, ultrasound and scans involving the use of radioactive materials (brain scans, lung scans, total body scans, etc.); and clinical procedures such as colposcopy and exploratory laparoscopy.

See also GYNECOLOGIC EXAMINATION.

diaphanography See TRANSILLUMINATION.

diaphragm 1. A muscle separating the abdominal and chest cavities.

2. A cup-shaped spring device that is inserted into the vagina along with spermicidal jelly or cream in order to prevent conception. It is *not* effective alone as a mechanical barrier to sperm, which can enter around its edges. Rather, it keeps sperm-killing material (see SPERMICIDE) in place over the cervix, so that sperm are killed before they can enter there. (Sperm do not survive for more than eight hours in the vagina because of its acid secretions.) In theory, the diaphragm, which requires a doctor's prescription to purchase, is one of the most effective and safest means of BIRTH CONTROL; when it is used properly its success rate is allegedly about 94%. However, it must be properly fitted, large enough to allow for expansion of the vagina during sexual excitement but not so tight that it is uncomfortable when the vagina returns to normal size. Further, the fit should be checked yearly, as well as after childbirth, abortion, or a weight loss or gain of 10 to 15 pounds (4.5 to 6.75 kilos) or more, since a woman's size can change. The diaphragm must be inserted properly each time, along with an adequate amount of active (not outdated) spermicide. It must be used for each act of intercourse and left in place for eight hours thereafter; additional spermicide must be inserted with an applicator if intercourse is repeated before eight hours are up. Because spermicide is effective for only six to eight hours, the diaphragm should not be inserted more

than two hours before intercourse. If more than two hours pass, it should be removed and fresh spermicide added before intercourse takes place. Given all these requirements, the actual effectiveness of a diaphragm in preventing unwanted pregnancy is far less than claimed, some studies saying only 80% or so.

The diaphragm itself consists of a flexible metal ring (spring) covered with rubber, taking the shape of a shallow dome. For insertion, spermicidal cream or jelly is placed inside the dome and all around the edges of the rim, about 1 tablespoon in all. Then, squeezing the diaphragm in one hand and spreading the vaginal lips with the other, the woman slides the diaphragm (cream or jelly side up) into the vagina, where it is held in place by spring tension. Its rim should rest behind the pubic bone, where it cannot be felt (except by touching), and the dome should cover the cervix. The diaphragm is easier to insert from a squatting position (or standing with one foot up on a chair). For women who have trouble inserting it, a plastic inserter, which looks somewhat like a crochet hook with a series of notches in it, is available for use with some kinds of diaphragm. The diaphragm is stretched onto the inserter, which is then put inside the vagina; once in, the diaphragm is released by giving the inserter a little twist, and it is withdrawn while

Inserting a Diaphragm

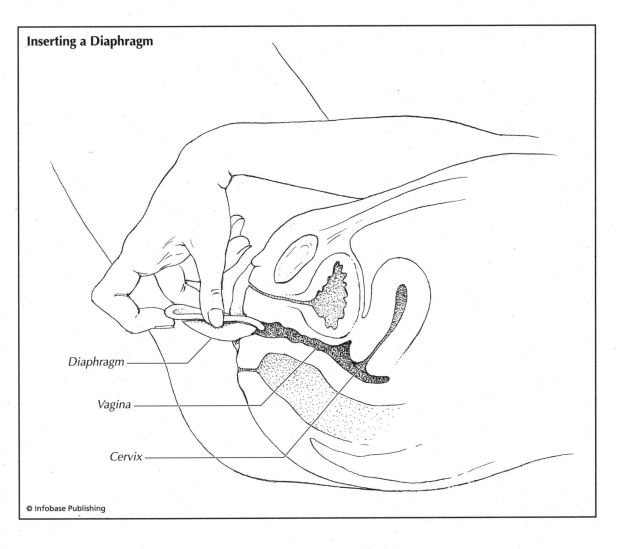

Diaphragm

Vagina

Cervix

© Infobase Publishing

the diaphragm remains in place. A diaphragm should not remain inside the vagina longer than 24 hours. After removing the diaphragm (eight hours after the last intercourse), it should be washed with soap and water, rinsed and dried (if desired, dusted with cornstarch), and stored in a container away from light. It should never be boiled and should be checked regularly for holes, either by holding it up to the light or by filling it with water and looking for leaks (especially near the rim). With regular care a diaphragm will last two years or so.

Diaphragms come in diameters of 50 to 95 millimeters (2 to 4 inches; most women require one between 70 and 90 millimeters) and with 1 of 3 types of rim: coil spring, flat spring and arcing spring (a coil with two rigid semicircles that form an arc shape when compressed). The coil spring fits women of average size and shape who have good vaginal muscle tone; the flat spring works best for women with a shallow pubic arch, with moderate descent of bladder or rectum (cystocele, rectocele) or with a uterus tilted forward more than average (anteverted). The arcing spring works best for women with poor vaginal muscle tone, a cervix that protrudes considerably, moderate descent of bladder or rectum, or extreme forward or backward tilt of the uterus (anteverted, retroverted). Very occasionally, however, women cannot be fitted properly, usually because they have a severely prolapsed uterus, or their vagina is either too tight (as in a virgin; it may take some months of regular intercourse for it to stretch) or too relaxed, or if the uterus is severely tipped. Occasionally, a woman's partner is allergic to either the rubber or the spermicide; in the latter case a different brand may solve the problem. For oral sex, many find that the spermicide tastes unpleasant.

A diaphragm can be used during menstruation, both for contraception and to collect the menstrual flow during intercourse. Occasionally the diaphragm may become displaced during intercourse, mostly in the position where the woman is on top of the man when his penis is withdrawn or when the penis is withdrawn and reinserted repeatedly. Sometimes women find that a diaphragm irritates their urethra and then contributes to infection (see URETHRITIS); such irritation usually occurs when the diaphragm rim presses on the urethra and

may indicate that the diaphragm is somewhat too large.

Devices like diaphragms have been in use for centuries. In the 18th century women sometimes inserted half of a squeezed lemon in their vagina over the cervix; presumably the acidity of the lemon juice helped kill sperm. The modern diaphragm was developed in the late 19th century in Europe. In the United States and Canada it was widely recommended by birth control clinics in the first half of the 20th century and, although briefly replaced in popularity by oral contraceptives and intrauterine devices in the 1960s, began to regain favor as women realized that its disadvantages and risks were considerably less than those of alternative methods of BIRTH CONTROL. See also CERVICAL CAP.

Dick-Read method   A method of PREPARED CHILDBIRTH devised about 1930 by an English obstetrician, Grantly Dick-Read, which involves education, correct breathing, relaxation techniques and exercises. It focuses on teaching a woman to relax during each uterine contraction as well as to turn inward and visualize the internal process of birth; in this respect it resembles Eastern techniques of meditation and differs from two other methods of prepared childbirth, the PSYCHOPROPHYLACTIC METHOD and the BRADLEY METHOD, which have largely replaced it. The breathing required is abdominal breathing (rather than the chest breathing advocated in the psychoprophylactic method) as well as light panting during the expulsion stage. A woman's partner is encouraged to be present during labor and delivery, mainly to give support. Dick-Read's method was the first of the prepared childbirth methods to become popular in America in the 1950s. He himself called it *natural childbirth*, a term now loosely used for any method of prepared birth.

diet   A regimen of food intake. A basic *normal diet* consists of a wide variety of foods that provide adequate amounts of all the essential nutrients; that is, a balance of carbohydrates, proteins and fats containing sufficient quantities of the essential vitamins, minerals and trace elements. In the

1990s the U.S. government replaced the format of its earlier nutritional guidelines with a Food Guide Pyramid, dividing the former four groups into five, and arranged from the pyramid's narrow top to the wide bottom to conform to the suggested level of intake. However, new findings concerning intake and other nutrients have called the government guidelines into question and have suggested new guidelines, described in the accompanying table. In addition to these figures, regular daily EXERCISE is recommended, at least 30 minutes a day and preferably 60 minutes. An important but often neglected element is dietary fiber, which helps prevent not only constipation but Type II diabetes. The simplest available source is cold cereals of various kinds (packages indicate precise fiber content).

At certain times of life, notably during adolescence, pregnancy and lactation, nutritional requirements are greater in terms of both total food intake (usually measured in calories) and increased need for particular nutrients. Even then, individual requirements vary according to body build, height and amount of daily exercise.

DIETARY GOALS FOR WOMEN[*]

Nutrient	Amount
Carbohydrate	45%–65% of calories (minimum 130 grams a day)
Fat[†]	20%–35% of calories
Omega-6 fatty acids	12 grams a day (women ages 19–50) 11 grams a day (women age 50 and over) 13 grams a day (pregnant or lactating women)
Omega-3 fatty acids	1.1 grams a day (women 19 and over) 1.4 grams a day (pregnant women) 1.3 grams a day (lactating women)
Protein	10%–35% of calories; 0.8 grams a day per kilogram of body weight
Added sugars[††]	No more than 25% of calories
Total fiber	25 grams per day (women ages 19–50) 21 grams per day (women age 50 and over)

[†]as little as possible saturated fat, cholesterol and trans fat
[††]Sugars incorporated in foods and beverages during production; major sources are soft drinks, fruit drinks, pastries, candies and other sweets.
[*]Report from Food and Nutrition Board, Institute of Medicine of the National Academy of Medicine

RECOMMENDED DAILY INTAKE[*]

Food energy	2,000 calories
Protein	44 grams
Dietary fiber	20 grams[†]
Total fat	65 grams[††]
Sodium	3,300 milligrams[†††] (maximum)

[*]For average moderately active women.
[†]National Cancer Institute and National Institute of Diabetes, Digestive and Kidney Diseases recommend 25 to 35 g.
[††]No more than 30% of total calories.
[†††]U.S. Nutrition Board recommends 2,300 mg. limit.

During the adolescent growth spurt (see PUBERTY) for girls from ages 10 or 11 to 15, for boys from 12 or 13 to 19, calorie requirements rise for both sexes. During this period most adolescents acquire almost half of their final adult weight. The precise amount needed depends on physical activity, but adolescent boys require at least 2,750 calories per day while girls need at least 2,200; participation in active sports may raise those amounts by 1,500 or more calories per day. (Adult men continue to require more calories than women simply because they usually are taller and have a heavier build.) After puberty, low-calorie diets, special athletic diets, strict vegetarian diets and other restrictive eating practices can impair fertility. The most common consequence is amenorrhea (cessation of periods), but sometimes anovulatory bleeding (menstruation without ovulation) results (see also CRITICAL WEIGHT).

During pregnancy the average woman needs 300 or so extra calories per day for proper nutrition. Protein in particular is important to nourish the growing fetus, and daily intake should be at least 65% higher (some say 100% higher) than before. Although clinicians routinely used to prescribe vitamin supplements, some now believe that a healthy pregnant woman eating a well-balanced diet composed of fruits, vegetables, meat, fish, eggs, whole grains and dairy products does not need any. However, unless she gets the CALCIUM equivalent of one quart (about one liter) of milk per day she may need a calcium supplement, and most authorities agree that she should also have supplements of IRON (aiming for a hemoglobin level of 12 to 16 grams per 100 milliliters of blood) and FOLIC ACID (folate). Some women lacking a certain enzyme may need extra vitamin B_{12} as well. Also especially

FOODS TO AVOID DURING PREGNANCY

- Raw fish and shellfish, a possible source of the parasite toxoplasma, which can cause fetal blindness and brain damage
- Large predatory fish such as swordfish, shark, king mackerel and albacore tuna (fresh or canned), which can contain risky levels of mercury
- Undercooked or raw meat, poultry and seafood
- Unpasteurized milk and soft cheeses (feta, Brie, Camembert, Roquefort, etc.) unless the label says it is made with pasteurized milk; may contain food-poisoning bacteria listeria, which can cause miscarriage, premature birth, stillbirth or fatal newborn illness
- Frankfurters and deli meats unless cooked until steaming hot
- Refrigerated patés, meat spreads and smoked seafood (unless cooked before eating; canned versions are safe)
- Soft-scrambled or lightly cooked eggs or foods containing them (homemade salad dressing, eggnog); cook eggs until white and yolk are firm to avoid salmonella poisoning
- Raw sprouts, including alfalfa, bean sprouts, clover
- Herbal teas and supplements; some, like black cohosh, can increase the risk of miscarriage
- Alcohol; limit to an occasional drink but no safe amount has been established

important are iodine, zinc, and vitamins A and D. Meat, chicken and fish are the best sources of iron and zinc, and fatty fish, egg yolks and fortified milk and orange juice are nearly the only dietary sources of vitamin D. For women who are lactose intolerant, yogurt with active cultures or lactose-reduced milk may be advisable. (See table under VITAMIN.)

Adequate liquid intake also is important, but alcoholic beverages in large amounts can be harmful to the baby. Safe levels have not been established, so many feel it is best to eliminate all alcohol during pregnancy (see ALCOHOL USE). Many clinicians also advise women to limit their intake of caffeine to no more than one or two cups of strong coffee a day and to discontinue their use of tobacco and nonessential drugs, including aspirin.

During lactation a woman may need 500 extra calories a day above her prepregnant level, mostly in the form of protein. The diet of the breast-feeding woman also should be high in calcium and the

B vitamins, with adequate fluids to replace what is lost through her milk. Some women find that if they eat certain foods their babies have more gas pains and colic; among the offenders often named are vegetables of the cabbage family (cauliflower, brussels sprouts, broccoli, cabbage), onions, garlic and chocolate. Others maintain that they can eat anything without ill effect on their babies.

With age, food requirements lessen; actually the total caloric intake needed to maintain weight declines by a small amount every year after the age of 20, by an estimated 5 to 10% each decade. By menopause only two-thirds as many calories are required to maintain weight, and after menopause, with the reproductive system no longer active, still fewer are needed. However, the need for calcium, vitamin D and the B vitamins continues to be great (some believe it is greater, since there is no longer much estrogen to help absorption of essential nutrients), and if the average woman must limit her total calories to 1,600 or so a day, she may need supplements of these nutrients to ensure adequate intake. The suggested level is 1,000 to 1,500 milligrams of calcium per day, along with 800 to 1,000 units of vitamin D (but no more, since higher amounts of D are toxic), along with a single B-complex supplement. Some women have found that vitamin E helps control HOT FLASHES, but there still is no conclusive evidence concerning its role, and it should not be used by women with hypertension (high blood pressure). Finally, certain substances should be restricted after the age of 50, notably CHOLESTEROL, which increases the risk of atherosclerosis, and sodium (salt; no more than 1,500 mg per day with an upper limit of 2,300 mg); the latter may call for a drastic reduction since the average American consumes 20 times that amount, which contributes to high blood pressure. (See MENOPAUSE; OBESITY.) Many also believe that alcohol and caffeine intake should be reduced greatly or eliminated.

During old age good nutrition becomes still more difficult to achieve. The elderly often are lonely and depressed, which diminishes their appetite and interest in taking care of themselves. They may have difficulty in shopping for food and preparing it; lose interest in preparing meals for themselves; lack teeth or have poorly fitting dentures, making it hard to chew healthful foods;

and live on a fixed income that limits their buying power. Consequently many older persons do not get enough protein, calcium, iron, vitamins, fiber or even total calories. Some gain weight on a diet high in carbohydrates but still are malnourished in terms of the proper nutrients. Capillary fragility, manifested in easy bruising and slow wound healing, is a common problem that can be helped by increasing vitamin C intake. Many physicians now recommend routine vitamin and mineral supplements for all elderly patients, on the assumption that they cannot get sufficient amounts of them without consuming far too many calories. Further, they suggest drastically lowering consumption of salt (1,300 mg a day after age 50, 1,200 after age 70), refined sugars and fats, in order to help prevent diabetes, hypertension and arteriosclerosis.

Vegetarianism, increasingly popular for numerous reasons (weight control; ethical qualms about animal products; lack of money; health considerations), poses some dietary problems. For vegetarians who eat both eggs and dairy products (*ovo-lacto vegetarians*), obtaining sufficient dietary protein and calcium may not be difficult. *Vegans,* who shun all animal products, must be careful to combine vegetable sources of protein (grains, legumes, nuts and seeds) in correct proportion so as to obtain usable protein. Although calcium is available from tofu with calcium salts, calcium-fortified orange juice and tahini, among other foods, and iron and vitamin B_{12} from fortified breads and cereals, it may be advisable to take supplements of these necessary nutrients, which are virtually absent in plant foods (vitamin B_{12} deficiency can cause pernicious anemia).

See also ANEMIA; VITAMIN.

diethylstilbestrol Also *DES.* A form of synthetic ESTROGEN developed in 1938 and widely used until about 1955 to prevent miscarriage. Although by then its effectiveness for this purpose was seriously questioned, it was used for almost 20 years longer, even after the U.S. Food and Drug Administration in 1971 warned against its use during pregnancy. The daughters of women who were given DES during pregnancy have shown a significant incidence of clear-cell ADENOCARCINOMA (see def. 2), a rare form of vaginal cancer—it appears in approximately 1 out of 1,000 DES daughters—as well as ADENOSIS (see def. 1) and other abnormalities of the reproductive tract. Further, some studies indicate that in their own pregnancies, DES daughters have higher rates of miscarriage and premature birth. Sons of DES mothers have shown a higher than normal incidence of genital and urinary abnormalities, and the mothers themselves are suspected of having a higher incidence of cancer of the breast and pelvic regions. Even more alarming, studies in research animals and laboratory-grown cells indicate that DES may damage the immune system, thus increasing the risk of developing such AUTO-IMMUNE DISEASES in DES daughters as a thyroid condition called Hashimoto's thyroiditis, pernicious anemia, myasthenia gravis, and possibly chronic fatigue syndrome and multiple sclerosis.

Today DES still is officially approved for use in a variety of other conditions, notably for treating certain advanced breast and prostate cancers, for "estrogen deficiency" in younger women, to suppress lactation in women not wishing to breast-feed and in the MORNING-AFTER PILL for birth control. It also is used as a growth stimulant in cattle and sheep, although in 1979 the FDA officially banned this substance from animal feed.

Because of the potential dangers to children born of DES mothers and the fact that anyone who gave birth after 1940 or was born after that date may unknowingly have been exposed to DES, certain guidelines have been developed. First, women suspecting that they may have received DES during pregnancy are urged to try to obtain their past medical records. Second, daughters of women who did receive DES are advised to have pelvic examinations every year beginning after their first menstrual period (or by the age of 14, whichever comes first) and also to have a checkup whenever they perceive unusual spotting, bleeding or heavy discharge. The examination should include a complete history, careful observation and palpation of vagina and cervix, a Pap smear and COLPOSCOPY of the vagina and CERVIX, including examination with an iodine stain (see SCHILLER TEST). Further, DES mothers are advised to perform monthly BREAST SELF-EXAMINATION and undergo annual breast exams by clinicians as well as annual pelvic examinations (including a bimanual examination and a Pap smear). Both DES mothers and daughters are advised to avoid when possible the use of estrogens for other purposes, such as oral contraceptives, menopausal estrogen replacement and the like. Finally, DES sons are advised to visit a urologist immediately following puberty to be screened for genital abnormalities that have been found in other DES sons, notably urinary problems, cysts, undescended testes (cryptorchidism) or underdeveloped testes, vas deferens blockage, low sperm count, abnormally shaped sperm or absence of sperm, and, as they get older, to be on the lookout for prostate cancer. Also see Appendix, Resources for DES.

dilatation and curettage   See D AND C.

dilatation and evacuation   Also *D and E.* A procedure that combines the traditional dilatation and curettage (or D AND C) with VACUUM ASPIRATION (def. 2) and is used chiefly to terminate pregnancies of 13 to 18 weeks, counting from the first day of the last menstrual period; technically it can be used up to 24 weeks but in practice it is not usually done after 18 weeks because the cervix would have to dilate too much in too short a time. It requires anesthesia, usually local (a paracervical block) or regional, and should be performed in a hospital or surgical clinic by a gynecologist. The cervix must be dilated more than for a D and C; often this is done with the aid of LAMINARIA, beginning 12 to 24 hours before surgery. A vacuum curet (suction tube) of the kind used in vacuum aspiration but with a larger bore (because more tissue must be removed) is inserted through the dilated cervix, and suction is applied to remove fetal and placental material; then forceps generally are used to complete the procedure, as well as a surgical curet to make sure all the tissue has been removed. Following surgery (sometimes during the procedure as well), most clinicians administer oxytocin to promote uterine contractions, which limits blood loss and returns the uterus to its normal prepregnant size. Dilatation and evacuation takes 15 to 45 minutes and usually does not require overnight hospitalization. If regional anesthesia is used, most patients experience sensations similar to those fol-

lowing vacuum aspiration, although the recovery period is somewhat longer and the patient usually is kept several hours for observation.

A rarely performed variant of dilatation and evacuation is the so-called *intact dilatation and evacuation,* or *partial-birth abortion,* which in the late 1990s became the focus of heated debate and was banned by a Supreme Court decision in 2007. In it the fetus is partly delivered, legs first, and its brains are suctioned out to permit easier passage through the birth canal. This procedure is carried out only if serious conditions in the mother or fetus warrant terminating the pregnancy. To avoid being prosecuted for violating the Partial-Birth Abortion Ban Act, which carries a two-year prison sentence, physicians at many hospitals inject the fetus with lethal drugs to be sure no live fetus is partially delivered. This procedure is generally done in abortions after 18 to 20 weeks' gestation and only with the patient's permission. The drugs used are either the heart drug dioxin or potassium chloride, a potentially poisonous salt. Not all abortion facilities engage in this practice.

See also ABORTION.

discharge, vaginal   Also *leukorrhea, vaginal secretions.* The normal secretions of the endocervical glands (located in the cervical canal) and Bartholin's glands, mixed with dead vaginal cells and bacteria normally residing in the vagina. These secretions normally are slightly acid, owing to lactic acid produced by the action of the DÖDERLEIN BACILLI.

The consistency of the cervical mucus changes during the menstrual cycle and therefore can be an indication of when ovulation takes place (see CERVICAL MUCUS METHOD). Normal vaginal discharge has practically no odor and does not cause itching, burning or other irritation. If such irritation occurs or if the discharge is smelly, copious, yellow, grayish green, cheesy or blood-specked, it usually signals the presence of an infection (see CERVICITIS; VAGINITIS).

discrete   Separate and distinct, a term used to describe lesions that are separated from one another.

diuretic Also *water pill*. A drug that acts on the kidneys to produce an increased output of sodium (salt) and water into the urine. It is used to treat disorders of the heart, circulatory system, kidneys or liver that result in excess fluid retention (edema, formerly called "dropsy"), especially hypertension (high blood pressure). Fluid retention also can be a problem with premenstrual tension (see DYSMENORRHEA, def. 5).

The principal diuretics are (1) thiazides and related drugs, such as chlorothiazide (under such brand names as Diufil, Aldocior and Diupres); (2) ethacrynic acid (Edecrin) and furosemide (Lasix), which are more powerful; and (3) carbonic anhydrase inhibitors, mild drugs used to treat glaucoma (acetazolamide, or Diamox).

Some thiazides, particularly chlorothiazide, developed in 1958, were for a time widely used to counter excess fluid retention in pregnancy, but in 1973 studies showed that they can damage both mother and fetus, and in 1976 the U.S. Food and Drug Administration required manufacturers to issue a warning concerning their many adverse side effects (loss of appetite, stomach irritation, diarrhea, constipation, cramping, jaundice, pancreatitis, hypertension and others).

HERBAL DIURETICS*

Simmer 1 tablespoon of herb
per cup of water for 20 minutes

Asparagus (*Asparagus officinalis*)†
Celery (*Apium graviolens*)† and celery seed
Cleavers, or bedstraw, or goosegrass (*Galium aparine*)
Cucumber (*Cucumis sativus*)†
Dandelion root and leaf (*Taraxacum officinale*)
Ground ivy (*Glechoma hederacea* or *Nepata glechoma*)
Hydrangea leaves or root (*Hydrangea*)
Juniper berries (*Juniperus communis*)
Parsley (*Petroselinum crispum*)†
Shepherd's purse (*Capsella bursa pastoris*)
Slippery elm (*Ulmus fulva*)
Wintergreen (*Gaultheria procumbens*), or partridgeberry

---

*Herbs, like synthetic drugs, have chemical constituents whose particular properties are what make them effective. However, like other drugs, they may contain allergens, and a person who is allergic to a particular substance can have an allergic reaction. Therefore herbs should be used with care.
†Eat as a vegetable.

Women who prefer HERBAL REMEDIES use infusions made from yarrow leaves (*Achillea millefolium*) or hibiscus flowers (*Hibiscus*), which are said to have diuretic properties. See also the accompanying table.

Döderlein bacilli Also *lactobacilli*. Rod-shaped microorganisms that live in the mucous membrane of the vagina and act on the glycogen of the vaginal walls, producing lactic acid. By breaking down the sugar that fosters the growth of yeast organisms, they help combat YEAST INFECTION. Oral antibiotics of various kinds, administered to fight other bacterial infections, often kill these helpful organisms as well, making a woman more susceptible to yeast infections.

See also YOGURT.

domestic abuse Also *abuse, intimate partner violence, IVP, violence against women*. Actual or threatened physical or sexual violence or psychological/emotional abuse of a woman by her intimate partner, including a current or former spouse, boyfriend or girlfriend. Physical violence includes RAPE as well as beating and other forms of assault. United States government statistics indicate that every 15 seconds a woman is beaten by her husband or boyfriend, and many women remain in abusive relationships. Domestic abuse can occur with both heterosexual and homosexual couples, and it is both a health and a mental-health problem. One study indicates that women victims of violence account for nearly 40% of all visits to hospital emergency rooms, and in more than one-third of these cases intimate partners were identified as the perpetrators. As a consequence of domestic abuse, women are more likely to need medical attention, take time off from work and spend more days in bed. Psychological consequences for victims of domestic abuse include depression, suicidal thoughts and attempts, lowered self-esteem, alcohol and other drug abuse, and post-traumatic stress disorder. Moreover, children in households where domestic abuse occurs not only are apt to become victims of it themselves, but also are at risk for mental-health problems and are likely to become abusers themselves. A recent study showed that women who suffer from domestic abuse have more headaches, chronic pain, gastrointestinal and gynecologic problems, depression and anxiety and injuries than other women, even long after the abuse has ended.

What should women in such situations do? During an attack, they are advised to protect themselves as best they can, to call for help or run to the nearest source of help, to call the police (or have someone else do so), to call their local crisis hot line to seek out a battered women's shelter in their area, and to get away as best they can. For resources that can help, see the Appendix.

donor egg An egg produced by a donor, fertilized by a man's sperm, either artificially or in vitro, and transferred to his partner's uterus, where gestation is completed. This form of assisted reproduction is used when a woman is anovulatory (cannot produce eggs or healthy eggs) but is able to sustain a pregnancy once a fertilized egg is implanted in her uterus. In some cases the eggs are taken from women who are undergoing LAPAROSCOPY for tubal ligation; the tube that is inserted through the abdomen for sterilization can be used to aspirate eggs from the ovary. These eggs are then fertilized in a laboratory container. In other cases an egg is fertilized inside the donor's fallopian tubes with the man's sperm through ARTIFICIAL INSEMINATION. The egg is washed from her uterus with a catheter inserted through the cervix before it has become implanted in the uterine wall and then is transferred to the body of the man's partner. For either technique, the donor is given hormone injections for about a week prior to egg retrieval, which increases the production of eggs from one per menstrual cycle to four or more (see FERTILITY DRUG). Donors also are usually required to undergo physical and psychological screening, blood tests, ultrasound and sometimes other tests. The timing of the procedure is based on the donor's menstrual cycle. Some religious groups oppose the procedure on moral grounds, and a few legal experts caution that it may raise the same question as surrogacy, that is, which woman is the child's legal mother.

Currently donor eggs are now used in 12% of all IN VITRO FERTILIZATION attempts and the number is growing. The major reason appears to be the rising birth rate among women in their 40s whose eggs cannot be fertilized as readily as those from a younger donor.

For sperm donor, see under SPERM BANK. See also SURROGATE MOTHER.

dorsal lithotomy The traditional position used for a gynecologic examination, in which the woman lies flat on her back on an examination table, with her knees drawn up, her legs spread and raised and her feet resting in stirrups for support. Because this position allows the clinician maximum visibility and ready access for a bimanual examination, it became the traditional position for childbirth, especially in hospitals. However, critics point out that it is actually less suited for efficient labor than positions where gravity can assist the process of birth, such as sitting up, squatting (see BIRTH STOOL) or lying on one side (see SIMS POSITION). It also places the weight of the pregnant uterus on the body's largest vein, the *vena cava*, so that the baby gets somewhat less oxygen during each contraction; further, it puts a strain on the perineum, increasing the need for EPISIOTOMY. Women with certain disabilities, such as SCOLIOSIS or arthritis of the hip, may find the dorsal lithotomy position very difficult or impossible for even a brief pelvic examination; for these women it may be preferable to perform an examination while they lie on one side with the uppermost leg lifted high (resting on the clinician's shoulder or held by an assistant).

douching Rinsing the vagina with water or some other solution. As a method of preventing pregnancy (douching after intercourse), it is considered less than 50% reliable (some authorities say 0%). Sperm can move quickly through the cervical opening into the cervical canal, beyond reach of the douche solution, within a minute or two of ejaculation, and can reach the fallopian tubes in as little as 10 minutes. Moreover, the pressure of the douching liquid may speed the sperm's progress. As a method of hygiene, comparable to bathing external areas of the body, douching is rarely necessary, and indeed by changing the relative acidity of the vagina it can encourage the growth of infection-causing organisms (see VAGINITIS) as well as help spread infection from the vagina up into the uterus and fallopian tubes. Women who feel unclean unless they douche are advised to do so no more than once a week, with only very gentle pressure (with a drainage bag at shoulder height or lower), using either plain warm water or 1 tablespoon white vinegar per quart of water. Douching should be avoided if pregnancy is suspected, after a D and C or abortion (for two weeks), after childbirth (for four to six weeks), and for three days prior to any gynecologic examination (because it may flush out organisms before they can be detected by the clinician).

Vaginal hygiene sprays sold over the counter often cause uncomfortable irritation and should be avoided; there is no clinical reason whatever for their use. Douching with antibacterial agents and home or over-the-counter remedies such as boric acid solution or vinegar and water is effective against some vaginal infections, but it is better to find out what organism is responsible for the condition before embarking on a course of douches.

doula   A person trained to work with doctors and midwives to give women emotional and physical support in planning for birth, during labor and, often, afterward. Working in a hospital or clinic setting, doulas do not actually deliver babies but remain with the mother for the entire labor. They may suggest different positions and breathing techniques to ease labor pain and comfort women who are frightened or anxious. They facilitate communication between the woman and her partner and her clinical care provider. They help her express her needs and desires and advocate for her when necessary. Following delivery, they may advise on breast-feeding, and many also assist mothers at home with their newborns, providing information and education on newborn care and sibling care, as well as emotional support.

The term *doula* comes from a Greek word meaning handmaiden or servant. Doula training consists of a minimum of a three-day course that covers the anatomy and process of labor along with techniques for providing emotional and physical comfort to the mother. In addition, a doula must attend at least three deliveries in order to be certified by Doulas of North America, an international organization that also provides training. (Also see resources in the Appendix.) However, many doulas have additional previous experience in the health care field. Research indicates that doula-attended births resulted in shorter labors, considerably less need for epidural anesthesia, pain medication and use of forceps, less delivery complications and far fewer Cesareans.

At this writing only about 1% of births in the United States are attended by doulas, but they are gaining wider acceptance by obstetricians and hospitals, and a growing number of insurance plans cover their services.

dowager's hump   Also *kyphosis*. Curvature of the upper vertebrae of the spine, giving a humped-back appearance. It is so called because it appears mostly in postmenopausal women, as a result of OSTEOPOROSIS.

Down syndrome   Also *Down's syndrome, mongolism*. A BIRTH DEFECT that usually is caused by the presence of an extra chromosome and is characterized by such abnormalities as mental retardation, retarded growth, poor muscle tone, a small, flat nose and slanting eyes (accounting for the older name, "mongoloid"), a protruding lower lip and small, broad hands and feet. In 80% of cases the extra chromosome comes from the mother, from whom the embryo thus gets 24 chromosomes that pair up with 23 from the father (see under GENETICS for further explanation). Most Down syndrome babies have three chromosomes in what would normally be a pair identified as number 21, so the disorder is also called *Trisomy 21*. About 3% of cases, however, are caused by translocation (genes out of order) and are hereditary, a defect that can be detected by KARYOTYPING.

Down syndrome is thought to be the most common form of mental retardation. It occurs in about 1 of every 600 babies born and is responsible for

DOWN SYNDROME

Age of mother	Incidence of
Under 20	1 in 2,500
20–29	1 in 1,500
30–34	1 in 850
35–39	1 in 280
40–44	1 in 100
Over 44	1 in 40

almost three-tenths of all cases of severe retardation in the Western world. Many Down syndrome babies suffer from serious heart defects as well, and, until recently, most died before reaching adulthood; those who did survive generally were institutionalized. Today it is recognized that Down syndrome children vary in intelligence level and that many, if their physical defects permit survival, can be educated sufficiently to manage adult life in some kind of supervised setting. Early intervention programs, begun as soon as one month after birth, have been found to promote considerable gains in a child's abilities.

The cause of Down syndrome is not known, but, because the frequency of Trisomy 21 increases in direct proportion to the age of the mother (see the accompanying table), it is strongly suspected that aging adversely affects the ova (eggs) in some way, a fact that has been demonstrated in other species of animal even though there is no direct evidence for human ova. Fortunately, the extra chromosome can be detected by AMNIOCENTESIS and CHORIONIC VILLUS SAMPLING, so that women who choose not to bear a baby with this defect may have the option of abortion. Blood tests of the mother, less invasive than either procedure, and performed earlier in the pregnancy, also have been developed. Tests performed during the first trimester are an ultrasound exam for nuchal translucency, which measures a fluid-filled space in the baby's neck, and blood tests for beta-hCG and pregnancy-associated plasma protein A (PAPP-A). Another test, performed during the second trimester, checks the levels of pregnancy-associated protein A, estriol, and human chorionic gonadotropin; it is called *triple screen* and, if levels are abnormal, is followed by amniocentesis. A variation is *quadruple screen*, which adds the hormone inhibin A to the markers

tested in triple screen. Although these tests may make it possible to avoid amniocentesis, which sometimes causes miscarriage, they also may yield false positive results, thus necessitating amniocentesis anyway, as well as missing some fetuses with Down syndrome.

Because the risk of Down syndrome rises with the mother's age, testing for it long was routine only for women aged 35 and older. However, most babies with Down syndrome are born to younger women simply because they give birth in far greater numbers. Therefore it is now recommended that screening for Down syndrome be offered to all pregnant women, regardless of age. As of this writing, noninvasive blood tests for this condition, expected to be very accurate, are under development.

See also AGE, CHILDBEARING; PRENATAL TESTS.

dropping See LIGHTENING.

drug use and pregnancy Practically all substances ingested by a pregnant woman—including tobacco smoke, alcoholic beverages, prescription drugs, illegal drugs and over-the-counter remedies such as aspirin and laxatives—have some effect on the fetus she is carrying. The placenta transports almost every substance the mother takes in to the unborn child. Therefore most authorities agree that no drug should be used during any stage of pregnancy (or while BREAST-FEEDING) unless it is absolutely needed, and then only in the smallest dose and for the shortest time possible. Habit-forming drugs such as *opiates* (opium, heroin, morphine, codeine, methadone) all can cause drug dependency in the baby, which will be born addicted and immediately begin to experience withdrawal symptoms. Tranquilizers and antidepressants have not been fully evaluated in terms of their effect on the fetus (except for a few, among them the disastrously damaging THALIDOMIDE). The phenothiazines— major tranquilizers such as Thorazine, Stelazine, Compazine and Mellaril—have caused infant death in test animals, and at least one has been connected with the development of jaundice in human babies. Librium and Valium, two common minor

TRANQUILIZERS, have caused skeletal abnormalities in animal fetuses and babies. The SSRIs (see ANTI-DEPRESSANTS) appear to be safer, but it is important to weigh the risks, which include possible malformations or other difficulties in newborns, against the benefits of preventing the danger of major depression. Some women reduce their dosage during pregnancy; others avoid antidepressants altogether during the first trimester, the period of fetal organ formation, and/or the end of the last trimester, to avoid newborn complications.

A recent study indicated that a sizable percentage of pregnant women are still prescribed medications with the potential to harm the fetus. The FDA classifies such drugs as category X, for which the risk to the fetus clearly outweighs any benefit, and category D, whose therapeutic benefits possibly outweigh the risks. Among drugs to be avoided are teratogens such as isotretinoin (Accutane), tetracycline antibiotics, the antifungal drug fluconazole, the antiepileptic carbamazepine, propylthiouracil and lipid-lowering drugs such as Lipitor. D and X drugs include estrogens, the heart drug atenolol, the barbiturate secobarbital and benzodiazepines (tranquilizers).

Other mind-altering or recreational drugs—LSD, mescaline, marijuana, cocaine, PCP or "angel dust," hashish—as well as amphetamines ("speed," diet pills, "uppers") and barbiturates (Seconal, Nembutal, sleeping pills) also reach the fetus, with varied effects. Even such a seemingly harmless remedy as aspirin can, especially when used in large doses in late pregnancy, disrupt the blood-clotting mechanism of both baby and mother, causing danger at delivery; it should be avoided throughout the pregnancy if possible. Frequent use of laxatives can interfere with the absorption of nutrients. Antibiotics also can damage the fetus: Tetracycline is known to cause permanent discoloration of the baby's teeth and also may affect bone growth. Penicillin, erythromycin and the cephalosporins are safe. Some sulfa drugs taken in late pregnancy can disturb the baby's liver function. Caffeine, present in coffee, tea, cola drinks and some pain relievers (usually together with aspirin), also may be implicated in birth defects and should not be taken in large quantities.

To avoid possible damage, a woman who discovers she is pregnant should, at her first prenatal care visit, discuss in detail any prescription medications and over-the-counter remedies she might use. Throughout her pregnancy she should be careful to remind other clinicians she may consult (including her dentist) that she is pregnant. On balance, use of an occasional aspirin or laxative is unlikely to cause any damage, but beyond such minimal use any drug taken during pregnancy always should be evaluated as to its risks versus its benefits.

dry eye Also *keratoconjunctivitis sicca.* A chronic dryness of the conjunctiva, the clear tissue that lines the eyelids and covers the eyeball surface. It affects both eyes, in which tears are inadequate or evaporate so quickly that the eyes constantly feel irritated and gritty, as if scratched by sand. In milder cases, the eyes become irritated in dry air (windy or sunny conditions, on airplanes and so on) or when focused for long periods while reading or watching television.

There are two types of dry eye. One is *aqueous deficient dry eye,* characterized by insufficient tear production. The other is *evaporative dry eye,* occurring when tears evaporate too quickly. An estimated 10 million Americans suffer from dry eye, the majority of whom are women, because many of the medical conditions that cause it occur more often in women. Among these conditions are SJÖGREN'S SYNDROME, hormonal disruptions during pregnancy and after menopause, rheumatoid arthritis, asthma, diabetes, lupus, thyroid disorders, Crohn's disease, acne rosacea, estrogen replacement therapy, glaucoma and blepharitis (chronic eyelid inflammation). Numerous medications also can cause the problem—antidepressants, decongestants, antihistamines, oral contraceptives, diuretics and beta-blockers, among others. Environmental factors also can be responsible, among them exposure to wind, sun, air pollutants (cigarette smoke); swimming in pool or seawater without goggles; working at a computer for long periods; or wearing long-wearing contact lenses. Aging also diminishes tear production, contributing to the problem.

Diagnosis is a simple test performed by an ophthalmologist. Treatment other than changing medications or reducing exposure to environmental factors includes frequent bathing of the eyes with artificial tears, which works for most patients.

Alternatives are gels and ointments, which are thicker than eye drops and last longer. Ointments, which tend to blur vision, are recommended for more severe symptoms and are used at night. All these are available over the counter. A newer prescription medication is cyclosporine A (Restasis) eye drops. The tear-making glands also respond to androgen, which may be used in eye drops. Evaporation of the tear film also may be reduced by plugging the drainage ducts in the eyes with tiny bits of silicone. In especially severe cases that do not respond to other treatment, the eyelids may be sewn partly shut to keep moisture in.

Patients are instructed to protect their eyes with wraparound sunglasses and to use gel at bedtime, especially when winter conditions—cold air, wind, dry indoor heat—can worsen the condition. Use a humidifier if you have dry heat in the house, turn car air vents away from your eyes and use artificial tears before air travel.

dry labor   Labor that occurs after the breaking of the membranes, that is, the spontaneous rupture of the AMNIOTIC SAC and release of the amniotic fluid. In most cases the sac does not rupture of its own accord until late in the first stage of LABOR, but occasionally it occurs very early in labor or prior to it. Sometimes it is broken by the clinician as part of INDUCTION OF LABOR or to strengthen uterine contractions. Actually, subsequent labor is not truly dry, since the cells lining the amniotic sac continue to secrete large amounts of fluid.

dryness, vaginal   See VAGINAL ATROPHY.

ductal papilloma   Also *intraductal papilloma*. A benign (noncancerous) tumor in the breast's system of ducts, which may produce both a mass (lump) in the breast and a serous (clear) or bloody discharge from the nipple. The serum secreted by papillomas tends to dam up in the duct and may become infected, leading to inflammation of the duct and surrounding tissue. Because such a tumor is hard to distinguish from a cancer, it nearly always is excised.

Duke's test   A blood test to discover if a woman has developed antibodies against her partner's sperm and therefore cannot become pregnant.

See SPERM.

dysfunctional bleeding, vaginal   Also *functional bleeding*. Heavy bleeding from the vagina with no discoverable cause, as opposed to bleeding that has a definite cause, such as a fibroid or some other lesion. Some authorities restrict the term "dysfunctional" to exceptionally heavy menstrual flow; others use it for any abnormal bleeding, either during a period or between periods (BREAKTHROUGH BLEEDING).

See also ANOVULATORY BLEEDING; ENDOMETRIAL HYPERPLASIA.

dysmenorrhea   **1.** Any physical or emotional discomfort associated with menstrual periods.

2. primary dysmenorrhea. Dysmenorrhea associated directly with menstrual periods rather than some underlying disorder.

3. secondary dysmenorrhea. Dysmenorrhea, usually spasmodic (see def. 4 below), that results from a specific condition or disorder, such as endometriosis, uterine fibroids, pelvic inflammatory disease or the presence of an intrauterine device (IUD).

4. spasmodic dysmenorrhea. Also *menstrual cramps*. Painful cramps, spasms of dull and/or acute lower abdominal discomfort, that occur on the first day of menstrual flow but sometimes some hours before the flow begins and/or on the second or subsequent days as well. The pain normally involves only the lower abdominal and genital area, but sometimes it is felt in the lower back, on the inner thighs and throughout the pelvis. Along with pain, some women experience nausea, vomiting, dizziness and fainting. Such cramps usually do not occur during the first year or two of menstrual cycles, appearing (if at all) only after ovulation becomes established. Possibly the shedding of endometrial tissue after ovulation causes stronger uterine contractions that, along with spasms of small arteries in the uterine walls, are the source of the pain. Cramps tend to lessen in severity after the age of 30. However, some women never (or hardly ever) experience spasmodic dysmenorrhea, and never enough to disable them even temporarily, whereas others continue to suffer from it monthly until menopause. In 5% or so of women the condition is severe enough to interfere significantly with their lives.

For some years physicians prescribed hormones, especially estrogens, to alleviate severe cramps, but more recent evidence indicates that the principal purpose served by such treatment, which is not without risk, was to eliminate ovulation; indeed, women taking oral contraceptives for birth control often find they no longer have menstrual cramps. More recently, increased levels of hormones called *prostaglandins,* which cause uterine contractions, have been suspected to be the underlying cause of most spasmodic dysmenorrhea, and treatment with antiprostaglandins or prostaglandin inhibitors— among them fenoprofen, ibuprofen, naproxen and mefenamic acid—has met with considerable success. Since these drugs also are commonly used as pain relievers, the results are not wholly conclusive. Further, they cannot be used by women with a history of ulcers or asthma, which these drugs might aggravate, or if there is a possibility of pregnancy (since they pass through to the fetus).

Women have long used a variety of home remedies for cramps. Heat tends to relax the spasms, and relief often is afforded by use of a heating paid or a hotwater bottle applied to the lower abdomen or deep-heating oil (such as tiger balm) rubbed into the affected area. Avoiding long periods of standing also helps. A hot bath (but not so hot as to provoke nausea or fainting) may ease the discomfort, along with drinks of warm broth or herbal teas (see discussion of herbal remedies below). Some women find a strong alcoholic drink helpful for relaxing uterine muscles. The deep breathing and back massage used in some methods of prepared childbirth may help, as do muscle-relaxing exercises such as the cobra, bow and pelvic rock of yoga. There is no need to avoid ordinary exercise, and some women actually find jogging or a game of tennis helpful. Orgasm also affords relief, probably by increasing blood circulation to the pelvis.

Good nutrition is important, and some women are helped by balanced supplements of calcium and magnesium in a 2 to 1 ratio (500 milligrams calcium, 250 milligrams magnesium), taken for a week before each period, and dolomite (which contains calcium and magnesium) taken every few hours (up to 6 pills per day) during the first and second days of a very painful period. Vitamins A, C and D are needed for good calcium absorption. A high-fiber diet (rich in whole grain, raw fruit and vegetables), with its natural laxative effect, may help relieve the constipation that often is associated with both spasmodic and congestive dysmenorrhea (see def. 5 below).

Among HERBAL REMEDIES used by women for cramps are: for mild cramps, an infusion (tea) of red raspberry leaves (*Rubus idaeus*), alone or with squaw vine or partridgeberry (*Mitchella repens*); for moderate cramps, capsules of cramp bark (*Viburnum opulus*) taken with red raspberry tea. Also used are infusions made from sweet or lemon balm (*Melissa officinalis*), chamomile (*Matricaria chamomilla, Anthemis nobilis*), mugwort (*Artemisia vulgaris*) or motherwort (*Leonurus cardiaca*).

If severe cramps do not respond to simpler remedies and there is no underlying disease causing them (see def. 3 above), a prescription for a stronger analgesic, such as codeine, or for antiprostaglandins may be needed.

5. congestive dysmenorrhea. Also *premenstrual tension, premenstrual syndrome, PMS.* A series of one or more symptoms that occur, alone or sometimes together, before the onset of a menstrual period, usually during the preceding week. The most common of them are edema (fluid retention, with bloating or swelling in the abdomen, breasts, fingers and ankles and accompanying weight gain), a dull ache in the lower abdomen, headache, backache, joint and muscle pains, skin lesions (especially acne), irritability, depression and fatigue. The occurrence of these symptoms more or less regularly before every (or nearly every) menstrual period and relief from them soon after menstrual flow begins are what pinpoint diagnosis.

The term *premenstrual tension* was coined in 1931 by Dr. Robert T. Frank. It is thought to occur to some degree in at least half (some say three-fourths) of all women of child-bearing age; in about 10% it seriously affects their lives, requiring time off from work or school. Extremely severe symptoms, especially extreme mood changes, are called *premenstrual dysphoric disorder,* or *PMDD.* The underlying cause of most of the symptoms may be the influence of estrogen on the body's salt and water exchange, with higher estrogen levels toward the end of the MENSTRUAL CYCLE inhibiting the normal flushing of sodium and water through the kidneys. The extra water then is redistributed into the body tissues, with resultant edema. Some researchers believe the adrenal hormone ALDOSTE-RONE may be responsible for fluid retention. The mood changes associated with congestive dysmenorrhea, which are as characteristic of the condition as fluid retention, also are most likely the result of biochemical factors, probably triggered by ovulation. Recent studies suggest that severe PMS is associated with lower than average levels of the neurotransmitter (brain chemical) serotonin. One study suggested that an obesity drug that affects this neurotransmitter, D-fenfluramine, may relieve symptoms. Another more recent finding is that serotonin-inhibiting ANTIDEPRESSANTS (SSRIs), such as fluoxetine (Prozac), sertraline (Zoloft), paroxetine (Paxil) or fluvoxamine (Luvox), begun on day 14 of the menstrual cycle and taken for 12 days, cut symptoms by 60%, especially the symptoms of depression, anxiety, mood swings and headache. Dosages are lower than those used to treat depression. Another medication is the anti-anxiety drug alprazolam (Xanax), taken for seven or eight days before a period begins. Still another approach uses GnRH (gonadotropin-releasing hormone) analogs, which induce a temporary, reversible menopause. Not only are they very expensive, but they cannot be used for more than a few months without compromising bone density. Still another drug is DANAZOL, which has severe side effects.

Before resorting to medication—and at this writing no drug has received Food and Drug Administration approval for treating PMS—it may be advisable to try some simpler remedies. Fluid retention may be minimized by reducing sodium intake (avoid table salt, carbonated drinks, soy sauce, MSG and very salty foods such as most cheeses and smoked meats and fish) and increasing the intake of potassium (found in ripe bananas, orange juice, peanuts and peanut butter) and calcium (milk and milk products). Reducing or elimi-nating caffeine, alcohol, fats and sweets during the premenstrual period may also alleviate symptoms. A high-fiber diet (whole grains, raw fruits and vegetables) helps counter the constipation often associated with the syndrome. Such constipation is thought to be caused by the shift of fluid from the bowel to the intestinal walls or by the effects of hormones on the muscles of the bowel. Daily aerobic exercise (running, brisk walking, cycling, etc.) also appears to be helpful, perhaps because of its tranquilizing effect. Recent studies indicate that calcium supplements—1,200 milligrams of chewable calcium carbonate a day—may help women. The symptoms that calcium seemed to relieve the most were food cravings, water retention, depression and mood swings, and back pain and cramping. It is not known how calcium works, but since women often do not get enough of this mineral in their diets, it seems advisable to try this simple remedy. In severe cases, however, more potent medication may be indicated, including oral contraceptives to halt ovulation, and, most extreme of all, GnRH agonists to stop the menstrual cycle entirely (and simulate menopause).

Some HERBAL REMEDIES used to relieve symptoms are infusions made from chamomile (*Matricaria chamomilla* or *Anthemis nobilis*), catnip (*Nepeta cataria*), hops (*Humulus lupulus*), motherwort (*Leonurus cardiaca*), mugwort (*Artemisia vulgaris*), skullcap (*Scutellaria lateriflora*), spearmint (*Mentha spicata*), sweet balm or lemon balm (*Melissa officinalis*) or valerian (*Valeriana officinalis*). An herbal compound made from the fruit of the chasteberry tree (*Vitex agnus castus*), found widely in southern Europe and western Asia, reportedly is helpful. Some women also report good results from using capsules of evening primrose oil, made from the seeds of the evening primrose (*Oenothera biennis*); they are available in health-food stores (follow directions on the bottle). In addition, some recommend taking 400 International Units of vitamin E twice a day up to 14 days before a period (alone or together with the primrose oil).

dyspareunia Painful vaginal intercourse. Pain in the vagina itself may be caused by a local disorder, such as irritation from a spermicide, a vaginal deodorant spray or the rubber of a diaphragm or condom, which subsequently is aggravated by the movement of the penis inside the vagina, or by a vaginal infection such as a yeast infection or trichomonas. If a woman has had little sexual experience, entrance into the vagina may be uncomfortable owing to an insufficiently stretched hymen, to fear or tension or to inadequate foreplay (sexual stimulation before actual penetration, which causes the vaginal walls to secrete lubricating fluids). Occasionally even considerable stimulation will not create enough fluid for lubrication. This is particularly common after menopause (see VAGINAL ATROPHY), during breast-feeding, immediately after a menstrual period and after radiation therapy for pelvic cancer. Often it can be relieved by using a water-soluble jelly, such as K-Y jelly, or a spermicidal cream, jelly or foam, or lubricated condoms. Pain from spasm of the vaginal muscles often can be corrected by therapy in which the woman learns to relax specific muscles (see VAGINISMUS). If the pain is deep in the pelvis, the cause may be a pelvic infection (such as pelvic inflammatory disease), endometriosis, ovarian tumors or cysts, or some other condition that should be investigated or treated by a physician. Sometimes COLPOSCOPY can determine the cause of dyspareunia. However, some women who have no specific disorder always experience pain when the penis hits the cervix; this can be avoided only by less deep penetration, which may be effected by a change in the woman's or the couple's position for intercourse.

dysplasia Also *cervical intraepithelial neoplasia, squamous intraepithelial lesions, SIL.* Mild to moderate abnormalities in the surface cells of the uterus (endometrium) and cervix. It is not certain whether or when such abnormalities are PRECANCEROUS LESIONS, and opinion differs as to whether they should be left alone (since some disappear spontaneously), treated conservatively or treated by surgery.

The surface, or epithelium, of the cervix is made up of several cell layers, and there is constant growth and development within the cervical epithelium. New cells are produced at the bottom layer, mature and move to the top, replacing old cells that are shed from the top. When precancerous cell changes occur, the maturation process is upset and there are more immature cells on the surface, along with unusually large or malformed cells. It is these surface cells that are picked up by a PAP SMEAR. With mild dysplasia, a significant number of young (immature) cells appear in the top layers of the epithelium (constituting a LSIL Pap smear), and with moderate dysplasia (HSIL smear) there is an even higher proportion of such cells. When there are few mature cells on the surface, the condition usually is called CANCER IN SITU, that is, a localized cancer without invasive (into neighboring tissue) propensities. With cervical cancer there are no mature cells on the top layer, which is now made up entirely of immature cells (see also CANCER, CERVICAL).

Dysplasia can result from infection or from oral contraceptives or other hormone therapy, environmental pollutants, radiation, profound emotional stress or any combination of these factors. Many authorities now believe that it is most often caused by the human papilloma virus (HPV), also responsible for genital warts and thought to account for most cervical cancers. In dysplasia the cervix may have a red bumpy (mosaic) appearance or leukoplakia (white patches), or it may show no overt signs at all. There rarely is any pain.

A Pap smear showing dysplasia usually calls for a second Pap smear, and if it confirms the diagnosis, COLPOSCOPY. (Some clinicians take needle biopsies—see BIOPSY, def. 3—of tissue from suspicious areas, but these may miss cancerous cells.) Before this technique became available, CONIZATION, which removes the entire surface of the cervix, was usually performed, but today this rarely is necessary for diagnosis. If dysplasia is confirmed by a colposcope-directed biopsy, treatment varies. If dysplasia is mild, it may consist of repeat Pap smears and/or repeat colposcopy, since the condition sometimes disappears spontaneously. If dysplasia is extensive and severe, treatment is aimed at eliminating the abnormal cells, usually by CRYOSURGERY, CAUTERIZATION or LASER SURGERY (which directs a destructive beam of light energy at the area of abnormality). Cryosurgery is not good for big lesions and produces a copious, unpleasant discharge that lasts up to three weeks. Lasers, which destroy tissue in 10 to 15 minutes, produce better results but are expensive. Another newer technique is LOOP ELECTROSURGICAL EXCISION PROCEDURE. Any of these procedures will kill the top layer of abnormal cells and usually, but not always, cure the dysplasia, which, however, may recur.

Surgical treatment of cancerous lesions consists of either conization or hysterectomy (removal of uterus and cervix), which are far more radical procedures. With severe dysplasia (cancer in situ) many authorities believe that either cryosurgery or cauterization is sufficient, but for women who want no children hysterectomy may be an appropriate choice, since it does away with the frequent follow-up examinations that are otherwise needed.

Some women who prefer far more conservative treatment have used herbal suppositories and douches as well as fasting, special diets and nutritional supplements in the form of vitamins and herbal teas. It should be emphasized that these, like more conventional treatment, should be followed up regularly with Pap smears to make sure the dysplasia is not progressing. One such treatment combines powdered squaw vine (*Mitchella repens*), chickweed (*Stellaria media*), slippery elm bark (*Ulmus fulva*), comfrey root (*Symphytum officinale*), golden seal root (*Hydrastia canadensis*), yellow dock root (*Rumex crispus*), mullen or mullein leaf (*Verbascum thapsus*) and marshmallow root (*Althea officinalis*),

mixed together with cocoa butter and formed into vaginal suppositories. Other treatments include a vegetarian diet supplemented with red clover (*Trifolium pretense*) tea and red raspberry (*Rubus idaeus*) tea; vitamin supplements containing A, B-complex, C and E; fasting for one to three days (unless there are contraindications); acidic douches of vitamin C or lemon juice or vinegar diluted with water. Yoga and meditation, especially with positive visualization (attempting to visualize the dissolving of abnormal cells and growth of healthy cells), have been used as well. Although skeptics may dismiss these treatments as fanciful, they apparently have helped some women and so cannot be discounted completely. On the other hand, their chief value may be as a form of PLACEBO, the dysplasia itself disappearing spontaneously and not as the result of any treatment.

dystocia Difficult labor or childbirth. It usually is due to three factors, either alone or, more often, in combination: ABNORMAL PRESENTATION (position) of the baby; too small a passage in the pelvis; and uterine dysfunction (see under PROLONGED LABOR).

dysuria Pain on urination, usually caused by a bladder or kidney infection.
See CYSTITIS, def. 1; PYELONEPHRITIS.

early pregnancy test Strictly speaking, any PREG-NANCY TEST made within a few days of the first missed period (or even before that). However, the term is usually reserved for various kinds of do-it-yourself test kits, which have been available in North American drugstores without prescription and at nominal cost since 1978. All of the kits currently available are urine tests that yield results in two hours. Positive results can be obtained as early as the first day after a missed period. When used precisely according to instructions, such tests are considered quite accurate. However, some of the kits instruct a woman who gets a negative result to repeat the test a week later (if her period has not begun in the meantime) and then, if the result is still negative and her periods do not resume, to consult a physician.

eating disorders See ANOREXIA; BULIMIA; OBESITY.

eclampsia Also (formerly) *metabolic toxemia of (late) pregnancy, toxemia.* An acute illness occurring after 24 weeks of pregnancy or just after childbirth that is characterized by severe convulsions and loss of consciousness, followed by coma. It may be fatal. The condition nearly always is preceded by PREECLAMPSIA, which often can be controlled, so that eclampsia usually can be prevented. Eclampsia occurs three times as often in women carrying a first child as in women who have borne other children. Approximately half of all cases develop before delivery (nearly always in the last trimester), one-fourth during labor and one-fourth after delivery (usually within 24 hours). Eclampsia occurs four times more often in multiple pregnancies than in single ones. It also is associated with ECTOPIC PREGNANCY and HYDATIDIFORM MOLE. Women whose mothers had eclampsia also are more likely to develop it.

Eclampsia is readily diagnosed by the onset of convulsions and coma. A convulsion can occur at any time, sometimes while the patient is sleeping, and is followed by coma of varying duration. Other signs are oliguria (decreased urinary output), high pulse rate, elevated blood pressure and temperature, proteinuria (protein in the urine), edema (fluid retention) and hyperreflexia (exaggerated reflexes). When eclampsia occurs during labor or after delivery, there may be only a single convulsion. More often, however, the first is followed by more convulsions, ranging from one or two in mild cases to as many as 100 in severe ones. The patient may recover consciousness between convulsions but sometimes does not, and, in severe cases, may die before awakening. If convulsions occur before delivery, labor generally begins soon afterward and progresses very quickly to completion, sometimes before anyone is even aware that the patient is having contractions. If convulsions occur during labor, the contractions rapidly become more frequent and much stronger, shortening the duration of labor. After delivery the condition usually improves within a day or so, although occasionally the convulsions resume and the second attack, usually occurring within two to four days, may be more severe or even fatal.

As with preeclampsia, the cause of eclampsia is not known, although many theories have been advanced. Prevention consists of treating preeclampsia. When eclampsia does develop, treatment is directed at stopping the convulsions with sedatives. The patient is hospitalized immediately and given medication to lower her blood pressure and increase urinary output. Although the delivery in itself may cure the mother, it is usually delayed (if possible) until she is free of convulsions and coma; nevertheless, some women go into labor spontaneously.

The risks associated with eclampsia are high for babies. Many succumb for lack of oxygen, from the heavy sedation required to control convulsions, from injury during too rapid a delivery and from prematurity. A woman who has had eclampsia once is more likely to develop it with subsequent pregnancies. Also, eclampsia may predispose a woman to the development of hypertension (high blood pressure) later in life (or it may simply signal the fact that she is already predisposed to develop it). Both these factors should be considered when another pregnancy is contemplated.

ectasia   See MAMMARY DUCT ECTASIA.

ectopic pregnancy   Also *tubal pregnancy.* The implantation and growth of a fertilized egg in some organ other than the uterus, usually in one of the fallopian tubes but occasionally (although quite rarely) in the ovaries, peritoneum or cervical canal. The condition usually is caused by distortion or damage of the fallopian tubes resulting from endometriosis, gonorrhea, pelvic inflammatory disease or some other disorder, exposure to diethylstilbestrol (DES), a previous ectopic pregnancy, tubal ligation, or past or present use of an IUD. Blocked by scar tissue, the fertilized egg cannot move down to the uterus, as it normally would, and remains in the tube, generally growing there for a period of two to three months. When the tube can no longer accommodate the enlarging embryo it ruptures, which may result in hemorrhage, a true medical emergency. Or, if the embryo is near the upper end of the tube, the muscular actions of the tube may push it into the pelvic cavity; if this occurs at an early stage of pregnancy, the embryo generally will be absorbed, giving rise to no further symptoms.

Diagnosing an ectopic pregnancy can be difficult. There may or may not be pain. There may or may not be a positive pregnancy test. Usually there will be at least one missed menstrual period, and then some slight bleeding and cramp-

ing pain. Some women continue to have periods, however, and experience no other symptoms of early pregnancy—morning sickness, enlarged or tender breasts, fatigue. Therefore the diagnosis of ectopic pregnancy often is not made until the tube ruptures. Danger signals are sudden sharp pain or persistent one-sided pain in the lower abdomen, shoulder pain, irregular bleeding or staining and abdominal pain following a very light period or a late period; these warrant seeking emergency treatment at once. If tubal pregnancy is suspected, blood tests should reveal if HCG (the hormone produced by the pregnancy) levels are increasing as they should in a normal pregnancy; if they are not, ULTRASOUND can establish the diagnosis.

Treatment depends on the extent of damage, the presence of infection in the area and the patient's age (whether she wishes to bear subsequent children), but a decision must be made quickly because of the danger of hemorrhage. In the past the affected fallopian tube usually was removed, but today practitioners often try to save it by removing the embryo through laparoscopy and repairing the tube. If the pregnancy is at an early stage, methotrexate, an anticancer drug administered by injection into the ectopic sac or by oral, intramuscular or intravenous means, may dissolve the embryonic tissue. Even if the tube cannot be saved, the adjacent ovary is spared if possible. When, however, the pregnancy has occurred in the only remaining tube (usually because the other was already removed for an earlier ectopic pregnancy) and this tube cannot be saved, hysterectomy (removal of the uterus) may be considered.

The occurrence of one ectopic pregnancy greatly increases the likelihood of another, since the underlying cause still may be present. Other predisposing factors are tubal surgery (see TUBEROPLASTY), gonorrheal infection, conception while an intrauterine device (IUD) is in place and conception while taking oral contraceptives.

edema   Also *fluid retention, water retention, bloating, dropsy* (obsolete). An abnormal accumulation of fluid in the body, specifically in the spaces outside the vessels of the circulatory system. The principal symptoms are swelling, particularly noticeable in the extremities (fingers, ankles), and weight gain. Mild edema is commonplace in women at certain times, especially premenstrually (see DYSMENOR-RHEA, def. 5) and during late pregnancy. It is not known just why or how the body accumulates more water at those times, but most likely the higher levels of estrogen and progesterone are a factor. Severe edema, on the other hand, is a symptom of a number of potentially life-threatening disorders, among them ECLAMPSIA in women who are pregnant or have just given birth, and liver, heart and kidney disease. Acute pulmonary edema, a complication of congestive heart disease, is a medical emergency requiring prompt treatment.

Edema commonly is treated with a DIURETIC, a class of drugs that aim to improve the function of vital organs whose impairment is causing the edema and/or to relieve the distress of symptoms. Such treatment nearly always is combined with the restriction of sodium (salt) intake in the diet, since high levels of sodium make the body retain water.

effacement   The process, during the last month of pregnancy and through the first stage of LABOR, of progressive thinning and shortening of the cervical canal from about 2 centimeters (⅘ inch) in length to none, the canal being replaced by a flat circular opening with almost paper-thin edges. The process takes place from above downward. As the muscular fibers around the internal cervical os (opening into the body of the uterus) are pulled up into the lower body of the uterus, the edges of the os are drawn up and become part of the lower body. In effect the tubelike canal is converted into a widely flaring funnel. As a result of BRAXTON-HICKS CONTRACTIONS, considerable effacement often takes place before true labor begins, and it continues throughout the first stage of labor, along with dilation (widening) of the external cervical os (opening into the vagina). Effacement is described in terms of percentage; that is, total thinning is described as 100% effacement, halfway as 50% and so on. Many women are 80% effaced by the time labor begins.

egg   See OVUM.

ejaculation   **1.** Also *coming* (slang). The release of seminal fluid from the PENIS, which is caused by a complex spinal reflex involving the contraction of the bulbar muscles at ORGASM (See also SEXUAL RESPONSE; SPERM.) Approximately 2 to 5 milliliters, or about 1 teaspoon, of seminal fluid are released in each ejaculation; the fluid is also called *ejaculate*.

2. premature ejaculation. A problem experienced by couples when the man rarely or never can delay ejaculation sufficiently for his partner to become fully aroused. The term actually is quite imprecise, because what may be too quick for one partner may be timely for another. In some cases, however, ejaculation occurs within a minute or two of achieving erection, which would be too fast for most partners.

Learning how to delay ejaculation can be accomplished by means of a simple maneuver called the *squeeze technique*, usually executed by the woman. As the man approaches ejaculation, he signals his partner, who then grasps his penis between the fingers, with the thumb on the underside of the glans and the first and second fingers held together on top, right at the coronal ridge (see under PENIS for an illustration); pressing the thumb and fingers firmly together for a few seconds causes loss of the desire to ejaculate (although the erection remains). By practicing this maneuver a number of times most men can learn to control ejaculation themselves. Use of a CONDOM also may help prevent premature ejaculation in men who find that it sufficiently lessens the exquisite sensitivity of the glans.

3. retarded ejaculation. Also *ejaculatory incompetence*. Inability to ejaculate while the penis is inside the vagina. For couples desiring children, this can be a cause of infertility. Most often the cause is psychological and requires SEX THERAPY or other counseling to be corrected.

4. retrograde ejaculation. A condition in which the seminal fluid flows backward into the bladder instead of out through the penis during ejaculation because the bladder sphincter does not close at the moment of ejaculation. The fluid eventually is eliminated in the urine. Retrograde ejaculation may occur after prostate surgery and often occurs in diabetics, paraplegics and men taking medication for hypertension. It causes no harm to the man; it does, however, lessen or eliminate the chances for impregnating a woman, since few or no sperm reach her vagina. Decongestant medication sometimes can control retrograde ejaculation, or it may be corrected by surgery.

5. split ejaculation. See under OLIGOSPERMIA.

electrocautery See CAUTERIZATION.

electrosurgical loop excision See LOOP ELECTROSURGICAL EXCISION PROCEDURE.

embolism The blockage of an artery by an *embolus*, which may be a blood clot (see THROMBUS), air bubble or some other material that has been transported through the circulatory system from elsewhere in the body. An air bubble (*air embolism*) can enter the bloodstream in the course of an intravenous infusion or by exposure to increased air pressure, as in deep-sea diving. A *fat embolus* sometimes forms following the fracture of a large bone, such as the hip. Among the most dangerous kinds of embolism is a *pulmonary embolism* (also called *thromboembolism*), in which a blood clot, usually originating in one of the deep veins of the leg or pelvis, lodges in an artery serving the lungs (pulmonary artery). A pulmonary embolism may be fatal, depending on the extent of the blockage and the person's general condition. It is a major complication of PHLEBITIS, whose treatment is directed primarily at preventing it; usually anticoagulants (anticlotting drugs) are given. A *systemic embolism* arises within the heart or an artery and is transported through arteries to the legs or elsewhere. If it cuts off the blood supply to an essential part of the brain—a *cerebral embolism*—it may cause permanent damage there.

See also ARTERIOSCLEROSIS.

embryo A fertilized egg, or ZYGOTE, that has begun to increase in size by cell division. Some authorities call the human fertilized egg an embryo as soon as the process of cell division has begun; others continue to call it an "egg" or "ovum" until four weeks

after fertilization, when organ development begins. Still others call it an "ovum" for about two weeks after conception, until it has become implanted in the uterine wall, and thereafter use the term "embryo." After the age of about six weeks (following fertilization), it is called a FETUS.

embryoscopy See under PRENATAL TESTS.

embryo transfer Also *embryo transplant*. The procedure of placing a living embryo inside a woman's uterus. The embryo may be the product of IN VITRO FERTILIZATION using her own egg and her partner's sperm, or it may be an embryo taken from the uterus of another woman, either already fertilized through artificial insemination or fertilized in a laboratory container outside the donor's body (see also DONOR EGG). A similar procedure, called *zygote intrafallopian transfer* or ZIFT, involves the transfer of one or more eggs fertilized in a laboratory container, each resulting in a zygote (a one-cell preembryo), back into the woman's fallopian tubes. From there they must make their way to the uterus and become implanted.

See also GAMETE INTRAFALLOPIAN TRANSFER.

emergency contraception Also *morning-after pill*. Any medication against pregnancy prescribed within 72 hours of unprotected intercourse, such as rape. The medication consists of high doses of the hormone progestin, taken orally and sold under the brand name Plan B. One pill is taken immediately, and a second pill 12 hours later. Successful in preventing pregnancy 99% of the time, it replaced an earlier regimen consisting of combined high-dosage estrogen and progestin, which often has severe side effects, mainly nausea and vomiting. That regimen, marketed as Preven, is also still available. Antinausea medication is usually prescribed along with it. It is 98% effective in preventing pregnancy. Emergency contraception works by delaying ovulation or preventing a fertilized egg from implanting in the uterus. It works even if taken as late as five days after sex, but generally within 72 hours is the recommended time. In 2006 the U.S. Food and Drug Administration ruled that consumers of all ages may purchase the drug without a prescription. It can be bought at any store that has a licensed pharmacist on duty or from Planned Parenthood (see Resources in the Appendix). Some doctors prescribe it in advance, along with birth-control pills, so that a woman is prepared in case she needs it.

Other possibilities for preventing pregnancy after unprotected intercourse are the insertion of a copper INTRAUTERINE DEVICE within days after unprotected intercourse, and MENSTRUAL EXTRACTION (def. 2).

emmenagogue   A drug, herb or other chemical agent administered to bring on a delayed menstrual period. Very strong emmenagogues also may bring on uterine contractions and, if a woman is pregnant, result in abortion (see under ABORTIFACIENT). Menstrual periods often are delayed in nonpregnant women, however, by illness, malnutrition or stress. To hasten the onset of a period when there is doubt about possible pregnancy, to eliminate premenstrual discomfort or simply for the sake of convenience, women have long resorted to a large variety of agents, principally herbs. Literally dozens of HERBAL REMEDIES have been used for this purpose, among them infusions made from a mixture of blue cohosh (*Caulophyllum thalictroides*), pennyroyal or squaw mint (*Mentha pulegium;* use plant only, for the oil is dangerous), rue (*Ruta graveolens*) and yarrow (*Achillea millefolium*); or a mixture of black cohosh (*Cimicifuga racemosa;* avoid in presence of low blood pressure), common tansy blossoms (*Tanacetum vulgare*) and motherwort (*Leonurus cardiaca*).

emphysema   See CHRONIC OBSTRUCTIVE PULMONARY DISEASE.

endocervical   Inside the cervical canal; see CERVIX. For endocervical curettage, see BIOPSY, def. 7.

endocervicitis   Inflammation of the cervix that affects the cervical canal, or endocervix. It is treated with locally applied antibiotics. If these are ineffective, cauterization (burning) or cryosurgery (freezing) may be necessary. See CERVICITIS.

endocrine   Also *ductless*. Literally, "internally secreting," referring to glands that secrete hormones and other chemical substances important for the maintenance of basic body functions directly into the bloodstream rather than through special ducts (as certain other glands do). The principal *endocrine glands* are the pancreas, the pituitary, thyroid, parathyroid and adrenal glands, the hypothalamus and the pineal body, and the gonads (or sex glands, that is, ovaries and testes) and placenta. There is a separate entry for each of them.

Together the endocrine glands make up the *endocrine system*, whose study, the field of *endocrinology*, dates only from the beginning of the 20th century. As a group, the endocrine glands are critically influenced by one another, in both their secretory ability and their control of many body functions, including the human reproductive cycle. Indeed, it is these interdependent relationships that account for changes in endocrine activity during a lifetime, governing puberty, conception, pregnancy, childbearing and menopause.

See also HORMONE.

endocrine therapy   See HORMONE THERAPY.

endometrial ablation   See ENDOMETRIAL HYPERPLASIA.

endometrial aspiration   See VACUUM ASPIRATION.

endometrial cancer   See CANCER, ENDOMETRIAL.

endometrial cyst   See ENDOMETRIOSIS.

endometrial hyperplasia   A thickening of the lining of the uterus (endometrium), which during a woman's menstruating years is normally thin, about half its thickness being lost each month in the menstrual flow. If the thickening occurs in one spot only, it forms a growth called a *uterine polyp* (see POLYP, def. 3); if it occurs throughout, it is called *hyperplasia*. In the monthly cycle, first estrogen and then progesterone cause the endometrium to thicken in preparation for implantation of a fertilized egg. If no egg is implanted, the thickened layer is sloughed off. (See MENSTRUAL CYCLE for a more detailed explanation.) In menstruation without ovulation, called ANOVULATORY BLEEDING, no progesterone is produced and the mechanism triggering the regular sloughing-off process is disturbed. Anovulatory cycles occur principally at menarche and menopause (when, in effect, the endocrine system is gearing up for reproduction and winding down for nonreproduction). At menarche, however, anovulation usually is too short-lived for endometrial buildup to progress to hyperplasia, which therefore is found chiefly in women undergoing unopposed ESTROGEN REPLACEMENT THERAPY or who continue to produce sizable amounts of estrogen in organs other than the ovaries (a process not fully understood). In all these instances, the underlying cause is persistent stimulation of the endometrium by estrogen in the absence of progesterone.

The main symptom of endometrial hyperplasia is heavy, prolonged bleeding; there is no pain. Diagnosis is by VACUUM ASPIRATION or D AND C, which in many cases also cures the condition simply by removing a sufficient quantity of endometrial tissue. If bleeding persists, in young women the administration of oral contraceptives containing both estrogen and progesterone or, in women of any age, of progesterone alone may correct the condition. However, while in younger women endometrial buildup is always benign (noncancerous), in menopausal and postmenopausal women the condition can be precancerous (see PRECANCEROUS LESIONS). Therefore, if the condition recurs following a D and C and the subsequent administration of progesterone does not correct it, many physicians recommend a prophylactic (preventive) hysterectomy (surgical removal of the uterus) to eliminate the risk of cancer entirely. A newer and more conservative technique is *endometrial ablation,* which uses a tiny viewing device and a roller-ball

electrode or cryotherapy (freezing) to remove the uterine lining. The procedure, done on an outpatient basis, takes about half an hour.

See also BALLOON ABLATION.

endometrial polyp   See POLYP, def. 3.

endometriosis   The appearance of tissue from the endometrium (lining of the uterus) outside the uterus, in such locations as on the ovaries or surface of the fallopian tubes, on the outer back wall of the uterus or in the pelvic space between the uterus and rectum. According to the National Institutes of Health, 5.5 million American women have endometriosis, most between the ages of 25 and 45 and most often in women in their 30s. Many begin getting symptoms before age 20, and the condition is increasingly being found in young women. It may also flare up during PERIMENOPAUSE. The principal symptoms are menstrual disturbances, most commonly extremely painful periods, and may progress to persistent pain. Some women also suffer pain, sometimes very severe, during vaginal sexual intercourse. There is, however, no true correlation between the severity of the pain and the extent of the disease. Further, nearly one-third of patients have no symptoms other than infertility. Also, the earlier stages of the disorder often are more painful than the later, more advanced stages, possibly because an increase in prostaglandins causes spasms.

The cause of endometriosis—why endometrial tissue migrates out of the uterus—is not known. One theory holds that during menstruation, some menstrual tissue (sloughed-off uterine lining) backs up through the fallopian tubes, implants in the abdomen and grows. Another holds that an immune-system hormone, interleukin-l, is secreted by white blood cells reacting to cells from the uterus that enter the abdomen during menstruation. Endometriosis then develops either because too many endometrial cells enter the abdomen, causing the immune system to overrespond to these cells, or because the immune system overresponds to even a normal number of such cells. Current research suggests that endometriosis may well be an immune-system disorder, but other researchers suspect exposure to environmental toxins, such as dioxin (used in herbicides and pesticides), is involved.

The course of the disease is better understood than the causes. Endometrial tissue outside the uterus is as responsive to hormone stimulation as that inside the uterus. During menstruation, when the uterine lining, which was built up in preparation for pregnancy, is shed, the endometrial tissue outside the uterus responds to hormones in the same way, by breaking down and bleeding. The blood is trapped in the pelvic cavity, and eventually a bloodfilled cyst—an *endometrial cyst* or *chocolate cyst* (so called because it is filled with old, dark, chocolate-colored blood)—can form.

At first the pelvic pain is felt only during menstruation, in the form of severe cramps. In time, however, chronic tissue inflammation leads to the formation of adhesions and scars, which surround and entrap the delicate reproductive organs. As endometrial tissue builds up and presses against them, pain may precede menstrual flow by as much as two weeks. The adhesions can be extensive enough to freeze the fallopian tubes, ovaries and uterus in place. Eggs are trapped in heavy shrouds of scar tissue, leading to infertility. As the disease advances, older endometrial cells die, leaving scar tissue in their wake.

Because the symptoms of endometriosis are similar to those of pelvic infection, the only certain diagnosis is by LAPAROSCOPY or exploratory surgery. Treatment varies but generally is directed at relieving pain and interrupting the menstrual cycle. Sometimes the administration of oral contraceptives (combined estrogen and progesterone) brings the condition under control. An intrauterine device, Mirena, releases a progestin, levonogestrol, and has been shown to ease cramps and can remain in place for five years but not without side effects (see also under CONTRACEPTIVE). Danazol, a synthetic male hormone that inhibits the release of FSH (follicle-stimulating hormone) and LH (luteinizing hormone) by the pituitary, can interrupt the MENSTRUAL CYCLE, suppressing ovulation and the mechanisms whereby the endometrium is built up. Treatment usually lasts from three to nine months, depending on the severity of the disease.

TELLTALE SIGNS OF ENDOMETRIOSIS*

- Extremely painful menstrual cramps that may worsen over time
- Chronic pelvic pain, also in the lower back
- Pain during or after sexual intercourse
- Intestinal pain
- Painful bowel movements or urination during menstrual periods
- Heavy menstrual bleeding
- Premenstrual spotting or bleeding between periods
- Infertility

*National Institutes of Health

Following treatment, however, the condition may recur. Further, danazol has such side effects as weight gain, acne, hair growth and deepening of the voice as well as causing unfavorable changes in blood cholesterol. Newer drugs called GnRH (gonadotropin-releasing hormone) agonists suppress FSH and LH production and inhibit ovulation and menstruation. Nafarelin (Synarel) is given as a nasal spray; leuprolide (Lupron) is injected daily or monthly; and goserelin (Zoladex) is an implant placed in the upper abdominal wall every 28 days. All of them have side effects similar to menopause, mainly hot flashes, decreased sex drive and vaginal dryness. Also, because they promote bone thinning, they can be taken for only six months, and symptoms frequently recur when they are discontinued.

None of these agents is curative but simply effects a temporary remission. Pregnancy can achieve this as well. However, 30 to 40% of all women with endometriosis are unable to conceive, even if they have normal periods, regular ovulation and unblocked fallopian tubes. Even mild forms of the disease interfere with fertilization, implantation or some other stage of the process. Some researchers believe that antibodies form against the misplaced endometrial tissue. These antibodies also attack the uterine lining itself, thereby causing the high rate of miscarriage (three times the normal rate) in patients who do manage to get pregnant. Endometriosis also poses a much greater risk of ECTOPIC PREGNANCY—16% as opposed to 1% in the normal population.

Although the precise way endometriosis causes infertility is not understood, a recently discovered connection with a protein called beta-3, believed to be necessary for the implantation of a fertilized egg in the uterine wall, may be implicated; it is apparently missing in women with even mild endometriosis. This discovery is expected to lead to a new test for the condition, which would require only an endometrial biopsy performed in a doctor's office (in contrast to laparoscopy, a more elaborate procedure).

For women who wish to bear children, surgery may be recommended. Conservative surgery, using laparoscopy, consists of removing patches of endometrial tissue by cauterization (burning), curettage (scraping) or laser surgery; it appears to restore fertility in about one-third to one-half of cases. During the same procedure the surgeon also may perform *uterine suspension,* which involves shortening or repositioning uterine ligaments to hold the uterus up and out of the cul-de-sac and thus prevent formation of adhesions. Sometimes the surgeon also will cut the major nerve plexuses that transmit pain to the brain so as to provide pain relief; this procedure, called *presacral and uterosacral neurectomy,* is readily performed by the laser. Most if not all of these procedures can be performed via laparoscopy, replacing the major abdominal surgery they formerly required.

If the adhesions are quite thick and the tubes are damaged but the woman still wants to become pregnant, major surgery (LAPAROTOMY) may be performed. Further, if the ovaries contain one or more chocolate cysts, they may be opened by laser, cleaned out, and repaired so as to restore normal function. If the symptoms are very severe, however, even after nine months or more of hormone therapy, and the patient is sure she wants no children, hysterectomy (removal of the uterus) may be considered.

Following menopause, endometriosis nearly always subsides. However, women with a diagnosis of endometriosis who can conceive and intend to bear children are urged to do so without delay, since until menopause the condition tends to be progressive (gradually worsens) and, even after conservative surgery, may recur. Endometriosis does not always disappear with menopause. Even after ovariectomy (so-called surgical menopause) endometriosis may persist if remnants of ovarian tissue remain in the pelvis.

See also ADENOMYOSIS.

endometritis An inflammation of the endometrium, or lining of the uterus. The main symptoms are pelvic or lower abdominal pain, a tender uterus (when a pelvic examination is performed) and a thick, foul-smelling, yellowish cervical discharge. Endometritis may result from irritation by an intrauterine device (IUD) or as a complication of an early (first-trimester) abortion. It nearly always responds to antibiotic treatment.

endometrium The lining of the UTERUS, a thin, pinkish, velvety mucous membrane. It consists of several layers: surface epithelium; glands that secrete a thin alkaline fluid which keeps the uterine cavity moist; blood vessels; and tissue spaces. In thickness it varies during each menstrual cycle from 0.5 millimeters to 3 to 5 millimeters, gradually being built up in preparation for pregnancy and, in the absence of fertilization, much of it being shed in the menstrual flow with some blood. After MENOPAUSE the entire endometrium atrophies, its epithelial tissue flattening, its glands gradually disappearing and the gland tissue becoming fibrous.

The endometrium is subject to a number of disorders and diseases, the most serious of which is cancer (see CANCER, ENDOMETRIAL). A common benign growth is endometrial POLYPS (see def. 3). Occasionally endometrial tissue begins to grow outside the uterus, a condition that can cause severe menstrual pain (see ENDOMETRIOSIS). Menstrual irregularities may lead to an over-buildup of endometrial tissue called ENDOMETRIAL HYPERPLASIA, which often can be corrected simply by removing some of the extra tissue by suction (see VACUUM ASPIRATION) or scraping (see D AND C). Both of these procedures also are used to diagnose endometrial cancer and other cell changes as well as to terminate a pregnancy.

engagement In childbirth, the descent of the baby's head so that its widest portion has passed through the pelvic inlet (the upper part of the pelvis). Engagement may not occur until the second stage of LABOR, that is, until the cervix has been fully dilated, or it may occur during the last few weeks of pregnancy, before labor begins. The latter happens in 90% of women pregnant for the first time. One way to tell whether the head is engaged is to locate its lowermost part in relation to the *ischial spines* (part of the woman's hipbones), which the clinician can feel in either vaginal or rectal examination or even by palpating the abdomen. Engagement demonstrates that the pelvic inlet definitely is large enough for the baby, but lack of engagement before labor begins does not necessarily indicate that the pelvis is too small. Engagement is the first of a series of movements made by the baby's head (provided the head is the presenting part, as it is in 95% of all deliveries) in the process of labor.

engorgement, breast   See LACTATION.

epidural anesthesia   Also *lumbar epidural block.* A kind of REGIONAL ANESTHESIA that numbs the lower half of the body and therefore is often used during childbirth. It involves injecting a local anesthetic, through a catheter, into a space between the ligaments of the bony vertebrae and the dural sac (which encases the spinal fluid and spinal column), thereby deadening pain from this level and lower but retaining motor function so that uterine contractions can continue although they will be slowed down. It can be given fairly early in labor, when the cervix is 4 centimeters dilated (of the total 10 centimeters required), provided the baby's head is well down into the pelvis, and, with the catheter remaining in place, it can be either repeated or infused continuously throughout the remainder of labor and delivery. Ideally, medication levels are kept as low as possible to minimize side effects. Adding small amounts of opioid drugs such as fentanyl to the injection reduces the amount of anesthetic needed by up to 75%. If continued through the second stage of labor (expulsion of the baby), the urge to push usually is not felt, making pushing less effective and often necessitating the use of FORCEPS or VACUUM EXTRACTOR. However, the use of the opioid lessens this effect, and further, the anesthetic can be allowed to wear off as the cervix becomes fully dilated.

Epidural anesthesia has definite disadvantages. It is difficult to perform, needing a highly skilled anesthetist to find just the right space for injection. It may not work correctly, with some nerves being blocked (all the nerves on one side, for example) and others not. If the needle is not in exactly the right position, some anesthetic may escape into the spinal fluid, which may cause a precipitous drop in the mother's blood pressure, dangerous to both her and the baby. (Intravenous fluids can be given to help control lowered blood pressure.) Bed rest is required to prevent displacing the epidural catheter. Because of potential problems, an anesthesiologist must watch the woman constantly, representing considerable expense if the labor is long. Further, epidural anesthesia often slows down labor; pitocin may have to be given to improve contractions. Because the mother feels no sensation whatever from the lumbar area down, she must be directed carefully to bear down for each contraction in expelling the baby. Finally, EPISIOTOMY and forceps or vacuum extractor are necessary more frequently when an epidural anesthetic is used. However, a recent study showed that combining epidural and spinal anesthesia did not significantly prolong labor, even when given at 2 centimeters dilation. Epidural anesthesia also is sometimes used for abdominal TUBAL LIGATION and CESAREAN SECTION, as well as CYSTOCELE repair, hip or knee replacement, and other surgical procedures on the lower body.

episiotomy   A surgical opening of the perineum made during the second stage of LABOR, when the baby is being pushed through the vagina, in order to avoid tearing of the delicate perineal tissues. An incision is made in the bottom of the vagina at the time the baby's head actually is being delivered; if the woman is not anesthetized, a local anesthetic usually is injected into the site to be cut, which extends from the vagina toward the anus. After delivery the cut is repaired with sutures (stitches), either the kind that are absorbed or a kind that fall out within two or three weeks. The site of the incision may be painful for a week or more until it heals.

Critics contend that episiotomies are performed too often, especially in hospital deliveries in the United States. In recent decades, however, the practice has declined, especially in leading teaching hospitals. One study found that in 1980 64% of vaginal deliveries in hospitals had episiotomies, a figure that shrunk to 39% in 1998, and today in some hospitals the surgery is performed on only 2 to 3% of women. Originally intended to avoid perineal tearing, it eventually was found to cause more lacerations and other complications. Perineal tearing, it is said, may often be avoided by performing PERINEAL MASSAGE (rubbing the area). Such massage, done daily for several weeks before the baby is due, as well as during labor and while the baby's head is crowning (begins to appear in the vagina), often allows the surface perineal tissue to stretch without tearing, although it cannot help the underlying muscle that also determines perineal elasticity. More important, tears often can be avoided by the birth attendant's gently controlling the advancing head and allowing it to emerge only between contractions (not during one).

erection   The condition of tissue that has become stiff and elevated in response to stimulation. Such tissue, called *erectile tissue,* contains numerous small arteries that dilate in response to sexual or other stimulation, causing engorgement (swelling). The swelling in turn blocks the flow of blood from the veins, thereby causing more engorgement. Engorgement causes the tissue to darken in color, increase in size and stiffen. In women, the prime areas of erectile tissue sensitive to sexual stimulation are the nipples, clitoris, inner labia and vaginal opening; in men, the penis, especially near its tip (the glans), is the most sensitive, but the nipples also are erectile. When sexual stimulation occurs, nerve endings in the penis release neurotransmitters. They cause the corpora cavernosa, two rods of spongy tissue that run the length of the penis, to relax and fill with blood from the penile arteries. The supply of extra blood fills a network of veins called sinusoids, which expand, closing off other veins that normally drain blood from the penis. The result is an erection.

Although other areas of the body respond to sexual stimulation, they do not become erect. Some erection of the penis is necessary for *intromission* (insertion of the penis into the vagina);

inability to have or maintain an erection is called IMPOTENCE.

See also SEXUAL RESPONSE.

ergot   A fungus that grows on rye and some other grains, and for centuries has been known to produce uterine contractions. In its pure form it is toxic, causing severe pain, convulsions, gangrene and death. However, an alkaloid isolated from ergot, ergonovine, can be used after childbirth to help the uterus contract and return to its normal size. Other ergot alkaloids have been used in mental illness, particularly for poor memory and confusion in the elderly, and ergotamine is useful in treating MIGRAINE.

erosion, cervical   See CERVICITIS.

ERT   See ESTROGEN REPLACEMENT THERAPY.

erythroblastosis   Also *erythroblastosis fetalis, Rh disease.* Hemolytic anemia of the fetus or the newborn baby, usually caused by Rh incompatibility.

See also RH FACTOR.

estrogen   General name for the principal female sex hormone, produced in women chiefly by the ovaries and placenta. In men some estrogen is produced by the testes. There are three principal forms of ovarian and placental estrogen—estrone, estradiol and estriol—and at least 17 minor kinds. At puberty production of a hormone, FSH, by the pituitary gland stimulates the development of egg follicles in the ovary, which produce estrogen. These increased levels of estrogen account for pubertal development: growth of the breasts, uterus, fallopian tubes and vagina; increase in layers of fat and their pattern of distribution, producing the characteristic female figure; slowdown and eventual ending of growth of the long bones (arms and legs, hands and feet); and growth of pubic and underarm hair. For the next 35 or 40 years, levels of estrogen rise each month during the MENSTRUAL CYCLE and drop if fertilization does not occur. During pregnancy estrogen production is taken over by the placenta and remains high until delivery. Some estrogen also is produced by a woman's adrenal glands and by adipose (fatty) tissue, which apparently converts androgens (male hormones) produced by the adrenal glands into estrogen. After menopause, when the regular monthly upsurge of ovarian estrogen stops, adrenal production and fatty-tissue release of estrogen continue (which may account for the fact that large, plump women often have fewer menopausal symptoms associated with estrogen decrease than small, thin women). Recent studies indicate that after menopause the ovaries may produce considerable quantities of estrone, but they do stop producing estradiol; any estradiol in circulation has been converted from estrone.

The discovery of estrogen dates from about 1915, and the first synthetic estrogen was produced some 15 years later. Both natural estrogen (often obtained from the urine of pregnant mares) and synthetic estrogen (made in the laboratory) are used in oral contraceptives to prevent pregnancy, to replace estrogen after surgically induced or natural menopause (see ESTROGEN REPLACEMENT THERAPY), to treat menstrual irregularities, to suppress lactation after childbirth and to treat some forms of cancer. Side effects from taking estrogen include nausea and vomiting (from too high a dosage), breast tenderness and enlargement (also in men), headache, vertigo (dizziness), fluid retention and irregular vaginal bleeding. Moreover, the administration of estrogen is considered a contributing cause in a number of disorders, especially blood clots, high blood pressure, stroke and some kinds of cancer, and its use therefore is controversial. Estrogen therapy of any kind is contraindicated if there is a personal or family history of cancer of the breast or pelvic organs or a history of thrombosis or high blood pressure. Further, it should be used only with great caution in the presence of obesity, gallbladder disease or diabetes. Also see the specific contraindications under ESTROGEN REPLACEMENT THERAPY and ORAL CONTRACEPTIVES.

See also SELECTIVE ESTROGEN-RECEPTOR MODULATOR.

estrogen-receptor assay A diagnostic test to determine whether a cancerous tumor's growth is dependent on estrogen. Some cancers of the breast are stimulated to grow by estrogen, and others are not. For those that are, chemotherapy (anticancer drugs) often is not very effective, but *endocrine manipulation*—changing the body's level of hormones—may help control the cancer. Such manipulation includes removing or inactivating organs and glands involved in estrogen production (ovaries, adrenal glands, pituitary gland) and administering large doses of hormone. The ovaries can be excised surgically, or their function can be ended by chemotherapy or radiation treatment, and the adrenals can be removed surgically (adrenalectomy). In 1981 researchers announced that their experience with the drug aminoglutethimide showed it cut estrogen production as effectively as adrenalectomy. Tamoxifen has a similar effect, as does megestrol acetate given with hydrocortisone. (Also see HORMONE THERAPY.) However, not all breast cancers are hormone-dependent, so it is important to establish whether they are before initiating such therapy. (Estrogen receptors are found in about 65 to 80% of breast cancers in postmenopausal women and 45 to 60% of cancers in premenopausal women.) The estrogen-receptor assay can be used not only to plan additional treatment after surgery but to help plan future treatment if the cancer recurs. The test itself is performed on the tumor tissue, taken by biopsy. If the hospital where the biopsy is taken is not equipped to perform the test (and many laboratories are not), it can freeze the tissue and send it to a laboratory that is. About two-thirds of patients whose tumors contain estrogen receptors (are estrogen-dependent) respond to endocrine therapy. Similar tests and treatments have been devised for progesterone-dependent tumors.

estrogen replacement therapy Also *ERT, hormone replacement therapy, HRT.* The use of estrogen—natural or synthetic, oral, by injection, in cream or suppositories, a vaginal ring, emulsion or gel applied to the skin or dermal patches—to "replace" estrogen no longer produced by the ovaries. It is used principally to relieve some of the symptoms of MENOPAUSE that occur either naturally or following surgical removal of both ovaries (which brings on menopause very suddenly). It is indeed effective against HOT FLASHES and VAGINAL ATROPHY, slows down bone resorption (see OSTEOPOROSIS) and apparently affords some protection against colorectal cancer. However, estrogen use may increase one's risk for developing potentially fatal blood clots, stroke, heart disease, endometrial cancer, dementia, gallbladder disease and breast cancer. Estrogen should never be used by women who have severe kidney or liver disease, phlebitis or a history of blood clots, heart attack, sickle-cell disease, estrogen-dependent cancer or vaginal bleeding for which no cause has been determined; it should be used only with caution by women who have had fibroids, endometrial cancer, migraine, high blood cholesterol, high blood pressure, stroke, asthma, gallbladder disease or seizure disorders.

Results of a study published in 2007 contradicted some earlier findings, which had been largely based on studies of older women. It suggested that younger women who have had hysterectomies and start taking estrogen while in their 50s apparently were 30 to 40% less likely to have blockage-causing calcium in arteries that lead to the heart than women who took placebos, although they still had slightly increased risks for stroke and breast cancer. Nevertheless, caution was still advised, since risks for stroke and blood clots remain with continued hormone use. However, women in their 60s and 70s who took hormone therapy were at increased risk for heart attacks.

The most appropriate candidates for estrogen therapy are women whose ovaries have been surgically removed at a relatively young age. Before beginning it, they are advised to have a thorough medical checkup, including a pelvic examination and a Pap smear, a breast examination and a mammogram, and tests investigating liver and thyroid function and blood sugar and cholesterol levels. After estrogen therapy is begun, regular checkups, including breast and pelvic examinations, are highly advisable.

To counter menopausal symptoms, therapy is usually begun when the symptoms become troublesome, but should not be continued for more than four to five years. Women with an intact uterus take either estrogen together with progestin (synthetic progesterone) or *unopposed estrogen*

ESTROGEN THERAPY SHOULD NOT BE USED IF ONE HAS

- Unusual vaginal bleeding
- Currently has or has had certain cancers, especially of the breast or uterus
- Had a stroke or heart attack in the last year
- Currently has or has had blood clots
- Currently has or has had liver problems
- May be pregnant

(estrogen alone). Since the latter puts them at risk for endometrial hyperplasia and potential endometrial cancer, they should have annual checks of the endometrium. When hormone replacement therapy is stopped, nearly all its benefits disappear, especially improvement in bone health, but a slightly higher risk for breast and other cancers persists for at least three years. These risks, however, are very small.

The most frequently used form of estrogen in the United States is *conjugated estrogen*, mixtures of several estrogens taken from the urine of pregnant mares (marketed as Premarin). Less potent natural estrogens synthesized in the laboratory—estradiol, estropipate and esterified estrogens—also are used. The mode of administration makes little difference; indeed, the estrogen in vaginal creams, suppositories and dermal (skin) patches is absorbed more readily than that in pills (because the liver apparently filters out a considerable amount of estrogen when it is taken orally). However, because the hormone in dermal patches is so readily absorbed, far less of it needs to be used than with oral estrogen for the same effect. The same is true of a vaginal ring (Estring) that is inserted into the vagina to counter dryness, which can be left in for 90 days. There also are combination dermal patches, which contain a progestin as well as estradiol, so as to avoid the risk of endometrial buildup.

Most authorities recommend that therapy aimed at preventing future disease be begun within a year or two after periods cease (and that those who take it to counter menopausal symptoms begin when the symptoms become troublesome). However, so far as protection against osteoporosis is concerned, ERT is still beneficial when begun years later, and protection continues as long as therapy is continued.

Because women are advised to take the lowest dose of estrogen that controls their symptoms, many low-dose products have entered the market, among them a spray that administers low-dose estrogen to the skin. Nevertheless, the ultimate safety of these products is not known. The North American Menopause Society has compiled a complete list of the products; it is available online at www.menopause.org/edumaterials/hormoneprimer.htm. Also, in January 2008 the FDA warned against the use of "bio-identical" hormone replacement therapy, consisting of pharmacist-concocted combinations of estrogen, progesterone and estriol (the last is not even proved safe or effective). They have not been adequately tested.

For women taking estrogen alone, it is often prescribed on a three-weeks-on, one-week-off schedule. In some women this gives rise to periodic vaginal bleeding resembling light menstruation—so-called withdrawal bleeding—usually near the end of the week without estrogen. For women taking both estrogen and progestin, one possible regime is estrogen taken for 25 days of the month and progestin taken for 10 to 14 days. Withdrawal bleeding then usually occurs at the beginning of the days when no hormone is taken. Others suggest somewhat different schedules, among them continuous daily estrogen and progestin as in *Prempro*, which combines Premarin with the progestin medroxyprogesterone acetate. In low dosage such a combination mostly avoids withdrawal bleeding (usually none after six months). Another option is a progesterone-infused intrauterine device (IUD), marketed as Progestasert, which, however, needs to be replaced annually. A recent study indicates that while progestin offsets some of estrogen's protection against heart disease, a natural form of progesterone called micronized progesterone, marketed as Prometrium, largely avoids this drawback. For women with surgically induced menopause (following ovariectomy), progestin is not needed, but the male hormone testosterone may also be prescribed.

Some women are unable to tolerate the side effects of estrogen therapy, which include headache, nausea, bloating, leg cramps, breast tenderness and engorgement, irregular vaginal bleeding and staining, and oversecretion of mucus (heavy vaginal discharge). Some of these are due to progestin. Lowering the dosage of either or both hormones may relieve these problems. All women on estrogen therapy who experience vaginal bleeding (other than the periodic few days of light withdrawal bleeding) should promptly consult a physician, since such bleeding is the only overt symptom of endometrial malignancy.

Hormone replacement therapy has become increasingly controversial as studies have found that its risks often outweigh its benefits. Even long-term unopposed estrogen for women without a uterus appears to increase the risk for ovarian cancer and stroke. It therefore seems wise to weigh one's own personal risk factors against the benefits before undertaking it. If undertaken at all, it is recommended to take the lowest dose of hormones for the shortest period of time to treat menopausal symptoms severe enough to interfere with the quality of life. The most recent research indicates it should be avoided, if possible, by women aged 60 and older. To avoid osteoporosis and colorectal cancer, lifestyle changes and other, well-tested medications are preferable. Both menopause and its aftermath can be managed in lower-risk ways: increased calcium intake and regular weight-bearing exercise to prevent osteoporosis, a healthy lifestyle to ward off heart disease, various medications for hot flashes and improved lubricants for vaginal dryness. Research is also being conducted about the benefits of *phytoestrogens*, substances in plant foods that have an estrogenlike activity. One kind, genistein, is most plentiful in foods derived from soybeans, such as roasted soybeans, textured vegetable protein and soy flour. However, considerable amounts of these foods may be needed to gain any benefit, and further, their long-term effect on heart disease and bone loss is not really known. Another source is flaxseed, which can reduce LDL (low-density lipoprotein, bad cholesterol) and relieve menopausal symptoms, but the data on it are still very sketchy. Herbal sources of phytoestrogens include black cohosh (*Cimicifuga raremosa;* in liquid or tablet form) and dong kwai (*Angelica sinensis*). Neither has been tested for safety or effectiveness. Some women cannot tolerate vaginal dryness, which can be treated with low-dose estrogen in cream, tablet or ring form. Their effects tend to be concentrated on the vaginal and surrounding tissues, and only small amounts are absorbed into the bloodstream (especially from creams). Nevertheless, their effect needs to be carefully monitored.

See also SELECTIVE ESTROGEN-RECEPTOR MODULATOR; VAGINAL ATROPHY.

eversion, cervical   See CERVICAL EVERSION.

excise   To cut out, to remove by surgery. Any such procedure is called an *excision*.

exercise   Physical exertion that is undertaken deliberately to promote and maintain good health as well as for recreation. Regular exercise is important for men and women throughout life, from infancy on. It improves blood circulation and muscle tone (including the muscle tone of the diaphragm and heart), enlarges lung capacity, benefits the digestive system and aids bowel function, contributes to good posture and a more vigorous appearance, lowers body weight and promotes relaxation and good sleep patterns. It also reduces the risk of breast and colon cancer and osteoporosis.

Women in particular are apt to neglect exercise at certain times of their life when it can be most beneficial. One such time is during pregnancy and following childbirth, when fatigue, fear of harming the unborn baby, and preoccupation and lack of sleep from caring for a newborn infant may prevent normal patterns of exercise. However, a program of simple exercises during and after pregnancy can greatly improve muscle tone and prevent some of the problems that can develop with the normal weight gain and loss involved in childbearing. It helps to counter some of the common pregnancy-related discomforts such as backache, bloating, constipation and swelling of the extremities. It also has profound psychological benefit, giving a woman control over her body while it is undergoing considerable changes and aiding relaxation. Moderate exercise has no adverse effects on the fetus. However, experts caution that after the fourth month one should avoid calisthenics done lying on one's back, as well as full sit-ups, double leg raises, and touching toes with knees straight, which all can strain the back. Women with pregnancy-induced hypertension, premature labor (in previous or present pregnancy), persistent bleeding or incompetent cervix should not exercise. Further, women should not exercise to the point of exhaustion but should stop when fatigued, breathless, dizzy or experiencing chest pain or pain in the back, hip or pubic area.

A special circumstance occurs when a pregnant woman is put on bed rest, which is estimated to occur for 700,000 women a year in the United States. It includes just about all women expecting multiple births, whose numbers have sharply increased in the past two decades. Although the American College of Obstetricians and Gynecologists no longer advises bed rest to prevent preterm births, physicians still routinely order it for women having contractions before 37 weeks, bloody spotting, high blood pressure or a history of preterm labor. However, a mild and gentle exercise program can avoid the deconditioning accompanying prolonged bed rest. It includes, with the doctor's approval, frequent circular motions with the ankles, bending the knees and pulling ankles toward the body and lifting light weights such as a soup can or a two-pound weight.

Another time when women are tempted to avoid or curtail exercise is during and after the menopausal years. It is precisely then that regular exercise—which need be nothing more complicated than regular brisk walks—can be of great benefit in maintaining cardiac (heart) function and delaying or offsetting the problems of bone loss (see OSTEOPOROSIS). Aerobic exercise, such as brisk walking, running, bicycling, cross-country skiing or swimming for 30 minutes three times a week, has such important benefits as reduced risk of heart attacks and diabetes. The Centers for Disease Control and Prevention recommend at least 30 minutes of moderate exercise on most days. It can consist of brisk walking one and a half to two and a half hours per week. Also, the half hour a day can be broken into 10- to 15-minute periods with the same benefit as exercising for 30 straight minutes. Stretching, recommended before one undertakes any vigorous exercise, helps lengthen tendons and muscles and increases the joints' range of motion.

Strength training and weight-bearing exercise help improve bone mass and increase muscle power; studies show that resistance training with weights benefits even very old and frail women. Strength training also improves balance, reducing the risk of falls and fractures.

Before embarking on a specific exercise program (other than brisk walking or swimming), women with any chronic condition, such as high blood pressure, as well as all women over the age of 45 who have been leading largely sedentary lives, are usually advised to have a general physical examination. Further, if they are considering a formal or strenuous exercise program, the clinician may advise a *stress test*, which measures pulse and blood pressure (sometimes also heart function by means of an attached electrocardiograph machine) during and/or immediately after increased levels of exertion. As a rule, all exercise programs should be started slowly and gradually increased in length and difficulty. Exceedingly vigorous programs of strenuous exercise may interfere with hormone production and the menstrual cycle, resulting in anovulatory cycles or amenorrhea and even some loss in bone density. Consequently, most clinicians suggest a policy of moderation, especially if a woman is trying to become pregnant.

A Chinese movement discipline that has become popular in the United States is *tai chi*, a low-impact way to improve strength, flexibility and balance. It has been found to be especially helpful for women aged 70 or older, reducing the risk of falling and also helping reduce blood pressure. Tai chi consists of a series of fluid movements, emphasizes relaxation and deep breathing and moves through a series of postures.

Exercise also is useful for those who wish to lose weight, both in using up some extra calories (although not as many as most people tend to believe) and in firming muscles after some body fat has been lost. It is estimated that brisk walking (a mile in 15 minutes) uses only about 5 calories a minute; bicycling, about 8 calories a minute; and swimming, 11 calories a minute.

See also ATHLETIC ABILITY, WOMEN'S; KEGEL EXERCISES.

face presentation In childbirth, the position of the baby when its face is the presenting or leading part as it descends into the birth canal. In this posture the baby's neck is sharply extended so that the top of its head virtually touches its back. Face presentation occurs about once in every 400 to 500 deliveries. If the mother's pelvis is normal in size and shape and the baby's chin is not extended too much, a vaginal delivery—either spontaneous or with some help from low FORCEPS—is possible in most cases. If the chin is severely extended, however, the baby's head becomes caught under the pubic bone (symphysis pubis) and cannot be delivered. The clinician may try to flex the face or it may flex spontaneously during the course of labor, but in stubborn cases a Cesarean section (surgical delivery) may be necessary.

fallen bladder See CYSTOCELE.

fallen uterus See PROLAPSED UTERUS.

fallopian tubes Also *oviducts*. A pair of narrow passages that are attached high on either side of the uterus and transport eggs to it from each OVARY. Each tube is 4 to 5 inches (10 to 12½ centimeters) long. It is quite narrow in the central portion—the outside about the diameter of a drinking straw, the inside that of a hair bristle—and flared at the trumpet-shaped open end near the ovary. This end is lined with *fimbriae*, tiny fingerlike projections that are constantly in motion. After ovulation (the monthly release of an egg from an ovary) their movement draws the egg from the ovary's surface into the tube, and the muscles in the tube walls

then contract, moving the egg down the tube toward the uterus. This action is further assisted by the waving motion of tiny hairs called *cilia*, which line the inside surface of the tube. If fertilization (the union of the egg with a sperm) takes place, it happens when the egg is about one-third of the way down the tube, a journey that must be made within 24 hours of its release from the ovary; thereafter the egg is no longer viable. Whether fertilization took place or not, the muscular contractions of the tube continue to move the egg into the uterus, which takes four to five days.

The principal functions of the fallopian tubes are to provide a hospitable environment for both sperm and eggs and to move eggs into the uterus. Occasionally the latter function fails (or is blocked) and a fertilized egg becomes implanted in the tubal walls and begins to grow there, a dangerous condition called tubal or ECTOPIC PREGNANCY. Without properly functioning fallopian tubes, conception cannot take place. Some women are infertile because their tubes are blocked by scar tissue or some other condition (see also TUBEROPLASTY). Indeed, scarring of the fallopian tubes is the single most common cause of infertility in young women. Blockage from abdominal adhesions or scar tissue may be caused by PELVIC INFLAMMATORY DISEASE, a ruptured appendix, gynecologic surgery (including Cesarean section) or postoperative infection, endometriosis, an ectopic pregnancy, bowel surgery or a postpartum infection. Fortunately, microsurgery and laser surgery may be able to repair the damage.

Women who do not want to bear children may have their tubes "tied," or closed off, so as to prevent conception (see TUBAL LIGATION). One surgical technique for such sterilization is *fimbriectomy*, the removal of the fimbriae, without whose action an egg cannot enter the tube.

The principal disease affecting the fallopian tubes is *salpingitis,* or inflammation and infection of the tubes, which may be caused by GONORRHEA, pelvic inflammatory disease, pelvic tuberculosis or as the result of an abortion, childbirth or intrauterine device. Cancer that originates in the fallopian tubes is rare, although it can spread there from the uterus or ovaries. Surgical removal of the fallopian tubes is called *salpingectomy.* It may be done in conjunction with HYSTERECTOMY or removal of an ectopic pregnancy.

false labor   The irregular contractions of the uterus that occur throughout pregnancy and can be mistaken, near term, for true labor. (See BRAXTON-HICKS CONTRACTIONS.) False labor may be perceived three or four weeks before actual labor begins, but it is differentiated from true labor because the contractions are relatively painless and intermittent, rather than increasing in intensity and regular. Also, they are felt chiefly in the lower abdomen, they do not become more frequent (the intervals between contractions remain long, rather than becoming shorter and shorter), they are not intensified by walking, and discomfort is relieved by mild sedation. In true labor, on the other hand, contractions occur with increasing frequency at regular intervals and are not affected at all by mild sedation. However, the only way to distinguish false and true labor with certainty is to examine the cervix, which after some hours of true labor shows progressive EFFACEMENT and dilation (widening).
See also CONTRACTION, UTERINE; LABOR.

false pregnancy   The appearance of some of the signs of pregnancy in a woman who is not pregnant. Among them are weight gain, breast enlargement, amenorrhea (cessation of menstruation), morning sickness (nausea) and, sometimes, sensation of fetal movements. However, the pelvic organs when examined are normal, and the uterus is unchanged in size from its nonpregnant state. Since such symptoms occasionally are associated with ECTOPIC PREGNANCY, a CORPUS LUTEUM cyst or a missed abortion (see MISCARRIAGE, def. 5), these conditions first must be ruled out. In their absence, false pregnancy is nearly always the result of a woman's desperate wish to conceive—although very occasionally it results from the opposite, that is, extreme fear of pregnancy—and often it can be managed with careful counseling on INFERTILITY and, if desired, treatment for infertility.

family planning   Planning for or preventing a pregnancy. Many American communities offer family planning services that offer contraceptive advice and care (including surgery for STERILIZATION), pregnancy testing and counseling, abortion and continuing gynecological care, as well as treatment for sexually transmitted disease and aftercare for rape victims. Family planning clinics may be located in a hospital (public or private) or in a freestanding facility. In most states information about local family planning clinics can be obtained by telephoning the Department of Public Health. Note, however, that for providing abortion facilities or information they are subject to the laws of the state in which they operate (see also ABORTION).
See also BIRTH CONTROL; CONTRACEPTIVE; GENETIC COUNSELING; NATURAL FAMILY PLANNING; PREGNANCY COUNSELING; RAPE.

fatigue   A feeling of excessive weariness that is both unrelated to an underlying illness and seems out of proportion to the amount of physical exertion and sleep a person has had. Fatigue is one of the most common complaints brought to physicians, and its cause is often very difficult to identify. It can be, of course, the symptom of numerous underlying disorders, ranging from low-grade minor infections to diabetes and cancer. Moreover, it often is symptomatic of an emotional problem of some kind, such as depression or anxiety. In women fatigue is sometimes related to fluctuation in hormone levels. Many women regularly experience intense fatigue at some point during their menstrual cycle, most often premenstrually, that is, just before the onset of a period, and/or during the first day or two of menstrual flow. Fatigue is a classic symptom of the early months of pregnancy as well as of menopause (particularly for women whose sleep is disturbed by hot flashes and night sweats). It also is a symptom of iron-deficiency ANEMIA.

Even though serious illness is the cause of prolonged fatigue relatively seldom, it cannot be overlooked, and anyone who feels drained of energy for weeks on end should have a thorough physical checkup. Treatment with sleeping pills, tranquilizers or strong stimulants (caffeine, alcohol and other drugs) should be avoided; in the long run such drugs are more likely to compound the original problem, and they can never eliminate its basic cause.

See also CHRONIC FATIGUE SYNDROME; INSOMNIA.

fat necrosis Death of a clump of fat cells, creating hard round lumps in the breast. Occurring most often in large-breasted, overweight women, and often around the site of a biopsy or injury, they are totally benign but should, like any breast lump, be checked by a health care provider.

See also FIBROCYSTIC BREAST SYNDROME.

fellatio Also *blowing, blow job, going down* (slang). A form of oral sexual intercourse in which the mouth (lips, tongue) is used to stimulate the partner's genitals.

See also CUNNILINGUS; ORAL SEX.

feminine hygiene See HYGIENE.

feminist health clinic See SELF-HELP.

feminist therapy Psychotherapy performed by a mental health specialist who incorporates the basic beliefs of feminism (women's rights) in her approach to treatment. In theory feminist therapists can be either male or female, but in practice nearly all are women. They do not use any special therapeutic method; rather, each uses whatever method of psychotherapy she prefers that also is compatible with feminist thinking. Although feminists hold a wide range of opinions and ideas, they share a number of fundamental beliefs that under-lie feminist therapy. Chief among them is the idea that the traditional role of women as passive and powerless, subordinate to and dependent on men (economically and emotionally), must be replaced so that they are (and feel they are) active, equal and autonomous. The feminist therapist therefore tries to help women understand the connection between their social conditioning as women and their present psychological situation. Unlike traditional psychotherapists, who usually focus on internal conflicts as the primary (or only) source of emotional distress, feminist therapists believe that social factors are largely if not entirely responsible for many women's emotional problems. Another central belief is that a therapist should not behave as a powerful authority figure who dominates or intimidates her client. Rather, she should help the client overcome the feelings of helplessness and dependency associated with traditional female roles and encourage her assertiveness and independence. To this end, feminist therapists may use such techniques as avoiding technical jargon, giving the client access to her own records and files and generally establishing a sense of equality between therapist and client. The client is encouraged to establish her own goals for therapy, rather than having the therapist set goals and standards for her. The use of group therapy, often recommended, also helps reduce a client's feelings of dependency on the therapist and at the same time helps her see what she has in common with other women in the group and elsewhere.

Feminist therapy grew out of the women's movement of the 1960s and represents a reaction against the influence of Sigmund Freud and his followers. The Freudians believe, among other things, that normal women are sexually less desirous or active than men, that they fulfill themselves best by childbearing (especially of male children) and that a woman's emotional problems often can be traced to unresolved childhood conflicts, such as unconscious envy of men for having a penis or the repressed desire to marry their fathers. The influence of these ideas, which few male psychotherapists today wholeheartedly accept, continues to be felt in culturally assigned sex roles, to which a woman traditionally is expected to adjust (or else be considered maladjusted, abnormal or "sick").

Like other psychotherapies, feminist therapy is most effective when client and therapist have a sound relationship in which the client trusts the therapist and feels respected and understood. To locate a feminist therapist, recommendations can be sought from friends or referrals from community health centers or consumer health groups. Some feminist organizations, such as the National Organization for Women, and some women's health clinics keep referral lists of professionals with a feminist orientation. The client herself should ask any therapist she is considering some basic questions about the approach she uses (behavioral, gestalt, psychoanalytic, etc.), her attitudes on whatever issues the client considers critical (sex roles, sexuality, divorce or abortion, for example), her fee, the estimated frequency and term of therapy (how many times a week and for how many months), her professional qualifications (training, certification, past experience) and whether she is available in case of emergency.

fern test See CERVICAL MUCUS METHOD.

fertility In women, the ability to become pregnant and carry a child to term. Fertility reaches its peak during a woman's mid-20s and then begins to decline, slowly in the 30s and more rapidly in the 40s. It ends completely with MENOPAUSE. In men, fertility is the ability to impregnate a woman. It reaches its peak in a man's early 20s and begins to fall off after the mid-20s, but the decline remains very gradual, and men in their 70s have been known to father children. However, recent research indicates that as men get older, from age 45 on, they face an increased risk of fathering babies with serious abnormalities, such as autism and schizophrenia. Also, analysis of sperm in healthy men found changes as they age, including lower sperm counts and increased fragmentation of DNA, which can lead to genetic defects. An estimated 15% of all North American couples have trouble conceiving.

In 2007 the FDA approved an at-home fertility screening test, a two-in-one test for men and women that assesses two basic markers for becoming pregnant. The male portion tests the ability of

FERTILITY IN WOMEN*

Age	Chance of live birth (%)
under 35	37%
38 to 40	21%
41 to 42	11%
over 42	4%

*Based on a large-scale study of women undergoing assisted technology such as test-tube fertilization using woman's own egg and partner's sperm.

sperm to pass through a liquid resembling cervical mucus and how many sperm can do so. The female portion measures the level of follicle-stimulating hormone on the third day of the menstrual cycle. See HOME MEDICAL TESTS for more details.

See also AGE, CHILDBEARING; INFERTILITY; SPERM BANK; SPERM BANK; STERILITY.

fertility drug Also *fertility pill.* One of several compounds that either induce ovulation or replace hormones in women who, for lack of them, cannot become pregnant. One of them, *clomiphene citrate,* marketed under the brand names Clomid and Serophene, is a synthetic compound that causes the hypothalamus to be stimulated so that it, in turn, stimulates the pituitary to release more FSH (follicle-stimulating hormone) and LH (luteinizing hormone) in order to induce ovulation (see MENSTRUAL CYCLE for an explanation of this process). Taken orally along with medroxyprogesterone (Provera), it succeeds in establishing ovulation in about 70% of the women treated with it. Provera is taken first to trigger a menstrual period, and then followed by clomiphene; in most cases ovulation occurs 5 to 10 days later and a menstrual period 14 to 16 days after ovulation. The conception rate is about that of normal couples, the best response occurring in women between the ages of 20 and 35. It generally is given for only four to six cycles. It has been used also to regulate highly irregular menstrual cycles and to correct progesterone deficiency that leads to ANOVULATORY BLEEDING, as well as to stimulate sperm production in men (see STERILITY). Clomiphene can adversely affect the cervical mucus, making it too thick for sperm to penetrate; this problem sometimes can be corrected by administering low-dosage estrogen. Side effects of clomiphene include hot flashes, abdominal bloating, breast tenderness, nausea and headache. In about 5% of cases, ovarian cysts and enlargement occur, which can be life-threatening.

Another drug, sometimes combined with clomiphene citrate, is HUMAN CHORIONIC GONADOTROPIN (HCG, found in the urine of pregnant women), which is given intramuscularly around the time of ovulation. It increases LH levels and helps the egg ripen for release. If these fail to establish ovulation, a stronger preparation, made from *human menopausal gonadotropin* (HMG) extracted from the urine of postmenopausal women, may be used. Sold under the trade name Pergonal, it is similar to human chorionic gonadotropin. Both are chemically similar to LH (and Pergonal also contains FSH). However, they can be used only under close medical supervision because they tend to overstimulate the ovaries, sometimes resulting in the formation of large ovarian cysts. Both are more expensive than clomiphene, and they tend to produce MULTIPLE PREGNANCY—not only twins but triplets, quadruplets and quintuplets, who have a much poorer chance of survival than single births. One way of overcoming this drawback involves IN VITRO FERTILIZATION in which newly fertilized eggs grown in laboratory dishes are kept for five days instead of three so that they are more mature and more likely to become implanted when transferred to the woman's uterus.

With Pergonal, estrogen assays and ultrasound should be performed regularly to detect multiple births and to avoid life-threatening complications. The treatment is demanding and extremely expensive, requiring daily injections, periodic blood tests, and ultrasound to monitor follicular development. If estrogen levels become very high and ultrasound shows numerous large egg follicles, Pergonal must be stopped at once. There are other side effects. The ovaries may become cystic and may hemorrhage or rupture, or they may twist, cutting off the blood supply (this is called torsion). The problem usually resolves itself, but hemorrhage or torsion may require surgical removal of an ovary. About 99% of women given Pergonal will ovulate and about two-thirds will conceive, usually within three cycles. Of these, about half bear one child, and about one-fourth of them have multiple births; of the rest, about 33% miscarry, compared to 15 to 25% among those who receive clomiphene.

Pure follicle-stimulating hormone (FSH), under the brand name Metrodin, and gonadotropin-releasing hormone (GnRH) agonists, under the brand name Lupron or Synarel, may be used to restore fertility when the hypothalamus is malfunctioning but the pituitary is functioning normally. Metrodin may have fewer side effects than Pergonal. The GnRH agonists are either intravenously injected or given by nasal spray. They do not result in multiple births or overproduction of estrogen. Other drugs used are bromocriptine, when infertility is due to high levels of prolactin in the blood (in non-breast-feeding women it appears to inhibit ovulation), and natural progesterone to cope with problems in the luteal phase of the cycle.

Early in 1982 the U.S Food and Drug Administration approved the use of HMG in men suffering from a pituitary deficiency that makes them infertile; in men, however, it appears to have no connection with multiple births or to produce any other side effects.

See also INFERTILITY.

KEY ELEMENTS FOR FERTILITY	
For women	**For men**
Ovulation	Hormones for sperm production
Favorable sperm-vaginal mucus interaction	Testicular function for sperm production
Fertilization	Post-testicular function for sperm transport (no blockage)
Tubal transport (no blockage)	Ejaculation of sperm
Embryo implantation	
Maintenance of pregnancy	

fertility monitor See under HOME MEDICAL TESTS.

fertilization Also *conception*. The mating of a sperm with an egg, involving the fusion of their nuclei, which results in a fertilized egg, or ZYGOTE.

In human beings fertilization takes place inside the FALLOPIAN TUBES. The sperm that survive the journey up the fallopian tubes surround the egg and strip away its outer layer of cells, bind to the zona pellucida and penetrate the space below. Then a single sperm fuses with the vitelline membrane and triggers a series of cellular changes that block the entry of other sperm. For an explanation of how both the mother's and father's characteristics are transmitted to their offspring, see GENETICS.

fetal alcohol syndrome   See ALCOHOL USE.

fetal cells in maternal blood   A recently developed test for birth defects that provides the same chromosomal information as amniocentesis and chorionic villus sampling but that may be performed at the end of the first trimester and yields results in only three days. Based on the finding that a few fetal cells can be found in the mother's circulation, it uses a special sorting process to isolate them and test them. Apart from being quicker, it presents almost no risk to either mother or fetus and is expected to replace the older tests as soon as enough medical centers become equipped to perform it.

fetal monitoring   Assessing the physical condition of a baby before and during labor and delivery. The oldest and simplest form of fetal monitoring is listening to the baby's heartbeat, which can first be detected about halfway through the pregnancy (between 16 and 20 weeks). It can be heard with the ear alone, but it sounds much clearer through a stethoscope, particularly a special obstetrical stethoscope with a metal headband that further amplifies the sound through bone conduction. It also can be detected by means of an ultrasound device called a Doptone as early as 11 to 14 weeks. The fetal heartbeat is a double beat like the tick of a watch and has a normal rate of 120 to 160 beats per minute. If during pregnancy or labor the heart rate slows down markedly and/or becomes irregular, it is a definite sign that something may be wrong with the baby.

The amniotic fluid also provides means of fetal monitoring; AMNIOCENTESIS is performed to discover severe genetic defects in midpregnancy. A simpler investigation can be made just before the onset of labor. Normally the fluid at this time is quite clear; if it is brownish green, it signals the presence of meconium (the baby's stool), which is passed when the baby is in distress. The amniotic fluid can be observed just before labor by passing a small viewing instrument through the cervix and observing whether it is cloudy or clear.

Most often, however, the term "fetal monitoring" refers to electronic devices used during labor and delivery to keep track of both the baby's heartbeat and the mother's uterine contractions. These devices augment or replace the older practice of listening to the heart through a stethoscope and manually feeling the abdomen during a contraction. Developed in the late 1950s, electronic fetal monitoring originally was used only in potentially abnormal births, when the mother had diabetes, severe heart or kidney disease, Rh-factor incompatibility or some other disorder associated with severe distress in a baby. When the monitor showed fetal distress, that is, a slowdown in heart rate, a Cesarean section would be performed. Today electronic fetal monitoring is used much more widely in North America, in some hospitals for as many as 75% of all births.

In *internal fetal monitoring* two electronic catheters are inserted into the vagina and through the cervix. One is attached to the baby's scalp and relays its heart rate, while the other lies between the fetus and the wall of the uterus and measures the rate and pressure of uterine contractions; the latter is rarely used, however, except for research. In *external fetal monitoring* two straps are placed around the mother's abdomen. One, around the upper abdomen, contains a pressure gauge to record contractions; the other, around the lower abdomen, contains a device to measure the fetal heart rate. Both kinds of monitor are connected to a machine that records the findings on a roll of paper. Not only can these devices show changes in the ordinary course of labor, but they can show how the baby's heart rate responds to artificially stimulated contractions. In the *contraction stress test* or *oxytocin challenge test* uterine contractions are stimulated either by nipple stimulation or administering the hormone oxytocin to the mother by intravenous infusion. Three moderate contractions within 10 minutes are considered adequate for showing how the placenta and the baby's heartbeat respond. If the contractions cause the heart rate to slow down, it is a sign that the baby is in distress and should be delivered at once.

Another device, a fetal oxygen monitor adopted by some in the 1970s, is inserted into the uterus to rest on the baby's cheek or forehead and is used in conjunction with fetal heart monitors. It was hoped that monitoring both the oxygen level and the heart rate would help decide if a baby needed to be delivered quickly. However, it was found to lead to higher rates of Cesarean and not to healthier babies, and in January 2006 the manufacturer discontinued the product.

In some centers the oxytocin challenge test has been replaced by the *Non-Stress Test* (NST), which uses the external fetal monitor to detect at least two fetal movements during a 20-minute period, each accompanied by a rise of 15 beats per minute in the baby's heart rate. (Some practitioners have different standards for a response, for example, a 15-beat acceleration of the fetal heart rate within 10 minutes.) Studies show that a baby responding in this fashion is in good condition and is likely to remain so for another seven days, provided there is no change in the mother's condition. If the test is nonreactive, that is, shows no fetal movement or no accompanying increase in fetal heart rate, then an oxytocin challenge test is performed.

Two newer devices are the *intrauterine pressure catheter* and the *fetal acoustic stimulator*. The first is used to determine the intensity of contractions in a woman whose labor is not progressing even though she has been given oxytocin (Pitocin) to strengthen contractions. It is inserted through the vagina into the uterus between the fetus and the uterine wall. The second is an instrument applied to the woman's abdomen; it uses sound waves to shock the baby, thereby markedly increasing the heart rate if the baby is healthy. Neither device has been used long enough to assess it for effectiveness or safety.

Supporters of fetal monitoring claim that the different patterns in the fetal heart rate cannot be discerned simply by a stethoscope and counting. Fetal monitoring provides a continuous record, and its simultaneous record of the pressure of contractions (with their possible effect on the fetal blood supply) permits more accurate correlation of these events. Moreover, if an internal fetal monitor indicates possible distress, it also permits taking a blood sample from the baby's scalp to determine whether it is being deprived of oxygen and whether labor should be allowed to continue or a Cesarean section should be performed. Supporters also hold that many babies have been saved from brain and other damage that would have resulted if a difficult labor had been allowed to continue.

Critics counter that fetal monitoring not only makes the mother uncomfortable but may compress the *vena cava* (a large vein) and thus compromise the uterine blood flow, interfere with efficient contractions and slow down labor. Further, internal monitoring may require artificial rupture of the membranes and cause injuries to the baby's scalp, the most common complication. For both internal and external monitoring, moreover, much of the information recorded may be misleading or be misinterpreted (for example, the mother's abdominal noises often are picked up as well), leading to unnecessary interference with a normal delivery. Certainly the increasing use of fetal monitoring in all births has been partly responsible for the increase in the performance of CESAREAN SECTION. Opponents of monitoring say there has been no difference in outcome for infants but there has been a higher rate of postpartum infection, presumably from the insertion of a foreign object into the uterus. Consequently most authorities suggest that internal fetal monitoring should be limited to high-risk births or instances where complications develop in the course of labor, and no kind of monitoring—external or internal—should be used merely as a matter of routine.

See also PRENATAL TESTS; UTERINE MONITORING.

fetal movement   Also *kicking*. The movement of the fetus inside the uterus, perceived as kicking, turning or flipping. Healthy fetuses are active, usually more so at certain times of day (frequently after the mother's meals), but they also have long intervals without movement when they are resting. Counting fetal movement is considered by some clinicians to be a simple assessment of fetal condition. They advise, beginning in the 34th week of pregnancy, counting the fetal movements at an active time (after a meal). Ten movements in an hour or less are considered healthy; if there are fewer, the woman is advised to repeat the procedure later in the day or evening. If fewer than 10 movements are felt in two hours, she is advised to call her practitioner, which also is advisable if she has not felt any movement all day.

fetoscopy A procedure in which an instrument called an *endoscope* is inserted inside the AMNIOTIC SAC in order to see parts of a fetus, withdraw skin or blood samples from it and determine whether it has certain disorders or defects. An exceptionally delicate operation, it is performed under local anesthetic some 15 to 20 weeks into a pregnancy. Usually ULTRASOUND (see def. 1) is used first to locate the fetus, placenta and umbilical cord. Then a small incision is made into the uterus through the abdomen and a narrow tube containing an endoscope is inserted into the amniotic sac. To obtain a blood or tissue sample, a tiny needle or forceps is inserted through the endoscope into the placenta.

Fetoscopy is much riskier for the fetus than AMNIOCENTESIS—it induces miscarriage in about 5% of cases, as well as ABRUPTIO PLACENTAE—and therefore is performed only when there is considerable risk of bearing a defective child. It enables not only discernment of gross visible defects in the limbs, eyes, ears, mouth and genitals but diagnosis of blood disorders such as hemophilia and thalassemia, as well as the 40% or so of cases of SICKLE-CELL DISEASE that are missed by amniocentesis. It also may be used to detect fetal levels of toxic substances or dangerous viruses or parasites to which the mother was exposed, as well as to administer medication directly to the fetus and perform minor surgery on it. A newer technique, embryoscopy, is considered safer (see PRENATAL TESTS).

fetus A name for a developing EMBRYO used either from six weeks after FERTILIZATION or from eight weeks on, depending on which authority one follows. By the end of the second month of development the fetus is about 1 inch (2.5 centimeters) long and weighs 1/30 ounce (slightly more than 1 gram). At this point centers of ossification (bone formation) appear throughout the skeleton, especially in the skull and long bones; the features of the head, which is quite large compared to the trunk, are well developed; the fingers and toes are present; and the ears form definite bumps on each side of the head. For subsequent fetal development, see GESTATION.

fibroadenoma Also *adenofibroma*. A benign (noncancerous) breast tumor, consisting of a firm, well-defined, movable, slow-growing, painless mass. It occurs most often in women between the ages of 15 and 35, in black women more than in white. Fibroadenomas are recognized easily on a mammogram (see MAMMOGRAPHY), but because they resemble breast cancer they can be diagnosed definitely only by biopsy and examination by a pathologist. Fibroadenomas are made up of connective tissue, duct and gland cells that have multiplied faster than normal. Some authorities believe that these tumors should be removed as a rule, but they feel that in teenagers it may be advisable to wait until the breasts are fully developed before surgery is performed. Others are more conservative and believe the tumors should simply be left alone. Newer techniques for removing such tumors avoid open surgery. They are preceded by biopsy to confirm that the tumor is benign. One, called *cryoablation*, uses ultrasound to locate the tumor, a local anesthetic to numb the area and a tiny incision through which a needle is inserted and liquid argon is used to freeze the tip of the probe. It forms a kind of ice ball that encompasses the tumor, which destroys the tissue. Usually two freeze cycles, with two periods of thaw, are employed. In 6 to 12 months the remains of the tumor is resorbed and disappears. Cryoablation takes 20 to 30 minutes and is a painless office procedure. The other technique uses radiofrequency heat or lasers to destroy all the proteins in the tumor.

See also FIBROCYSTIC BREAST SYNDROME.

fibrocystic breast syndrome Also *breast lumpiness, fibrocystic changes*. The most common benign (noncancerous) disorder of the breast, characterized by the formation of lumps or cysts in one or both breasts. Because it is so common, occurring to some extent in 60 to 90% of all women, it is no longer considered a disease, nor is it necessarily associated with a higher risk of developing breast cancer. There are three main types of benign breast lump. Most are either FIBROADENOMAS or cysts, which are small fluid-filled sacs. The latter occur most often in the breasts of women between the ages of 35 and 55, when levels of estrogen and progesterone are relatively high. Indeed, it is estimated that between 15 and 30% of all women have such cysts during those years. The third kind, called *pseudolumps*, comprise generalized lumpiness, FAT NECROSIS, or an ABSCESS or GALACTOCELE.

Cysts, unlike cancerous growths, are movable, spherically shaped, fairly soft and subject to rapid changes in size. Often they are associated with nodules or other lumps of the breast; they usually occur multiply (not singly) and in both breasts. Some cysts are painful, and others are not. Their formation appears to be directly related to estrogen: Cysts rarely appear after menopause, when estrogen levels are much lower, and they often become firmer and more tender just before a menstrual period, when estrogen levels are high. Some women find temporary relief by lowering their salt intake during the premenstrual days or by taking a mild diuretic. Others have benefited from eliminating caffeine (in chocolate, cola, coffee, tea). Although a cyst is, strictly speaking, harmless, a large one usually is subjected to *needle aspiration*, that is, it is drained with a needle syringe; if it refills after such drainage it is surgically excised. The fluid and tissue withdrawn are always examined by a pathologist in order to rule out malignancy.

Formerly general breast lumpiness was called fibrocystic breast disease, and patients were long considered to have a greater risk for developing breast cancer. It now is believed, however, that only certain lesions are linked to increased risk, specifically cell changes called *atypical ductal hyperplasia*. Nevertheless, a biopsy (either needle aspiration or surgical) is indicated to determine whether a lump is benign or a solid and possibly malignant tumor. Cysts usually can be differentiated from solid tumors with ultrasound or on a mammogram (see MAMMOGRAPHY).

Treatment of benign breast lumps now ranges from leaving them alone to surgically excising them, that is, lumpectomy (see MASTECTOMY, def. 7). Abscesses should be drained by a clinician, who may also prescribe antibiotics to treat the underlying infection. If repeated biopsies have shown lumps to be benign, a conservative course may be best.

See also CANCER, BREAST.

fibroid Also *fibromyoma, leiomyoma, myoma*. A benign (noncancerous) growth of the uterine wall that occurs only after puberty. It may occur singly or, often, in numbers. Fibroids are extremely common. Some 20% of all women over 35 have at least one fibroid, and they are far more common in black women than in white. Their growth apparently is stimulated by estrogen, and consequently they shrink and even disappear entirely after menopause.

Fibroids range in size from a small bean to a large grapefruit or larger; a large fibroid can weigh 20 pounds (9 kilos) or more. The symptoms of a fibroid include a palpable lump in the abdomen, heavy and prolonged menstrual periods (but, usually, no bleeding between periods) and a feeling of fullness. Sometimes there is urinary frequency owing to pressure on the bladder. Usually there is no pain, but sometimes, if fibroids press on the ureters or rectum, there may be quite severe pain, and severe pain also occurs if a tumor degenerates, that is, twists and cuts off its own blood supply.

Small fibroids that cause minimal symptoms require no treatment at all. Larger ones that cause little or no discomfort also may be ignored. Often it is less their size than their location that makes them require treatment. In terms of location, there are three kinds of fibroid. An *intramural* or *interstitial fibroid*, the most common kind, lies deep in the uterine wall. Often it produces an enlarged uterus and causes heavy bleeding during menstruation, with cramps if the fibroid is degenerating. A *subserous (subserosal) fibroid* lies outside the body of the uterus; occasionally it causes heavy bleeding into the abdomen. A *submucous (submucosal) fibroid*, the least common kind, lies under the endometrium (uterine lining), which is pushed into the uterus as the fibroid grows. It nearly always causes heavy bleeding, even when very small, and may become pedunculated (form a stemlike part by which its body is connected to the uterine wall). Intramural and subserous fibroids rarely require treatment unless they are very large or are pressing on the bladder or bowel. Submucous fibroids are more apt to require treatment because they cause such severe menstrual problems.

Diagnosis is based on pelvic examination, but because a fibroid may be difficult to distinguish from an ovarian cyst (see CYST, def. 6), it may be necessary to investigate via LAPAROSCOPY (viewing through a small abdominal incision); a submucous fibroid usually cannot be detected by examination alone (the uterus simply feels enlarged) but must be verified by ultrasound or biopsy.

In the removal of a fibroid, called MYOMEC-TOMY, the surgeon usually tries to leave the uterus intact, especially in women who still want to bear children. Subserous fibroids sometimes can be removed via laparoscopy, making an incision in the uterus and cutting out the fibroid. Larger tumors may be shrunk by *myolysis,* which uses a laser or electric needles. Small fibroids inside the uterine cavity can sometimes be removed by a laser or electric knife, a technique called *hysteroscopic resection.*

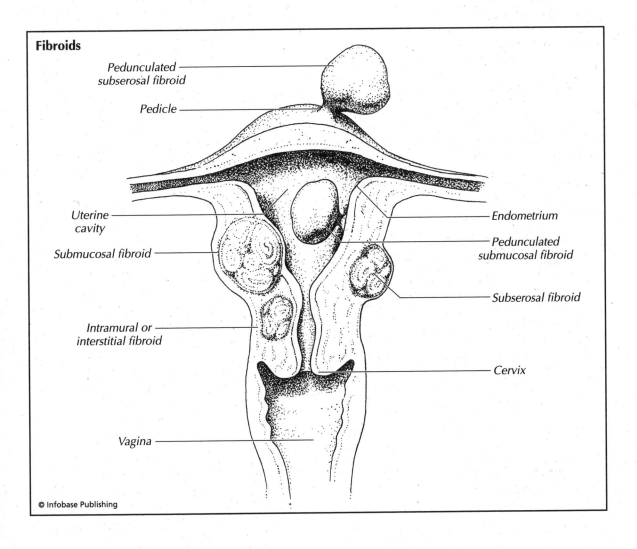

Fibroids

Pedunculated subserosal fibroid

Pedicle

Uterine cavity

Submucosal fibroid

Intramural or interstitial fibroid

Vagina

Endometrium

Pedunculated submucosal fibroid

Subserosal fibroid

Cervix

© Infobase Publishing

A new procedure is *uterine artery embolization,* or *uterine fibroid embolization (UFE),* a method of reducing fibroids by obstructing their blood supply. Minimally invasive, this technique has succeeded in postmenopausal women as well as younger ones. Before the procedure the pelvic area is imaged (preferably with MRI) to rule out other causes of symptoms and pin down the size, location and type of fibroids involved (the kind that grow on a stalk do not respond well to this procedure). Generally considered safe and effective, it takes less than an hour and requires no general anesthesia. The main side effects are cramping and abdominal pain immediately afterward, which usually disappear in a few hours. A catheter is inserted through a small incision in the groin and threaded into the femoral artery and up to the blood vessels supplying the fibroid. Through it tiny plastic particles are inserted, closing off those vessels. Deprived of blood, the fibroid shrinks, but the uterus continues to receive blood flow from surrounding areas. Another new technique, called *radiofrequency ablation,* uses a needle electrode inserted laparoscopically through a small incision in the abdomen into the fibroid. Using radio waves, the electrode generates heat and destroys the fibroid, which is reabsorbed by the body. The largest fibroid so treated was more than four inches in diameter, a size traditionally treated with HYSTERECTOMY. Another technique approaches the artery through the vagina to apply a clamp, which may need to be in place only a few hours to treat the fibroid.

Yet another technique, approved in 2004, is completely external; it involves pointing a sharply focused beam of high-intensity ultrasound energy at the tumor, which is located via an MRI scan. The procedure, called *focused ultrasound,* lasts two to three hours in an outpatient setting and requires virtually no recovery time. Although it spares the uterus, it is intended only for women who do not plan to have children. Also, the technique cannot be used for fibroids close to sensitive organs such as the bowel and bladder. However, a major study of the treatment indicated that while it gave patients considerable symptom relief, the fibroids may return in as little as six months, and more research is needed. Still another alternative is *endometrial ablation,* used to treat ENDOMETRIAL HYPERPLASIA, which removes both fibroids and the endometrium.

For women nearing menopause, when estrogen levels are declining, hormonal therapy may be an option. A low-dose oral contraceptive or DepoProvera injected every three months may stop excess bleeding. Or GnRH agonists (antiestrogens) like leuprolide (Lupron) or nafarelin (Synarel) may stop bleeding, reverse anemia and temporarily shrink fibroids, either sufficiently to halt problems or to enable easier myomectomy. Severe bleeding from fibroids can give rise to ANEMIA, which must be treated with iron supplements.

If already present before conception, fibroids tend to grow during pregnancy, when estrogen levels are high. Despite such growth, which can be very rapid during the early months (sometimes the tumor fills the entire pelvis), they rarely interfere with pregnancy because they usually move out of the pelvis (most often up into the abdomen). When this occurs a normal vaginal delivery is quite feasible. When fibroids remain in the pelvis, however, the baby may have to be delivered by Cesarean section. Also, a fibroid may interfere with the placenta, and the closer it is to the placenta, the greater the chance of its causing bleeding during the pregnancy. Women who have fibroids should avoid using an INTRAUTERINE DEVICE, since a distorted uterine cavity has a greater tendency to bleed.

For another benign uterine growth, see POLYP, def. 3.

fibromyalgia   Also (formerly) *fibrositis.* A condition characterized by muscle aches and stiffness, especially around the neck, trunk and hips, as well as restless sleep and consequent fatigue. It differs from similar conditions in that pressing down on specific tender points where muscles join tendons elicits extreme pain. (Similar disorders, such as rheumatoid arthritis, do not respond in this way.) A finding of at least 11 such tender points (out of a possible 18) and widespread pain and fatigue for at least three months establishes the diagnosis, which at this writing cannot be confirmed by any laboratory tests. The condition affects an estimated 2 to 4% of Americans, most of whom are women between the ages of 20 and 50. The cause is not known, but fibromyalgia may be an autoimmune disease, perhaps related to chronic fatigue syndrome. Some researchers are investigating it as a sleep disorder; morning stiffness and feeling tired after a good rest are common, as are frequent headaches. Other researchers believe it is related to depression or some other mental disorder, or that it reflects an abnormality in one of the neurotransmitters (brain chemicals), such as serotonin. Since the cause is not understood, treatment is largely palliative. Cortisonelike drugs and anti-inflammatory agents in high doses are not beneficial. Low doses of an antidepressant or a muscle relaxant, however, may help return sleep patterns to normal. In addition, small doses of analgesics such as acetaminophen and nonsteroidal anti-inflammatory drugs (aspirin, ibuprofen, naproxen) may afford relief. In 2007 the FDA approved pregabalin (Lyrica), the first approved drug to treat the condition. However, it has numerous side effects, among them sedation, dizziness, dry mouth, edema, weight gain and impaired motor function and concentration. The drug is approved for doses of either 300 mg or 450 mg daily; the higher dosage afforded greater relief from pain but was associated with more side effects. Another drug, not yet approved by the FDA for fibromyalgia at this writing, is gabapentin (Neurontin). It is approved to treat pain related to postherpetic neuralgia (an aftermath of shingles) and so may be prescribed off-label, but it may have serious side effects. Still another medication found effective for pain relief is methadone, a narcotic used principally to combat drug addiction. It, too, has side effects and must be carefully monitored.

For patients preferring other measures for severe pain, pain clinics may help patients learn such forms of pain control as biofeedback, hypnosis and behavior modification. Cognitive behavioral therapy, a form of psychotherapy that focuses on how thoughts influence feeling and behavior, may be helpful in teaching patients adaptation techniques. Regular mild physical activity, such as swimming or bicycling, apparently counteracts muscle pain (which worsens when the muscles get out of shape). Various dietary treatments have been tried, but none has proved to be effective. See also Resources in the Appendix.

fibromyoma   See FIBROID.

fibrosis, cystic   See CYSTIC FIBROSIS.

fimbria, fimbriectomy   See FALLOPIAN TUBES.

fissure   See ANAL FISSURE.

fisting   See ANUS.

fistula   An abnormal narrow pathway between some body cavity and the outside skin or another body cavity. A *vaginal fistula* may connect the vagina and bladder (*vesicovaginal fistula*) or the vagina and rectum (*rectovaginal fistula*). The principal symptom of the former is leakage of urine from the vagina; for the latter it is leakage of gas or fecal matter (or both) from the vagina. Most vaginal fistulas are caused by injury of some kind, frequently inflicted during Cesarean section, hysterectomy or some other surgical procedure. Small vaginal fistulas may close spontaneously. If they do not, they require surgical repair. An *anal fistula* usually leads from the anal canal to an opening in the skin near the anus, from which fecal matter may leak. Anal fistulas rarely heal by themselves and nearly always require surgical repair.

See also MAMMARY DUCT FISTULA.

fluid retention   See EDEMA.

foam, contraceptive   See SPERMICIDE.

folic acid   Also *folate*. A B vitamin produced by plants and yeast that protects against NEURAL TUBE DEFECTS, can reverse some anemias and appears to lower the risk of heart disease. Recent studies indicate that folic acid supplementation reduces the risk of stroke by 18%, and a study of more than 11,000 postmenopausal women concluded that those with the highest folate intake from foods and/or supplements had the lowest incidence of breast cancer during a follow-up period of more than nine years.

The best sources are liver, certain fortified cereals, dark green leafy vegetables (especially raw, since cooking can deactivate folic acid), asparagus, some nuts and seeds, and dried beans. Deficiency of folic acid is linked to neural tube defects, a serious form of birth defect, as well as megaloblastic anemia. In 1998 the Food and Nutrition Board distinguished between folate in food, called *dietary folate equivalent (DFE),* and its synthetic counterpart, folic acid. As a supplement, folic acid is absorbed about twice as well as folate is. A supplement of 400 micrograms (mcg) of folic acid supplies more than 665 mcg of DFE.

See also VITAMIN.

follicle, ovarian   A small group of cells in the ovary that surround an egg. Each month, during the *proliferative* or *follicular stage* of the MENSTRUAL CYCLE, follicle-stimulating hormone (FSH) produced by the pituitary gland causes a few of the ovarian follicles to grow and secrete estrogen. In time all but one (or two) atrophy and disintegrate. The surviving one, called the GRAAFIAN FOLLICLE, matures and eventually is stimulated by another hormone, luteinizing hormone (LH), to move to the surface of the ovary, rupture and release an egg. This process is called OVULATION. After ovulation the cells of the ruptured follicle cluster together, and a yellow pigment, lutein, accumulates in them. The follicle, now called a CORPUS LUTEUM, continues to produce estrogen but, under the influence of LH, also produces progesterone. If the egg that was released is not fertilized, during the last days of the menstrual cycle LH levels decline markedly, so the corpus luteum can no longer function (secrete either estrogen or progesterone) and disintegrates. Sometimes a follicle does not disintegrate and instead remains as a fluid-filled sac, or cyst (see CYST, def. 6).

follicle-stimulating hormone   See FSH.

forceps   Also *obstetrical forceps.* A two-bladed instrument, resembling a pair of tongs, that is used to extract a baby. The blades are inserted into the vagina separately and articulated after being placed in position to grasp the baby's head. The most important function of forceps is traction (pulling), but they also can be used for version (turning), especially if the baby is in POSTERIOR PRESENTATION.

Forceps procedures are classified according to where the baby's head lies at the time the blades are applied. *Low forceps* are applied after the head has reached the perineal floor; *midforceps* are applied sooner but after ENGAGEMENT has taken place; *high forceps* are applied before engagement. Today high forceps are practically never used, and even midforceps are becoming rare, a Cesarean section usually being regarded as safer. To a large extent the VACUUM EXTRACTOR, which uses suction, has replaced forceps.

foreskin   See PREPUCE.

fragile X syndrome   A form of mental retardation caused by a chromosomal abnormality, named for the appearance of the X chromosome under a microscope. (The tips of two of its four arms seem to be hanging by a thread). Most individuals with this form of retardation, which affects males twice as often as females, have a long narrow face, large protruding ears, and, in males, large testicles. In addition, they tend to have loose elbow and finger joints, crowded teeth, and flat feet. However, not every individual with this chromosomal defect is mentally retarded. As with Down syndrome, after which fragile X is the most common form of congenital mental retardation, the chromosomal defect can be detected in a woman through a simple blood test, and during pregnancy, prenatally through amniocentesis and chorionic villus sampling; nevertheless, detection here does not constitute a reliable diagnosis or outlook.

fraternal twins   See MULTIPLE PREGNANCY.

frequency, urinary   An urgent desire to void more often than usual, with no increase in the amount of urine voided. It is a common symptom of pregnancy, especially in the early months (until the 10th or 12th week) and again during the weeks preceding delivery. It can be particularly annoying at night (*nocturia*), since it may require two or three trips to the bathroom each night. In early pregnancy frequency usually is caused by anteversion of the uterus (a kind of forward tilt), which irritates the bladder; in the late stages it is caused by pressure from the enlarged uterus and presenting part of the baby on the bladder.

Urinary frequency also may be caused by pressure from a FIBROID; it is the chief symptom of urinary and kidney disorders (see URETHRITIS; CYSTITIS, def. 1); and it may be aggravated by a fallen bladder (see CYSTOCELE).

See also URINARY INCONTINENCE.

frigidity An older name for female SEXUAL DYSFUNCTION, specifically the inability to achieve orgasm. Until the mid-20th century little or nothing was done for this condition, but today an estimated 90% of women who seek treatment are helped. Present-day sex therapists believe that the term *frigidity* implies a permanent condition and so prefer the terms *preorgasmia* or *dysfunction*.

See also SEX THERAPY; VAGINISMUS.

frozen section See BIOPSY, def. 1.

frozen shoulder Also, *adhesive capsulitis*. A syndrome of increasing stiffness and pain in the shoulder, sometimes becoming severe enough to interfere with using the affected shoulder and arm. Its precise cause is unknown, but it affects three times more women than men. It is thought to be the result of inflammation in the shoulder capsules (fibrous tissues surrounding the joint) that cause adhesions limiting movement. Treatment consists of exercises to increase range of motion and anti-inflammatory medication. In extreme cases that do not respond to conventional treatment within 12 to 18 months, steroid injections or surgery to cut the adhesions may be required. The sooner treatment is begun, the sooner the condition may be cured.

FSH Abbreviation for *follicle-stimulating hormone*, a hormone produced by the pituitary gland. In women it stimulates growth of the follicles in the ovaries (see FOLLICLE, OVARIAN) and in part is responsible for the expulsion of a mature egg (see OVULATION) and the manufacture of estrogen in the ovaries. In men FSH contributes to the maturation of sperm cells.

See also MENSTRUAL CYCLE.

functional bleeding See DYSFUNCTIONAL BLEEDING, VAGINAL.

fundus See UTERUS.

galactocele Also *milk cyst*. A CYST in the breast that is caused by blockage of one of the lactiferous (milk-secreting) glands.

galactorrhea The spontaneous flow of breast milk in a woman who has not recently given birth.

See AMENORRHEA-GALACTORRHEA SYNDROME; LACTATION; POLYGALACTIA; PROLACTIN.

gallbladder A pear-shaped sac in the rear upper quadrant of the abdomen, underneath the liver, whose main function is the collection of bile. Bile, which is secreted by the liver and assists in various digestive processes, is transported from the gallbladder through bile ducts to the duodenum, part of the small intestine. The gallbladder is subject to a very common disorder, the development of *gallstones*, which occur in 10% of all American adults—20% over the age of 40 and twice as often in women as in men. Gallstones, technically called *biliary calculi*, are abnormal concretions made up of crystals that precipitate out of bile; they are made up of cholesterol, bile pigments and calcium. Higher levels of estrogen, during puberty or pregnancy, or from oral contraceptives or estrogen replacement therapy, contribute to their formation. High levels of triglycerides, nearly always present in cases of diabetes, also increase the risk, as does obesity (but only in women).

Gallstones may give rise to no symptoms at all, but usually they cause upper abdominal discomfort, bloating, belching and intolerance to certain foods (especially fatty foods). The pain usually takes the form of an "attack," that is, a fairly sudden episode of acute discomfort, generally after a fatty meal or at night. Many individuals with gallstones experience no attacks or only a single one; others suffer repeated episodes. Because gallstones can lead to serious complications, severe or repeated attacks call for prompt treatment. However, because similar pain can be caused by peptic ulcers or other digestive conditions, diagnosis by ultrasound is indicated. It finds only 40 to 70% of stones trapped in bile ducts, so if acute cholecystitis (gallbladder infection) is suspected, *cholescintigraphy,* scanning involving a radioactive injection that is nearly 100% accurate, may be required.

For patients whose gallstones are relatively small, urosodiol, a naturally occurring bile acid that helps dissolve cholesterol, may dissolve those gallstones made of cholesterol. This oral medication may take as long as two years to work, and further, gallstones are likely to recur within five years. A newer drug used in this way is chenodiol, which, however, has troubling side effects. Another method is the dissolution of gallstones by *lithotripsy* (shock-wave therapy), a procedure in which the stones are bombarded with shock waves from outside the body. This procedure often does not require general anesthesia and involves a very brief hospital stay. If the stones cannot be dissolved by any of these methods, surgical removal of the gallbladder, called *cholecystectomy,* may be indicated. Since the late 1980s, laparoscopic surgery (see LAPAROSCOPY) has largely replaced conventional open surgery, which requires a 5-inch abdominal incision. Instead, several small holes are cut in the abdomen, a laparoscope is inserted (which allows a close-up view of organs and surrounding tissues on a video monitor), and the gallbladder is removed with surgical instruments inserted in the other holes. Recovery is quicker because no major abdominal muscles are cut, and many patients spend only a day or two in the hospital and return to work much sooner. Occasionally, complications such as bleeding occur, and the surgeon will have to convert the procedure to open surgery and make an abdominal incision. The most recent experiments involve gallbladder removal through the vagina (or the rectum in men), but the technique is considered experimental and has not been approved.

gallstones See GALLBLADDER.

gamete intrafallopian transfer Also *GIFT*. A kind of EMBRYO TRANSFER for women whose fallopian tubes are intact but who are infertile as a consequence of unknown or uncorrectable factors associated with endometriosis, cervical mucus problems, immunologic problems or others (see also INFERTILITY). The procedure is similar to IN VITRO FERTILIZATION up to the point where the woman's eggs are retrieved by means of laparoscopy. However, instead of being mixed with sperm in a laboratory container, the eggs are loaded into a catheter together with sperm obtained earlier and are inserted through the laparoscope, which is still in place in the fimbrial opening of the fallopian tube. Once in the tube, sperm and egg mingle just as they would following intercourse, and fertilization occurs more or less naturally. In a slightly different version called *zygote intrafallopian transfer (ZIFT)*, fertilization of the egg by sperm takes place in the laboratory.

Gardnerella vaginalis See VAGINOSIS.

gastric bypass See OBESITY.

gastroesophageal reflux disorder Also *chronic heartburn, GERD*. A backflow of acid stomach contents into the esophagus, causing the sensation of heartburn or upper abdominal or chest pain, or belching that leaves an acid taste. Affecting women more often than men, it is thought to afflict about one-third of all Americans at least once a month, and 10% on a daily basis.

Mild reflux is part of the normal digestive process. As food is swallowed and propelled toward the stomach, the lower esophageal sphincter relaxes, allowing it to pass through. Once food is in the stomach, the sphincter closes, but before it is fully closed some reflux can occur. Usually the amount is too small to be noticed. When it is more severe, however, its effects are perceived as heartburn and the other aforementioned symptoms. They usually occur within an hour of eating and are most pronounced when one lies down, bends or stoops, increasing pressure on the abdomen. Overweight and advanced pregnancy have a similar effect, as do acidic foods, nonsteroidal anti-inflammatory drugs (NSAIDs) or infection. In some individuals reflux may actually inflame the lining of the esophagus, a condition called *reflux esophagitis*. Occasionally this may give rise to scarring or narrowing of the esophagus, making it hard to swallow.

For most women, avoiding large meals and eliminating irritating foods (chocolate, coffee, tea, citrus fruits, high-fat foods, alcohol) and cigarette smoking are sufficient treatment. Not eating for at least three hours before going to bed and raising the head of the bed 6 to 8 inches should mitigate nighttime symptoms. Over-the-counter antacids such as Tums, Maalox or Mylanta help neutralize stomach acids. Histamine blockers such as cimetidine (Tagamet), famotidine (Pepcid), nizatidine (Axid) or rantitidine (Zantac) in low dosages also may help. Stubborn cases may need stronger prescription medications. Finally, in the most severe cases, a new class of drugs that block acid secretion in the stomach almost completely—lansoprazole (Prevacid) and omeprazole (Prilosec)—have largely eliminated the need for corrective surgery that in effect creates a new valve around the lower esophagus. Other brands of these drugs include Nexium, Protonix, Pantoloc, Prilosec OTC and Aciphex, as well as generic omeprazole. However, long-term use of high-dosage *proton pump inhibitors*, as these acid-blocking drugs are called, is associated with the development of polyps and atrophic gastritis (irritation of cells lining the stomach), and also a doubled risk of hip fractures in older patients.

A recent study indicates that severe heartburn, occurring on a daily basis over a long period, can cause a precancerous condition in the lining of the esophagus that may progress into a very serious and often incurable cancer. Therefore anyone who has heartburn two or more times a week should consult a clinician, perhaps a gastroenterologist, who may wish to assess possible damage through an endoscope and biopsy. In cases of premalignancy, the esophagus can be surgically removed and replaced with sections of intestine or stomach. Newer treatments use lasers to destroy abnormal cells, but they are still experimental.

Gaucher's disease   A hereditary disease that, like TAY-SACHS DISEASE, is characterized by the lack of an enzyme enabling the body to break down and eliminate the accumulation of certain fats in the cells. Also like Tay-Sachs disease, it is a recessive-gene disorder (see BIRTH DEFECTS) and is most common in Jews of European ethnic origin, among whom an estimated 4 to 5% are carriers. If both parents are carriers, there is a 25% risk that any child of theirs will have the disease and a 50% chance that the child will be a carrier. However, a test can determine if one is a carrier for the disorder, which helps a carrier decide if he or she is willing to risk having children with another carrier. Also, AMNIOCENTESIS or CHORIONIC VILLUS SAMPLING can determine the presence of Gaucher's disease in a fetus. Efforts at massive genetic screening are hoped to reduce incidence of the disorder, as they have for Tay-Sachs disease.

The disease is named for Philippe Gaucher, a French physician who discovered it in 1882. Unlike Tay-Sachs, it is not invariably fatal. Fatty substances tend to accumulate in the liver, spleen and bone marrow, causing gross enlargements of the affected organs, painful swelling, of the joints, brittleness of the bones and malfunction of bone marrow, causing severe anemia. There are three basic forms of the disease. Type I, the most common, usually does not give rise to symptoms until adulthood; Type II, the acute infant form, is the most severe and usually ends in death within a year; Type III, the juve-

nile form, arises sometimes during childhood and usually is slowly progressive. Enzyme replacement therapy at first produced encouraging improvement in relatively few patients, but a substitute enzyme produced from human placental tissue, alglucerase, appears to help all Type I patients to some extent (depending on the length and seriousness of their illness).

gender identity   **1.** A person's physical identification with a particular sex. For most individuals there is never any question about which sex they belong to, but in persons with a congenital abnormality, such as TURNER'S SYNDROME or KLINEFELTER SYNDROME, characteristics of both sexes are present, and a decision must be made as to whether the child should be brought up as a boy or a girl.

See also TRANSSEXUAL.

2. A person's emotional identification with a particular sex, leading him or her to seek out sexual partners of the same or the opposite sex, or sometimes both.

See BISEXUAL; HETEROSEXUAL; HOMOSEXUAL.

gene   See GENETICS.

gene therapy   Treating genetic disorders by replacing or correcting the genes that cause them; that is, placing beneficial genes into the cells of patients. Advances in biotechnology have made it possible to trace the genes implicated in many diseases to their chromosomal locations. (See GENETICS for more about genes, chromosomes and DNA.) Once such a gene is identified, molecular copies of the gene can be made for use in treating the disorder. The most difficult problem with gene therapy has been finding a way of getting healthy genes to the cells that need them. Generally they must be delivered by a vehicle called a *vector*. To date a variety of vectors have been tried, mainly infectious agents such as a retrovirus (a virus containing DNA's cousin, RNA, which has a knack for attaching itself to a cell's genome) and an adenovirus (such as the one that causes the common cold, tried on patients with cystic fibrosis). The virus is made harmless by deleting some or all of its genes, splicing the therapeutic gene into the remaining material and mixing it with human cells. Sometimes, however, the body's immune system rejects the viral vector as a foreign invader and causes inflammation, swelling and other harmful reactions. To date only very few such attempts are showing success. One is an engineered retrovirus (which invades only cells in process of dividing) that attacks brain tumors; it works by sensitizing the tumor cells to a herpes drug that is then administered and kills them. However, this treatment has troublesome side effects. Another method is delivering a missing enzyme to children with a rare inherited immune-system disorder via mouse leukemia viruses, helping them produce the essential enzyme. Gene therapy is still in early experimental stages, but eventually, it is hoped, it will enable treating or correcting genetic disorders in the womb, before a baby is born.

genetic counseling Professional advice concerning the probability and implications of transmitting a hereditary disorder within a family and the alternatives available. The process usually begins with determining the reason for seeking such advice. Some couples already have a child with a birth defect. Others know they have a potential problem (as shown by a blood test or ultrasound, for example) or have a family member who is affected. Women over the age of 35 may wish advice concerning the chances of giving birth to a child with a chromosomal defect (see also AGE, CHILDBEARING). Others may be concerned about the effects of their exposure to environmental hazards, and still others may have a history of HABITUAL MISCARRIAGE.

The first step in genetic counseling is formulating a complete family history and personal medical history for both parents, which systematically reviews all past and present medical problems. The individual's (and couple's) age, nationality or ethnic background, habits, diet, hobbies, education and vocation all are included, as well as information about former marriages, family illnesses and abortions. Possible exposure to infection and hazards such as X-rays, drugs and toxic chemicals is investigated. This careful review is followed by a detailed physical examination; if

needed, specialists of various kinds are consulted. Specific laboratory tests, including biochemical and cytogenic studies, may be performed. Among these are *metabolic screening,* with an amino acid chromatogram; *urinary screening* if there is more than one retarded child in the family; and *chromosome analysis* based on a simple blood test. (See also KARYOTYPING.) Sometimes physical examination and laboratory tests may be carried out on close relatives as well.

When all the relevant information has been gathered, the counselor tries to determine if there is a genetic problem or one caused by a known environmental factor; if it is the former, he or she tries to establish the mode of inheritance. The conclusions then are reviewed with the concerned individual or couple, the mode of inheritance and recurrence risks are fully explained and various options (ARTIFICIAL INSEMINATION, AMNIOCENTESIS and others) are considered.

Genetic counseling, which is available principally at major hospitals and medical centers, is time-consuming and expensive. However, many couples who are at risk find it less costly than bringing into the world a child who cannot survive or perhaps may never function as a self-sufficient adult.

An estimated 12 million Americans currently carry traits due wholly or partly to defective genes or chromosomes, and although some defects, such as color blindness, are a very minor handicap, others are exceedingly serious. Some 40% of all infants who die do so because of hereditary disorders; of all surviving newborn babies, 15% have one or another genetic disorder. Indeed, it is estimated that every individual carries five to eight genes for genetic defects, and each couple has a 3% risk of bearing a child with a birth defect, which may be as minor as a birth mark or very major. When a serious condition is suspected, genetic counseling may prevent at least some of the tragedy.

See also BIRTH DEFECTS; GENETICS; PRENATAL TESTS.

genetic disorders   See BIRTH DEFECTS.

genetics The science of heredity. It is named for the basic unit of heredity, the *gene*, a blueprint for making a particular protein. There are an estimated 100,000 human genes; the complete set is called the human *genome*. In human beings genes are located on 23 pairs of *chromosomes*, in effect strands of genes, which are present in the nucleus of each body cell. The chromosomes are filled with tightly coiled strands of a chemical called *DNA* (for deoxyribonucleic acid; see also NUCLEIC ACID), whose structure was discovered only in 1953. Genes are segments of DNA that contain instructions to make proteins, the building blocks of all cells.

Within a few years of this discovery, genes from a toad were transplanted into bacteria and functioned there, an experiment marking the birth of a new science, *recombinant DNA research* or *genetic engineering*. Soon scientists learned how to cut, splice and transplant genes almost at will, as well as how to make synthetic genes (from laboratory chemicals), read the messages of the genes and even devise new genetic messages. In 1966 came another major advance, the complete translation of the genetic code embodied in the structure of DNA, showing how the sequence of DNA subunits spells out instructions for building proteins. (Proteins, the main constituents of all body cells, have thousands of forms and functions; they may be hormones such as insulin, structural elements such as collagen, or vital enzymes.) Since then there has been a steady stream of breakthroughs that have profoundly affected the field of medicine: the transplant of genes to correct cell deficiencies in, for example, regulating cholesterol; the discovery of *oncogenes*, aberrant genes linked to cancers; the identification of dozens of genes connected with inherited defects and diseases, enabling them to be detected prenatally; the development of vaccines against such diseases as cholera by manipulating the genes of the organisms that cause the disease; and the manufacture of insulin, human growth hormone and similar substances produced by the body.

Some knowledge of genes had existed prior to these discoveries from the experiments of Gregor Mendel (1822–84), an Austrian monk and botanist, and Luther Burbank (1849–1926), an American horticulturist and plant breeder. The basic principles were used in selective breeding of plants and animals. It was known that genes are present in chromosomes and that each gene governs a different trait, such as flower color, in the organism. The genes are arranged on the chromosome in linear order, and a given gene normally occupies the same position on its chromosome in each cell within the living organisms of its species. The chromosomes in a cell occur in pairs, each of which has genes for the same trait. However, although the pairs of genes govern the same trait, they are not necessarily identical; thus a plant can have one gene for blue flowers and another for white. When there are a number of possible genes for a given trait, some are usually *dominant* over others, which are said to be *recessive*. For example, blue may be dominant and white recessive; therefore a plant with one gene for each will have blue flowers but one with two genes for white will have white flowers. (Mendel's theories were based on garden peas, but human beings are more complicated, and even a simple trait such as eye color can involve not just one gene but the interaction of several.) Since some genes are associated with specific diseases, such as sickle-cell disease, or with a tendency to develop certain disorders, such as diabetes, whether they are dominant or recessive is important in determining the chances of their being transmitted to offspring.

The traits an organism inherits from its parents are governed by the way their genes are passed down. In normal cell division, called *mitosis*, each chromosome (and therefore each gene) is duplicated before the cell divides, so that each of the two new or "daughter" cells receives an identical set of genes. Sexual reproduction, however, involves the fusion of two special cells called *gametes*, the egg cell of the mother and the sperm cell of the father. In order for offspring to have the correct number of chromosomes (and genes) for their species, each gamete must provide *half* that number. Therefore, in a chromosome-reducing process called *meiosis*, the pairs of chromosomes are separated, with one member of each pair going to a particular egg or sperm. Thus the parent with one trait for blue flowers and one for white can give either of them to his sperm (or her egg). The second gene for flower color will come from the other parent. In human cells, which normally have 46 chromosomes, 23 come from each parent.

Most inherited traits come from individual genes or combinations of genes. An individual's sex, however, was long thought to be determined by entire chromosomes. The sex chromosomes are the only ones in which the two members of the pair may differ: Every female carries two female, or X, chromosomes, but every male carries one female, X, and one male, or Y, chromosome. During meiosis the male parent's sperm receives either an X or a Y chromosome, while the female parent's egg receives an X chromosome. The offspring that receives the Y chromosome from the male parent becomes a male (XY), while the one receiving the X chromosome from the male parent becomes a female (XX). Actually, it is a *particular* gene or genes on the Y chromosome that is responsible for maleness, a discovery that accounts for formerly baffling abnormalities of sex determination.

Genes for certain traits other than sex are located on the X chromosome. When a male offspring inherits such a trait on his X chromosome, there may be no matching gene on the Y chromosome, so that trait will invariably be shown. A female offspring, on the other hand, has two X chromosomes, so even if she inherits such a trait it may be masked by another, more dominant gene for the same trait on the other X chromosome. For this reason certain characteristics, called *sex-linked* or *X-linked characteristics*, appear far more often in men than in women; among them are red-green color blindness and the blood-clotting disorder hemophilia. (See BIRTH DEFECTS for other examples.)

Normally, children resemble one or another of their parents or grandparents in most of their basic physical features. Occasionally, however, a totally new characteristic appears, one that cannot be traced back even several generations. In effect there has been a sudden accident, resulting in a changed gene or genes. Such a change is called a *mutation*, and the organism showing the change is a *mutant*. Usually just a gene is affected, but sometimes the change affects a chromosome. In either case the changed genetic material is passed on to that organism's offspring. Mutations can be present at birth, or they may arise from DNA-copying errors as aging cells divide, or they can be caused by environmental factors, some of which have been identified although many still are unknown. With the development and use of many new chemicals and the increased use of high-energy radiation, mutations have become far more common. They have been produced experimentally in test animals by means of exposure to high doses of X-rays, gamma rays, extremely high temperatures and a growing variety of chemical agents. Most mutant genes are recessive—the offspring with dominant ones do not survive—so in effect they are masked by the normal gene of their pair. They do not appear until two parents with the same mutant genes have offspring. The disorder that results from such mutations depends on the kind of protein involved and the nature of the defect. In cystic fibrosis, for example, a faulty ion-conducting protein results in the formation of thick mucus that obstructs the lungs.

See also GENE THERAPY; GENETIC COUNSELING; PRENATAL TESTS; SEX DETERMINATION.

genetic testing The use of DNA tests for mutations in specific genes in order to determine whether persons with a family history of hereditary disorders are likely to develop them. Such tests can be performed before birth and, with in vitro fertilization, even before an embryo is implanted in the uterus (see PRENATAL TESTS). Further, tests are now available for determining whether one is a carrier for hemophilia, muscular dystrophy or some other genetic disease that one might pass on to one's children, or for whether one is likely to develop a particular disorder, such as Huntington's disease, later in life. Tests are available for the mutant BRCA1 and BRCA2 genes responsible for some breast and ovarian cancers, for the particular ApoE genes involved in Alzheimer's disease, the gene defect responsible for Huntington's and so on. Genetic testing raises a number of issues. Not every individual wants to know if he or she will, for example, develop Alzheimer's in old age. Furthermore, test results may make health insurers reluctant to insure individuals genetically at risk for diabetes or breast cancer or some other disorder. Although present law forbids insurers to deny insurance on the basis of a pre-existing genetic disorder, the law may change; also, it does not prevent insurers from charging higher rates for what they consider greater risk.

See also GENETIC COUNSELING.

genital herpes See HERPES INFECTION.

genitals Also *genitalia*. The external reproductive organs. In women the principal external organs also are called the pudendum or VULVA; in men they include the PENIS and SCROTUM.

genital warts See CONDYLOMA ACUMINATA.

German measles See RUBELLA.

gestation Also *term*. The period of development of human beings and other animals whose young grow inside the mother's body from conception until birth. For the mother this period is called PREGNANCY. The average duration of gestation of the human fetus is nine months. However, since most women cannot tell exactly which act of intercourse was responsible for a given pregnancy (and, even if they could, there is some variation in the length of gestation from individual to individual), gestation is calculated in terms of menstrual age, that is, counting from the *last menstrual period* (LMP), even though that may precede conception by two weeks or more. Thus the average gestation is nine and one-third months, (or 40 weeks, or 280 days), and the date of delivery is calculated by adding exactly nine months and seven days to the first day of the LMP. A baby born close to this time is described as *full term*; a baby born before about 36 weeks' gestation is usually PREMATURE, and one born after 42 weeks' gestation is usually POSTMATURE.

Although the exact time for each stage of development also varies among individuals, and the size of fetuses varies considerably, the general sequence is roughly the same and is as follows (for a white North American baby):

WEEK 4   Implantation has occurred; egg barely visible to naked eye (see IMPLANTATION).

END OF WEEK 8   Embryo measures 22 to 24 millimeters (⁹⁄₁₀ inch) long, weighs 1 gram (.07 ounce); fingers and toes appear; ear buds seen on head.

END OF WEEK 12   Fingers and toes fully formed, have nails; external genitals appear; fetus measures 7 to 9 centimeters (3½ inches) long, weighs about 14 grams (½ ounce). In another week or two risk of miscarriage becomes very small.

END OF WEEK 16   Fetus is 13 to 17 centimeters long (6 inches), weighs about 100 grams (3½ ounces).

END OF WEEK 20   Downy hair (lanugo) covers body; fetal movements have been felt for several weeks; heartbeat sometimes heard; fetus weighs more than 300 grams (10 ounces).

WEEK 24   Fetus weighs about 600 grams (20 ounces); skin wrinkled; if born, half to two-thirds may live if given special care.

WEEK 28   Length 37 centimeters (14 inches), weighs more than 1,000 grams (2.2 pounds); skin is red, covered with *vernix caseosa*, a white, cheesy substance. If born and given special care, more than half survive.

WEEK 32   Weighs 1,700 grams (3½ pounds), length 42 centimeters (16 inches); if born, has fairly good chance of survival with special care.

WEEK 36   Length 47 centimeters (18 inches), weighs 2,500 grams (5½ pounds). Has good chance of survival if born.

WEEK 40   Fully developed newborn baby. Average length 50 centimeters (20 inches), weighs 3,100 to 3,400 grams (7 pounds); smooth skin still covered with *vernix caseosa* (black babies are dusky bluish red, not yet dark-skinned).

giant cell arteritis Also *cranial arteritis, Horton's disease, temporal arteritis*. A chronic inflammation of certain large blood vessels, called *temporal arteries*, such as those on the upper front sides of the head near the temple. Inflammation causes them to narrow, often leading to persistent headache as well as vision and hearing problems. Occurring mostly after the age of 50, the condition appears twice as often in women as men, but only rarely in black women. The cause is not known but is thought to be linked to aging as well as to a genetic predisposition in persons of northern European heritage. Onset usually is slow but may be quite sudden. Typical symptoms are severe headache, scalp tenderness and visual disturbances. Often a physical examination will reveal the abnormal artery. A blood test will reveal an elevated ESR (erythrocyte sedimentation rate), and sometimes a biopsy of the artery (which can be done under local anesthesia) is required for definitive diagnosis. Treatment consists of large doses of corticosteroids, which reduce swelling and avoid damage to the artery supplying the optic nerve. Untreated, the disorder can progress to blindness. Improvement usually occurs within 72 hours of treatment. However, steroid therapy must continue until the ESR returns to normal and usually must be continued to some degree for 18 to 24 months. Giant cell arteritis frequently appears in conjunction with another disorder, POLYMYALGIA RHEUMATICA, suggesting they are closely related.

ginseng Also *American ginseng, manroot, flower of life, fountain of youth root.* An herb, *Panax quinquefolium* (or *Panax ginseng*), the root of which has been used in many primitive cultures as well as in ancient and modern China and in the former Soviet Union, as a general tonic to help the body adapt to heat stress and reduce sweating, to prevent numerous infectious diseases and to treat impotence. More recently it has been suggested as a remedy for the HOT FLASHES of menopause. It contains saponins, compounds that interact with neurotransmitters and may counteract the effects of stress. It should *not* be used by women with high blood pressure. Currently there are no reliable controlled studies showing that ginseng is an aphrodisiac or that its effects are similar to those of estrogen. Nevertheless, it is widely available in American health-food stores and pharmacies, both the root itself and an assortment of powders, instant teas, capsules and liquid concentrates made from it. American ginseng and Asian ginseng are slightly different plants, distinguished as

Panax quinquefolium and *Panax schinseng (chinensis);* another close relative is Siberian ginseng, *Eleutherococcus senticosus.* Still another related plant is dong kwai (*Angelica sinensis* or *polymorpha*), which has been recommended for relief of menstrual cramps, menopause and other gynecologic conditions. It apparently contains compounds that dilate the blood vessels or prevent muscle spasms. There is no scientific evidence of its effectiveness. It also contains chemicals that increase the skin's sensitivity to sun and so should not be taken in high doses. As with all HERBAL REMEDIES, it is important to remember that, while some may be just as effective as inorganic drugs, they also can give rise to allergic reactions and undesirable side effects. Moreover, since information about herbs is based largely on hearsay and the experience of others, determining proper dosages for effectiveness and nontoxicity is more difficult.

GnRH Abbreviation for *gonadotropin-releasing hormone,* a substance produced by the hypothalamus that stimulates the pituitary to produce LH (luteinizing hormone) and FSH (follicle-stimulating hormone; see under MENSTRUAL CYCLE for further explanation) and possibly also prolactin. GnRH has been isolated and synthesized in the laboratory. At least three forms of so-called GnRH agonist have been approved for treating ENDOMETRIOSIS. It also is being used experimentally to shrink fibroid tumors and to halt abnormal vaginal bleeding. GnRH acts by producing a reversible menopause. Earlier names for it were FRH (follicle-releasing hormone) and LRH (luteinizing-releasing hormone).

See also MALE CONTRACEPTIVE.

goiter See THYROID.

gonad Sex gland. In the human female the gonads are the ovaries, in the male, the testes.

See also OVARY; TESTES.

gonadotropin A hormone that controls the functions of a sex gland, or gonad. Two such hormones are produced by the pituitary gland, follicle-stimulating hormone (FSH) and luteinizing hormone (LH). Their production in turn is controlled by the hypothalamus by means of gonadotropin-releasing hormone (GnRH). (See MENSTRUAL CYCLE for further explanation.) Another pituitary hormone, prolactin, inhibits production of the gonadotropins and so sometimes is called an *antigonadotropin*.

See also HUMAN CHORIONIC GONADOTROPIN.

gonorrhea   Also *GC, clap, dose, drip, strain* (slang). The second most commonly reported SEXUALLY TRANSMITTED DISEASE in North America today (after CHLAMYDIA INFECTION), usually transmitted by sexual intercourse (vaginal, anal or oral). It is caused by a bacterium, the gram-negative gonococcus *Neisseria gonorrhoeae*. Outside the body the gonococcus dies within seconds, so the disease cannot be spread by towels, toilet seats or other objects touched by an infected person. It thrives only in mucous membrane, the moist lining of the mouth, throat, urethra and cervix. In men symptoms appear 1 to 14 days after the sexual contact, and in women 7 to 21 days, but *no* symptoms whatever occur in about 80% of infected women and perhaps 20% of infected men. If symptoms do appear, in women they tend to consist of a greenish or yellow-green vaginal discharge and very occasionally irritation of the vulva; in men they consist of burning on urination and a urethral discharge, usually white, but sometimes yellow or yellow-green. Both men and women may have a sore throat if infection is by oral sex, as well as tender enlarged lymph glands in the groin. Anal gonorrhea (infecting the anus) rarely gives rise to any symptoms, although occasionally there may be discomfort or itching in the area or an anal discharge of pus and sometimes blood. Gonorrhea also can affect the eyes, in adults usually from contact with the urethral discharge of an infected man and in newborn babies while the baby is passing through the infected mother's birth canal. The principal complication of gonorrhea in both men and women is sterility.

Diagnosis of gonorrhea requires examination and testing of mucus from the cervix, penis and, if oral or anal contact are possibilities, the mouth, throat and anus. (In women the anus always should be checked because infection may spread there from the vagina.) With speculum inserted in the vagina, the clinician takes a sample of cervical secretions, since the cervix is usually the first site of infection. A bimanual pelvic examination also should be performed to make sure the fallopian tubes are not infected. The kind of laboratory test performed on the mucus is important as well. The commonly used Gram stain, which shows up many kinds of bacterium, fails to reveal the gonococcus in 40 to 60% of women; a bacteriologic culture, in which the bacteria are allowed to grow and multiply in a nutrient jelly, is far more accurate.

Treatment of gonorrhea consists of a very large dose of an antibiotic, given orally or injected. The former drugs of choice, penicillin and tetracycline, have been replaced by other drugs because of the emergence of resistant strains of gonococci. Further, chlamydia is so often found along with gonorrhea that a course of oral antibiotics against it is advisable. Currently recommended treatment consists of a single injection of ceftriaxone (alternatives are oral cefiximine, cirofloxacin or ofloxacin; the last two should not be taken by pregnant women), plus a one-week course of doxycycline given orally. The latter is contraindicated for pregnant women, who instead are given a one-week course of erythromycin. Patients allergic to these cephalosporins should be given one injection of spectinomycin, a drug not available in the United States. Further, patients are urged to abstain from sexual activity until a cure has been confirmed by testing one week after treatment (and preferably again after two weeks). If the test is positive, checking for resistance to antibiotics is advisable so that another treatment can be substituted. Unfortunately, new resistant strains of the gonococcus have been appearing. Some authorities believe that oral contraceptives give rise to an ideal environment for gonococcal growth and therefore must be avoided while an infection is being treated; others disagree. An IUD (intrauterine device) must always be removed once gonorrhea is diagnosed.

Untreated gonorrhea in women may lead to infection of the fallopian tubes (salpingitis) or generalized PELVIC INFLAMMATORY DISEASE, which develops in half of all women not treated for 8 to 10 weeks. These infections in turn can produce scar tissue that causes infertility and also increases the risk of ECTOPIC PREGNANCY. Symptoms of *gonorrheal salpingitis* may begin with a menstrual period that is longer and/or more painful than usual, with pain developing on one or both sides of the lower abdomen within a few days. In acute cases the pain becomes severe, the temperature rises to about 102 degrees Fahrenheit, and there may be headache, nausea and vomiting. In some women the infection is less acute, marked only by dull aching in the lower abdomen, pain during or after intercourse or pelvic examination, backache and low fever (99 degrees Fahrenheit). Other possible complications are *gonococcal ophthalmia* (eye infection), usually only in babies born of infected mothers, which requires very prompt treatment with silver nitrate or penicillin eye drops to prevent blindness, and *septicemia* (blood poisoning), which may give rise to an *arthritis-dermatitis syndrome*. Septicemia more commonly occurs in women and homosexual men who have had gonorrhea for months without any other symptoms. Spread of the bacteria in the bloodstream causes fever (100 degrees to 104 degrees Fahrenheit), chills, loss of appetite, general malaise, and stiffness or pain in several joints. In about 3% of cases *gonococcal arthritis* may develop, affecting the knees, wrists, fingers and hands, ankles and elbows. In about half of such cases a characteristic and painful skin rash (dermatitis) develops also, usually on the arms, hands, legs and feet and especially around affected joints. Though the rash may heal by itself in a few days, new joint pains tend to develop. Intravenous antibiotic treatment must be given without delay to avoid permanent joint damage.

In pregnant women gonorrhea may lead to miscarriage or tubal infection in the early months. After the third month the infection usually is confined to the lower genital tract, but, as noted, the baby may become infected during delivery.

Gonorrhea has been known since ancient times. The mode of its transmission was not recognized until the late Middle Ages. The slang name "clap" (from *clapoir*, "bubo") was introduced by the French in the 14th century. The gonococcus was identified in 1879. The first significant worldwide gonorrhea epidemic occurred during and after World War I. Incidence fell between wars but rose drastically again during World War II and dropped again after the war when penicillin came into widespread use. In the early 1960s incidence again began to climb, especially among the American armed forces in Southeast Asia. During the 1960s strains of gonococcus resistant to penicillin began to develop, so the disease became much more difficult to cure. At this writing about 360,000 cases a year are being reported in the United States, but the actual occurrence is thought to be two to four times higher. Moreover, penicillin-resistant forms of the disease have been increasing; a new strain of the gonococcus produces a penicillin-destroying enzyme called penicillinase. This form of gonorrhea is called PPNG (for *penicillinase-producing* Neisseria gonorrhoeae).

gossypol   See MALE CONTRACEPTIVE.

gout   A painful inflammation of joints caused by defects in uric acid metabolism. Contrary to older opinion, women contract gout as often as men, but usually a decade or so later than men, who mostly contract it after age 60. Women patients tend to have a larger number of coexisting medical conditions and receive diuretics more often, probably because diuretics are used to control hypertension, more common in women than men over age 50. Both diuretics and hypertension predispose a person to gout. Gout most often affects the joints in the feet, although it can also affect ankle, knee, wrist, or elbow. An attack typically occurs without warning, often at night. The joint becomes inflamed and the skin over it appears red or purplish, tight and shiny, and fever may develop. The first few attacks usually affect only one joint and last a few days. However, if the disorder progresses, untreated attacks last longer, occur more often and may affect several joints. Treatment focuses on relieving pain by controlling the inflammation. Nonsteroidal anti-inflammatory drugs (NSAIDs) are the first line of approach. Colchicine has long been used but can have serious side effects. Corticosteroids may be needed to reduce inflammation in those who cannot tolerate other drugs. Preventive measures for recurrence are losing weight (many patients are overweight), avoiding diuretics, blood thinners and low doses of salicylates such as aspirin.

Avoiding alcoholic beverages and certain foods, such as anchovies, asparagus, consommé, herring, meat gravies and broths, mushrooms, mussels, all organ meats, sardines and sweetbreads is also beneficial. For severe and intractable cases, drugs that lower uric acid levels in the blood may be used.

Graafian follicle The one ovarian FOLLICLE (sometimes, but rarely, there are two) that develops to maturity during each ovulatory menstrual cycle and eventually breaks through the wall of the ovary and releases a mature egg cell (ovulation). It is named for Reinier de Graaf, who discovered it in 1672. Before ovulation takes place, this one follicle may occupy as much as one-fourth of the entire volume of the ovary and measure up to 1.5 centimeters (½ inch) in diameter. Since at puberty there are an estimated 75,000 immature egg cells in each ovary, it is obvious that the Graafian follicle grows many times larger than the others.

The Graafian follicle consists of two primary layers of cells, the *granulosa,* which surround the mature egg in the center, and the *thecae interna,* which surround the granulosa and are the prime repository and producer of the hormone estrogen. After the egg ruptures through the ovarian wall, the Graafian follicle in effect collapses in on itself. The space left by the egg is filled with blood, and a new structure, the CORPUS LUTEUM, is formed.

Gram stain A special staining method used on tissue samples to help identify certain organisms under the microscope. It is used to detect GONORRHEA, for which it is not very reliable, and TRICHOMONAS.

granuloma inguinale A SEXUALLY TRANSMITTED DISEASE that occurs mostly in tropical countries; a few hundred cases are found in North America each year, mostly in the southern United States. It is caused by an organism called *Donovania granulomatis* (for its discoverer, Charles Donovan) or *Calymmatobacterium granulomatis,* which is thought to be a bacterium. It probably is transmitted by sexual intercourse but is not highly contagious, and many persons exposed to infected partners never contract it. Men are more apt to get it than women. Symptoms, which appear from three days to four months after contact, consist of a painless bump or blister appearing on the genitals, thighs, groin or near the anus. It soon becomes an open sore, raised, rounded and bleeding readily. It does not heal but grows larger and somewhat painful. Neglected, it can extend to the thighs, lower abdomen and buttocks, making the whole area raw and open to infection by other organisms. The sore area itches, burns and exudes a foul smell. Diagnosis is made by taking a bit of tissue from the edge of a sore; under a microscope it will reveal the organisms. Treatment consists of tetracycline for 10 to 20 days; for women who are pregnant or those allergic to tetracycline, streptomycin, erythromycin or another antibiotic, taken for 30 days, usually is effective. All patients should be followed up every three months for one year to make sure the disease has been totally eradicated.

Graves' disease See THYROID.

gravida A woman who is pregnant.

growth and development The progressive increase in size (height and weight) and the maturation of certain organs and physiologic functions that mark the changes from infancy to adulthood. The rate of these changes and their total extent vary enormously among individuals and depend on numerous factors: heredity, diet, general health and others. Despite such variation, broad guidelines have been developed to differentiate normal growth and development from that influenced by diseases and deficiencies. Standardized growth charts represent one such guideline. Another is the progressive development of the fetus (see FETUS; GESTATION). During adolescence the development of certain secondary sex characteristics, notably the growth of the breasts and of pubic hair, tends to occur in certain stages, which are used for similar guidelines to assess normal development.

See also PUBERTY.

growth spurt   See PUBERTY.

guided imagery   See VISUALIZATION.

gynecologic examination   A physical checkup that includes special attention to the pelvic area and breasts in order to detect any abnormalities at an early stage and/or to treat an existing disorder. It may be performed by a GYNECOLOGIST, a family physician (general practitioner, family practitioner or internist) or a nurse-practitioner specializing in this area. It is highly desirable for all women to have such checkups at regular intervals, but there is some disagreement concerning how often. Most authorities agree that the first checkup should take place between the ages of 16 and 19, but earlier if a girl is sexually active before 16 or is about to become sexually active or has not yet begun to menstruate. Thereafter, some procedures should be carried out once a year, whereas others need to be performed only every two or three years, until the age of 40, when the guidelines change again.

A thorough gynecologic examination includes (1) taking of history; (2) the physical examination itself; (3) certain tests; and (4) a discussion with the clinician concerning his or her findings and recommendations for the future. *History taking* consists of a discussion with the clinician of a complete history of the patient's health and that of her immediate family. Among the topics covered are age, number of pregnancies and their outcomes, chief complaint and present illness (if any), menstrual history, contraceptives used (past and present), previous gynecologic problems, general medical history (including certain illnesses in parents, grandparents and siblings), hospitalizations and surgery, medications currently used (including alcohol, smoking, drug use), any previous adverse reactions to drugs and any past use of DES (diethylstilbestrol) by the patient or her mother.

The *physical examination* should include measuring height, weight, temperature, pulse and blood pressure. Many clinicians also listen to the heart and lungs with a stethoscope, check the inside of the throat and mouth and examine the neck for tender lymph nodes and thyroid enlargement. (For women using or planning to use oral contraceptives, heart and lung examinations are mandatory.) The breasts should be examined for lumps, tenderness, nipple discharge, dimpling or puckering and any other signs of a possible tumor (see BREAST SELF-EXAMINATION).

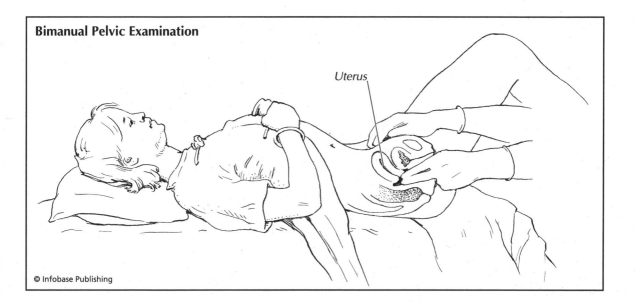

Bimanual Pelvic Examination

Uterus

© Infobase Publishing

The *pelvic examination*, with the patient in DORSAL LITHOTOMY position unless some disability makes that impossible, includes both external and internal pelvic organs. The external genital area is checked first, including labia, pubic area, clitoris, anus and urethra, for lumps, sores, growths, discoloring, discharges or lice. Both BARTHOLIN'S GLANDS and SKENE'S GLANDS are palpated to detect lumps. It is followed by an *internal examination* (before which the patient should empty her bladder). A metal or plastic SPECULUM is inserted into the vagina so that the vaginal walls and cervix can be inspected for redness, swelling, unusual discharge or irritation. At this time specimens for laboratory tests are collected, the clinician simply inserting a swab or spatula through the speculum to remove tissue shreds for a PAP SMEAR, gonorrhea culture or wet smear (see the discussion of tests below). After removing the speculum (or before inserting it)—the exact order of procedures varies with different clinicians—the clinician performs a *bimanual examination*, inserting two fingers of one hand into the vagina and placing the other hand on the abdomen. In this way he or she can check the position, size, firmness and mobility of the uterus, locate the fallopian tubes and ovaries (and feel any lumps there) and inspect the entire abdominal area for tenderness and lumps. Some clinicians ask the patient to bear down (as for a bowel movement) to check for relaxed muscles or a prolapsed uterus. Next comes a *rectovaginal examination* in which the clinician keeps one finger in the vagina and inserts another into the rectum, both to check the wall between rectum and vagina and to feel the pelvic organs from this angle. Finally, there should be a *rectal examination*, in which one finger is inserted into the rectum only to check for growths or other abnormal conditions there.

The pelvic examination usually is not painful, although it can be uncomfortable. Urinating immediately beforehand helps, but douching should be avoided during the preceding 24 hours (preferably 72 hours), so as not to hide discharges or other symptoms. The speculum is much easier to insert if the woman's muscles are relaxed; open-mouth deep breathing helps many women to relax more. If insertion still seems quite painful, the clinician should be asked if a smaller speculum is available or if the one being used can be adjusted. Most women can be examined quite readily, even if they have never had vaginal intercourse or even never used tampons. (The clinician cannot tell from an examination whether a woman has had sexual experience.) Women who find pelvic examination agonizingly embarrassing or are unsure about a new clinician's attitude may find it helpful to ask a friend or a patient advocate (see under PATIENTS' RIGHTS) to accompany them on their visit.

Among the *laboratory tests* generally performed are a *urine test* for protein, sugar and blood (recommended annually); a *Pap smear* for cervical cancer (formerly recommended annually for all women, now recommended once every three years for women who have had two negative tests in succes-

GOOD NUMBERS FOR PHYSICAL EXAMINATION

- Blood pressure: 120/80 mmHg or less
- Blood glucose (fasting): Under 110 mg/dL
- Total cholesterol: 200 mg/dL or less
- LDL (low-density lipoprotein): 100 mg/dL (less if there are cardiac risk factors)
- HDL (high-density lipoprotein): More than 50 mg/dL
- Triglycerides: Less than 150 mg/dL
- TSH (thyroid-stimulating hormone): 0.2–4.7 mcl/ml
- BMI (body mass index): 18–24.9
- Waist circumference: Less than 35"
- Bone density (T-score): No less than under 1 SD

sive years but more often in high-risk women); a *gon-orrhea culture* (some clinicians do it routinely, others only when exposure is suspected); a blood count for anemia (some do it routinely once a year, others do not). Other tests, usually performed only when they are specifically indicated, include syphilis test; tests for vaginal infection (usually only in the presence of symptoms); urinalysis or urine culture (if infection is suspected); stool test (for blood); BLOOD TESTS for cholesterol, triglycerides and other substances; and a mammogram (see MAMMOGRAPHY).

After completing the physical examination and tests, most clinicians sit down with the patient to discuss their findings, prescribe medication and/or contraceptives (if needed), answer questions and schedule future visits if necessary and/or the next checkup.

See also PRENATAL CARE.

gynecologist A physician who specializes in women's health. This specialty is frequently combined with OBSTETRICS, which includes all aspects of childbirth (prenatal care, delivery and postpartum care); such a specialist is called an *obstetrician-gynecologist* or *ob-gyn*. A board-certified gynecologist has had three years of residency in obstetrics and gynecology and may have had two additional years of fellowship training in a subspecialty, such as gynecologic oncology (cancer of the reproductive organs). He or she also has passed special examinations. In the United States about 65% of all board-certified gynecologists are men. Although the number of women physicians has been growing rapidly, the increase has been slower in surgical specialties, of which ob-gyn is one.

Although gynecologists have studied general medicine as well, like other specialists they tend to focus on the particular areas they know best. Therefore a woman who uses a gynecologist for routine health care, such as physical checkups, should make sure that her examinations include regular measurements of blood pressure and blood and urine tests and not only pelvic and breast examinations. Routine gynecologic care also can be performed by internists (physicians who specialize in internal medicine), family practitioners and general practitioners (GPs). They are able to perform standard breast and pelvic examinations but are both less experienced in and less highly trained for more specialized gynecologic care. Many authorities believe that routine or primary care is best carried out by a practitioner who is not specifically trained as a surgeon (as most gynecologists are).

See also SELF-HELP; SURGERY, UNNECESSARY.

habitual miscarriage Also *habitual abortion*. The spontaneous loss of three consecutive pregnancies by MISCARRIAGE. The causes lie either in the fetus, which may have some genetic abnormality or other defect, or in the mother or father. Conditions affecting the mother include endocrine abnormalities (in the thyroid or adrenal glands, progesterone deficiency or diabetes, for example); a structural abnormality in the UTERUS, such as an INCOMPETENT CERVIX; ENDOMETRIOSIS; or genital HERPES INFECTION or some other infection. Women whose mothers were given the hormone DIETHYLSTILBESTROL while pregnant with them may be more likely to miscarry than untreated women, but this theory has not been satisfactorily verified. Smoking, heavy alcohol use and caffeine consumption (more than 10 cups of coffee a day), and various drugs (hormones, antibiotics, antihypertensives) may contribute to early pregnancy loss. Exposure to certain industrial chemicals (copper, lead, sulfur, etc.) also may be linked to miscarriage, and several recent studies have implicated long exposure (more than 20 hours a week) to video display terminals (CRTs). In some women the cause may lie in an immunologic reaction that makes their body reject a fetus as foreign tissue. Called an *allo-immune disorder*, it occurs when the parents are very similar genetically, and the woman's immune system fails to make antibodies against a rejection action of the immune system. This condition sometimes can be corrected by transferring to the woman some of her male partner's white blood cells to stimulate the production of the needed antibodies. In other cases clinicians try to treat the woman with immunoglobulin, a blood product pooled from thousands of donors and used to regulate abnormal responses of the immune system. This treatment is very expensive and critics maintain there is not sufficient proof of its efficacy to warrant its use, but apparently it has worked for some women.

In the approximately 5% of American women of childbearing age who have two or more miscarriages for which no cause can be found, recent research indicates that a susceptibility to form blood clots due to genetic flaws is responsible for some cases. The flaws consist of one of two mutations, Factor V Leiden and prothrombin, the two most common causes of a tendency to develop blood clots. Therefore, it is recommended that women who have had two or more miscarriages undergo blood tests for the genetic mutations, even if they have no history of blood clots.

In another disorder, *antiphospholipid syndrome*, the woman produces antibodies that trigger formation of blood clots in the placenta that cut off nutrients to the fetus. Treatment consists of one baby aspirin a day during pregnancy to thin the mother's blood; in severe cases a stronger blood-thinning drug, heparin, or the immune-suppressing steroid prednisone may be used. For *luteal phase defect*, in which the woman does not produce sufficient progesterone to maintain an early pregnancy, vaginal suppositories containing progesterone may help.

Another field of investigation is abnormalities in sperm caused by environmental factors, such as exposure to toxic substances, which also are linked with a high risk of miscarriage. One agent so implicated is vinyl chloride.

The duration of pregnancy at the time of miscarriage is often a clue to the cause. Up to about 12 weeks it tends to be a genetic or hormonal abnormality; thereafter it tends to be a structural one. For repeated miscarriage during the first 13 weeks, tests should begin with a complete physical examination of the woman and testing for disorders such as diabetes, heart disease, lupus and thyroid problems. Often treating an underlying disorder will result in a healthy pregnancy. Tests also should include genetic and CHROMOSOME studies of both parents, a thyroid function test, and an endometrial biopsy (see BIOPSY, def. 8) timed so as to investigate hormone deficiency after ovulation, such as luteal phase defect (see under IMPLANTATION). If the results of all these studies are negative, a hysterosalpingogram (special X-ray of uterus and tubes) may be performed. Habitual miscarriage later in pregnancy calls for careful examination of the uterus and cervix by X-ray and other techniques to check for abnormalities associated with 5 to 10% of recurrent miscarriages, among them scarring, a double uterus or malformations from prenatal exposure to DES (such as an incompetent cervix).

Until recently it was commonly believed that women who miscarry three consecutive times will almost inevitably miscarry again. More recent studies indicate that the risk of a fourth miscarriage is only about 25%; that is, there is a 70 to 80% chance that the fourth will be a perfectly normal pregnancy. Such spontaneous cures of whatever condition caused the previous miscarriages are not fully understood, but it is suspected that they result from the self-correction of some delicate hormonal feedback mechanism that had gone amiss.

hair loss Also *alopecia.* The thinning or falling out of scalp hair, which is affected to some extent by hormonal changes that are not completely understood. For many women hair loss is attributable to the inherited condition *androgenetic alopecia,* with higher androgen (male hormone) levels, which causes them to have diffuse hair loss all over their heads. Hair loss can also result from physical or psychological stress, including severe illness, surgery and some medications (chemotherapy drugs, blood pressure drugs and others). Called *toxic alopecia,* it is usually temporary and subsides when the causative factor is removed. When round irregular patches of hair on the scalp are suddenly lost, the condition is called *alopecia areata* and is thought to be an autoimmune disorder; it can be treated with corticosteroids.

Some women experience loss of scalp hair when they take oral contraceptives. Since a common cause of such hair loss is an underactive thyroid gland (hypothyroidism), this condition should first be ruled out. Thereafter, switching to another kind of oral contraceptive may solve the problem. Other women experience hair loss when they stop taking oral contraceptives; usually this is a temporary condition, probably caused simply by the change in hormone levels, and is self-correcting within a few months. Pregnancy sometimes affects hair growth and also hair texture. Also, many women experience considerable *thinning* of scalp hair after delivery; again, it usually is a temporary condition that is self-correcting. After menopause, most women experience some thinning of both scalp and pubic hair, and sometimes an increase in facial hair. These changes are most likely caused by a relative increase in androgen levels compared to estrogen levels, which are lowered. Still another possible cause of hair loss is anemia, which should be ruled out by means of a simple blood test. The drug minoxidil (Rogaine) has been approved to treat hair loss, mainly by slowing it, but it does not achieve regrowth. Available without prescription, it is used in a lower dose for women than for men. Also, it must be used continuously or its effect wears off. Hair transplants are another option, but an expensive one. They work best when hair loss is concentrated at the crown. See also Resources in the Appendix.

Halsted radical mastectomy See MASTECTOMY, def. 2.

Hashimoto's thyroiditis See THYROID.

headache A general term for moderate to severe pain in the head, which can be a symptom of numerous disorders but generally does not require medical attention unless it occurs often enough to be considered chronic and/or is severe enough to be disabling. The headache accompanying a cold or other infectious disease normally subsides when the disease does and usually responds to aspirin or other over-the-counter remedies. Severe and recurrent headache, however, may be caused by a tumor or other brain lesion; by a serious infection, such as meningitis or encephalitis; by infections of the eye, ear, nose, mouth, sinuses or teeth; or by allergy. The most common kinds of recurrent headache, whose causes often are very difficult to determine, are those caused by various vascular disturbances, that is, disturbances of the blood flow to the head. Among these are the *cluster headache,* found 20 times more frequently in men than in women; the *tension headache,* in which tense muscles of the head, face and neck cause blood vessels to constrict spasmodically; *toxic metabolic headache,* caused by a toxic state (overindulgence in alcohol—the typical "hangover" headache—as well as lead, arsenic, morphine or carbon monoxide poisoning); *hypertension headache,* caused by complications from high blood pressure; and MIGRAINE, caused by arterial spasm. Headache also may be a side effect of ORAL CONTRACEPTIVE or other medication. A change to a different kind of oral contraceptive may help, but if the headache is of the migraine variety oral contraceptives should be discontinued at once and another form of birth control substituted.

Numerous drugs, both prescription and over-the-counter, as well as psychotherapy have been used to fight chronic headache, with mixed success. In fact, some studies show that overuse of over-the-counter medications like acetaminophen (Tylenol) and ibuprofen (Advil) actually can cause chronic daily headache because constant intake of the drug interferes with the brain's pain-control pathways. One promising nondrug approach is *biofeedback,* in which patients are taught to increase the blood flow to the head. Another approach is learning relaxation exercises, which can be used whenever a stressful situation arises. Some researchers believe poor nutrition can cause sufficient physical stress to produce chronic tension headache and suggest that eating foods rich in calcium and the B vitamins may be helpful. Another form of self-treatment is acupressure, which consists of pressing an index finger firmly on certain pressure points of the body and slowly rotating the finger for 20 to 30 seconds; this may relieve the headache within a minute or so. Sometimes a cold pack placed on the forehead alleviates the pain (because cold constricts blood vessels); it should work in about five

minutes. Many HERBAL REMEDIES have been used for headache, among them teas made from dried rosemary (*Rosmarinus officinalis*), skullcap (*Scutellaria laterifolia*), hops (*Humulus lupulus*), passion flower (*Passiflora incarnate*), peppermint (*Mentha piperita*), or valerian (*Valeriana officinalis*), or massaging the forehead and temples with peppermint oil. Native Americans once treated headache with a tea brewed from the bark of a willow tree. Willow bark, available in powder form from health-food and herbal dealers, contains salicin, a compound the body converts to salicylic acid, which is the active ingredient in aspirin.

health care proxy An advance care directive assigning a close relative or friend to make decisions about one's medical treatment when one is unable to do so oneself, in case of a persistent coma or stroke or in the late stages of Alzheimer's disease or congestive heart failure. All 50 states have some type of legislation permitting durable power of attorney for health care; the person may be called a health care agent, surrogate or proxy. The directive must be in writing, signed by both parties and witnessed by two independent persons. The proxy is informed of one's wishes concerning artificial nutrition and hydration, and being connected to life-support machinery when recovery is unlikely. A form provided by the state health department is generally available from a physician or a local hospital. A health care proxy differs from a *living will,* a treatment directive made out by oneself; it generally cannot cover all the eventualities that might occur.

hearing loss See DEAFNESS.

heart attack See ARTERIOSCLEROSIS.

heart disease See ARTERIOSCLEROSIS; CONGESTIVE HEART FAILURE.

heart failure See CONGESTIVE HEART FAILURE.

Hegar's sign   An early physical change of the reproductive tract in pregnancy and therefore a useful presumptive sign in its diagnosis. Just above the cervix at the bottom of the corpus (body) of the uterus is a tiny area called the *isthmus*. In early pregnancy this area, just a few millimeters long, feels softer than either the cervix or the corpus. This softness, called Hegar's sign, is readily detected by the clinician during bimanual pelvic examination, because the area is easily compressed between the two hands.

height loss   Also *shrinkage*. A reduction in height, particularly occurring after menopause. Studies show that the average woman aged 43 will thereafter lose about 0.1% of her height annually. Thus a woman who was 5 feet 6 inches tall in her youth may be just over 5 feet 3 inches at age 80. Although height loss may be due to OSTEOPOROSIS, when spinal fractures in weak, demineralized bone cause sometimes fairly considerable height loss, other factors influence less dramatic shrinkage. Weak muscles make one tend to sag, and poor posture can contribute to such muscle atrophy. The vertebrae become flatter and wider after age 50, and the spinal disks, pads of fibrous tissue between the vertebrae, wear thin with time. Both phenomena result in a gradual compression of the spinal column. Height loss can be minimized by regular weight-bearing exercise (walking, dancing, jogging), which helps maintain muscle and bone, and by improved posture.

hematuria   The presence of blood in the urine, usually symptomatic of a urinary infection (most often urethritis or cystitis) but sometimes of a more serious condition, such as a tumor of the bladder or kidney, kidney stones, cysts or sickle-cell disease. The urine is reddish or brownish, depending on how much blood is present and on the chemical makeup (especially the acidity) of the urine itself. Because it may signal a serious problem, hematuria always calls for careful diagnosis to identify the underlying cause.

hemochromatosis   An excess of iron in the blood. A genetic disorder whose symptoms in women surface mainly after menopause, this buildup of iron can result in debilitating and even life-threatening problems. Symptoms include chronic fatigue, joint pain, loss of libido, abdominal pain and grayish or bronze skin color. If not diagnosed and treated, the disease can lead to congestive heart failure and severe liver and pancreas damage. If the disorder is suspected, blood should be tested for iron storage. Treatment involves repeated drawing of blood, which can be performed in a doctor's office or blood bank, as often as twice a week until iron is depleted and thereafter several times a year. Alcohol and foods high in iron, such as liver and red meats, should be avoided.

Hemochromatosis is caused by a mutation in a gene, most often C282Y, that helps regulate iron absorption. Individuals who inherit a copy of the gene from both parents are likely to develop the disorder. Carriers inherit only one mutated gene and probably do not develop it but can, of course, pass it on.

hemophilia   A hereditary bleeding disorder that is due to a lack of or abnormality of some of the chemical factors that make blood coagulate (clot). It is a sex-linked recessive gene disorder (see under BIRTH DEFECTS and GENETICS for further explanation) passed on by mothers to their sons. Depending on which clotting factor is defective, there are various kinds of hemophilia, the most common of which are hemophilia A (abnormal Factor VIII) and hemophilia B (abnormal Factor IX). The former accounts for more than four-fifths of all cases in the United States. The disease usually is detected early in life, when symptoms such as hematomas (internal blood clots) and hematuria (bloody urine) appear. In some cases superficial cuts and wounds heal slowly, but in others serious hemorrhages result from trivial injuries or mild exercise, and hemarthrosis (bleeding into the joints) develops. There is no cure for the disease, but it can be controlled by administering the missing clotting factor. Factor VIII is present only in quite fresh plasma and has a short shelf life. However, it can be precipitated from plasma by freezing and can be stored frozen in blood banks. Therapy depends on the severity of the bleeding; internal hemorrhage into a large area, for example, may require transfusion at least twice a day for several days. In recent years home-care programs have been developed whereby the missing factor can be self-administered by the patient at home or injected by a family member.

Hemophilus vaginalis   See VAGINOSIS.

hemorrhage, vaginal   Heavy uncontrollable blood flow from the vagina, frequently but not always originating in the uterus. Unlike heavy MENSTRUAL FLOW, it tends to come in spurts, irregularly, rather than at a steady rate. The most common causes in adult women are MISCARRIAGE or an ECTOPIC PREGNANCY. Following childbirth, a POSTPARTUM HEMORRHAGE may occur when the uterus does not contract sufficiently after delivery or a portion of the placenta or fetal tissue is retained. It also may occur, for similar reasons, following abortion. During labor, hemorrhage can be caused either by ABRUPTIO PLACENTAE or by PLACENTA PREVIA.

Like uncontrolled bleeding elsewhere, vaginal hemorrhage constitutes a medical emergency and must be dealt with promptly, by stopping the bleeding, restoring blood volume (by blood transfusion) and combating shock.

hemorrhoid   Also *piles.* A VARICOSE VEIN in the anus or lower rectum. It is caused, like other varicosities, by increased pressure that weakens the wall of a vein, destroying the valves that keep blood moving back to the heart and ultimately causing blood to pool in places. The causes of such increased pressure include constipation (and hence straining to defecate), prolonged coughing or sneezing, obesity, pregnancy and abdominal tumors. The principal symptom is bleeding, usually noticed after a bowel movement. Since such bleeding also can be caused by polyps or tumors elsewhere in the gastrointestinal tract, it is very important to rule out serious conditions. Physicians can look for internal hemorrhoids through a lighted tube called an *anoscope.* To rule out cancer or other bleeding sources, it may be necessary to inspect the lower portions of the colon via sigmoidoscopy, using a longer, flexible

lighted tube, or to view the entire colon via colonoscopy. After ruling out more serious conditions, the diagnosis of hemorrhoids can be confirmed and treatment begun.

Hemorrhoids may occur outside or inside the anus. *External hemorrhoids* are small, soft, purplish skin-covered mounds that become more prominent with straining at stool. They are rarely painful unless they thrombose, that is, form a clot. The hemorrhoid then may become inflamed, break down, bleed profusely and be extremely tender, especially during defecation. After a few days the clot is absorbed and the swelling subsides. *Internal hemorrhoids* generally occur in clusters and are covered by a thin layer of mucous membrane. Passage of a hard stool may cause them to ulcerate and bleed; frequently they also cause itching and leakage of mucus from the anus. If the fibrous attachments that hold them in place are weakened, they will slide out, fill with blood and prolapse (protrude through the anus).

Small hemorrhoids that cause only slight occasional bleeding and otherwise are not troublesome need no treatment other than identifying and removing the underlying cause; those that appear during pregnancy often disappear after delivery. Constipation often can be relieved by a high-fiber diet and increased intake of liquids. For internal hemorrhoids that cause pain on defecation, use of a stool softener may help. Also, the anal area always should be cleaned very gently to avoid irritating it further. Sitz baths frequently help relieve discomfort, and cold packs applied to the buttocks can reduce swelling. Over-the-counter creams can help reduce friction and, if they contain a topical anesthetic, reduce inflammation. Itching can be relieved by dabbing the anal area with witch hazel. The use of suppositories and any local manipulation of the affected area should be avoided. If these measures fail and the bleeding is sufficient to cause ANEMIA, or if the pain is disabling or the itching intolerable, internal hemorrhoids often can be treated with one of several office procedures: surgical banding (to cut off the blood supply to the swollen tissue); injection sclerotherapy (injecting a liquid into mucous membranes above the hemorrhoid, which causes the tissue to scar and shrink); cryotherapy (freezing); or infrared photocoagulation (whereby infrared heat waves kill the hemorrhoid tissue). Laser therapy has been used but appears to be no better than these simpler treatments. A thrombosed external hemorrhoid can be lanced to remove the blood clot, affording immediate relief.

External hemorrhoids give rise to pain, swelling and itching. Itching, however, often is caused by an allergic reaction to local over-the-counter anesthetic agents that are promoted for hemorrhoids. A topical cream with cortisone to help itching and a nonallergenic anesthetic to relieve pain, available by prescription, is preferable. However, large external skin tags that remain after symptoms have disappeared may have to be removed surgically if they present a hygiene problem.

A more invasive option is stapled hemorrhoidopexy for treating bleeding or prolapsed internal hemorrhoids. A stapling device anchors the hemorrhoids in their normal position. Usually performed under general anesthesia as outpatient surgery, it need only be done once. Large protruding hemorrhoids or those that do not respond to these treatments may require hemorrhoidectomy, in which a narrow incision is made around both external and internal hemorrhoids and the swollen blood vessels are removed. While more painful, requiring general anesthesia and longer healing, it usually cures 95% of cases.

HERBAL REMEDIES for hemorrhoids include infusions made of dandelion root (*Taraxacum officinale*), chicory root (*Cichorium endiva*), cascara sagrada (*Rhamnus purshiana*), Oregon grape root (*Berberis aquifolium*) or licorice (*Glycyrrhiza glabra*), which all are drunk as a tea, or direct insertion into the rectum of an infusion of witch hazel leaves (*Hamamelis virginiana*), bayberry bark (*Myrica cerifera*) and goldenseal (*Hydrastis canadensis*).

hepatitis An inflammation of the liver caused by one of several viruses. The means of transmission and the long-term effects differ from virus to virus, but all can cause a temporary liver disease weeks after the initial exposure. Several principal viruses have been identified. *Type A* is spread mainly by fecal contamination of food, water and shellfish, and also can be transmitted through direct or indirect oral-anal contact during sexual intimacy. Within two to four weeks it causes mild to severe liver inflammation, with nausea, pain, dark urine, lightened stools and jaundice. There is no treatment, but patients usually recover on their own within six months. Two vaccines are available.

Type B (or *hepatitis B*), considered a SEXUALLY TRANSMITTED DISEASE, is spread through blood contact with virus-containing bodily fluids, most commonly in sexual intercourse but also in transfer of blood (transfusion, needle sharing, maternal transmission to a fetus). It causes liver disease one to three months after initial infection, but 90 to 95% of persons fight off the virus and recover in a few months. Others become carriers who show no symptoms but have a higher risk of cirrhosis, a degenerative liver disease, or liver cancer. Carriers have a permanent ability to infect others, and, since it is highly contagious, it may be spread through a shared toothbrush or razor, or possibly even kissing where there is an exchange of saliva.

Type C (hepatitis C) was called non-A, non-B until the virus was identified in 1989. It causes most post-transfusion and some other infections, and also is transmitted through sexual activity and blood (see further discussion below). *Type D* usually appears in conjunction with Type B, which makes it more severe, and *Type E* appears in conjunction with Type A.

Hepatitis B, as Type B is often called, has become a fast-spreading venereal disease of enormous concern, not only because of its severe long-term consequences for the patient but because many individuals infected with it become lifetime carriers. In the 1990s 50% more cases were reported than in the 1970s because of transmission by intravenous drug abuse and homosexual activity. Today, though the number of cases in the United States seems to have stabilized (about 300,000 a year), the incidence of the disease worldwide continues to rise. There is a preventive vaccine, which must be administered in three doses over a six-month period (the second dose a month later, the third six months after the first) and which is 95% effective. The Centers for Disease Control now recommends that the vaccine be given to all newborn infants at birth as well as to older children and adolescents. It also recommends screening pregnant women and vaccination for adults at increased risk of infection. Although universal vaccination has not yet been achieved and is expensive, it is cheap compared to the costs of the disease. Meanwhile, condoms do afford protection against sexual transmission of the virus, much as they do against AIDS.

At present no medication is completely effective in curbing liver damage from chronic infection or in ridding the body of an entrenched infection. Avoiding alcohol is highly recommended. Alpha-interferon, an immunity-enhancing drug, has helped some patients but is not considered curative and is very expensive. The AIDS drug lamivudine (Epivir), administered in smaller doses than for AIDS, appears to target an enzyme important for the virus's reproduction and thus affords some protection against liver damage, but it is not curative and has not been studied long enough to indicate how long it must be taken.

Prevention is particularly important for newborns, who can contract the disease during birth and can become chronic carriers for the rest of their lives. Therefore all pregnant women should be tested for hepatitis B virus, so that babies who need it can be treated immediately after birth. Many children who carry it eventually—sometimes decades later—develop illnesses such as hepatitis, cirrhosis and, in up to 25%, liver cancer. Only about 5% contract the infection while in the uterus; most are exposed during delivery. For maximum protection, the vaccine and gamma globulin are given during the first 12 hours of life; this has proved about 90% effective but is much less so with even a few days' delay. Additional vaccine is then given at ages one month and six months.

At this writing some 4 million Americans are believed to have hepatitis C, considered the leading blood-borne infection in the country. Many harbor the virus without experiencing symptoms, but symptoms can appear decades after infection. They generally include fatigue, nausea, poor appetite, muscle and joint pain and tenderness in the right upper abdomen. Over time, serious liver damage can occur. Some 60% of them are thought to have been infected through sharing needles with drug users; for the rest the source of infection may be a blood transfusion received before 1992, when the blood supply was not screened for the virus, or engaging in high-risk sexual practices, or in health care workers a prick from a needle containing infected blood. A combination of the antiviral drug ribavirin with interferon (marketed as Rebetron) appears to curb recurrence of hepatitis C more than interferon alone does; a newer version, peginterferon (Peg-Intron), also taken with ribavirin, is even more effective. However, these drugs are very expensive and can have severe and even life-threatening side effects. They cannot be taken by pregnant women. In 1999 the Food and Drug Administration approved a home kit to test for hepatitis C. Available without prescription, it contains a lancet to prick the finger and filter paper to collect a drop of blood. The user sends the sample to a laboratory for analysis, and test results are reported within 4 to 10 days. If positive, counseling or referral to a physician is available.

Hepatitis E is considered rare in the United States, but some studies suggest it has infected 5% of Americans. It is potentially fatal, especially in the third trimester of pregnancy, and can cause miscarriage, stillbirth and serious illness in newborns. Spread by fecal contamination of water, it is common in Mexico and some African and Asian nations. There is no specific treatment for it.

herbal remedies Also *herbalism*. The use of plants to relieve or cure a variety of disorders, a practice that is thousands of years old. Herbal medicine was and is practiced in virtually every part of the world and became the basis of early European pharmacology. The ancient Greek physician Hippocrates left a valuable description of herbs in use in his time, some of which are still popular today, and Dioscorides (first century A.D.) wrote a *materia medica* listing more than 500 plants. Printed herbals appeared soon after printing was invented, and their circulation enabled anyone who wished (and could read) to medicate him- or herself. Unlike other kinds of treatment, herbal remedies require no special skills or costly apparatus. As medicine became a formal profession, surgery (including bloodletting) and the use of chemical substances (such as arsenic and mercury) began to replace the use of medicinal plants. Nevertheless, the practice of herbalism survived, mostly passed down by word of mouth. In America colonial women learned the uses of New World plants from Native Americans, and African blacks brought with them knowledge of their traditional remedies. By the mid-20th century, however, herbal medicine had fallen into disrepute. Drug companies manufactured more and allegedly better chemical remedies, often synthesizing some of the organic compounds (in effect, copying nature in the laboratory). About 1970, interest in herbalism revived in America, in part due to the women's movement, with its emphasis on women's right to control their own bodies, and in part to the advocates of vegetarianism and "natural" foods. Actually, herbal medicines are more "natural" only in that their preparation is simpler and their ingredients are wholly organic. Chemically they can be identical with, and just as toxic as, human-made inorganic compounds.

Herbal medicines are prepared from the flowers, roots, leaves, stems, seeds or bark of plants. They may be inhaled, applied to the skin as a salve or ointment, inserted as a suppository or ingested as a tea or tablet. Often different herbs are combined for maximum effect. Because herbs may cause adverse reactions and do not work equally well for everyone, it is wise at first to use only one herb at a time (avoiding herbal teas that blend numerous plants) and in a small dose. Once it is fairly certain there will be no bad reaction, one can gradually increase dosage and add other herbs.

Like most plants, herbs have both common and scientific names. Because common names often vary and sometimes one name is used for several different herbs, every herb mentioned in this book is identified by its scientific name.

Herbs can be extremely effective medications. The leaves of the foxglove plant were used to treat heart disease long before their active ingredient, digitalin, was isolated, and digitalis is still an accepted remedy for heart patients. Herbs act on the body in the same ways as manufactured medications do and potentially are just as dangerous—indeed, in some respects more dangerous, because potency and dosages are less exact (whereas the amount and quality of active ingredients in a pill or capsule generally are closely controlled). Herbal remedies can cause serious side effects or extreme allergic reactions, and with

HARVESTING AND DRYING HERBS

1. Select disease-free plants. Be sure no pesticides were used.
2. Pick leafy stems on the morning of a dry, sunny day, after dew has dried from plants.
3. For *air drying,* place a bunch of freshly picked herbs upside down. Tie a perforated paper bag around them to protect from light and to catch any leaves that drop. Hang in a dry area with good air circulation. When completely dry, strip leaves from stems and store in airtight jars in a dark place.
4. For *oven drying,* strip freshly harvested leaves from stems and spread on a baking sheet. Put in oven set at lowest temperature, leaving oven door ajar. Check and stir often. Leaves are thoroughly dry if they crumble when rubbed between the fingers. Store in airtight jars in a dark place.

some used on a regular basis, there may even be withdrawal symptoms when their use is discontinued. Many healing plants also have toxic qualities, so that overdoses of them can have drastic effects. Experts advise particular caution with, or even total avoidance of, herb mixtures (teas) containing lobelia (*Lobelia inflata*), sassafras (*Sassafras albidum*), wormwood (*Artemisia absinthium*), comfrey (*Symphytum officinalis*), tonka bean (*Dipteryx odorata*), penny-royal (*Mentha pulegium*), pokeroot or pokeweed (*Phytolacca americana*), burdock (*Arctium lappa compositae*), ephedra (*Ephedra sinica* and other species—also called ma huang), yohimbe (*Pausinystalia yohimbe*), chaparral (*Larrea divaricata*) and senna (*Cassia senna*).

It must be emphasized that **herbal remedies are not a substitute for professional medical attention for any acute illness or persistent ailment.** Further, it is important to tell your clinician of any herbs you take lest they interact with prescribed drugs. It is especially important to do so when facing surgery, because herbs can alter surgical outcomes. According to one study, eight in particular do so: echinacea and St. John's wort may interact with and lessen effectiveness of immunosuppressant drugs; kava and valerian can magnify the effects of anesthesia; garlic, ginseng and ginkgo can pose a bleeding risk; and ephedra increases blood pressure and heart rate, posing a cardiovascular risk (the FDA recently banned it as a dietary supplement).

Herbs can be bought dried from herbalist suppliers, and the more common ones are also available in health-food stores, sometimes in the form of capsules. It is important to use a reliable supplier whose stock is adequately fresh. Look for standardized preparations to be certain of getting the same product with each bottle bought. In 1998 the U.S. Pharmacopeia published the first American standards for the potency of nine herbs, including chamomile, feverfew, St. John's wort and saw palmetto. Therefore, also look for the letters *NF* (national formulary) on the label, indicating that the manufacturer adheres to those standards. The best way to obtain fresh herbs is, if possible, to pick one's own; many grow wild in gardens, fields and city lots. They can then be dried, either by hanging in bunches in a well-ventilated place or by drying in a barely warm oven (but taking care oven temperature is never higher than 35 degrees Celsius, or 94 degrees Fahrenheit). They should not be dried in sunlight. Once dried, herbs may be stored in bags, jars or tins and can be expected to keep for about three years.

To prepare them for use, most herbs are made into an *infusion* or *tea*, usually 1 teaspoon of dried herb (3 teaspoons of fresh) per cup of boiling water. Roots usually are simmered over low heat for 15 minutes; with leaves or flowers the boiling water is poured over the herb, covered and allowed to steep (brew) for 10 to 20 minutes. For a remedy using both roots and leaves, simmer the roots first; then pour, with their water, over the leaves or flowers and let steep. All are strained before use. An infusion will keep for a day or two if stored in a cool, dark place.

Specific herbs used medicinally are mentioned in this book under the following entries: ABORTIFACIENT; ALZHEIMER'S DISEASE; ANALGESIC; ANEMIA; ANTI-DEPRESSANTS; BREAST-FEEDING; CERVICITIS; CYSTITIS; DYSMENORRHEA; DYSPLASIA; EMMENAGOGUE; GINSENG; HEADACHE; HEMORRHOID; HOT FLASHES; HYPERTENSION; INSOMNIA; IRRITABLE BOWEL SYNDROME; LACTATION; MASTITIS; MENSTRUAL FLOW; MIGRAINE; OBESITY; PELVIC INFLAMMATORY DISEASE; PERIMENOPAUSE; SITZ BATHS; TRICHOMONAS; VAGINITIS; YEAST INFECTION.

hereditary disease   See BIRTH DEFECTS.

heredity   See BIRTH DEFECTS; CHROMOSOME; GENETICS; NUCLEIC ACID.

hermaphroditism   Also *pseudohermaphroditism*. A congenital condition that can affect both men and women in which structural characteristics of both sexes appear in one person. The particular characteristics affected are those that ordinarily determine sex: chromosomal arrangement (see CHROMOSOME), external genitals, internal genitals and gonads (sex glands). A *male hermaphrodite* may have testes but external genitals resembling a woman's vulva. A *female hermaphrodite* may have ovaries but the chromatin structure of a man. In *true hermaphroditism*, which is extremely rare (only a few hundred cases have ever been reported), both ovaries and testes are present.

All hermaphroditism results from defects in fetal development. One kind of female hermaphroditism is known to be caused by administering progesterone to the mother in order to prevent miscarriage. Treatment of hermaphroditism usually involves hormone administration and surgery to make both the external and internal sex organs conform to the sex with which a child can most closely identify.

See also TRANSSEXUAL.

hernia, umbilical   An outward bulge of the navel that is caused by a weakness in the abdominal wall. Far more common in women than in men, such hernias often are associated with previous pregnancies as well as with obesity. They usually have no effect on subsequent pregnancies. Umbilical hernias also occur in newborn babies in which, after the skin of the navel heals, there usually is still an opening in the deeper muscular layers of the abdomen. When the baby cries, a small portion of intestine is pushed through this hole, making the navel protrude more. Such hernias heal of their own accord, although when they are large it may take months or even several years. No treatment is needed, but surgical repair may be done for the sake of appearance.

herpes infection   Also *genital herpes, herpes genitalis, herpes simplex II*. A disease of the genital organs caused by the herpes simplex virus 2 (HSV2). Unknown until the mid-20th century, genital herpes is now one of the most common SEXUALLY TRANSMITTED DISEASES in North America, especially in women, who contract it far more than men. (It is now thought to afflict one of every five Americans older than age 12.) The virus is closely related to another herpes virus, Type 1 (HSV1), which usually causes "cold sores" or "fever blisters" on the lips and in the throat, and sometimes eruptions that affect the eyes (*herpes simplex keratitis*), stomach or brain. Type 2 nearly always affects the genital area. Types 1 and 2 can be distinguished from one another by laboratory tests, but the symptoms of infection are the same for both, and occasionally Type 1 has been found in genital sores and Type 2 in mouth sores. The virus cannot survive outside human cells and is believed to be transmitted by vaginal, anal and oral-genital sexual intercourse. However, some persons whose sexual partner(s) are not infected somehow contract the infection anyway. Possibly they had a long-standing infection that became active years later. In order to infect a new host, the virus must attach to skin cells. Symptoms usually develop in 2 to 20 days, the average being 6 days. The principal symptom of infection is the appearance of one or several groups of small, painful, itchy blisters along the vulva and genital mucous membranes; the area most affected is the labia (vaginal lips), but the clitoris, outer part of the vagina, anal area and cervix also can be involved. The blisters are moist and grayish in color, with red edges. Men are affected most commonly on the glans, foreskin or shaft of the penis and, in homosexual men, around the anus. The blisters soon rupture to form soft, extremely painful open sores on a reddish base, covered by a grayish yellow secretion. (On the cervix, however, the sores are painless.) In women the sores can spread so as to involve the entire surface of the labia. There also may be inflammation and swelling around the urethra (and consequent pain when urinating), and irritation and ulceration of the cervix, causing a vaginal discharge and staining. In addition to these local symptoms, with a primary (first-time) infection, when the patient does not have antibodies, there is usually a low fever, general malaise and swollen tender lymph nodes in the groin.

The first attack is usually the most severe. Untreated, the outbreak usually clears up by itself in two to three weeks. However, it frequently recurs, because the virus remains dormant in the body, residing in the nerve cells. Consequently the body's immune system cannot dispose of it. It may remain dormant permanently or may give rise to infection again and again, at rates that typically vary from once or twice a year to once or twice a month. When infection does recur, subsequent attacks are usually milder and shorter-lived than the first one, probably because some antibodies have been built up. There appears to be more risk of recurrence during menstruation, ovulation and pregnancy (all involving higher hormone levels) as well as with gonorrhea, heat, emotional stress, tension, fever or a general rundown physical condition. Recurrence also may be limited to certain triggering factors, notably trauma to the skin that can occur through kissing, rubbing, and, for oral herpes, sunburn, shaving, dental work, smoking and contact with particular foods. To avoid spreading the infection, patients should always use condoms and avoid sexual contact entirely during a flareup, when lesions appear.

Herpes infection is more uncomfortable than dangerous except for two factors. First, women who have had herpes infections may be more susceptible to cervical cancer and therefore are urged to have a PAP SMEAR at least yearly. The infection also may be associated with precancerous lesions on the vulva. Second, a baby may become infected while passing through the birth canal of a mother with active herpes, and some babies may become infected before labor begins, while still in the uterus. Premature babies seem to be especially susceptible to such infection, which can quickly spread to the brain, leading to brain damage, blindness and even death. A primary (first-time) infection in the mother during pregnancy appears to be more dangerous to the baby than a second or subsequent attack. To prevent infection of their babies, pregnant women with herpes infection may be advised to have a CESAREAN SECTION, so that the baby does not pass through the birth canal. Of course, if infection has already spread through the placenta before labor begins or if the membranes have been ruptured for more than two hours, such surgery is useless. A baby usually shows signs of infection within four to seven days, although in severe cases it may be evident immediately. Treatment for such infants is difficult, since the only drugs effective—primarily antiviral drugs or experimental drugs—may have toxic side effects.

Diagnosis of herpes is often missed because the sores resemble those of two other venereal diseases, SYPHILIS and CHANCROID. In all cases of multiple genital sores, therefore, herpes should be suspected. To test for the virus, a smear of secretions from the sores is put on a slide and fixed as for a Pap smear or a Tzanck smear; in the presence of herpes virus, characteristic changes in the nucleus of cells usually are seen. The virus also can be grown in the laboratory, but this test is costlier and not widely available. Blood tests are not accurate if they are performed *after* (rather than during) an initial attack because the results are unclear. None of these tests detects the difference between Types 1 and 2, but the site of infection often indicates which is responsible.

At this writing there is no permanent cure for herpes. However, three oral antiviral drugs—acyclovir (Zovirax), famciclovir (Famvir) and valacyclovir (Valtrex)—can suppress symptoms, especially if used at the beginning of an outbreak, help sores to heal more quickly and suppress recurrences. Acyclovir in ointment form may help heal the lesions but does not prevent recurrence. For those who have frequent recurrences (more than six a year) the drugs taken in low daily doses may suppress the outbreaks. Long-term effects, however, are not known, so their use should be limited to one year. In 2006 the FDA approved a vaccine against HUMAN PAPILLOMA VIRUS (HPV), which protects against two variants of the virus that are responsible for 90% of herpes cases.

To relieve discomfort of a severe outbreak, simpler remedies include wet dressings of cool water, ice or wet teabags, and cool sitz baths with or without baking soda added to help relieve itching and pain, along with oral analgesics, such as aspirin and codeine. Because the mucous membranes affected by herpes are very sensitive—far more so than skin—caution is advised in applying any topical agent, lest it cause even more irritation. Also, it is important to avoid self-infection (spreading the virus to another part of the body) by washing one's

hands frequently. Among the herbal remedies for herpes are compresses with an infusion of cloves, peppermint oil and clove oil. Cotton underwear (or no underpants) and loose clothing promote healing, as does keeping the genital area clean and dry with normal bathing. Some authorities believe a diet rich in certain nutrients, especially vitamins C, B-complex, and B_6, along with zinc and calcium, and the daily use of kelp powder (one capsule a day) and sunflower seed oil (one tablespoon a day) help prevent recurrence. The Herpes Resource Center (see Appendix) and its local branches around the nation offer authoritative up-to-date information to herpes patients.

The viruses causing herpes are closely related to several other organisms: varicella, which causes chicken pox; herpes zoster, which causes shingles, a painful infection of the sensory nerves that results in inflammation of the skin along their pathways; Epstein-Barr virus, which causes infectious mononucleosis; and cytomegalovirus, which may give rise to no symptoms in healthy children and adults but can cause severe birth defects when a pregnant woman becomes infected and can be a life threatening infection in AIDS patients.

heterosexual Also *straight* (slang). Describing a male-female sexual relationship or a person who prefers a sexual partner of the opposite sex.

See also HOMOSEXUAL.

high blood pressure See HYPERTENSION.

high-risk pregnancy A term used for pregnant women who have a chronic disease or some other condition that makes pregnancy more dangerous for them and/or their babies. Among the chronic diseases associated with such a risk are DIABETES, HYPERTENSION (high blood pressure), heart disease, kidney or lung disease, liver disease, SICKLE-CELL DISEASE or related blood disorders, any form of CANCER, alcoholism (see ALCOHOL USE) and drug addiction (see DRUG USE AND PREGNANCY). In addition, certain infections in the mother can have serious effects on her baby, especially RUBELLA, genital HERPES INFECTION, AIDS, SYPHILIS, and GONORRHEA.

Blood incompatibility (see RH FACTOR) represents a risk. Finally, there is increased risk to the baby if the mother is either over 35 or in her early teens (see AGE, CHILDBEARING), has had difficulty with previous deliveries, is known to have a small pelvis, is obese, or is known to be carrying more than one fetus (see MULTIPLE PREGNANCY). In all these instances prenatal care must be more frequent and more cautious, and the woman is urged if possible to be in reach—during the last trimester particularly—of a medical center that specializes in high-risk obstetrics and special intensive care for the newborn.

During pregnancy, hypertension, common especially among obese women, older women and black women, can compromise the flow of blood through the placenta, resulting in smaller babies. Also, hypertension carries the risk of kidney damage, which can be life-threatening to both mother and child. The normal heart and kidneys must work considerably harder during pregnancy; for disease-damaged organs the overload may be too great. Pregnancy itself can induce hypertension in women whose blood pressure previously was normal (see PREECLAMPSIA). Cancer anywhere in the pelvic or abdominal area is particularly dangerous; CANCER IN SITU of the cervix can be treated conservatively during pregnancy, as can breast cancer, although extra efforts must be made to shield the fetus from damaging radiation exposure during either diagnosis or treatment. Marked OBESITY is dangerous to both mother and baby. The majority of obese women develop some obstetric complication, especially hypertension, diabetes, kidney disease, wound complications and thromboembolism (blood clots). Women who smoke heavily are more likely to bear undersized and premature babies than women who do not, and their risk of MISCARRIAGE, PLACENTA PREVIA and ABRUPTIO PLACENTAE is also higher.

hirsutism   In women, excess body hair distributed as it is normally found in men, especially on the face, chest and abdomen below the navel. Occasionally a hereditary trait, hirsutism more often is caused by excess production of androgens (male hormones) by the adrenal glands (ADRENOGENITAL SYNDROME), a tumor of the adrenals, CUSHING'S SYNDROME, or an abnormality in the ovaries, such as POLYCYSTIC OVARY SYNDROME. Depending on the cause, hirsutism is treated with medication and/or electrolysis or other forms of hair removal. Several drugs are effective, but hair usually grows when they are discontinued. When excess hair is caused by polycystic ovary syndrome or insulin resistance, metaformin, which increases insulin sensitivity, may work. Oral contraceptives, which stabilize hormone balance, also may be effective. GnRH (gonadotropin-releasing hormone) antagonists, which suppress ovarian hormone production (including androgens), are sometimes used. Finasteride (Proscar), which treats prostate enlargement in men, has been used to treat both hirsutism and balding in women (see also HAIR LOSS) and appears to have few side effects. The diuretic spironolactone (Aldactazide) works similarly well but has side effects. Neither of the last two should be taken by pregnant women, nor should they take bromocriptine, used to treat prolactin overproduction. None of these has been approved for treating hirsutism.

A safer avenue is hair removal. Shaving works (it does not change the texture, color or rate of hair growth). Depilatories in cream, gel or lotion form contain calcium thioglycolate, which breaks down the structure of hair; they often produce minor irritation. Tweezing is painful, and hairs reappear after a few weeks. Also painful are waxes, which like tweezers remove the entire hair from its follicle and have longer-lasting results than shaving or depilatories; they should not be used on skin that is irritated or cut, over varicose veins, moles or warts, or around genital areas. Electrolysis requires a skilled operator who uses a wire needle inserted into the hair follicle; an electric current travels down it and destroys the hair root. (A newer technique, still being studied at this writing, involves a tweezers epilator that grasps a hair and sends a current down it to kill the root.) The newest kind of hair removal uses a laser; one kind, the ThermoLase Softlight, has been approved for this purpose. After a black solution is applied to the area and penetrates the hair follicles, the laser scans the area and the black pigment absorbs the laser light, which destroys the hair follicles. It may, however, cause scarring, redness and other changes in skin color.

HIV   Also *human immunodeficiency virus*. The virus that causes AIDS. Several hundred strains of the virus exist, each slightly different. HIV-1 causes AIDS in North Americans; HIV-2 has been found in both AIDS patients and healthy individuals in different parts of the world. HIV is a retrovirus, meaning it can alter the genetic material of cells so that the virus's genes become an integral part of the cell. About 20% of persons infected with HIV (see AIDS for how one becomes infected) feel ill within two to eight weeks, but most have few or no symptoms. Symptoms include fever, fatigue, joint or muscle pains, sore throat, or headache, mood changes and problems with thinking or balance. Antibodies to the virus appear in the blood within three to six months of infection (but may not appear for as long as 18 months). Thus there can be healthy carriers of HIV; the virus is not active in them but can be transmitted to others via blood, sperm, vaginal secretions and possibly also breast milk. Diagnosis is by means of an *HIV antibody test,* a blood test involving a small blood sample (usually taken from the arm); it yields results in several weeks. A negative result may mean that antibodies have not yet developed, and therefore the test usually should be repeated after some months; a positive result often calls for counseling to help cope with its implications, especially for women who are sexually active, who are pregnant or considering pregnancy, or who wanted to breast-feed. A newer test is the OraQuick Rapid HIV-I Antibody Test. It uses a pinprick of blood and results are seen in 20 minutes. In 2004 the Food and Drug Administration approved the first HIV test that uses saliva instead of blood; it delivers results in 20 minutes. A urine test uses urine instead of blood but is less accurate than a blood or saliva test.

Unlike antibodies to many other infectious agents, HIV antibodies do not confer immunity. Although not everyone who tests positive will develop AIDS, general health measures are very important for HIV-positive individuals. Eating well, getting enough sleep and avoiding harmful substances (tobacco, alcohol and other drugs) are important. Donating blood should be avoided, and safe sex (see chart under AIDS) is mandatory to avoid infecting one's partner. Regular Pap smears should be done, since cancer of the cervix is a hazard, as well as screening for tuberculosis and sexually transmitted diseases. A general physical exam and CD4 + lymphocyte count every three to six months is highly recommended to evaluate the need for treatment. AZT (zidovudine), the antiviral drug first used only to strengthen the immune system in AIDS patients, now is recommended for healthy HIV-positive persons whose CD4 + count is dropping.

holistic medicine   See ALTERNATIVE MEDICINE; NATUROPATHY.

home birth   Also *home delivery.* Delivering a baby at home rather than in a birth center, clinic or hospital. Such deliveries were the norm until about 1900, when the use of anesthesia for childbirth and hospitalization became accepted practice in most industrialized countries, including Canada and the United States. By 1950 hospital births were the general rule. About the only exceptions were those women too poor to seek prenatal care of any kind and those whose babies came too early or too quickly to permit transport anywhere. About 1970, with the fast-rising cost of health care and the increasingly elaborate technology of childbirth, some women began to view home birth as a good alternative. By 1980 there were a number of organizations, some composed of physicians and other health care professionals and many more of lay persons, devoted to the promotion of safe childbirth at home. Some offered a variety of services, including instruction for lay persons to deliver babies at home without outside assistance and prepackaged equipment kits with plastic sheets and bed pads, syringes, cord clamps, sterile scissors and other items needed for labor and delivery. Most women who plan to have babies at home (still a considerable minority in the United States) choose to have professional supervision of some kind, by either a midwife or a physician, or at least some kind of professional backup service.

Home birth has both risks and benefits. For the 5% of births that are not normal—that is, where complications of some kind arise—they clearly represent a greater risk than would be involved in a hospital. Among the most common complications are ABNORMAL PRESENTATION of various kinds, a disproportionately large baby (relative to the size of the mother's pelvis), hemorrhage from PLACENTA PREVIA or ABRUPTIO PLACENTAE, PROLONGED LABOR, and fetal distress from a PROLAPSED CORD or other causes that are not detected because of inadequate FETAL MONITORING.

Although there is conflict between those who oppose home birth for any woman and those who feel it is the only natural (and therefore desirable) way to have a baby, most knowledgeable supporters agree that no woman characterized as a HIGH-RISK PREGNANCY (representing 10 to 15% of all women) should seek home birth deliberately. Further, critics maintain that even low-risk pregnancies can become high risk without warning during labor, since this is the most stressful time for the baby. Advocates of home birth, on the other hand, point out that most births are normal and that at home the parents can remain in control of the delivery, friends and family (including siblings) can be present and become intimately involved with the new family member from the start, the medical expense is minimal, and in a relaxed, familiar atmosphere labor tends to progress faster and medication of various kinds may be avoided. If a qualified birth attendant cannot be present, there should at the very least be some emergency backup for reviving an infant, recognizing and controlling excessive bleeding in the mother, assessing signs of fetal distress and evaluating the condition of mother and baby immediately after delivery. In addition, oxygen should be available as well as standby transportation to a hospital, preferably one that has been contacted beforehand so that in an emergency there will be prompt admission and treatment.

See also BIRTHING ROOM; MIDWIFE; PREPARED CHILDBIRTH.

home medical tests Lab tests that are available over the counter to test for a number of conditions. The earliest such test marketed in the United States was the PREGNANCY TEST, based on a urine sample, and it was followed by a test for OVULATION. In recent decades many more such tests have been devised. There are several kinds of glucose monitor, or glucometer, to check blood glucose in DIABETES patients. Among them are the Life-Scan One-Touch, Prestige IQ, Glucometer, Accu-Chek and Gluco-Watch. All of them involve pricking a finger and squeezing a drop of blood onto a special strip that is inserted into the measuring device. Patients with Type I diabetes are advised to monitor blood-sugar levels three to four times a day; those with Type II diabetes who take insulin also should monitor two to four times a day. Patients whose diabetes does not require insulin can benefit from testing themselves periodically. Monitors also need to be checked periodically for accuracy.

Among the newest tests is one for fertility screening for both men and women. Called Fertell, it was approved by the FDA in 2007 and became available midyear. For men, the test measures the concentration of motile sperm; for women, it measures a hormone considered a marker for egg quality. The test for men requires a semen sample and assesses the ability of sperm to swim through a solution similar to cervical mucus and counts the number able to do so. Results are available in 80 minutes. The female test is a urine stick, much like that in home pregnancy tests, that measures the level of follicle-stimulating hormone (FSH) on the third day of the menstrual cycle. An unusually high level indicates that the egg quality is low. Results are available in 30 minutes. The tests mainly screen for possible problems but do not show all fertility-related difficulties. However, they do provide an early warning to couples to see a physician if they want a pregnancy.

Another test is a fertility monitor, which helps increase a woman's likelihood of becoming pregnant. A urine test, it measures levels of LH, or luteinizing hormone, which is released by the pituitary gland in a surge approximately 24 hours before ovulation. Detecting this surge in LH permits timing intercourse or artificial insemination with donor sperm during the most fertile time of a woman's menstrual cycle. Half a dozen different brands are available over the counter.

Fecal occult blood testing, to check for colorectal cancer, detects tiny amounts of blood in a stool sample. The test uses cards that are treated with guaiac, which reacts with blood, and are prepared at home with three consecutive stool samples. They are then sent to labs for analysis. Although this test can have both false negative and false positive results, it is still recommended to be performed annually, since the more accurate sigmoidoscopy and COLONOSCOPY are performed at much longer intervals.

Testing for blood clotting needs to be performed monthly for patients who take anticoagulants (blood thinners) such as warfarin (Coumadin) following heart attack or stroke, or with atrial fibrillation. Too much anticoagulant can cause internal bleeding; too little increases the risk of dangerous clots. The standard test to measure the balance between the two uses a system called the international normalized ratio. A home test, ProTime Microcoagulation System, obtains this ratio or the time it takes blood to clot (prothrombin time) using a drop of blood from a finger prick. The device is expensive but may be covered by insurance.

Blood pressure monitors have become very common. The most accurate devices are digital; the least accurate are those that use a finger to check pressure. Before using a monitor, it should be calibrated at the doctor's office and checked against a reading taken with a mercury sphygmomanometer. Blood pressure should be taken while sitting down, one hour after waking and before bedtime on alternate days. It is advisable to take three readings one after the other, using the same arm, and average the results. (See HYPERTENSION.)

A home test for allergy, My Allergy Test, screens for 10 common allergens, including dust mites, mold, ragweed, cat dander, milk and wheat. It can indicate whether over-the-counter allergy medication is needed.

There are home tests for CHOLESTEROL, but to date they have not been found accurate and test only total cholesterol; a urine test for PERIMENOPAUSE; a blood test for HEPATITIS C; and tests for HIV. There also are several new *genetic tests*, to screen patients for various genetic disorders, such as the ability to metabolize drugs. Most tend to predict susceptibility to a certain disease, and although these tests are regulated by the Food and Drug Administration, it is not known how reliable they are. Such tests generally involve either a cheek

swab or a small amount of blood. The sample is sent to a laboratory for analysis, with results reported in two to four weeks.

Although home tests can be helpful indicators, it is not advisable to rely on them exclusively to make decisions about illnesses or treatments.

homeopathy Also *homeopathic medicine.* A medical system based on treating disease by using minute, highly diluted doses of the very substances that, in large doses, can cause similar symptoms. Invented by an 18th-century German physician, Samuel Hahnemann, it relies on the principle that like cures like, that is, a medicine's power to cure comes from its ability to produce symptoms in a healthy person that are like those caused by the disease itself. It is based on the belief that symptoms are signs of the body's attempt to throw off disease, and it seeks to strengthen the body's ability to do so. Homeopathic practitioners begin by asking for an extensive description of symptoms, including such seemingly irrelevant ones as "Do you crave sweet or salty foods? Do you lose your temper easily?" The practitioner then forms a "symptom picture," focusing especially on the most uncommon ones, and chooses a remedy from one or more of some 2,000 possible substances. These substances are used in enormously diluted form and tiny amounts, so that the active ingredient is barely present. Often such treatment is administered as a sugar pill that has absorbed the prepared solution. In the United States, homeopathic remedies are exempt from the testing required of other drugs. Nearly all are classified as over-the-counter drugs, limited by law to treat acute conditions that usually resolve without treatment.

Homeopathy is considered the practice of medicine and therefore is subject to licensing; that is, it can be performed legally only by professionals who are licensed to prescribe drugs. Physicians and osteopaths may practice it in all states, although in some they must be specifically licensed to practice homeopathy. In some states chiropractors, naturopaths, dentists, nurse practitioners and other providers can practice homeopathy, depending on their license. There are no uniform standards for learning homeopathy, and consequently the mere fact of being trained in it does not confer the legal right to practice it. Nevertheless, many individuals with *no* formal health care training practice homeopathy. Further, even licensed providers come from widely diverse backgrounds, such as acupuncture, nursing, herbalism and nutritional therapy. Some medical physicians also practice homeopathy, but they are a minority.

The principal risk in relying on homeopathic remedies is missing out on effective medical treatment. For example, by using over-the-counter remedies for a disorder such as "bladder irritation" a person may delay seeking treatment for a bladder infection that can progress to serious kidney infection. Also, no scientific basis for homeopathy's effectiveness has been discovered. Nevertheless, individuals with conditions for which conventional treatment has been useless—conditions such as insomnia, colds, muscle soreness—claim that homeopathic remedies have given them relief.

homocysteine   A naturally occurring amino acid that in high levels is linked to an increased risk of heart disease and heart attack. Excessive levels can lead to the formation of blood clots, osteoporosis and other bone abnormalities, and eye problems. Apparently some individuals lack the enzymes needed to process this substance in their bodies. To help them do so, a medication called betaine anhydrous (Cystadane) was introduced in 1997. Also found in such foods as beets, spinach, seafood and cereals, betaine is generally prescribed along with vitamins B_6 and B_{12} and folate, all of which aid in processing homocysteine. However, it should not be taken by women who are pregnant or breast-feeding.

homosexual   Also *gay* (slang). Describing a sexual relationship in which both partners are of the same sex or a person who prefers a sexual partner of the same sex.

See also HETEROSEXUAL; LESBIAN.

honeymoon cystitis   See CYSTITIS, def. 1.

hormone   In human beings, a chemical substance produced by a gland that serves to stimulate and control vital bodily functions. Acting as a kind of chemical messenger, hormones are carried to various organs and tissues by the bloodstream. The most important hormones regulate growth, sexual development and reproduction, the composition of the blood, metabolism, the transmission of messages in the nervous system and the production of other hormones as well as still other functions not yet completely understood. Some hormones, such as insulin, are necessary to maintain life.

The discovery of hormones and their functions is quite recent. The word *hormone* was coined in 1902, when the first hormone was identified. As hormones began to be synthesized in the laboratory, they came into increasing use to treat disorders associated with their lack, as in DIABETES and ESTROGEN REPLACEMENT THERAPY, as well as to prevent pregnancy (see ORAL CONTRACEPTIVES) and to treat some diseases not directly related to hormone deficiency, such as the use of cortisone to treat arthritis. (See also HORMONE THERAPY.)

Most hormones are produced by ENDOCRINE glands, and sometimes all hormones are classified according to where they are produced—pituitary hormones, ovarian hormones, adrenal hormones and so on. Another way of classifying hormones is by the functions they affect, as sex hormones, gonadotropins (sex gland-stimulating hormones), metabolic hormones and so on. Still another way of classifying hormones is according to their chemical makeup, which for a few of them still is not known. Chemically there are two basic kinds of hormone: the *steroids*, which are derived from cholesterol and include the sex hormones and hormones produced by the adrenal cortex, or corticosteroids; and those based on single amino acids or strings of amino acids, called *protein* or *polypeptide hormones*, which include insulin and thyroxine. The chief steroid hormones are the androgens (principally testosterone and androsterone), estrogens and progesterone. Although androgens usually are produced by the testes, estrogen and progesterone by the ovaries and the corticosteroids by the adrenals, these same organs can make any kind of steroid hormone and sometimes do. The principal protein hormones are human chorionic gonadotropin

(HCG), produced by the placenta during pregnancy, and follicle-stimulating hormone (FSH), luteinizing hormone (LH), prolactin, oxytocin and somatotropin (growth hormone), all released by the pituitary gland. Prolactin and oxytocin normally do not occur in men, although in certain diseases they may do so. The so-called gonadotropic (gonad-stimulating) hormones function in both sexes; in men FSH stimulates sperm production and LH stimulates testosterone production.

Most of the body's hormones are intimately interconnected. For example, FSH and LH stimulate a woman's ovaries to produce estrogen; the anterior pituitary gland in turn is stimulated to produce FSH and LH by gonadotropin-releasing hormone (GnRH), produced by the hypothalamus. When estrogen levels drop, the hypothalamus is stimulated to produce release factors to stimulate the pituitary to produce FSH and LH to stimulate the ovaries, and so on. A similar feedback system is involved in the production of testosterone in men as well as many other hormones. There are separate entries for the most important hormones.

See also HYPOTHALAMUS; MENSTRUAL CYCLE; PITUITARY GLAND.

hormone cream   See VAGINAL ATROPHY.

hormone replacement therapy   Also *HRT.*
See ESTROGEN REPLACEMENT THERAPY.

hormone therapy   Also *endocrine therapy.* The administration of natural or synthetic hormones or the removal of hormone-producing organs to treat a disease, deficiency or other disorder. Although the term *hormone therapy* technically applies to, for example, the insulin given to insulin-dependent diabetics (see DIABETES) or danazol to treat ENDOMETRIOSIS, today it most often is applied to hormone treatment of cancers. Among the earliest kinds of hormone therapy was the removal of the ovaries and adrenal glands of women with breast cancer, thereby greatly reducing the body's estrogen-making capacity. This treatment always induced menopause and sterility, with varying degrees of

such menopausal symptoms as hot flashes, vaginal dryness and accelerated bone loss (leading to osteoporosis). Today *ovarian ablation,* using surgery, radiation or chemicals to halt ovarian function, still is used to some extent.

Many tumors now are tested routinely for estrogen receptivity (see ESTROGEN RECEPTOR ASSAY); when they are found to be dependent on estrogen, as many breast cancers are, an antiestrogen or estrogen antagonist such as *tamoxifen,* a synthetic hormone, is given. Tamoxifen is effective only when a tumor is estrogen-receptor positive, not if it is estrogen-receptor negative. (Combining tamoxifen with CHEMOTHERAPY greatly improves the prognosis for postmenopausal women with advanced cancers.) Similar treatment is available for progesterone-dependent cancers.

Tamoxifen (Nolvadex), on the market since 1978, is an early *selective estrogen-receptor modulator (SERM),* which acts much like estrogen in some tissues, such as the uterus and bones, but blocks estrogen's effect in others, such as the breast. Also called a designer estrogen, it has been found to reduce significantly the rates of recurrence and death from breast cancer in women of all ages and whether or not the cancer spread to axillary lymph nodes, as well as halving the risk of new cancers in the other breast. Moreover, tamoxifen also reduces the risk of breast cancer by approximately 45% in women at high risk for the disease. The drug, however, is a mixed blessing. In women over 50 it doubles the risk of developing endometrial (uterine) cancer and also increases the chance of blood clots developing in the veins and lungs. (These side effects do not appear to occur in women under 50.) Minor side effects include hot flashes, a vaginal discharge, nausea or vomiting, and weight gain. The drug should not be taken by women who are pregnant, who are at risk for blood clots (owing to hypertension, obesity, diabetes or cigarette smoking) or who are on oral contraceptives or estrogen replacement therapy. The drug's benefits, it is believed, still outweigh this risk, but women taking it (or who took it in the past) are advised to be vigilant for symptoms of endometrial cancer (bleeding between periods or after menopause, or unusual vaginal discharge) and receive regular gynecological checkups to monitor endometrial buildup. At this writing, it is recommended that the drug be taken for no longer than five years. Another SERM that acts in a similar way is raloxifene (Evista), which helps prevent osteoporosis and appears to avoid the risk of developing endometrial hyperplasia (and uterine cancer). It, too, can increase clotting and induce hot flashes. In 2004 a large study revealed that women who took tamoxifen to prevent recurrent breast cancer for two and one-half years and then switched to a newer drug, exemestane (Aromasin), cut their chances of developing another tumor by one-third and experienced fewer side effects. The most serious risk of Aromasin and other aromatase inhibitors is bone loss, which in postmenopausal patients at risk for osteoporosis might be offset by additional calcium supplements. Also in 2004, the Food and Drug Administration approved the use of letrozole, a drug originally used against advanced breast cancer, to prevent recurrence in women treated for early forms of the disease. Prescribed for postmenopausal patients who completed five years of tamoxifen, it cuts the risk of recurrence by half. The chief side effects are hot flashes and arthritis.

Cancers of the endometrium and prostate also may be hormone-dependent. Some kinds of thyroid cancer respond to replacement doses of THYROID hormone, which prevents the release of thyroid-stimulating hormone and other thyrotropic hormones, and corticosteroids have been used successfully in treating some kinds of leukemia and lymphoma. Finally, corticosteroids often help counter the nausea and vomiting induced by chemotherapy and so may be useful as additional therapy.

Other synthetic hormones for treating breast cancer also are being investigated. One is the contragestive RU-486, which works in breast cancers that contain a progesterone receptor (it blocks progesterone action). Its side effects may include nausea, vomiting, fatigue and skin rashes.

See also HORMONE. For hormone replacement therapy, see ESTROGEN REPLACEMENT THERAPY.

hospice   A facility or system of medical care for dying patients. In Europe, especially in Great Britain, the hospice often is a residential facility in a pastoral setting where the terminally ill may live out their days in peaceful surroundings. Such hospices are based on the medieval "hospitality houses" from which the term is derived, shelters maintained by religious orders that took in strangers, travelers and the indigent sick.

In the United States, the first hospice began accepting patients in 1974. At first it provided only comprehensive home care so that a dying person might be kept pain-free and comfortable in his or her own familiar surroundings, amid family and friends, for as long as possible. Such care includes home nursing visits and the services of a homemaker or part- or full-time home health aide as well as backup from a nearby hospital or nursing home in case the patient's condition becomes unmanageable at home or the family needs a respite from caring for a dying relative. In addition, it includes special arrangements for social services and psychological and pastoral counseling for both the patient and family members. Today some American hospices offer residential facilities as well, but the number of patients they can accommodate is still very small, and most programs offer only home care. Hospice care is available in some hospitals too, where it takes forms ranging from a special ward set aside for terminal patients to a team whose members—doctors, nurses, social workers—are available to visit dying patients anywhere in the hospital and to train and assist other hospital staff in their care.

Medical care for the dying is palliative, directed at making a person as comfortable as possible and often including the use of alcohol and addictive drugs to ease pain. Essentially, hospice care provides an alternative to impersonal high-technology intensive care in a hospital, where patients may be kept alive by means of machinery even when there is no hope for recovery. In contrast, the hospice concept emphasizes the quality of life at the expense, perhaps, of duration, and at much lower financial cost. It has become sufficiently attractive for some medical insurance companies in the United States to plan insurance coverage for hospice care, and Medicare is the primary payer for hospice care in approximately 80% of cases, with care most often provided in the patient's home. A new development is the establishment of perinatal hospice programs for babies born with a fatal condition. A collection of services often associated with a hospital rather than offered in a stand-alone facility, they cater to women pregnant with a baby having a lethal problem as well as to newborns with such problems. They may arrange birthing lessons for women who do not wish to be in classes with those carrying a healthy child, advise how to tell siblings their new baby will not live beyond a few days, and if the baby does live for more than a few days, teach the family how to care for him or her. As in the adult hospice program, perinatal hospices give palliative care to ease discomfort but do not offer aggressive intervention such as feeding tubes and surgeries. For locating hospice care, see the Appendix.

hospitalist   A physician who provides care only in a hospital setting. Hospitalists have completed medical school and postgraduate training in internal medicine, family practice, or pediatrics. They may work directly for a hospital or as part of a managed-care organization, multispecialty practice, or other group. The fastest growing medical specialty, hospitalists today work in about half of American hospitals. If your primary-care physician is turning over your in-house care to a hospitalist, he or she will share your records and other information so that the hospitalist will know your medical history, health condition, and preferences. Upon admission, the hospitalist will examine you, coordinate all your tests and treatments, and visit you daily. Upon discharge the hospitalist prescribes the medication you will need and sends a summary of your hospital records and treatments to your primary-care physician. The advantage of using a hospitalist over a primary-care physician is that it frees primary-care physicians from hospital visits and lets them focus on in-office care. The advantage to hospitals and patients appears to be lower costs and shorter lengths of stay, but no definitive research results are yet available.

hot flashes   Also *hot flushes, vasomotor instability.* A sudden sensation of heat that passes over the upper body, usually from the chest up over the neck and face, which actually may become flushed

and sweaty, and which often is followed by copious perspiration and chills. The single most common symptom of PERIMENOPAUSE and MENOPAUSE, hot flashes of varying frequency and severity occur in an estimated 60 to 80% of women. A hot flash may last from a few seconds to several minutes and may occur as seldom as once or twice a year or as often as six times an hour. Hot flashes occur at night as well, although often a woman is aware of them only after waking up soaking wet from the subsequent sweat (so-called *night sweats*). (See also INSOMNIA.)

Hot flashes actually are the rapid dilation of surface blood vessels, believed to be caused by a disturbance of the hypothalamus (which controls body temperature), in turn caused by hormone imbalance. After menopause, as the body adjusts gradually to lower estrogen levels, hot flashes usually subside. Typically they begin to occur about the time when menstrual periods begin to deviate from their normal pattern and continue until after periods have ended (although a few women continue to experience them for 10 or more years after the last period). They also occur, often more suddenly and more severely, in women whose ovaries have been surgically removed (see OOPHORECTOMY).

Hot flashes can occur with or without obvious signs of their presence (red face, drops of perspiration). For a few women they are very severe indeed, sometimes accompanied by numbness of the hands and feet, shortness of breath, a feeling of suffocation, palpitations, dizziness and even fainting. They are greatly eased by ESTROGEN REPLACEMENT THERAPY, which, however, has numerous risks. Some women find relief with a cream containing natural progesterone (as opposed to synthetic progestin), applied on the arms, legs and other body parts. Available over the counter, it has been considered less potent than progesterone pills, but a recent study showed that women using one popular brand, Pro-Gest, had the same blood levels of progesterone as those using pills, with attendant risks.

Medications found effective by some women are clonidine (Catapres), used to treat high blood pressure but giving rise to possible side effects such as drowsiness, dry mouth, constipation and insomnia; megestrol acetate, a synthetic progesterone used to treat breast cancer, and small amounts of the antidepressants gabapentin (Neurontin), venlafaxine (Effexor-XR) or fluoxetine (Prozac); they, too, may have unpleasant side effects. Other approaches are supplements of vitamin E (either alone or combined with vitamin C and calcium supplements). However, vitamin E must be used very cautiously by women who have diabetes, rheumatic heart disease or high blood pressure, and no one should take more than 600 International Units per day without medical supervision. Acupuncture helps some women. Various HERBAL REMEDIES have been recommended for hot flashes, among them licorice root (*Glycyrrhiza lepidota*), which contains a substance chemically similar to estrogen, and sarsaparilla (*Smilax officinalis*), which contains one similar to progesterone; ginseng root (*Panax quinquefolium*) and dong kwai (or dong quai or tang kuei; *Angelica sinensis*), long used in China (see GINSENG); and red raspberry leaf (*Rubus idaeus*) tea. Allegedly, some women also have found relief with black cohosh (*Cimicifuga racemosa*); the roots and rhizomes (underground stems) are ground and taken in tablet, capsule or liquid form. In the United States it is marketed as the brand RemiFe-min, but other brands containing black cohosh in the form of teas and tinctures, creams and pills, also are available. How it works (and whether it will work) is not understood. It appears to be safe for most women, but some have developed severe liver problems, so it may be wise to monitor liver function. Moreover, a number of recent studies indicate that black cohosh does not actually help hot flashes or other menopausal symptoms, suggesting that it may work only as a placebo for those women reporting relief. A wild yam cream that contains a phytoprogesterone, diosgenin, has helped some women; marketed as PhytoGest and Yamcom, it is not regulated and its contents vary, some creams containing little of the active ingredient. Some claim relief from consuming soy protein (20–50 grams per day) in foods such as soy milk, protein bars, powder drinks, soybeans and tofu. Soy contains isoflavones; soy supplements are not recommended because they contain much higher isoflavone levels than foods and could pose a risk to breast cancer survivors. A simple but effective palliative for a hot flash is a cold-water compress applied to the face. Women are also advised to limit or avoid caffeine, alcohol, spicy foods, hot liquids, and synthetic fabrics in clothing and bedsheets.

hot flush   See HOT FLASHES.

HPV   See HUMAN PAPILLOMA VIRUS.

HRT   See ESTROGEN REPLACEMENT THERAPY.

human chorionic gonadotropin   Also *HCG*. A group of hormones produced during pregnancy by the placenta. Their presence in urine therefore is a good indication of pregnancy, and indeed most kinds of PREGNANCY TEST are based on this finding. Their function is not entirely understood, but they have properties similar to luteinizing hormone (LH) and follicle-stimulating hormone (FSH), and they are believed to maintain the CORPUS LUTEUM during the early weeks of pregnancy. Injecting HCG into an ovary that has been sufficiently stimulated by FSH induces ovulation, and therefore HCG sometimes is used to treat infertility. It also has been used to stimulate sexual development when the pituitary gland fails. Various tumors also have been found to secrete HCG, producing high blood levels of this substance in men as well as in women.

human menopausal gonadotropin   Also *HMG*. A synthetic compound used to replace the natural pituitary hormones, luteinizing hormone (LH) and follicle-stimulating hormone (FSH) (see MENSTRUAL CYCLE for explanation). It is used to induce ovulation in women who do not respond to clomiphene citrate as well as to stimulate estrogen production in women with a malfunction of the pituitary or hypothalamus. In men it is used to stimulate sperm production. In the United States it is sold under the brand name Pergonal.

See also FERTILITY DRUG.

human papilloma virus   Also *HPV*. A slow-growing virus that infects skin and mucous membranes. It can cause certain kinds of wart, including

CONDYLOMA ACUMINATA, and is also associated with DYSPLASIA and cervical cancer.

More than 100 types of HPV have been identified, and about 15 of them cause nearly all cases of cervical cancer. Most HPV infections show no outward symptoms and often cannot be detected in a Pap test. A new vaccine, Gardasil, approved in 2006, protects against four forms of HPV, two that are implicated in 70% of cases of cervical cancer and two that account for 90% of cases of genital HERPES. A recent study indicated that the vaccine protects against additional strains of the virus. An estimated 20 million Americans—one in four women aged 14 to 59—are infected with HPV, and more than 6 million new HPV infections occur annually. The vaccine, licensed for use in girls from nine to 26 (but recommended for girls aged 11 or 12), is given in three doses over six months, the first two doses one month apart, and the third dose five months later. Some states have considered making it mandatory.

The vaccine is expensive, costing about $360. It may cause some temporary side effects, mainly pain, itching and swelling at the injection site and possible fever, nausea and dizziness. It may not be given to women who are or may be pregnant or to those allergic to its ingredients. The vaccine may also be of benefit to boys and men, who can spread HPV infection to women, and also because the virus can cause cancer of the penis and anus. The last is a particular concern to gay men, but at this writing no conclusive study has been made as to whether it will protect gay men from cancer. In 2008 another version of the vaccine, to be marketed as Cervarix, was awaiting FDA approval.

Recent research has implicated the virus in other kinds of cancer. HPV-16 can cause oral cancer, often transmitted through oral sex. However, only one-third of the more than 100 strains of HPV have been linked to cancer, and even those trigger cancer only in a fraction of infected individuals.

For HPV test, see under CANCER, CERVICAL.

husband-coached birth   See BRADLEY METHOD.

hyaline membrane disease   Also *respiratory distress syndrome, RDS.* A potentially fatal condition that affects infants, particularly PREMATURE infants, who lack a chemical called *surfactant,* which lines the lungs and keeps the small sacs, or alveoli, open. Without surfactant, the airways in effect collapse every time the baby exhales, and as a result the infant cannot get enough oxygen. The signs of the disease include cyanosis (blue color), flaring or enlargement of the nostrils and a grunting noise with each breath, a very rapid breathing rate and a caving in of the sternum (breastbone) with each breath, all indications of the baby's efforts to get more air. Hyaline membrane disease is a leading cause of death in newborn infants, with death usually occurring within 72 hours of birth. For severely afflicted babies the death rate is 30%. Treatment consists of incubation (because body temperature tends to be low), administering oxygen under positive pressure and giving antibiotics to prevent development of pneumonia. The maturity of the lungs can be detected before birth by AMNIOCENTESIS, which sometimes is performed in order to determine whether a baby is ready for Cesarean delivery.

hydatidiform mole   Also *hydatid mole, molar pregnancy.* An abnormal development of embryonic tissue (specifically the PLACENTA) resulting in the formation of a grapelike cluster instead of a fetus. It is distinguished from a normal pregnancy in that the uterus grows far more rapidly, there is vaginal bleeding in the third or fourth month (ranging from spotting to profuse hemorrhage) and no fetal heartbeat or movement can be discerned. Severe nausea and vomiting often occur, and eventually grapelike molar tissue is discharged through the vagina. If suspected, ultrasound can reveal the condition and diagnosis can be confirmed by the presence of exceptionally high levels of HUMAN CHORIONIC GONADOTROPIN (HCG) in the blood or urine at three and one-half months or so. Although 80 to 90% of such moles are benign (noncancerous), they are considered potentially malignant because they occasionally give rise to a cancer called CHORIOCARCINOMA. Treatment is directed at expelling the mole, which often occurs spontaneously near the end of the fourth month. If it does not, a D AND C is performed, usually by means of suction (vacuum aspiration) followed by some scraping (curetting) to make sure all of the molar tissue has been removed. Most often chemotherapy, consisting of methotrexate, is administered. The patient usually is checked for HCG levels in the blood until there have been negative levels for one year. Further, oral contraceptives often are prescribed for one year, provided there are no contraindications for them, in order to prevent conception. After one year of negative HCG levels, it is safe to attempt another pregnancy.

hydramnios Also *polyhydramnios.* An excess amount of amniotic fluid (see also AMNIOTIC SAC). In general, more than 2,000 milliliters (ml) of fluid at term (9 months) is considered excessive, the normal amount being about 1,000 ml. In rare cases as much as 15 liters (quarts) of fluid have been found. In most instances, the increase in amniotic fluid progresses gradually over the course of the pregnancy and so is called *chronic hydramnios.* In some cases, however, the amount increases very suddenly and the uterus becomes grossly distended in a matter of days; this is called *acute hydramnios.* In both kinds the fluid is chemically the same as that found normally.

The cause of hydramnios is not known, but frequently it is associated with fetal malformations, especially of the central nervous system and gastrointestinal tract. It also tends to occur more often in multiple pregnancies and in mothers with diabetes. The symptoms of hydramnios result chiefly from the pressure exerted by the overdistended uterus on neighboring organs. Breathing becomes difficult. Fluid retention is common, especially in the legs, vulva and abdomen, which become very swollen. If there is any doubt about the diagnosis, ultrasound will reveal the condition. If hydramnios is extreme, the outlook for the baby is poor. In addition to its connection with congenital defects, many of which are life-threatening, hydramnios tends to lead to premature labor. That, together with problems experienced during labor, lead to an overall death rate (both before and after birth) of 50% or more.

There is no treatment for the condition. Bed rest and sedation may make the mother more comfort-able but do not slow down fluid accumulation. The use of diuretics and restriction of fluid and salt intake also have no effect. Sometimes AMNIOCENTESIS—to draw off some of the excess fluid—is performed, either through the cervix or abdominally. However, this procedure itself is not without risk, and it often initiates labor, even when only a little of the excess fluid is removed.

hydrosalpinx A large, fluid-filled, club-shaped FALLOPIAN TUBE, closed at the fimbriated end (closest to the ovary), thus making it impossible for an egg from that ovary to enter the tube. It usually is the result of GONORRHEA, which causes inflammation and infection in the tube. As the pus from the infection is absorbed, hydrosalpinx results. Often the condition is bilateral (affecting both tubes), making the woman infertile. Treatment is aimed at early detection by pelvic examination; confirmed by HYSTEROSALPINGOGRAPHY, it may then be surgically corrected.

hygiene The science of health and practices such as cleanliness, which help preserve it. Regular use of soap, water and toothbrush generally suffice to keep the body clean. Body odor comes mostly from perspiration and can be controlled by daily bathing of those areas where it is most likely to be concentrated, chiefly the armpits and pubic area. Hair removal on the underarms and legs is not related to health but to appearance. Armpit hair does trap perspiration odors, and regular shaving minimizes that, but otherwise it is purely cosmetic. The use of underarm DEODORANTS also helps, but they should not be used in the pubic area lest they irritate the very sensitive skin there.

The vagina does not ordinarily need to be washed or douched. Its normal secretions, menstrual flow and seminal fluid all are alike in that they are not "dirty." Strong odors in the pubic area tend to be those trapped by the pubic hair, which simply requires regular washing. If strong odor persists despite washing, it can be a sign of vaginal infection and should be investigated. Use of "hygiene sprays" inside the vagina should be avoided; they frequently cause allergic reactions and, should a woman using them be pregnant, they can harm the baby. Wiping after a bowel movement should always be done from front to back, to avoid contaminating the vagina with fecal matter, which can contain bacteria harmful to it.

See also DOUCHING.

hymen Also *maidenhead*. A thin elastic membrane, about ⅛ inch (0.3 centimeter) thick, that partly covers the introitus, or vaginal opening. In most young girls and women who have never had vaginal intercourse, the hymen partly blocks the opening, allowing menstrual flow to pass through. The size and shape of the hymen vary enormously. It can be stretched by the use of tampons or with the fingers, as well as by physical exercise that causes stretching in that area, such as gymnastics, ballet or horseback riding. Consequently it is not possible to tell from examining the hymen whether a woman has ever had vaginal intercourse. During the first vaginal intercourse the hymen may rupture, if it has not done so earlier, tearing at several points. The edges of the tears then heal, and the hymen may remain permanently divided into two or three sections. There may or may not be slight bleeding (occasionally severe bleeding) when it is ruptured; thus the presence or absence of such blood also does not signify virginity. Occasionally the hymen is very resistant to tearing and may require a small surgical incision (*hymenotomy*) or even removal (*hymenectomy*) before vaginal intercourse can take place. Even rarer is the condition called *imperforate hymen*, in which the membrane completely blocks the vagina so that menstrual flow cannot pass through; this condition requires minor surgery for correction.

hyperbilirubinemia See NEONATAL JAUNDICE.

hyperemesis gravidarum See MORNING SICKNESS.

hypermenorrhea Also *menorrhagia*. Exceptionally heavy bleeding during regular menstrual periods. (See MENSTRUAL FLOW.)

hyperplasia, endometrial See ENDOMETRIAL HYPERPLASIA.

hypertension Also *high blood pressure*. Elevation of arterial, systolic and/or diastolic blood pressure, occurring either alone and called *primary* or *essential hypertension* or as the by-product of kidney disease or some other condition, called *secondary hypertension*. About 27% of American women aged 18 to 74 have high blood pressure; the figure rises with age, for about 70% of women aged 65 to 75 have hypertension. This figure includes about 25% of white women and almost 39% of black women; by age 65 almost 80% of black women have hypertension. Even women who have never had high blood pressure may develop it during pregnancy (see PREECLAMPSIA). It can develop rapidly in the last trimester, posing danger to both mother and fetus. Women are at even greater risk after menopause. More than half of all women over age 55 have high blood pressure, and after 65 women are more likely to develop it than men. In this age group, 83% of black women have it, compared to 66% of white women.

There usually is no warning symptom of hypertension until a person suffers one of its complications, most commonly a heart attack, stroke (cerebral vascular accident) or kidney disease. The only way to discover the disease is to measure the *blood pressure;* that is, the pressure of the blood on the walls of the arteries, which in turn depends on the energy of the heart action, the elasticity of the arterial walls (which decreases with advancing age) and the volume and viscosity (thickness) of the blood. There are two components to blood pressure. The first, the *maximum* or *systolic pressure,* is the pressure that occurs with the contraction of the left ventricle (the lower chamber of the left side of the heart, which pumps oxygenated blood out to the tissues of the body). The second, the *minimum* or *diastolic pressure,* is the pressure when the ventricle dilates and refills with blood (when the heart is at rest). Blood pressure is measured with a *sphygmomanometer,* an instrument containing a column of mercury, or a similar device. During contraction (systole) the pressure in a healthy adult may, for example, support a column of mercury

120 millimeters high (expressed as 120 mm Hg), and during relaxation it supports a column only 80 millimeters high. That individual then would be said to have a blood pressure of 120/80 ("120 over 80"), the 120 signifying systolic pressure and the 80 diastolic pressure. With age the elasticity of the arteries may be reduced, so that they resist the flow of blood and greater pressure is required to keep blood flowing. New guidelines published in 2003 defined normal blood pressure as less than 120/80 and established a new category called *prehypertension* (see the accompanying table). Prehypertension does not call for treatment in the absence of diabetes, kidney disease or another cardiovascular risk factor, but does call for preventive lifestyle changes. Mild hypertension usually is defined as a diastolic pressure between 90 and 104, moderate between 105 and 114, and severe 115 or higher. In adults a pressure consistently higher than 140/90 also is considered hypertensive. In the elderly, some clinicians regard higher levels as normal; others do not.

There is no known cure for primary hypertension, but treatment can modify its course; secondary hypertension is treated by eliminating the underlying cause. Without treatment there is great risk of developing a serious, and possibly fatal, complication. The greatest dangers are CONGESTIVE HEART FAILURE and stroke. The extra pumping needed may cause the left ventricle to fail entirely, or the increased pressure may cause some smaller blood vessel to burst. In the brain this releases blood that presses on and damages brain tissue, causing a cerebral hemorrhage or stroke; see CEREBRAL VASCULAR ACCIDENT. Another frequent complication is kidney disease.

BLOOD PRESSURE EVALUATION*

mm Hg.	Condition
115/75 to 119/79	Normal
120/80 to 139/89	Prehypertension
140/90 to 159/104	Stage I hypertension
160/105 to 179/114	Stage II hypertension
180/115 or higher	Stage III hypertension

*According to guidelines of the National High Blood Pressure Education Program of the National Heart, Lung and Blood Institute

LIFESTYLE CHANGES TO PREVENT HYPERTENSION

- If overweight, lose weight and maintain healthy body-mass index.
- Eat lots of fruit, vegetables and low-fat dairy foods.
- Reduce salt intake to 1 level teaspoon (1,300 mg after age 50, 1,200 mg after age 70) per day or less.
- Engage in aerobic physical activity for 30 to 45 minutes per day on most days.
- Take no more than one alcoholic drink (5 ounces wine or 12 ounces beer) per day.
- Have blood pressure checked once a year, more often if you have diabetes.

General measures for treating hypertension include weight control (obesity definitely contributes to the disease and, further, creates a greater workload for the heart) and physical exercise (30 to 45 minutes of aerobic exercise on most days). Smoking should be avoided and salt intake restricted to 1 teaspoon (1,300 mg after age 50, 1,200 mg after age 70) a day. A diet high in fruits, vegetables, whole grains and low-fat dairy products is recommended for both prevention and treatment of mild (Stage I) hypertension. Alcohol should be limited to one drink per day. Potassium (3.5 milligrams a day) is also important. These measures may be sufficient to control Stage I hypertension, provided there are no complications, such as kidney disease, or high-risk factors, such as a strong family history of hypertension and heart disease. Antihypertensive drugs, when required, usually must be continued for life. Mild hypertension has long been treated with an oral DIURETIC drug, which stimulates the kidneys to increase elimination of salt and water and thereby reduces the blood volume; it also relaxes the walls of the smaller arteries, allowing them to expand and thus reducing the need for such high pressure to pump blood through them. Moderate and severe hypertension usually are treated with a variety of newer drugs, each of which has different side effects. *Beta-blockers* work by blocking the effect of the hormone adrenaline on the heart, so that the heart slows down and does not have to work as hard. They are especially useful for patients who have suffered heart attacks and those whose hearts chronically malfunction. They are not recommended for patients with chronic lung disease or for extremely active individuals. Possible side effects are insomnia, slow pulse, asthmatic attacks and impotence. The beta-blockers include propanolol, metropolol, atenolol, bisoprolol and timolol. While beta-blockers do reduce blood pressure, a recent study indicated they are not as effective as other drugs with fewer side effects and should not be used as a first-line treatment for hypertension; diuretics should remain the first-line treatment. The *calcium-channel blockers* prevent the entry of calcium into small blood vessels, making them relax. They include diltiazem, isradipine, nisoldipine and verapamil. Among their side effects are headache, palpitations, constipation and edema. The *angiotensin converting enzyme (ACE) inhibitors,* which include captopril, enalapril, lisinopril, moexipril, quinapril and trandolapril, block the production of angiotensin II, a hormone that constricts the blood vessels; their main side effect is a persistent cough. A newer class of antihypertensive drugs are the *angiotensin II receptor antagonists,* which work much like the ACE inhibitors. Currently on the market are valsartan, losartan, telmisartan, candesartan, eprosartan and irbesartan. In addition, there are vasodilators, which dilate blood vessels in a different way; they are usually added as a second drug when another alone does not lower blood pressure enough. Herbalists say that a tea brewed from the leaves and stem of hyssop (*Hyssopus officinalis*) has an antihypertensive effect.

With treatment most persons with uncomplicated hypertension can lead relatively normal lives. Women who desire to bear children must remember that hypertension makes pregnancy risky for both mother and child, but if the mother's blood pressure can be maintained within a normal range, by close prenatal supervision, restriction of sodium (salt) intake and regular medication, the prognosis for both is quite good.

Secondary hypertension, which affects about 7% of all hypertensive patients, can normally be reduced by eliminating the cause. Such conditions as hyperthyroidism and adrenal tumors often can be treated with hormone therapy. Certain medications constrict blood vessels and cause blood pressure to rise. Among them are phenylpropanolamine in appetite suppressants (and in the herbal remedy ephedra) and pseudoephedrine in cold and allergy medications. Discontinuing or limiting their use can correct the problem. Oral contraceptives, formerly associated with high blood pressure, today contain much smaller amounts of estrogen and progestin, and the risk of hypertension is very low.

In recent years blood-pressure monitors for home use have been greatly improved since the earliest, quite unreliable models came on the market. Often they work better at home, where the patient is relaxed, than in the doctor's office, where feelings of stress may affect the reading. For those at risk for hypertension, regular monitoring may afford more protection. It is a good idea to check the reading of a home monitor against a medical office unit to make sure of its relative accuracy.

See also HOME MEDICAL TESTS.

For pregnancy-induced hypertension, see PREECLAMPSIA.

THE DASH DIET*

Grains and grain products: 7 to 8 servings a day /(1 serving = ½ cup of whole grain cereal or one slice whole grain bread)

Vegetables: 4 to 5 servings a day (1 serving = 1 cup raw or ½ cup cooked vegetables)

Fruit: 4 to 5 servings a day (1 serving = 6 oz fruit juice or 1 medium-sized fruit)

Dairy: 2 to 3 servings of low fat or nonfat products a day (1 serving = 8 oz of milk or 1 cup yogurt)

Meat, poultry, fish: 2 or fewer servings a day (1 serving = 3 oz cooked fish; choose lean cuts of meat and fish with omega-3 fats like salmon)

*DASH stands for Dietary Approaches to Stop Hypertension

---

hyperthyroidism See THYROID.

hypnotherapy A method of inducing a trance-like state characterized by extreme suggestibility in order to help patients relax, recall repressed memories, control pain or overcome addictions such as smoking. Invented in the mid-19th century, the process of *hypnosis* induces a state somewhere between sleeping and waking. Some prefer to describe it as a condition of deep relaxation and focused concentration. It has been used by psychotherapists to help patients recall suppressed events, by dentists and surgeons to deaden pain, and as a mode of alternative medicine to help such conditions as headache, skin disorders and chronic colitis. Another use for it, sometimes called *hypno-birth*, is a kind of self-hypnosis so that childbirth occurs in a trancelike, deeply relaxed state. Invented by Marie Mongan in 1989, it is taught in a series of lessons, mostly by hypnotherapists and midwives. It allegedly reduces the pain and duration of labor enormously, and at least one practitioner claims it cut his rate of Cesarean sections from 25% to 1%.

A recent study showed that women who were hypnotized immediately before a breast biopsy or lumpectomy needed less sedation and anesthesia during the surgery and felt less pain, nausea, fatigue, discomfort and emotional distress afterward.

At present few states have certification or licensing requirements for hypnotists or hypnotherapy. Consequently those considering it should take care to choose a trained hypnotist, one certified by a state-approved school of hypnosis. See Resources in the Appendix.

hypoglycemia Also *low blood sugar*. A rare condition in which the level of blood glucose is too low for normal functioning. It occurs when the body's system for regulating the amount of glucose in the bloodstream is disturbed owing to a tumor of the pancreas, liver disease, surgery in the gastrointestinal tract, prolonged starvation or severe widespread infection. It also may occur in premature babies or in infants or toddlers who have a serious disease or who have been poisoned.

The symptoms of hypoglycemia involve the central nervous system and range from loss of alertness and fainting to coma and convulsions. Also, as the body tries to compensate for the lack of glucose, there may be adrenergic symptoms (from increased adrenaline production), such as jittery feelings, increased perspiration and rapid heartbeat. Treatment of hypoglycemia requires eliminating the underlying causes, although glucose must be administered as well to mitigate the symptoms. Because these symptoms also appear with other disorders, diagnosis consists of a blood test taken *during* the time symptoms occur. (Oral glucose tolerance tests are not reliable.) If blood glucose is less than 45 milligrams per deciliter and the symptoms disappear when blood sugar is raised by administering glucose, the diagnosis of true hypoglycemia is confirmed.

Another form of hypoglycemia is called *reactive* because it occurs after eating. The symptoms include hunger, sweating, tremor, anxiety, rapid heartbeat, headache and fatigue—all symptoms that can be associated with a low level of blood sugar and that also occur when a diabetic takes an overdose of insulin. Formerly this condition was thought to result from an overabundance of insulin; however, several studies showed that many who experienced it actually have normal blood sugar levels. Nevertheless, physicians often treat these patients as if they had alimentary hypoglycemia (due to previous stomach surgery)—that is, with a low-carbohydrate, high-protein diet and frequent small meals instead of three large ones a day. Even though neither diagnosis nor treatment is well founded, many patients find they improve with the diet, indicating that perhaps it works as a placebo or that they simply cannot tolerate a high intake of sugar. A simple solution for those who find that eating relieves the symptoms is to keep some fresh fruit or fruit juice on hand.

hypomenorrhea Exceptionally light bleeding during regular menstrual periods.

See also MENSTRUAL FLOW.

hypophysectomy Surgical removal of the PITUITARY gland, a treatment sometimes used for breast cancers whose growth is stimulated by estrogen (see ESTROGEN-RECEPTOR ASSAY). Since the pituitary is the controlling organ for the adrenal glands and ovaries, which in turn produce most of the female body's estrogen, removing it eliminates a hormone-dependent tumor's source of growth. A patient's response to previous hormone therapy is a factor in determining whether the procedure will succeed in arresting the cancer. Current statistics indicate that more than half of the patients who had responded favorably to oophorectomy (removal of the ovaries) could be expected to improve after hypophysectomy, and that figure is even higher (70%) for postmenopausal women who have had previous hormone therapy.

hypothalamus   A part of the brain that is considered part of both the ENDOCRINE system and the central nervous system. Adjacent to the posterior pituitary gland, the hypothalamus produces two hormones that travel through the posterior pituitary and are released into the bloodstream: *oxytocin,* which influences labor (in childbirth) and milk production, and *vasopressin,* which constricts the blood vessels, raises blood pressure and also influences the uterus and kidneys. The hypothalamus also controls the synthesis and release of hormones by the anterior pituitary gland, producing gonadotropin-releasing hormone (GnRH), causing the pituitary to secrete LH (luteinizing hormone) and FSH (follicle-stimulating hormone), which in women make the ovaries produce estrogen and progesterone (see under MENSTRUAL CYCLE for further explanation). Levels of estrogen and progesterone in turn influence hypothalamic activity in a kind of feedback system, along with stimuli from the central nervous system. It is these stimuli that account for the fact that thoughts and feelings can affect the endocrine system (see LET-DOWN REFLEX for an example). In men LH and FSH maintain the sex glands and sperm formation, but not on a cyclical basis.

Other substances released by the hypothalamus are *corticotropin-releasing hormone,* which influences production of ACTH and of adrenal cortisol (see ADRENAL GLANDS); *prolactin-inhibiting factor* (PIF), arresting the release of PROLACTIN; *growth-hormone releasing hormone* and *thyrotropin-releasing hormone,* stimulating the secretion of these hormones by the pituitary; and *dopamine* and *somatostatin,* which inhibit various hormones. There appear to be additional hypothalamic functions, which are not yet fully understood.

hypothyroidism   See THYROID.

hysterectomy   Surgical removal of the uterus. A *total hysterectomy* involves removal of the body of the uterus and the cervix; a *supracervical hysterectomy* (formerly called a *subtotal,* or *partial, hysterectomy*) leaves the cervix intact. A hysterectomy as such does not involve removal of the fallopian tubes or ovaries and consequently does not bring on menopause since it does not stop ovulation or estrogen production by the ovaries. It does, however, preclude child-bearing, and it puts an end to menstruation. Surgical removal of the ovaries, or OOPHORECTOMY, and of the fallopian tubes, or SALPINGECTOMY, can be and often is performed along with hysterectomy; in that case the operation is technically known as a *total abdominal hysterectomy and bilateral salpingo-oophorectomy* (abbreviated TAH and BSO) or, in lay terminology, a *complete hysterectomy.* "Bilateral" means both ovaries and both tubes, "unilateral" means only one; "abdominal" refers to the fact that the incision is made through the lower abdomen, distinguishing it from a vaginal hysterectomy, where the uterus and cervix may be removed through an incision inside the vagina (see below).

Hysterectomy was first performed by Dr. Robert Battey in 1872 and by 1975 it was the second most widely performed operation of any kind in the United States (after the D AND C), with 725,000 hysterectomies performed in that year (and 1,070,000 D and Cs). Together these made up 10% of all surgery performed, and it was estimated that if this rate continued, about half the women in the United States would have their uterus removed by the time they reached the age of 70. In 1977, at a hearing before a congressional committee investigating unnecessary surgery, critics within the medical profession said that perhaps 40% of all hysterectomies performed were questionable, and of those done in 1975 only 20% could be justified as treatment for cancer and other life-threatening conditions. In the next few years it was discovered that seeking a second opinion after hysterectomy was proposed greatly reduced the number of operations performed. By 1992 about 580,000 hysterectomies were being performed each year, a reduction thought to result from stricter peer review in hospitals, activism among consumers of health care and technological advances that provide alternative treatments, such as BALLOON ABLATION. However, the numbers again were rising (615,000 in 2005), and many experts believe the number of hysterectomies performed is still much too high. Some states now have an informed-consent law requiring surgeons to inform patients of any discomfort or risks that may accompany or follow hysterectomy as well as any known available and appropriate alternatives.

There are certain clear-cut indications for hysterectomy, when the operation may be necessary to save a woman's life: (1) to stop severe uncontrollable bleeding (hemorrhage); (2) as a last resort for severe infection, such as the bursting of an abscess secondary to PELVIC INFLAMMATORY DISEASE; (3) to remove a malignant tumor (cancer) from the vagina, uterus, fallopian tubes or ovaries. In addition, a hysterectomy sometimes may be necessary as part of surgery required to correct a life-threatening disorder elsewhere in the abdominal cavity, in the bladder, rectum or intestines.

A second category of indications for hysterectomy is less clear-cut, the need for surgery depending on the severity of the condition. Among these are (1) severe and recurrent attacks of pelvic inflammatory disease; (2) extensive ENDOMETRIOSIS or ADENOMYOSIS with disabling symptoms that do not respond to hormone therapy (especially when the disease is so widespread that pregnancy is very unlikely or the woman is past childbearing age); (3) uterine FIBROIDS that are very large and/or pressing on other organs and/or causing recurrent, very profuse menstrual periods, and/or showing sudden marked growth, and that have not responded to hormone therapy, and are not suitable for myomectomy (removal of the fibroid only); (4) when both ovaries must be removed (bilateral oophorectomy); (5) the presence of PRECANCEROUS LESIONS; (6) prolapse of the uterus, bladder or rectum that is severe enough to interfere with bladder or bowel functions and is not correctable by lesser surgery.

Hysterectomy should *not* be undertaken for pelvic pain or backache, irregular periods, menstrual cramps, small fibroids, uterine polyps or ovarian cysts until alternative, lower-risk treatment has been tried. It probably should not be done for moderate prolapse of the bladder, rectum or uterus, for which there are other alternatives. Further, unless a woman faces an acute emergency (as with a massive hemorrhage) where immediate treatment is imperative, she is well advised to get at least one more opinion from a second clinician concerning the best course of treatment for her. Finally, hysterectomy should *never* be done for sterilization alone (TUBAL LIGATION is easier, cheaper and safer) or to eliminate the risk of uterine cancer when no disease is actually present. (See also SURGERY, UNNECESSARY.)

Where hysterectomy is the appropriate treatment, the kind of surgery performed depends on a number of factors. In women past menopause, removal of the ovaries often is recommended, since they may no longer produce hormones and can possibly become cancerous. However, not all agree, since postmenopausal hormone production does not cease completely. Ideally the decision is made by the woman herself. In women who are still menstruating regularly and whose ovaries are not diseased, oophorectomy is far more controversial. Advocates say that in women over 40 in particular the ovaries will soon cease functioning and present a risk of cancer and therefore should be removed; they are less dogmatic concerning younger women. Opponents point out that ovarian cancer is rare and surgically induced menopause is a violent shock to the endocrine system, often resulting in severe menopausal symptoms. Further, some authorities believe that the ovaries continue to supply significant amounts of hormone even after menopause. ESTROGEN REPLACEMENT THERAPY, which can mitigate the shock of surgical menopause, may be risky, and in the presence of any estrogen-dependent cancer it is definitely contraindicated.

The choice between abdominal and vaginal hysterectomy generally is easier to make. *Vaginal hysterectomy* is preferred whenever possible, if there are not too many adhesions (scar tissue) and no very large fibroids. The principal advantages are a hidden incision (and therefore no visible scar) and faster healing. The disadvantages are that the operation is more difficult to perform, especially if adhesions are present; it is harder for the surgeon to see where he or she is working (although use of a laparoscope may overcome this; see below); there is more risk of injury to the bladder and urethra; and there is danger of shortening the vagina more when the incision is closed, making for painful intercourse. There is also a 50% greater risk of postoperative infection, which can, however, be offset by administering antibiotics both before and after surgery. The procedure is straightforward. After anesthesia (general or regional), the patient is placed in the same position as for pelvic examination (see DORSAL LITHOTOMY). The surgeon makes an incision inside the vaginal wall near the cervix, the uterus is gradually cut free from the pelvic structures to which it is attached by ligaments and blood vessels and it is removed through the vagina. The surgeon then repairs each layer of the incision and closes it. In a laparoscopically assisted vaginal hysterectomy, the surgeon makes three or four small incisions in the abdomen through which are inserted a fiberoptic viewing device or camera and surgical tools. The ligaments are severed and the uterus is removed through the vagina. This procedure is more expensive and takes three hours instead of two, but enables examining the abdominal cavity for endometriosis and scar tissue.

Abdominal hysterectomy is always chosen when a fibroid is too large to remove through the vagina and when there are many adhesions from previous pelvic infection or previous surgery. The principal advantage is that the surgeon can see the entire abdominal cavity. The disadvantages for the patient are a longer recovery period, more postoperative pain (because the abdominal muscles must be cut and then must heal) and a higher probability that adhesions will develop. Two kinds of incision are used, either a vertical (midline) incision extending from the pubic bone toward the navel or a curved transverse incision below the pubic hairline, extending up on both sides toward the hipbones. The transverse incision allows the scar to be partly or wholly hidden by pubic hair, but the vertical incision affords the surgeon better visibility and more room in which to operate.

Hysterectomy is major surgery, requiring hospitalization for three to five days and four to eight weeks for full recovery (one to two days' hospitalization for the vaginal procedure and two to four weeks for recovery). After the patient is anesthetized, the incision is made into the abdomen and the bladder is separated from the uterus so that it will not be injured. The ligaments connected to the uterus are divided, the blood vessels clamped

and tied and the vagina is cut from around the cervix and uterus. The uterus is removed, with or without the cervix, tubes and ovaries. The vagina is nearly always shortened somewhat. Often an *appendectomy* is performed at the same time. A hysterectomy for cancer may be still more extensive. In a *radical hysterectomy* (also called *Wertheim procedure*) the surgeon removes the pelvic lymph nodes and ligaments and the upper portion of the vagina, along with the cervix and uterus. Even in this extreme procedure, however, the ovaries, if they are definitely not involved, may be left intact.

Although the risk of death from hysterectomy is fairly low, that of complications is quite high. Some 30 to 40% of women have postoperative infections that require treatment, and, though antibiotic treatment alone often is sufficient, some do develop large abscesses that require further surgery. Hemorrhage occurs during surgery in about 15% of cases, requiring blood transfusion, and heavy bleeding may occur, most often one to two weeks following surgery, when the internal sutures begin to dissolve. The risk of blood clots developing in the pelvic or leg veins is increased by surgery on the pelvic organs. Such clots can break off and travel to the lungs; called pulmonary emboli, they can be life-threatening. Problems with the urinary tract are common during the first few postoperative weeks, with about half developing bladder or kidney infections. Danger signs after the patient returns home, any one of which should be reported to the surgeon immediately, are fever (over 100 degrees Fahrenheit oral); pain not relieved by medication given when leaving the hospital; bright red vaginal bleeding with large clots (small ones alone are common) or bleeding that soaks one or two pads per hour; constipation (more than three days without a bowel movement); persistent bladder discomfort, bloody urine or inability to urinate; pain, swelling, tenderness or redness in a leg; chest pain, cough, difficulty in breathing or coughing blood; odorous and/or copious vaginal discharge.

In addition to the above-named complications, fatigue and minor discomfort affect most women for some weeks. Some women feel weepy. They also may experience HOT FLASHES even if their ovaries were not removed; the reason is not known, but presumably their hormone balance is upset temporarily by surgery. Recovery time varies, depending on the individual's age and general physical condition. Most women return to regular activities in four to six weeks, but some recuperate much more slowly. In some women extreme fatigue and depression may persist for as long as a year or more after surgery. Premenopausal women whose ovaries have been removed will experience some or all of the symptoms of MENOPAUSE caused by greatly lowered estrogen levels.

After a complete hysterectomy (with removal of the ovaries) estrogen replacement therapy is usually given, most often estrogen alone. However, recent findings have shown it is not without serious risk, and therefore should be administered for as short a time as possible. And it may not be used at all by some women.

Many women tend to gain weight postoperatively, chiefly because they are so much less active during the period of recuperation. Such weight gain can be avoided by reducing caloric intake. Conditioning exercises will help retone muscles flabby from inactivity and usually may be begun four to six weeks after surgery. Vaginal sexual intercourse usually may be resumed after six weeks. Some women experience a change in their sexual functioning. The removal of uterus and cervix leaves less pelvic tissue to become engorged during sexual arousal. There no longer can be any sensation of expansion in the uterus nor the contractions of the uterus normally felt during orgasm. These changes may be very apparent to some women and scarcely noticeable to others. In contrast, other women may experience increased sexual response, especially if prior to surgery intercourse was painful or conception was an unacceptable risk. In women whose ovaries also are removed, the consequent loss of estrogen may make the lining of the vagina thinner and less readily lubricated, making intercourse more difficult and sometimes uncomfortable. (See VAGINAL ATROPHY.) Estrogen relieves such dryness but, as indicated above, is not without risk and cannot be used by all women.

The drawbacks of hysterectomy are, for many women, partly or entirely offset by the relief following surgery that has eliminated a previously painful (and sometimes life-threatening) disorder, along with the nuisance of menstruation and the risk of pregnancy. Thus, although some women feel a profound sense of loss, others (and sometimes even the same women) regard it as a relief from the burden of illness, menstruation and unwanted pregnancy.

hysteria, conversion Also *conversion disorder, hysterical neurosis, hysteria syndrome.* An emotional disorder that is expressed as (or "converted into") a severe bodily dysfunction without any physical cause. It occurs far more often in women than in men. It may take the form of *paresis* (partial paralysis) or *complete paralysis* (inability to move) of a limb that is physically quite healthy, or perhaps loss of sight when nothing organic is wrong with the eyes. Other common manifestations are *aphagia* (inability to swallow food or water), *aphonia* (inability to tense the vocal cords to utter sounds, although the person usually can whisper), sensory disturbance (loss of vision or sensation) and pain. Such symptoms, crippling as they may be, often are accompanied by a seeming indifference to them, which psychiatrists call *la belle indifference* (French for "beautiful unconcern").

Conversion hysteria was first described by the Greek physician Hippocrates, who believed it to be caused by a uterus that somehow became detached and moved around inside the body, obstructing the particular area in which the symptoms appeared. Indeed, *hysteria* comes from *hysterikos,* the Greek word for "uterus." The condition was described by Sigmund Freud, who added the term "conversion" and believed that it expressed a repressed psychological conflict, usually one of a sexual nature. For example, repressed guilty feelings about masturbating might be expressed as paralysis of the hand used to masturbate. Most modern psychiatrists have broadened this concept to include psychological conflicts other than sexual ones. Treatment is directed at uncovering the underlying cause, which, when recognized and acknowledged by the patient, usually eliminates the symptoms.

hysterosalpingography The injection of dye and subsequent X-ray study of the uterus and fallopian tubes, usually to determine whether a woman's inability to become pregnant is caused by a uterine abnormality, or tubal blockage or dilation (HYDRO-SALPINX). Sometimes the process of forcing dye through the tubes will dislodge material blocking them. The procedure, usually performed in the outpatient X-ray department of a hospital or in a radiology clinic, involves the injection of special dye through a small tube inserted into the cervix. The radiologist watches on an X-ray screen as the dye fills the uterus and is forced up into the fallopian tubes, revealing abnormalities in shape as well as any obstruction in these organs. A second X-ray may be required 24 hours later. By then the dye will have spread throughout the pelvic area, and a residue of dye near the end of either fallopian tube may indicate scar tissue near the ovary, which may be obstructing the passage of an egg into the tube.

Hysterosalpingography involves some discomfort, usually resulting from the dilatation of the cervix to allow insertion of the dye. Also, the cervix usually must be held steady by means of a clamp (tenaculum; see under D AND C), which may cause cramping and pinching when it is first applied. The procedure, which is best performed after a menstrual period but before ovulation, is accurate in detecting tubal obstruction in about 75% of cases. Its chief drawback is that it delivers a high dose of radiation to the ovaries, and therefore many clinicians consider the minor surgery of LAPAROSCOPY safer. Others, however, consider it less invasive.

hysteroscopy   The insertion of a visualizing instrument, called a hysteroscope, through the cervix into the uterus. It is used to locate and remove, by means of a special forceps attachment, an INTRA-UTERINE DEVICE (IUD) that has perforated the uterine wall. It also can be used to effect TUBAL LIGATION by means of a cauterizing instrument that is passed through the scope to coagulate the tubal openings, as well as in conjunction with surgical instruments to remove uterine adhesions and/or a FIBROID. Further, it is used for diagnostic purposes similar to a D AND C, to which it is superior in that the entire endometrium can be seen on a video monitor, allowing a view of polyps, fibroids or a blockage of the fallopian tubes. Usually an outpatient procedure, it requires local anesthetic and oral painkillers, and the aftereffects are similar to those of a D and C. If carbon dioxide is used, there may be some shoulder pain afterward as the gas seeps into other tissues, but it is usually of brief duration.

hysterosonography   See POLYP, def. 3.

hysterotomy   Surgery through the uterine wall to terminate a pregnancy of 16 to 24 weeks. It resembles the surgery of CESAREAN SECTION, with the fetus and placenta being removed through a small incision in the uterus. In some cases the fetus is alive when removed, but usually it dies very quickly because it is too immature to sustain life. The complications and mortality rate of hysterotomy are high enough to make it a dangerous procedure, far more so than AMNIOINFUSION for a second-trimester abortion, so that it should be used only for women whose medical problems rule out safer methods.

iatrogenic disorder Any disorder directly resulting from medical treatment. Until modern times it was commonplace for physicians and surgeons to do more harm than good, and today medical care itself still is sometimes responsible for new illness. Among the most common iatrogenic disorders today is postoperative infection following HYSTERECTOMY, which apparently afflicts anywhere from one-fourth to one-half of women undergoing the procedure.

See also SIDE EFFECT.

identical twins See MULTIPLE PREGNANCY.

idiopathic Having no known cause. Menstrual irregularities often are idiopathic.

ileostomy A permanent surgical opening on the abdomen, where the ileum section of the small intestine, through which solid wastes (feces) are eliminated, is brought to the surface. Usually the entire colon and rectum are removed. The end portion of the ileum is brought through the abdominal wall to form a *stoma* (opening), usually on the lower right side of the abdomen. An appliance (bag) must be worn over the stoma at all times to collect feces and control odor. With a somewhat different procedure—the *Kock internal reservoir* operation—the diseased portion of intestine is removed and an internal sac is fashioned from some of the tissues; this sac, or reservoir, collects fecal matter, which the patient must remove with a catheter four or five times a day. This method avoids the use of an appliance but can be used only in certain patients.

About 80% of all ileostomies are performed for ulcerative colitis, a chronic inflammation of the colon characterized by bloody diarrhea. Usually ileostomy is performed only when medical treatment over a period of time has failed to control the condition. Other indications are birth defects, familial polyposis (the formation of numerous polyps that may become cancerous), injury, cancer, and Crohn's disease, or regional enteritis, a chronic inflammation of unknown cause that most often affects the lower ileum. The ileostomy substitutes for the elimination functions formerly performed by the colon.

Ileostomy involves major surgery and a period of recovery and readjustment afterward. It need not interfere with leading a normal life; only a job that requires very heavy lifting may be contraindicated lest the stoma be injured. Sexual function in women is not impaired at all, and sexual potency in men only rarely (see also under OSTOMY). Bathing or showering can be done, with or without the appliance in place. Although a low-residue diet usually is recommended for the first few weeks after surgery (including only easily digested foods and no raw fruits or vegetables), in most cases a largely normal diet can be resumed fairly soon. Some, although not all, persons have excessive gas following ileostomy; it usually can be relieved by eliminating certain foods entirely and by chewing all solid foods slowly and thoroughly.

immune system See IMMUNITY.

immunity The body's state of resistance or lack of susceptibility to a disease or disorder, usually due to the presence of antibodies against the causative agent (see ANTIBODY). Immunity may be congenital, acquired from the mother and present at birth (but then usually not long-lasting), natural (resulting from an infection that produces antibodies) or induced by immunization (vaccination).

The body's *immune system* is a complex network of cells and organs organized into sets and subsets that communicate with one another to defend the body against invasion by bacteria, viruses, parasites and fungi. Able to distinguish between the body's own cells and foreign cells, this network responds to triggers called *antigens* (foreign substances such as a virus, part of a virus, tissue or cells from another person). Sometimes the immune system errs and attacks part of the body's own cells, which happens in so-called AUTOIMMUNE DISEASES. In other instances it responds to seemingly harmless substances such as ragweed pollen, resulting in *allergy*. The immune system's chief agents are *lymphocytes*, small white blood cells (see LYMPH) that travel throughout the body via the blood vessels or their own system of lymphatic vessels. Of these, the main immune cells are B cells, which secrete antibodies that ambush circulating antigens but cannot penetrate target cells; T cells, which direct and regulate the immune response, binding to target cells and triggering other immune activity; natural killer (NK) cells, which attack any foe; and phagocytes, large white cells that can swallow and digest microbes and other foreign particles. Immunity to disease is conferred because whenever T and B cells are activated, some of the cells become "memory cells"; that is, the next time the same antigen attacks, the immune system is set to demolish it.

There is considerable variation among individuals in their immune response. For example, some women may have a single eruption of genital HERPES INFECTION even though the virus remains dormant in their bodies for life, while others suffer recurrent attacks. AIDS undermines the immune system so that the body eventually succumbs to one or another major infection or disease.

immunization   See under VACCINE.

immunotherapy   Treatment of cancer that attempts to stimulate the body's immune system to produce cancer-fighting cells. For example, a strain of tuberculosis bacillus used to vaccinate human beings has shown some ability to kill cancer cells when administered in conjunction with levasimole, a drug used to treat certain parasitic infections. Another approach to immunotherapy uses actual tumor cells, or extracts from them, that are treated in various ways (by radiation or chemicals) and then reinjected into patients. Still another approach uses antibody cells from experimental animals that are fused in the laboratory with cancer cells, enabling them to grow indefinitely. These hybrid cells then are made to reproduce by cloning and are injected into cancer patients.

Among promising developments is *interferon*, a protein produced in the body by natural killer cells of the immune system in response to invading viruses and bacteria. Discovered in 1957, it is named for its ability to interfere with virus reproduction. It also attacks cancers, interfering with their metabolism (growth), and/or encourages various body cells to destroy them. It comes in three forms: alpha, beta and gamma; human beings carry 12 genes to make alpha-interferon, which is produced by B-lymphocytes, and one gene each for the other two forms. In 1986 alpha-interferon became the first commercial cancer drug developed through genetic engineering (see under GENETICS) that was approved by the U.S. Food and Drug Administration. It works against genital warts (condyloma acuminata), hepatitis B and some cancers, including Kaposi's sarcoma in AIDS patients.

Another promising agent is *interleukin-2* (IL-2), an immune-system activator. When synthesized and mixed with lymphocytes in the laboratory and then injected into a cancer patient along with more IL-2, it transforms the lymphocytes into cancer-cell killers. Immunotherapy research is advancing rapidly. However, at this writing it is still largely experimental.

imperforate hymen   See HYMEN.

implant, contraceptive   See CONTRACEPTIVE.

implantation   Also *nidation*. The attachment of the fertilized egg, or zygote, to the endometrium (wall of the uterus), which takes place 7 to 10 days after fertilization. During that period the fertilized egg travels through the fallopian tube into the uterus. It then penetrates the soft uterine lining by means of enzymes that break down the endometrial tissue. The outside layer of cells forms tentacles called villi, which dig into the endometrium and start to draw nourishing elements from it. By about the 12th day after fertilization a rudimentary PLACENTA has begun to form at the site of implantation, and in the next week or two the zygote begins to develop a circulatory system whereby nutrients and oxygen from the mother's body will be absorbed by the fetus through the thin-walled villi. Some women experience slight vaginal staining, called *implantation bleeding,* around the time of implantation, owing to the formation of new blood vessels there.

For implantation to succeed, it is necessary, after ovulation, for the CORPUS LUTEUM to produce progesterone, which stimulates the development of the endometrium so as to provide the egg with needed nutrients. When this stimulation fails to occur, a condition called *luteal phase defect,* the embryo may not implant or it may fail to thrive. Luteal phase defect is found in 3 to 5% of infertile women and accounts for an estimated one-third of recurrent early miscarriages. It sometimes can be corrected by administering progesterone at precisely the right time in the cycle.

impotence   Also *male erectile dysfunction.* In men, a SEXUAL DYSFUNCTION that occurs during the excitement phase of sexual response, in which the man loses his ERECTION. A man may have difficulty in achieving or maintaining an erection with his partner, or he may lose the erection during penetration, or he may lose it after penetration but before ejaculation. Impotence does not affect libido or the ability to have an orgasm.

Temporary impotence affects practically every man at one time or another; it can be caused by fatigue, anxiety, fear, grief, overindulgence in alcohol or drugs or some other transient condition, and rarely persists long enough to require treatment. Long thought to be largely psychological, impotence today is believed to have a physical basis in as many as 85% of cases. Organic causes include such diseases as diabetes, severe circulatory problems (advanced atherosclerosis), multiple sclerosis, Parkinson's disease, epilepsy, severe arthritis, severe liver or kidney disease, spinal cord injury, congestive heart failure, chronic lung disease, extreme obesity, and cancer of the prostate, bladder or rectum. Heavy cigarette smoking and excessive alcohol consumption frequently impair potency. Impotence also may be a side effect of numerous drugs (certain heart and blood pressure medications, ulcer drugs, psychoactive drugs, antidepressants, antihistamines, hormonal drugs, methadone, amphetamines, marijuana, heroin, etc.). *Potency*—the ability to have and sustain an erection—is not impaired by masturbation or too frequent intercourse; conversely, there is no physical reason for male athletes to avoid sex before an important competitive event. Most prostate surgery does not affect potency, although afterward men may experience retrograde ejaculation (see EJACULATION, def. 4). Age also does not necessarily affect potency, although it may lengthen the time needed to achieve erection and nearly always lengthens the time of recovery after ORGASM.

Anything depriving the penis and clitoris of oxygen—vascular problems, sexual abstinence, sleep deprivation, lack of exercise, smoking, diabetes, injuries—contributes to impotence. Among the treatments currently used are self-injection with a drug—a combination of papaverine and phentolamine, or alprostadil, a synthetic form of prostaglandin E-1—into the penis, which is usually painless, relaxes arterial muscles and lets blood flow into the penis, resulting in a firm erection. Alprostadil may also be inserted into the urethra by means of an ultrathin applicator. The most common problems are mild pain or a slight burning sensation while waiting for the drug to take effect (10 to 20 minutes) and scar tissue formation with frequent use (more than two or three times a week over time). A less common but more dangerous problem is *priapism,* a prolonged erection (lasting three to four hours). It calls for immediate injection of epinephrine by a physician. Another medication is sildenafil (Viagra), introduced in 1998. In convenient pill form but expensive, it works 30 to 60 minutes after taking it by increasing blood flow to the penis and keeping it there. About 70% of those who take it achieve an erection sufficient for intercourse. Minor side effects include headache, flushing, indigestion, stuffy nose and temporary changes in visual perception. However, it must *never* be taken by anyone taking nitrate medications (such as nitroglycerin by heart patients) and only with caution by those taking high blood pressure medications. Approved for use in men, Viagra also is being used in trials by some women who suffer from SEXUAL DYSFUNCTION but to date has not proved effective. Two newer oral drugs are vardenafil (Levitra) and tadalafil (Cialis). The former is similar to Viagra, with the same side effects, but can be taken with food (Viagra requires an empty stomach). Cialis has the advantage of remaining effective for up to 36 hours. Other medications that have been used are oral versions of phentolamine, yohimbine and testosterone. The first two are less effective than Viagra and the last can cause unpleasant side effects. Other drugs are inserted or injected into the penis to widen the arteries supplying blood.

Other avenues of treatment are a mechanical vacuum device that puts negative pressure on the penis and draws blood into it, with a tight rubber band applied to the base holding the erection in place; or, for irreversible organic impotence (and as a last resort), a surgical *penile implant*, which simulates a normal erection, can be bent easily and worn in a normal position under clothing, and enables intercourse but does not guarantee fertility.

See also SEX THERAPY; SEXUAL DYSFUNCTION.

impregnation   See ARTIFICIAL INSEMINATION; FERTILIZATION.

incest   A sexual relationship between two persons who are so closely related that marriage between them would be prohibited by law and/or cultural taboo. The most common such combinations are parent and child, and brother and sister. A child born of two such closely related parents is far more likely to have serious birth defects.

incompetent cervix   Also *incompetent cervical os*. In pregnancy, the dilation of the cervix during the sec-

ond trimester (fourth to sixth months), followed by rupture of the amniotic membranes and expulsion of the fetus, which is nearly always too immature to survive. Generally neither bleeding nor pain occurs, so there is little or no warning of the condition. The cause is not known, but since it rarely happens in a first pregnancy it is believed to result from injury to the cervix during a previous delivery or during a D AND C or other surgical procedure. Exposure to diethylstilbestrol (DES) also may be responsible. Moreover, it tends to recur with each subsequent pregnancy, making incompetent cervix one of the more common causes of HABITUAL MISCARRIAGE. Treatment consists of reinforcing the cervix with sutures that, in effect, tie it into closed normal position. This procedure usually is performed between the 14th and 18th week of pregnancy, before the cervical os has dilated to 4 centimeters (11/2 inches). The sutures must be removed before the onset of labor, usually during the 38th or 39th week, unless Cesarean delivery is planned (in that case they can be left in place). In the majority of cases this procedure will prevent miscarriage. If, however, it fails, the sutures must be removed as soon as there are signs of imminent miscarriage, lest the cervix be injured (see MISCARRIAGE, def. 2 and 3).

incomplete miscarriage   See MISCARRIAGE, def. 4.

incubation period   The time lapse between the moment an infectious agent invades the body and the first appearance of symptoms and signs of infection. In the common infectious diseases of childhood, it varies from about three to five days for scarlet fever to as long as two to three weeks for rubella (German measles). The incubation period is not identical to the period of *communicability*, that is, the period during which another person exposed to the patient can become infected. Measles, for example, can be communicated to another person two to four days before a rash has appeared, but the incubation period ranges from 7 to 14 days.

induction of labor   Also *induced labor*. Stimulating uterine contractions in order to start or speed up labor and delivery. There are three principal means of inducing labor, sometimes used together: (1) Applying a hormone jelly (Preppidil gel or Prostaglandin gel) to the cervix to ripen it and thereby produce contractions; it can be repeated after four to six hours; (2) rupturing the membranes (also called AMNIOTOMY) and administering the hormone oxytocin; done only when the cervix is *ripe*, that is, more than 50% effaced (see EFFACEMENT) and sufficiently dilated to admit an index finger easily (2 centimeters, or ¾ inch); in absence of any of these conditions, labor probably will not begin or, even if contractions do begin, labor is likely to be prolonged (see PROLONGED LABOR); (3) administration of oxytocin (Pitocin) alone—see below.

If the cervix is not ripe and labor needs to be induced because of PREECLAMPSIA or some other serious condition, occasionally it can be helped to dilate more by *stripping the membranes*. However, this can be done only if the cervix is already dilated enough to admit the clinician's index finger. When it is, the clinician places a finger between the cervix and membranes and rotates the finger around the cervix to loosen the membranes. This may cause the cervix to dilate more quickly, but sometimes not for several days.

The third principal means of induction is by administering OXYTOCIN (Pitocin), usually as an intravenous drip. Again, this procedure is effective only if effacement of the cervix has occurred and the cervix is dilated at least 3 (some say 4) centimeters. If labor has begun and the baby is in good position (not in any ABNORMAL PRESENTATION), the intravenous drip is carried on for as long as 8 to 10 hours if necessary, along with careful checking of the fetal heartbeat (see FETAL MONITORING) and constant observation of uterine contractions. If there is fetal distress or the contractions become too strong, a Cesarean section may have to be performed. Sometimes, if oxytocin does not take effect within eight hours, it may need to be repeated two or three times, each on a different day, a process called *serial induction*.

The principal danger of oxytocin is that it can induce contractions strong enough to rupture the uterus and/or kill the baby. Because of this potential danger, there are definite contraindications to its use. Oxytocin should *never* be used when there is any mechanical obstruction to vaginal delivery (that is, any contraction of the mother's pelvis or malposition of the baby). It should not be used if the baby appears to be very large (weighs more than 4,000 grams, or 8.8 pounds). It should not be used in a woman who has had five or more children, because her uterus will tend to rupture more easily than those of women with fewer deliveries. Some counsel that it should not be done in women who have had a previous Cesarean section. Finally, it should not be used unless the baby is judged to be in good condition, based on a regular heart rate and absence of amniotic fluid stained with MECONIUM. (A dead fetus, on the other hand, is not a contraindication.) Nevertheless, the number of inductions of labor has soared since 1989, and many of these (some say as many as 40%) are elective inductions, performed for the convenience of mother and physician.

Even if oxytocin is harmless for the mother (other than creating more discomfort from very strong contractions), it can damage the baby. Because it speeds up contractions as well as strengthening them and shortens the interval between contractions, the baby may be deprived of oxygen. Similarly, during delivery, if the cord descends the birth canal first (PROLAPSED CORD) or is somehow compressed, the baby may get insufficient oxygen. Lack of oxygen can lead to irreversible brain damage.

Because of these risks, induction of labor should be performed only when delaying labor is just as (or more) dangerous. It was long held that if the

---

FOR SAFE INDUCTION OF LABOR*

- Make sure fetal lungs are mature
- Fetal heartbeat has been documented for 20 weeks by a stethoscope or 30 weeks by Doppler test of gestational age
- Reliable tests showed presence in mother of human chorionic gonadotropin at least 36 weeks ago
- Fetus is judged to be at least 39 weeks old from ultrasound measurement of length, obtained at 6 to 12 weeks of pregnancy
- Medical personnel should carefully monitor uterine contractions stimulated by Pitocin
- Screen for fetal fibronectin, whose presence shows labor may begin soon

*Recommended by American College of Obstetricians and Gynecologists

membranes rupture spontaneously but regular contractions have not begun within 24 hours (or began, but then stopped), there is considerable danger of infection, justifying the induction of labor. This view is increasingly being challenged in the belief that it is quite safe to wait for labor to start on its own. However, if there is Rh incompatibility (see RH FACTOR) or if the fetus has already died inside the uterus or there are other complicating factors, rapid delivery may be safer than waiting. Since 1978 the Food and Drug Administration has opposed *elective induction* of labor—performed for the clinician's and/or the mother's convenience—and holds that oxytocin must never be used for this reason. Nevertheless, it is estimated that one in five pregnant women has her labor induced, though it is not certain how many such inductions are elective.

Recently the American College of Obstetricians and Gynecologists approved the use of a test to determine the presence of fetal fibronectin, or fFN, a protein thought to act like a uterine glue. If it seeps into the vaginal tract from mid-pregnancy on (weeks 24 to 34 of gestation) it signals that membranes are breaking apart and labor may begin soon. If it is not present, labor is not likely to begin and induction probably should be postponed.

inevitable miscarriage　See MISCARRIAGE, def. 3.

infection　The invasion of the body by microorganisms, such as bacteria and viruses, that multiply and damage its cells and tissues. Many such organisms normally reside in the body—in the abdominal and uterine cavities, in the lungs, on the skin and elsewhere. However, they are prevented from multiplying to the extent that they can cause damage by the activity of mucus and other natural body substances that kill some of them, as well as by bacteria-fighting white blood cells. Occasionally, however, such organisms do overcome the body's natural defense system and an infection results.

The overall process of bacterial infection is similar no matter what kind of organism is involved or where it attacks. Bacteria are nourished by the very fluid or tissue they attack and produce waste products that are released into these same tissues. White blood cells are sent into the area to defend it. The area becomes warm, red and swollen, both from increased circulation and from the accumulation of pus (made up of dead bacteria, dead white cells and fluids). The bacterial waste products meanwhile enter the bloodstream and exert a poisonous effect on the body, which may be manifest in fever, chills and generalized aches and malaise. Meanwhile some normal cells are being destroyed, either directly by bacteria or indirectly by the excessive swelling and poisonous bacterial wastes. Even after the bacteria are eradicated by drugs such as antibiotics, body tissues may take some time to heal completely and some may never return to normal, being replaced by so-called *scar tissue*.

Virus-caused infections, which range from the common cold to HERPES INFECTION, are not susceptible to antibiotics. Effective antiviral agents still are few in number, and those that do work often produce adverse reactions and undesirable side effects; therefore, patients who receive them require careful monitoring. However, vaccines against a number of virus infections have been developed, and they have been used so successfully that in some areas these infections have virtually disappeared; among them are vaccines for smallpox, yellow fever, measles, mumps, rabies, poliomyelitis and rubella (German measles).

The principal kinds of infection that attack women in particular are vaginal infections (see VAGINITIS), urinary infections (see CYSTITIS), breast infections (see MASTITIS) and infections of the pelvic organs (see ENDOMETRITIS; PELVIC INFLAMMATORY DISEASE). In addition, sexually active women are vulnerable to various SEXUALLY TRANSMITTED DISEASES.

See also ABSCESS; IMMUNITY.

infertility　Inability to become pregnant after one year of regular unprotected intercourse, a condition that affects an estimated 10% of American couples. In *primary infertility* there has been no preceding pregnancy; *secondary infertility* follows one or more pregnancies. In approximately 40% of cases the cause lies in the man and most often is poor SPERM production; in another 40% of cases the cause lies in the woman; and in the remaining 20% the cause is either a combination of factors in both or is never determined. In women common causes of infertility are hormonal dysfunction so that ovulation does not take place or the eggs produced are not viable; blockage in the FALLOPIAN TUBES so that the eggs cannot enter or pass through them, usually owning to scar tissue resulting from PELVIC INFLAMMATORY DISEASE or ENDOMETRIOSIS; malformation of the uterus or fallopian tubes; disorders affecting the cervix so that sperm cannot move up through it, because or either local inflammation or hostile secretions; an immunologic reaction, resulting in the production of antibodies to the partner's sperm; and inability to remain pregnant (see HABITUAL MISCARRIAGE).

A number of medications also may compromise fertility. Hormones, antibiotics and antihypertensive drugs can prevent embryo implantation. Painkillers such as aspirin and ibuprofen can, at midcycle, suppress ovulation, as can antidepressants, hallucinogens and alcohol. Sometimes simply stopping these drugs restores fertility.

Determining the cause of infertility is the province of the fertility specialist, or *sterologist*. Reproductive endocrinology and fertility now constitute a certified subspecialty of the American Board of Obstetrics and Gynecology. Often these physicians are affiliated with a university fertility research program, an infertility clinic or an in vitro fertilization center, and they are skilled in microsurgery techniques. To locate such a physician, contact your local chapter of RESOLVE, Inc., a national organization devoted to helping infertile couples (see the Appendix), your county medical society or a nearby fertility clinic.

An infertility workup begins with a careful history and physical examination of both partners, including blood and urine tests. Among the routine tests usually made are semen analysis (see SPERM); BASAL BODY TEMPERATURE charts or an endometrial biopsy (see BIOPSY, def. 8) to find out if and when the woman is ovulating; a SIMS-HUHNER TEST to check the cervical mucus; one of various tests to determine if the fallopian tubes are obstructed (see HYSTEROSALPINGOGRAPHY); blood tests to measure hormone levels; checking if sperm is inhibited by the presence of VARICOCELE; and a test for sperm incompatibility (see DUKE'S TEST), which usually is performed last because it is least likely to be correctible.

If the partner's semen analysis is normal but the cervical mucus test shows few or no sperm, different timing, techniques and positions for intercourse may be suggested. If none of these is effective, ARTIFICIAL INSEMINATION with either the partner's sperm or, if semen samples show insufficient healthy sperm, a donor's sperm may be considered.

In the woman, cervical mucus consistency can be changed by estrogen therapy and cervical infections cured by antibiotics or other treatment. Also, artificial insemination involving insertion of the partner's sperm directly into the uterus may overcome problems in the cervix. Ovulation can be induced or improved by treatment with clomiphene citrate or human menopausal gonadotropin or other medications (see FERTILITY DRUG). Uterine fibroids preventing the egg's implantation in the uterine wall may be corrected by surgery. Sometimes obstructed tubes can be opened by using a balloon catheter similar to those used to clear blocked arteries, or corrected by surgery (see TUBEROPLASTY). Often, however, they cannot be reconstructed successfully; then an embryo transplant procedure may be needed to result in a successful pregnancy (see IN VITRO FERTILIZATION). Antibody formation against the partner's sperm sometimes is reduced by using a condom for intercourse for a period of six months, during which time the antibody level may decline markedly; if this measure does not help, artificial insemination directly into the uterus normally will. However, while far less expensive than IN VITRO FERTILIZATION, intrauterine insemination or ovulation induction, alone or in combination, achieve pregnancy only between 5 and 15% per cycle.

A recent study found that consuming whole milk instead of skim or low-fat products may decrease the risk for infertility caused by failure to ovulate. The study found that an extra eight-ounce serving of whole milk every day cut the risk of failure to ovulate by 50%. However, more research is required before this result prompted a recommendation to consume whole-milk foods to women trying to become pregnant.

See also OLIGOSPERMIA; STERILITY.

inflammation   The body's protective response to injury or destruction of its tissues by microorganisms such as bacteria, a foreign body (such as a splinter), poison or some other trauma. In effect the body walls off the injured tissue (and, sometimes, the agent causing the injury) from the rest. The classic signs of inflammation are pain, heat, redness, swelling and loss of function. Not all these signs are present with every inflammation. The presence of inflammation does not necessarily signal INFECTION, but neglected inflammation often will become complicated by infection.

inflammatory bowel disease   Chronic inflammation of the lining of the intestines, speeding up the normal passage of food and causing diarrhea. Poor food absorption can cause weight loss and nutritional deficiencies, and inflammation and erosion of the intestinal lining causes ulceration or fissures that can bleed, resulting in bloody stools. The two principal forms of inflammatory bowel disease are *Crohn's disease* and *ulcerative colitis,* and more than half of patients with them are women. Ulcerative colitis can affect any part of the large intestine. Crohn's typically affects the lower part of the intestine but can also produce inflammation in any part of the colon and digestive system, from the mouth to the anus.

The cause of inflammatory bowel disease appears to be a bacterial trigger that sets up an uncontrolled immune response in susceptible individuals. Besides bloody diarrhea, symptoms include weight loss, abdominal pain and cramps, bloating and constipation. Because these are so similar to IRRITABLE BOWEL SYNDROME, a disorder that affects muscle contractions in the colon, as well as to various gastrointestinal infections, diagnosis requires ruling out other conditions. Inflammatory bowel disease tends to be chronic and characterized by repeated flare-ups. There is no definitive cure, so treatment is aimed at reducing inflammation and relieving symptoms. Medications include anti-inflammatory and antidiarrheal drugs as well as immune-system modulators. Two drugs are now approved for moderate and severe Crohn's disease. One is Remicade (infliximab) a monoclonal antibody, to which not every patient responds, and those who

do respond can build resistance to it over time. The other is Humira (adalimubab), approved earlier for other disorders that seems to work well in Crohn's. Approved for limited use in Crohn's is the arthritis drug Cimzia (certolizumab pegol). Still another possible medication is the multiple sclerosis remedy Tysabri (natalizumab). However, it was withdrawn from the market after being linked to a rare brain infection, and then in 2006 was approved for very limited use. In extreme cases surgery may be indicated to repair intestinal narrowing or obstruction, and some cases of ulcerative colitis may require ILEOSTOMY.

inflammatory breast cancer   See CANCER, INFLAMMATORY BREAST.

infusion   See HERBAL REMEDIES.

inherited disorder   See BIRTH DEFECTS.

injectable contraceptive   See DEPO-PROVERA.

insemination   The EJACULATION of semen into the vagina.

See also ARTIFICIAL INSEMINATION; SPERM.

insomnia   Also *sleeplessness.* Persistent lack of sleep or disturbed sleep patterns. A very common complaint, it is associated with a number of physical and emotional disorders. Insomnia also is common in late pregnancy, when it may be difficult to find a comfortable sleeping position or one that is comfortable for more than a couple of hours at a time. The safest solution is to make up for sleep loss by napping briefly whenever possible during the day and to avoid all sedatives (even mild ones should not be taken without consulting one's clinician). Insomnia also is common during perimenopause and menopause, particularly if sleep is interrupted by nighttime hot flashes and sweats. Estrogen therapy can alleviate such insomnia, but whether it does so because it relieves the hot flashes or because it actually alters sleep patterns is not known; the former is more likely. According to a recent study, from age 45 on, women have more insomnia than men do and continue to do so for the rest of their lives, indicating that hormone status is probably related to sleep quality. Sleeplessness or disturbed sleep also may be caused by physical pain (discomfort is usually worse at night, partly because there are fewer activities to serve as a distraction), increasing age, emotional distress of various kinds (anxiety, stress, depression) and shifting to a different time pattern or zone (jet lag, usually temporary). Older people tend to need less sleep and often experience interrupted sleep; this is thought to be perfectly normal, since metabolism in general slows down with advancing age. Worrying is a time-honored cause of wakefulness. Also, severe depression can cause a person either to sleep excessively or to awaken very early (several hours before the accustomed time) and be unable to fall asleep again.

Most medications for insomnia are hypnotic sedatives that depress brain function. The principal *sleeping pills* are barbiturates (phenobarbital, amobarbital, etc.), nonbarbiturates (bromides, chloral hydrate and others), antihistamines (most nonprescription pills are of this class) and benzodiazepines (TRANQUILIZERS). All of them involve some risk of habituation and tolerance (needing ever larger doses to be effective), and some are addictive. They should be used, therefore, in only the smallest possible amounts for the shortest possible time, and never without medical supervision. A newer class of sleeping pills, sold only by prescription, are nonbenzodiazepines. They include eszopiclone (Lunesta), zolpidem (Ambien) and zaleplon (Sonesta), and are rapidly replacing benzodiazepines. With the latter, people develop tolerance and must keep increasing dosage for the same effect. Benzodiazepines also can cause rebound insomnia (a recurrence of insomnia after stopping the drug) and other withdrawal symptoms, such as nightmares. Nonbenzodiazepines are less likely to cause tolerance or withdrawal symptoms. Lunesta has been approved by the FDA for as long as six months of nightly use. Other drugs in this class are approved only for 35 days or less. Before considering medication, it is advisable to try such old-fashioned and much safer approaches as vigorous exercise (outdoors if possible) on a regular basis but not within three hours of bedtime; using the bed for nothing but sleep or sex; going to bed only when one feels sleepy; taking a warm bath (but not too hot) and/or drinking a glass of warm milk or mild herb tea before going to bed; and avoiding cola, coffee, tea and other caffeine-containing drinks after 4 P.M. When one does have trouble sleeping, getting out of bed to do something productive or pleasant—writing a letter, reading, doing a chore—may relieve some of the anxiety often experienced with wakefulness. Some HERBAL REMEDIES taken for their soothing, sedative effect are teas brewed from camomile leaves and flowers (*Matricaria chamomilla*) or catnip (*Nepata cataria*). Valerian root (*Valeriana officinalis*) is widely used for this purpose in Europe, but lack of regulation and quality control in the United States means one should exercise caution with this product. Other supplements such as tryptophan and melatonin are also potentially hazardous.

insufflation, tubal   See RUBIN TEST.

intercourse, sexual   Broadly speaking, any kind of sexual contact. In practice, the term most often means coitus, involving a man and a woman.

See also anal sex, under ANUS; ORAL SEX; ORGASM; SEXUAL RESPONSE.

interferon   See IMMUNOTHERAPY.

interstitial-cell-stimulating hormone   Also *ICSH*. Another name for luteinizing hormone (LH), which in men triggers the growth of interstitial cells in the TESTES and stimulates their production of testosterone.

interstitial cystitis   See CYSTITIS, def. 2.

intraductal cancer in situ   See CANCER IN SITU.

intraductal papilloma   See DUCTAL PAPILLOMA.

intrauterine device   Also *IUD.* A device made of plastic, metal or some other material that is inserted into the uterus and allowed to remain there for months or years in order to prevent pregnancy. It is a reversible contraceptive—that is, once it is removed a woman can become pregnant if she wishes—but it differs from other reversible methods such as the diaphragm in that it must be both inserted and removed by a trained clinician, usually a physician or nurse-practitioner. It is not known exactly how the device prevents pregnancy. It does not prevent ovulation, nor does it always prevent conception. One kind of IUD, TCu-380A (Paragard), contains copper, a material that helps prevent pregnancy, although it is not known exactly how; it is known that copper causes an inflammation of the endometrium (uterine lining), to which the body's response may somehow damage sperm or interfere with fertilization and/or implantation. Another kind, Progesterone T (Progestasert System), releases synthetic progesterone (PROGESTIN), which helps prevent sperm from entering the cervix by altering the cervical mucus.

Before the insertion of an IUD, a woman should have a checkup that includes a careful history to make sure she has no reason not to use such a device. **No IUD should be used by women who have any of the following conditions:** pregnancy or suspected pregnancy; a previous ECTOPIC PREGNANCY; abnormal anatomy, such as a double uterus or very small uterus; PELVIC INFLAMMATORY DISEASE or a history of several severe pelvic infections; GONORRHEA or any other SEXUALLY TRANSMITTED DISEASE or the possibility of exposure to one; a positive test for HIV (which causes AIDS); one or more fibroid tumors large enough to distort the shape of the uterus; vaginal bleeding from unknown causes; a history of heavy menstrual bleeding and/or severe menstrual cramps; active cervical infection (cervicitis) or an abnormal PAP SMEAR; endometrial disorders, especially ENDOMETRIOSIS or ENDOMETRIAL HYPERPLASIA; heart disease; diabetes; liver disease; anemia, leukemia, clotting disorders or sickle-cell disease; current use of cortisone-type drugs or anticoagulants. Further, copper-containing IUDs should not be used by women allergic to copper.

In addition, clinicians are reluctant to insert an IUD in young women (under 25) who have had no children and have numerous sexual partners because of their increased risk of contracting a sexually transmitted disease. At the least, such women should have a gonorrhea test (since gonorrhea often has no symptoms in women) before an IUD is inserted. Indeed, many clinicians feel that no childless premenopausal woman should use an IUD because of its association with subsequent infertility (see below).

A woman considering an IUD should first have a checkup to learn more about it and any contraindications she may have. The checkup should include a pelvic examination to ensure that her organs are normal, and tests for gonorrhea and chlamydia (which can be symptomless). Once the decision to use an IUD is made, it can be inserted any time during the menstrual cycle provided she is sure she is not pregnant (therefore *during* a menstrual period is a good option, since IUDs in pregnancy are dangerous; see below). Some clinicians say it can be inserted immediately after an abortion, but others believe it then increases risk of uterine rupture, heavy bleeding and infection. It is safe to insert during the first menstrual period following abortion. It can be inserted as early as eight weeks following vaginal delivery of a baby, even if the woman has not yet resumed menstruating, and three months after delivery by Cesarean section. Occasionally an IUD is inserted for EMERGENCY CONTRACEPTION, that is, within seven days of unprotected intercourse, to avoid pregnancy. However, this should be done only after a single instance of unprotected intercourse, because the insertion of an IUD after implantation of a fertilized egg can lead to serious damage. Some clinicians consider it too risky a procedure to perform.

There are several types of IUD. Copper IUDs are made of plastic with a wire or band of copper partially covering them; the TCu-380A (Paragard) lasts for 10 years, but other copper IUDs must be changed more often. The Progestasert, which releases progesterone, must be changed every year because the supply of the hormone is used up in that time. Progesterone helps reduce heavy menstrual flow experienced by some women. Another progestin-releasing device approved in 2000, Mirena, can remain in place for five years. Possible side effects, which usually disappear within four months of insertion, include breast tenderness, nausea, headache and mood changes.

An IUD can be inserted in a doctor's office, clinic or the outpatient department of a hospital. A pelvic examination is performed first to investigate the position of the uterus, and a long, thin measuring instrument called a uterine sound is inserted through the cervix to the top of the uterus, to measure its length. (Local anesthesia can be used if the cervix is tightly closed but prolongs the procedure.) The sound is withdrawn, the IUD loaded into its inserter, and a stop is positioned on the inserter at the distance indicated by the sound. The loaded inserter then is passed into the uterus until the stop-mark reaches the cervix. The device is released by means of a plunger mechanism, and the inserter is withdrawn, leaving the IUD in place with its attached strings extending into the vagina.

The IUD is effective against pregnancy immediately. Most failures occur during the first six months of use, so it is advisable to use a backup contraceptive during that period. Among the most common problems associated with an IUD is spontaneous expulsion of the device from the uterus, which happens most often during the first three months after insertion. Therefore women are advised to check for the IUD strings inside the vagina once a week; if she feels something hard or can't find the strings, the IUD is not in place and she should return to the practitioner. Further, a follow-up examination is recommended within three months of insertion.

The insertion process ranges from being moderately uncomfortable to quite painful, with bleeding and cramping. After insertion, tampons and vaginal intercourse should be avoided for the remainder of that menstrual cycle. The cramps gradually diminish. If they remain severe for more than 24 hours and/or there is fever, there may be an infection, and the clinician should be contacted immediately. Thereafter, most women find periods are heavier and longer than before, with more cramps as well. Also, many IUD users experience staining between periods, especially at midcycle; such

bleeding should always be checked lest it be caused by some other disorder. BREAKTHROUGH BLEEDING after an IUD has been in place three months or longer often is an early sign of pelvic inflammatory disease.

Another complication is perforation, which happens most often during insertion. A puncture is made into the abdominal cavity (usually by the sound) and in time the IUD slips out of the uterus and into the abdomen, where it may cause no problem (unless it is copper-releasing) but can no longer, of course, prevent pregnancy. Absence of the strings protruding from the cervix therefore usually means either that the IUD has been expelled into the vagina or that it has moved elsewhere out of the uterus, and for this reason regular checking of the strings is important.

If the IUD remains in position, it is very effective in preventing pregnancy: 99% for the copper IUD and 98.5% for progesterone. This means if 100 women used it for a year, no more than one of them would become pregnant. For those who do become pregnant with an IUD in place, the consequences can be serious. The likelihood of miscarriage is very high—about 50%—and if infection is present, the situation can be very dangerous. Therefore, if a woman with an IUD skips a period or has other signs of early pregnancy, she should see her clinician very soon to rule out pregnancy; if she also has symptoms of infection, she should see someone immediately. If she is pregnant, the IUD should be removed within 24 hours to prevent infection, whether she intends to continue the pregnancy or not.

Another considerable risk is that of ectopic pregnancy, which can be life-threatening. It is not known whether IUDs actually increase the risk of ectopic pregnancy or if they simply are less effective in preventing it. In any case, the incidence in IUD users appears to be considerably higher than average.

Apart from pregnancy, the principal complication of the IUD is a much higher incidence of pelvic infection, so much so that the use of IUDs is considered a leading cause of infertility due to pelvic inflammatory disease. Such infections range from mild to severe and can become life-threatening. Some studies indicate that infection often occurs during or soon after insertion, and administering an antibiotic at the time of insertion helps prevent that.

Signs of infection therefore should be attended to promptly; they include abdominal pain or tenderness, pain during vaginal intercourse, fever or chills and unusual vaginal bleeding or discharge (see also PELVIC INFLAMMATORY DISEASE). Infections of the cervix (cervicitis) also tend to occur more frequently in IUD users. Because of these complications and the side effects (chiefly more menstrual cramps and heavier flow), about half of the women who use IUDs have them removed within two years of their insertion.

Removing an IUD can be done anytime, although at midcycle it is possible that pregnancy from recent sexual intercourse could occur. Removal is quicker and less painful than insertion, and if the woman wishes to continue IUD use, another can be inserted at once.

Putting something inside the uterus to prevent pregnancy allegedly was first done by ancient camel drivers who inserted pebbles into their animals to prevent them from becoming pregnant on a long desert trek. Modern IUDs date from the early 1900s and a variety of materials have been used, ranging from silkworm gut to silver wire. Plastic IUDs were marketed in the late 1950s, copper was added a decade later and progestin in the 1970s. Since their development, a number of devices have been taken off the market. One was the Dalkon Shield (in 1974), which was linked to the deaths of a number of women and was thought to be responsible for uterine infection, septic abortion and hysterectomy in more than 2,000 others. Since then IUDs have been used much less in the United States but continue to be very popular elsewhere, especially in Asia.

intrauterine polyps   See POLYP, def. 3.

introitus   An opening, specifically the opening of the VAGINA, which occupies the lower part of the VESTIBULE. It varies considerably in size and shape. In virgins it is hidden by the overlapping LABIA minora; when exposed, it may appear to be almost completely blocked by the HYMEN.

intromission   See ERECTION.

inverted nipple   See NIPPLE.

in vitro fertilization   Also *IVF, test-tube baby.* A procedure in which a number of eggs are removed from a woman's ovaries after they have been stimulated by a FERTILITY DRUG and are then fertilized outside the body by sperm from her partner or a donor. (*In vitro* is Latin for "in glass" and refers to the laboratory dish originally used for this purpose.) Sometimes a DONOR EGG is used instead of the woman's own. The embryos are allowed to divide in a protected environment for two or three days and then the healthiest looking ones are reinserted into the woman's uterus. Because not all will be successfully implanted, practitioners traditionally transfer several in hopes of at least one implant. (Also see below.) The first pregnancy begun in this way and successfully brought to term took place in England, where the first "test-tube baby" was born in 1978. In 1980 the first North American clinic for this purpose was opened in Norfolk, Virginia, and in the next decade more than 200 in vitro centers opened in the United States. However, the success rate of different clinics is highly variable, so women considering in vitro fertilization should investigate resources with care (see accompanying box; also see under infertility in the Appendix). Further, the procedure is quite expensive—approximately $8,000 per attempt—and rarely is covered by medical insurance. Nevertheless, approximately one in 80 to 100 births in the United States now result from IVF.

By law, all IVF clinics in the United States must report outcomes to the Centers for Disease Control and Prevention, and national and clinic-specific outcomes are available on the Internet (www.cdc.gov/ART/ART2003/index.htm). At this writing, the most recent statistics date from 2003, but they will be periodically updated.

Before IVF, most couples will have had a standard infertility evaluation, including semen analysis; assessment of the female reproductive tract by transvaginal ultrasound or a similar process; and tests to detect ovulation. The best candidates for achieving pregnancy in this way are women

QUESTIONS TO ASK ABOUT AN IN VITRO CLINIC

- How long has it been operating, and how many babies have been born?
- How is the success rate calculated? Does it include older couples and those with male infertility problems?
- How many in vitro cycles are performed each year? (Centers performing 100 or more tend to have higher success rate.)
- Do quoted costs include medications? ultrasound examinations?
- Is the clinic a member of the Society for Assisted Reproductive Technology of the American Fertility Society (which sets standards)?

in their 20s or early 30s whose only reproductive problem is blocked fallopian tubes and whose partners have a normal sperm count (unless donor sperm is to be used). The effect of a woman's age on the outcomes of IVF with her own eggs is striking. The rate of live births in women up to age 34 is between 40 and 49% per embryo transfer. After that the live-birthrate declines by 2 to 6% for each one-year increase in age. By age 43 it is only 5% and at this age 50% of pregnancies conceived with IVF result in miscarriage. Often a couple must undergo psychological tests and counseling to make sure they are prepared for the emotional stress that accompanies the procedure. The woman then is given FERTILITY DRUGS so that a number of ovarian follicles will mature (instead of just one per cycle). Follicle development is monitored by transvaginal ultrasound. When conditions are deemed to be optimal, an injection of HUMAN CHORIONIC GONADOTROPIN will trigger ovulation in about 36 hours. Eggs are retrieved through the vagina by means of ultrasound-guided aspiration of follicular fluid. The mature eggs are placed with the partner's sperm in a culture dish, which is then put into an incubator for another 36 hours or so. In most IVF procedures today eggs are fertilized by intracytoplasmic sperm injection, in which a single sperm is injected into the egg using a thin glass pipette. (Also see below). Multiple embryos are cultured, often for three days or five days, before being inserted by catheter into the woman's uterus. Good-quality embryos not transferred may be frozen. (A newer technique, ZIFT, inserts the embryo directly into a fallopian tube; see GAMETE INTRAFALLOPIAN TRANSFER.) Progesterone then is administered to support a pregnancy. Within 10 to 14 days one can tell if pregnancy has occurred. An estimated 10 to 15% of women reach this point. For those who do not, the procedure may be repeated.

Different clinics and practitioners have developed numerous modifications of this basic procedure. For example, some frequently put several embryos (two to eight) in the woman's uterus to increase implantation rates, a practice that has led to an increase in multiple births. One method of dealing with this is *selective reduction*, that is, terminating one or more fetuses to improve the odds that some will survive and be healthy; however, few women are able to accept this procedure. Another practice, called *blastocyst transfer*, is to transfer only five-day-old embryos, or blastocysts (possible only with the development of better growth media). A recent study showed that a *single embryo transfer* resulted in nearly as many live births as transferring two embryos and greatly reduces multiple births. In vitro fertilization also allows testing of embryos for a serious hereditary disorder, such as Tay-Sachs. Called *preimplantation genetic diagnosis*, it involves testing the DNA of the embryo's cell for the harmful gene, so only healthy embryos will be transferred to the woman's uterus.

If sperm have difficulty penetrating the egg, it is possible to treat the sperm with salt solutions or albumin in the laboratory, helping remove the outer coat, or to make a small opening in the outer egg wall, or zona pellucida (*partial zona dissection*) to increase chances of sperm penetration, or even to insert the sperm inside the egg using a hollow needle (*intracytoplasmic sperm injection,* or *ICSI*). After fertilization takes place, some clinics freeze additional embryos (if the couple permits) for use if the initial cycle fails. Babies conceived via in vitro fertilization run the risk of lower birth weight, sometimes dangerously low, as well as a greater risk of a major birth defect diagnosed by age 1 than naturally conceived infants. Also, in the case of women expecting more than one child, the risk of PREECLAMPSIA may double.

Even when women become pregnant on a first attempt, about one-fourth of these pregnancies end in miscarriage; the success rate in achieving pregnancy is estimated to be at best 30% with three attempts. Beyond three or four cycles the rate does not appear to improve much. The reasons for failure vary, ranging from selection of good candidates and judgment on when to retrieve eggs to technical skill in retrieving eggs, bringing egg and sperm together, and transferring the embryos. In view of all these variables, it is prudent to investigate the success rate of any clinic one is considering (see table).

A newer method, called *in vitro maturation (IVM)*, involves the collection of immature egg cells. Instead of priming a woman with fertility drugs so that the egg cells mature, immature eggs are removed and made to mature outside the ovary. Success hinges on both locating them and stimulating them to mature. The follicles containing such eggs are located by means of ultrasound, and the eggs are plucked out with a specially designed needle. A cell-culturing procedure then ripens them in one or two days in the laboratory, where they subsequently are doused with sperm and fertilized. Because it eliminates drugs, curtails testing and reduces doctors' fees, this method is far less expensive. Still newer is a technique called *cytoplasmic transfer* or *ooplasmic transfer.* Here an egg is taken from both an infertile woman and a fertile donor, and sperm is taken from the infertile woman's mate. A small amount of the donor egg's cytoplasm is removed and injected into the infertile woman's egg, along with sperm. Another version of this technique, called *nuclear transfer,* involves placing a cell such as a skin cell from an older woman and placing it inside a younger woman's egg, whose original DNA was removed. Theoretically the new cell will divide to become a cell more successful in leading to pregnancy. To date this method has succeeded in animals, but it has not been approved by the U.S. Food and Drug Administration for use by humans.

Some couples frustrated by unsuccessful in vitro fertilization have turned to *embryo adoption.* Some women undergoing successful IVF have an excess of frozen embryos, which then are implanted in the infertile woman.

A recent and still controversial development is the use of in vitro fertilization to impregnate postmenopausal women. Using donated eggs and the sperm of either their partner or another donor and implanting the embryo inside the woman's uterus, healthy children have been born to women in their 50s. Most in vitro clinics do not accept patients over the age of 40, because their eggs are old and the success rate for them is minimal. Donor eggs greatly increase the odds. However, there still are health risks—increased risk of diabetes, obesity, high blood pressure and other complications of pregnancy in the mother, which in turn can harm the fetus. There also are ethical and social concerns.

See also DONOR EGG; SPERM BANK.

involution, uterine   The return of the uterus to its prepregnant condition following pregnancy. It begins almost immediately after delivery of the baby, even before expulsion of the placenta (see under LABOR), and is aided by continued uterine contractions for about 48 hours after delivery. From a 2-pound (0.9 kilo) mass of muscle immediately after birth, it changes back into a smooth, hard, gourd-shaped organ. By the end of a week it weighs 1 pound and has descended to about 2 inches (5 centimeters) above the pubic bone. Soon afterward it sinks within the pelvis and can no longer be felt by merely palpating the abdomen. The process of shrinkage progresses more rapidly when a woman breast-feeds. It continues until, after five or six weeks following delivery, the uterus is again the size and shape of a pear, weighing about 2 ounces (56 grams). The growth in the uterus during pregnancy consists of an increase in size of each individual muscle fiber, which in turn must shrink again during involution. This process of growth and involution takes place with each pregnancy, making the uterus unique among body organs.

iron   See ANEMIA; DIET.

irradiation   See RADIATION THERAPY.

irregular periods   A widely varying MENSTRUAL CYCLE, with menstrual flow occurring at very irregular intervals, for example, 21 days, then 42 days, then 35 days, then 28 days, and so on. This condition frequently occurs in girls during their first two or three years of menstruating and in women approaching menopause. It is caused by hormone imbalance, particularly lack of progesterone in the absence of ovulation (see ANOVULATORY BLEEDING). Irregular periods also can be caused by stress, emotional problems, crash reducing diets, thyroid disturbances, iron or platelet deficiency (see ANEMIA), any serious illness, and a variety of pelvic lesions ranging from endometrial hyperplasia to cancer.

See also BREAKTHROUGH BLEEDING; OLIGOMENORRHEA; POLYMENORRHEA.

irritable bowel syndrome   An abnormally active lower bowel, leading to such symptoms as periodic diarrhea or constipation, sometimes occurring alternately, abdominal bloating and distention, and changes in stools. It is an aggravating condition, and no organic cause for it has yet been identified. Further, because its symptoms are similar to those of numerous other conditions, including INFLAMMATORY BOWEL DISEASE, diagnosis is difficult. Nevertheless it affects 25 million to 45 million Americans, some two-thirds of whom are women.

Diagnosis involves ruling out physical illnesses such as endometriosis, ulcerative colitis, infection and colon cancer. A careful history of diet, medications, sleep and exercise habits and emotional distress should be followed by a physical exam, laboratory tests (including one for lactose intolerance and a stool sample) and sigmoidoscopy. Emotional state definitely plays a role, anxiety or intense anger increasing intestinal contractions and even triggering diarrhea.

Treatment focuses on relieving discomfort and adjusting bowel habits. A high-fiber, low-fat diet is often recommended, and gas-producing foods such as cabbage should be avoided. A bulk-producing product such as psyllium may be recommended for constipation, and loperamide (Imodium) or another agent to relieve diarrhea. Foods that trigger gas and bloating should be avoided: among them are beans, bananas, carbonated drinks, dairy products and cruciform vegetables (cabbage, cauliflower and broccoli among others). Two drugs alter the action of the neurotransmitter serotonin in the colon. One, alosetron (Lotronex), worked for the severe diarrhea-predominant syndrome, but some women suffered such severe complications that the manufacturer withdrew the drug from the market; it was later restored, but only under a tightly controlled prescribing program. For severe constipation, tegaserod maleate (Zelnorm) was often helpful but in March 2007 it, too, was withdrawn from the market owing to serious side effects. A few months later it was restored, under a new restricted access program but was discontinued in 2008 and can be used only in life-threatening cases. In 2008 the FDA approved Amitiza (lubiprostone) for women aged 18 or older. At this writing it is the only available prescription medication for severe constipation. The most common side effects are mild to moderate nausea and diarrhea.

Several other serotonin-modulating medications are now being studied. For alternating diarrhea and constipation, polycarbophil (Fibercon, Equalactin, Mitrolan) may be effective. Antispasmodic drugs such as dicyclomine (Bentyl) or hyoscyamine (Levsin) may ease bowel spasms and pain, and antianxiety drugs or an antidepressant may ease emotional stress. An herbal remedy is peppermint, in the form of a tea or enteric-coated peppermint oil capsules; however, extreme caution is needed, since as little as 12 drops of pure, uncoated peppermint oil can produce heartburn and cardiac arrhythmias. The tea is probably safe, as are capsules that contain 0.2 to 0.4 milliliters of peppermint oil, with a maximum dosage of three capsules a day. However, people with gastroesophageal reflux disease should avoid peppermint oil, which can worsen reflux symptoms. Some patients have found relief with PROBIOTICS, live bacteria taken in capsule or powder form or in yogurt. They help restore bacterial balance in the intestine. Two that have shown promise in relieving such symptoms as gas, bloating and diarrhea are *Lactobacillus plantarum*, marketed as Culturelle, and *Bacillus infantis*, sold as Align.

itching   Also *pruritus*. An irritating sensation of the skin that is relieved by scratching. Although itching may be a symptom of skin disease as well as other disorders in both men and women, two kinds affect only women. One occurs during the latter months of pregnancy, when some women develop intense itching, sometimes accompanied by jaundice. Also called *cholestasis of pregnancy*, it is caused by the effects of increased hormone levels on liver function and disappears completely after delivery. However, it is apt to recur in subsequent pregnancies and also if an estrogen-high oral contraceptive is later used. The other, itching of the vulva and vagina, is common in VULVITIS and VAGINITIS, which may be due to inflammation and infection from a variety of causes, as well as from dry skin and membranes (see VAGINAL ATROPHY). The itching from YEAST INFECTION often spreads to the area around the anus as well. Treating the underlying causes of infection usually cures the itching, but sometimes a topical cortisone ointment must be used for a time to clear up the skin involved.

IUD   See INTRAUTERINE DEVICE.

jaundice   See NEONATAL JAUNDICE.

jelly, contraceptive   See LUBRICANT; SPERMICIDE.

karyotyping   A genetic study to diagnose problems leading to habitual miscarriage and possible birth defects. Chromosomes from a woman's tissue, usually white blood cells scraped from the lining of the mouth, are photographed, the photographs are enlarged and the chromosomes cut out and arranged according to size and structure on a chart called a *karyotype*. This process may reveal various chromosomal abnormalities, such as the fragile X trait responsible for a common form of mental retardation (see FRAGILE X SYNDROME).

See also CHROMOSOME.

Kegel exercises   Also *pelvic floor exercises*. Exercises to strengthen the pubococcygeous muscle of the pelvic floor in order to reduce sagging, prevent URINARY INCONTINENCE, strengthen orgasmic response and prepare for and recover from childbirth. Named for their inventor, Arnold Kegel, an American physician, they consist of alternately contracting (tightening) and relaxing the pelvic floor muscles. To locate the right place, place one finger in the vagina and contract the muscle around your finger; if you're uncertain, ask your clinician to do this. The contraction will be felt mostly in the anal area. Hold each contraction for 3 to 5 seconds and rest the same amount of time between them. Work up to 10-second contractions, performing them 30 to 40 times a day (they can be divided into groups of 10, done at various times of day). It may take some weeks to experience improvement. For stress incontinence, it is helpful to do a Kegel just before coughing or sneezing to prevent leakage. For urge incontinence, do one when experiencing the urge to void but no toilet is available.

For those unable to manage Kegels on their own, a probe can be placed inside the vaginal canal to electrically stimulate Kegels. It can be used either at home or in a clinician's office. At home, two 15-minute sessions a day are recommended.

keratosis   See CANCER, SKIN; SKIN CHANGES.

Kerr incision   See CESAREAN SECTION.

Klinefelter syndrome   A congenital condition in which a male has three chromosomes, X, X and Y, instead of one X and one Y chromosome, and therefore usually is sterile. Klinefelter syndrome occurs in about 1 of every 500 to 1,000 live male births and, being a chromosomal defect, may be detected with AMNIOCENTESIS or CHORIONIC VILLUS SAMPLING. Although the condition is widespread, the symptoms and characteristics resulting from having an extra chromosome are uncommon, and many men live out their lives without ever knowing they have the chromosomal abnormality. Those that do generally have a rounded body type, tend to be overweight and quite tall, occasionally have breast enlargement, lack of facial and body hair, small testes, and weakly developed secondary sex characteristics (deep voice, beard, pubic hair, chest hair). There is a much higher than normal incidence of learning problems, especially language disabilities. However, administration of testosterone at the onset of puberty can diminish these symptoms, and also the emotional difficulties experienced by some individuals, and should be continued for life. Further, special education can help overcome the learning difficulties. For those who develop embarrassingly extreme breast growth at puberty, breast reduction surgery may be an option. In most cases XXY males do not produce enough sperm to father a child. However, no individual should automatically assume infertility without further testing, for a small percentage of such individuals are fertile.

knee problems Pain and stiffness owing to injuries to the anterior cruciate ligament (ACL), meniscus, tendons or patella. Women are more susceptible than men to serious injuries to the ligaments that hold the knee together and to chronic problems involving the kneecap (patella) and the cartilage (menisci) that cushion the contact between the upper and lower leg bones. The woman's wider pelvis creates a sharper angle where the leg bones meet, making for alignment problems for the kneecap. Women tend to land from jumps with their knees inward, which stresses the ACL, ligaments and cartilage. Also, the notch through which the ACL passes is narrower in women than in men, making it more susceptible to tearing. Further, women's ligaments tend to be more lax than men's, and the muscles that support the knee may not be as strong as they should be.

For women who engage in sports like basketball, soccer, tennis and skiing, the most common injury is to the anterior cruciate ligament, a tough band of connecting tissue in the center of the knee that is its main stabilizer. It can be injured by a fall, twist or direct blow. A torn ligament is extremely painful, and the knee swells and is unstable. If it does not heal, it may be repaired by arthroscopic surgery or even be replaced with tissue from another area or a cadaver. Similar pain and swelling is the hallmark of a torn meniscus, one of several small cartilage discs that pad the junction of the upper and lower leg bones. It can be torn by a sudden twist or repeated squatting. Arthroscopic surgery can either repair damage on the outer edge of the meniscus or remove injured tissue from its inside. A very common problem in women especially is chondromalacia patella (Latin for front-of-the-

knee pain), or runner's knee. Often modifying activities that cause pain and doing special exercises to strengthen muscles so that they counteract tight ligaments solve the problem, but if these are ineffective surgery can correct it. The patella's underside is lined with cartilage, which is highly susceptible to wear and tear. Again, with arthroscopy surgeons can shave away cartilage to smooth the undersurface and, if the kneecap is off center, clip bands of tissue that hold it tight in the proper position. The patellar tendon is also subject to injury; patellar tendinitis, or "jumper's knee," is caused by repetitive high-impact activities such as basketball or aerobics.

Both meniscus and tendon injuries are first treated with RICE—that is, rest, ice, compression and elevation. For tendinitis, steroid injections around the inflamed tendon may be helpful.

While arthroscopic knee surgery involves only several pencil-width incisions through which the surgeon views and repairs the damage, it still is surgery and requires a recovery period and rehabilitation. Prevention is a better route by far. Keeping one's weight down places less stress on the knees even for simple walking. Also, women athletes, unlike men, rely more on their quadriceps (front thigh muscles) to stabilize the knee than on the stronger hamstrings behind the thigh. Exercises to stretch and strengthen the hamstrings so as to maintain good muscle balance in the legs can help avoid ligament tears. Stretching muscles around the knee before exercise is important, as are properly fitting shoes. If knee pain is a problem, do not rely on painkillers, knee supports and ice to continue active sports but rather consult an orthopedic surgeon or other specialist in this field. Instead of surgery, he or she may prescribe special exercise, special supports and possibly orthotic shoe inserts.

In some women knee problems are the result of osteoarthritis or rheumatoid arthritis. With the former, cartilage is roughened, and small bits of it may be floating within the joint. It can be arthroscopically smoothed and removed. With the latter, the painful synovial lining of the joint can be removed. (See illustration accompanying RHEUMATOID ARTHRITIS.)

A last resort is surgical replacement of the knee with a prosthesis, most often done in cases of severe OSTEOARTHRITIS. Several newer options exist. One is a kidney-shaped disc made of a composite, cobalt chrome, inserted between the knee bones; it may help for a time but not for severe osteoarthritis. Traditionally, *total knee replacement (TKR)* has been used, but although it relieves pain and improves function, recovery tends to be slow and painful. A newer technique called *small incision (TKR)* or *mini-incision TKR* avoids cutting the quadriceps tendon and flipping the kneecap; it allows quicker recovery, less pain and less scarring, but it is less widely available.

Kronig-Selheim incision   See CESAREAN SECTION.

K-Y jelly   See LUBRICANT.

labia Also *labium* (sing.). A Latin word meaning "lips," referring to two sets of tissue folds that serve to protect the vaginal opening. The outer, larger pair of labia, or *labia majora* (*labium majorus,* sing.), are composed mostly of fatty tissue and correspond to the scrotum in men. Extending back from the MONS VENERIS to the perineum, they vary considerably in size and appearance, but on the average they are 7 to 8 centimeters (3 inches) long, 2 to 3 centimeters (1 inch) wide and 1 to 1½ centimeters (½ inch) thick. In children and virgins they usually lie close together, completely concealing what lies underneath, whereas in women who have borne one or more children they often gape widely. Their outer surface is dry, covered with skin and, after puberty, with hair. Their inner surface is moist, has little or no hair and is richly supplied with sebaceous (oil) glands. After menopause the labia majora gradually shrink in size.

The inner pair of labia, or *labia minor* (*labium minus,* sing.), are two flat, firm, reddish folds that extend down from the clitoris. At their upper end each labium minus divides into two separate folds that form the prepuce (foreskin) surrounding the CLITORIS. They, too, vary greatly in size and also in shape. Before childbearing they usually are hidden by the labia majora, but afterward they may project beyond them. Their outer covering looks more like mucous membrane (like the inside of the mouth) than skin. They are hairless but have many sebaceous glands and some sweat glands. The interior is supplied with numerous nerve endings and so is extremely sensitive.

labor Also *accouchement, childbirth, confinement, parturition.* The process of giving birth to a baby, the actual birth being called *delivery.* In nearly all animals whose young are conceived and carried inside the mother's body, labor begins spontaneously after a more or less fixed period of time (GESTATION), when the baby is mature enough to survive in the outside world but still small enough to make its way out of the mother's body. What exactly triggers the onset of labor, in human beings or other animals, is not known.

Labor is quite literally physical work, that is, the generation of motion against resistance. The forces involved in labor are the muscles of the UTERUS, diaphragm and abdominal wall, opposed by resistance to the baby's passage by the structures of the BIRTH CANAL. Contractions of the uterine muscles, aided by hormonal changes, cause the cervix to soften, thin out and dilate to allow the baby through it. This process usually takes up most of the time of labor. Continuing contractions of the uterus and abdominal muscles then propel the baby through the bony birth canal. The muscles of the pelvic floor force the baby's head to rotate and extend as continued pressure from above expels the baby. This pressure often results in considerable molding of the baby's head in order to permit its passage.

Labor is divided into three stages. The *first stage,* which begins with the first perceived uterine contraction and ends with the full *dilation* of the cervix to a diameter of 10 centimeters (also called 5 fingers, since it is about the width of the average man's fingers held closed), involves both uterine contractions against the cervix or, if the membranes have already ruptured and separated, the pressure of the baby's presenting part against the cervix (see also AMNIOTIC SAC; DRY LABOR). During this stage of labor the cervical canal is flattened and shortened to the point of disappearing altogether (see EFFACEMENT). Some clinicians subdivide the first stage into a *prodromal* (latent and early) phase, with cervical dilation up to 4 centimeters, and an *active* phase, with dilation up to 8 centimeters.

The *second stage* of labor, or stage of expulsion, begins with the complete dilation of the cervix and ends with the expulsion of the baby (delivery). During this stage the baby descends—slowly but surely with a first baby, more rapidly in subsequent births—as it is pushed downward by the uterine muscles with the help of the abdominal muscles and the diaphragm. The amniotic membranes usually rupture during this stage if they have not done so already. In a head-first, or vertex, delivery, the baby's head begins to distend the vagina and vulva and eventually *crowns,* that is, appears in the vaginal entrance. Then the head, followed by the rest of the baby, is delivered. In a breech presentation the lower pole of the baby—that is, feet and legs

or buttocks—leads the way, followed by the trunk, shoulders and head; this requires more active effort from the mother, since the head is the largest part of the baby, and also is more hazardous to the baby, because its oxygen supply may be compromised by pressure of the umbilical cord between its body and the birth canal. (See also BREECH PRESENTATION; PROLAPSED CORD.)

The *third stage* of labor involves the separation of the PLACENTA from the uterine wall and its expulsion. As the baby is born, the uterus shrinks to fit its diminishing contents. During the process the placenta is forced down until it separates from the uterine wall and is pushed out. The remaining amniotic membranes are stripped out along with the placenta, partly by the continuing uterine contractions and partly by traction exerted by the placenta. Some women cannot push the placenta

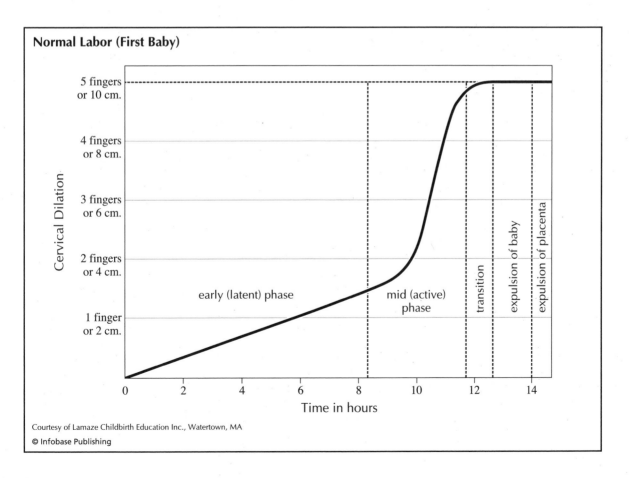

Normal Labor (First Baby)

Cervical Dilation

- 5 fingers or 10 cm.
- 4 fingers or 8 cm.
- 3 fingers or 6 cm.
- 2 fingers or 4 cm.
- 1 finger or 2 cm.

early (latent) phase

mid (active) phase

transition

expulsion of baby

expulsion of placenta

Time in hours

0   2   4   6   8   10   12   14

Courtesy of Lamaze Childbirth Education Inc., Watertown, MA

© Infobase Publishing

out of the vagina, but they can be assisted simply by pressure of the birth attendant's hand over the fundus (top of the uterus), which stimulates the uterus to contract more.

The average duration of the first stage of labor with a first baby is about 9 to 15 hours, and with subsequent children about 7 hours, but there is marked variation among individuals, and the position of the baby also affects the time (see ABNORMAL PRESENTATION; PROLONGED LABOR). Toward the end of the first stage of labor, when the cervix is dilated about 8 centimeters, the contractions become much stronger and longer, with less relaxation between them; this period is called the *transition* and often is accompanied by any of various symptoms, particularly nausea, vomiting, trembling and irritability. However, the transition rarely lasts longer than half an hour with a first baby. The average duration of the second stage is one to three hours with a first baby and 20 minutes or less with subsequent births. In the third stage, placental separation rarely takes more than two or three minutes, and placental expulsion about five minutes more. The reason for faster labor in multiparas (women who have given birth previously) is that the cervix, once dilated in labor, offers less resistance the next time; the same is true of the pelvic floor, which tends to be more relaxed. Labor also tends to proceed faster than normal when the membranes have ruptured before labor has begun, which occurs in about 12% of all cases, lasting on the average about 10 hours with first pregnancies and six hours with subsequent ones.

See also ANESTHESIA; CONTRACTION, UTERINE; FALSE LABOR; INDUCTION OF LABOR; PREPARED CHILDBIRTH.

labor, induction of   See INDUCTION OF LABOR.

lactation   The production of milk by the breasts, which is controlled by two hormones, prolactin and oxytocin. Prolactin is secreted by the pituitary gland. Except after delivery of a baby or under other special circumstances, it is inhibited (suppressed) by another substance, prolactin-inhibiting factor (PIF), secreted by the hypothalamus. After childbirth PIF is not produced and so prolactin

is released, stimulating the ACINI to secrete milk. As the baby suckles, more prolactin is released and more milk is produced, a process that continues until BREAST-FEEDING is discontinued. If a woman decides not to breast-feed, however, milk production will stop within a few days after delivery provided that her breasts are not stimulated by suckling. Binding the breasts, restricting fluid intake or administering estrogen, all measures formerly used to stop milk production, are not effective; only the lack of suckling stops lactation. Further, the use of estrogen for this purpose is associated with a higher incidence of blood clots. Stimulation from suckling also makes the posterior pituitary gland release oxytocin, the same hormone that stimulates uterine contractions during labor. It is oxytocin that is responsible for the LET-DOWN REFLEX, which squeezes milk into and through the ducts in the breast.

The preparation of the breasts for lactation begins during pregnancy, when high levels of estrogen and progesterone cause the growth of breast ducts and maturation of glandular structures. Because of the increased glandular mass, a pregnant woman's breasts enlarge significantly. During the second trimester of pregnancy the cells of the acini are stimulated to produce *colostrum,* a protein-rich yellowish fluid that also contains minerals, vitamin A, nitrogen and antibodies. Colostrum continues to be produced until two or three days after delivery, when lactation begins; it is the baby's first nourishment. If lactation is suppressed by lack of suckling, colostrum production also ceases.

After delivery the production of pituitary prolactin increases rapidly, and milk is secreted on the third or fourth day after delivery. At this time the bulk of the breasts increases considerably, by as much as one-third, a phenomenon called *engorgement.* It may be accompanied by some discomfort (tenderness and pain) that generally disappears by itself within one or two days, particularly if breast-feeding is begun. Allowing the baby to nurse very briefly and/ or manually expressing a little of the fluid can give some relief. If the mother decides not to breast-feed, firm breast support, ice bags and mild analgesics will afford relief until engorgement subsides.

For centuries women have used HERBAL REMEDIES either to increase or to decrease their milk supply. An infusion of borage seeds and leaves (*Borago officinalis*) or fennel (*Foeniculum officinale*) eaten raw as a vegetable or fennel seeds steeped into a tea supposedly increases the flow of milk. To decrease the milk supply and assist weaning, teas made from cinnamon sticks or the powdered spice or from common sage (*Salvia officinalis*) have been used.

Normally prolactin is released only after childbirth. However, tumors of the pituitary gland, the estrogen in oral contraceptives and certain drugs can interfere with prolactin regulation, so that breast milk is produced without the stimulus of suckling (see AMENORRHEA-GALACTORRHEA SYNDROME). Also, severe emotional or physical stress can affect the hypothalamus and interfere with its production of PIF. Occasionally lactation has been induced deliberately in women who have not recently given birth—or, in rare cases, in women who have never been pregnant—in order to breast-feed an adopted child. Also, milk production can sometimes be reestablished after a long interruption owing to early weaning or a separation of mother and baby. Such lactation usually is induced by stimulation through suckling, massage and pumping the breasts by hand or with mechanical or electric breast pumps.

lactobacilli See DÖDERLEIN BACILLI; YOGURT.

lactose intolerance A diminished ability or total inability to break down lactose, the principal sugar in milk and milk products. From birth on, an enzyme called lactase breaks down lactose into glucose and galactose in the small intestine. After the age of two, however, the ability to digest lactose declines, and undigested lactose causes intestinal gas and diarrhea. These symptoms usually do not occur until late childhood or adolescence. A number of diagnostic tests are available to detect the condition, among them a blood test, a hydrogen breath test and a stool acidity test, the last used mostly in infants and young children. Dealing with this chronic condition is not too difficult. Some individuals space their lactose consumption over time, allowing four hours or so between drinking,

for example, a glass of milk. Eating lactose-containing products with other foods may help. Milk with added enzyme supplements, such as LactAid, is tolerated by many individuals. Eating yogurt and aged cheeses may also help, since they contain lactase-producing bacteria. For the severely lactose-intolerant, avoiding dairy products may be the only choice, and then one should make up for the lack of calcium and riboflavin through a varied diet and possibly also a calcium supplement.

Lamaze method See PSYCHOPROPHYLACTIC METHOD.

laminaria A species of seaweed that is very useful in dilating the cervix before a D AND C or other procedure requiring the insertion of instruments through it. When wet, laminaria expands to a diameter three to five times greater than when dry. One or two thin rods of laminaria are inserted into the cervical canal, where, during the course of six hours or so, they absorb moisture from cervical mucus and gradually swell, thereby very gradually widening the cervical canal. A mild cramp or two may be felt when the laminaria are first inserted, but thereafter there usually is little or no discomfort when they swell, making this method, unlike other ways of dilating the cervix, practically painless. After insertion it is important to avoid douching, use of tampons, vaginal intercourse or anything else involving putting something into the vagina.

laparoscopy The insertion of a long, narrow optical instrument through a ½-inch to 1-inch (1¼- to 2½-centimeters) incision in the abdominal wall just below the navel (hence the nickname "belly-button operation") in order to obtain a panoramic view of the pelvic organs and structures. It is used for purposes of diagnosis (diagnostic laparoscopy) and/or surgery (operative laparoscopy). It can detect adhesions (scar tissue), ovarian cysts, blocked fallopian tubes, ectopic pregnancy, endometriosis and other sources of acute abdominal and pelvic pain as well as causes of infertility. It also is used for sterilization and other surgical procedures. The injection of two or more liters (quarts) of carbon dioxide or nitrous gas into the abdomen lifts the abdominal wall up and away from the underlying bowel, exposing the uterus and fallopian tubes. Specially designed instruments then can be passed through the laparoscope to remove a wandering IUD (see INTRAUTERINE DEVICE), diagnose a tubal pregnancy or endometriosis, collect biopsy samples, remove adhesions or growths or perform a TUBAL LIGATION. When the laparoscopy is completed and the gas removed from the abdomen, the tiny incision can be closed with a single absorbable suture (stitch) and covered with a Band-Aid (hence another nickname, "Band-Aid surgery").

As a diagnostic aid laparoscopy can avoid a larger incision and major surgery (see LAPAROTOMY). For sterilization (tubal ligation) it requires more skill of the clinician than an abdominal procedure, although it is easier for the patient. It is easier to perform immediately after childbirth, but the American College of Obstetrics and Gynecology now recommends waiting eight weeks after delivery. Only regional anesthesia is needed, although general anesthesia often is used. A tiny incision is made at the lower border of the navel and through it a long, thin needle is inserted into the abdominal cavity. The needle is attached to a tube connected to a source of either carbon dioxide or nitrous oxide, which is pumped in until the abdominal wall is lifted up and away from the bowel. (With regional anesthesia, the woman may feel a sense of bloating.) Then a large metal instrument, a *trocar*, encased in an electrically nonconductive sleeve, is inserted through the incision into the abdomen; the trocar is removed and the sleeve left. The laparoscope, which includes a powerful light and an electrocauterizing forceps, is then inserted through the sleeve. (Some surgeons insert the instruments through a single incision, but many prefer to make a second small incision just above the pubic bone for the operating scope.) After each fallopian tube is located and grasped with the forceps, the current is activated from the cautery machine (usually by foot pedal) and, in repeated bursts, coagulates the tube. The surgeon then makes sure there is no bleeding, releases the gas from the abdomen by opening a valve on the sleeve and manually compressing the abdomen, removes the instruments and closes the incision.

When the procedure is being performed for diagnostic or therapeutic (treatment) purposes, it is essentially the same as tubal ligation up to the point of cautery. To determine if there is tubal blockage, a dye may be injected via a cannula inserted through the vagina and cervix into the uterus. To remove adhesions or growths by electrocautery or laser, or to collect biopsy samples or to aspirate fluid, another small puncture is made in the uterus through which the appropriate instruments are inserted. A D AND C also may be performed in this way.

Regardless of the anesthesia used, the woman may leave the hospital within eight hours, and the dressing may be removed the next day. The patient may even have vaginal intercourse on the same day if she wishes. The principal discomfort felt is chest and shoulder pain caused by a residual pocket of gas in the abdomen, which stimulates a nerve that refers the pain to the chest and shoulder. Such pain usually lasts three to five days but can persist for a week. Air travel should be avoided for several weeks, however, because pressure changes may affect the residual carbon dioxide, causing pain.

Originally used for gynecologic procedures, in the late 1980s the procedure began to be widely used for abdominal and urological procedures, such as removing a diseased gallbladder or repairing a bulging varicocele, as well as in some orthopedic surgery. While enabling much less extensive cutting, quicker recovery and shorter hospitalization than the major procedures it replaced, laparoscopy is not without risk and should be performed only by an experienced clinician. Possible complications include a major drop in blood pressure during surgery, bleeding, hernias at the wound site, peritonitis and infection severe enough to cause abscess formation. Excess carbon dioxide accumulation can lead to cardiac arrest, a rare complication that can be avoided by limiting the amount of gas instilled and by constant monitoring of the heart rate. Also, the instruments can damage internal organs, perforating the stomach or intestine or injuring the bladder or blood vessels. The principal postoperative complication suffered by some women following laparoscopy in the pelvic area (and thought to result from it) is subsequent heavy menstrual bleeding; in a few it is heavy enough to call for repeated D and Cs and even hysterectomy (removal of the uterus).

Laparoscopy should not be undertaken in women with intestinal obstruction, extensive abdominal cancer, tuberculosis or a serious heart condition. Laparoscopy can be performed in women with an UMBILICAL HERNIA, but the incision should be made at least 2 inches (5 centimeters) lower than usual, farther away from the navel (umbilicus). Finally, for women in their late 40s, close to menopause, laparoscopy for sterilization may not be worth the risk, since their chances of becoming pregnant are fairly small and safer contraceptive measures are available.

See also MINILAPAROTOMY.

laparotomy Abdominal surgery that is performed either for exploratory purposes or to treat certain disorders. It is used to diagnose a suspected serious condition such as ectopic pregnancy, an enlarged ovary that might be cancerous or severe pelvic infection with suspicion of pelvic abscesses, or to assess the spread of some pelvic cancers. It also may be used to treat endometriosis that cannot be dealt with using LAPAROSCOPY or hormonal therapy, to correct uterine displacement, to remove a fibroid tumor, to reverse a tubal ligation, to free the pelvic organs from adhesions or to repair or resect the ovaries. Laparotomy may be used to perform a uterine suspension (tighten the ligaments so that they hold the uterus and ovaries up out of the cul-de-sac), perform an appendectomy and/or perform presacral and uterosacral neurectomies (cut nerve fibers to eliminate severe pain). Laparotomy is performed under general anesthesia, through a crescent-shaped incision made above the pubic hair in the lower abdomen. The hospital stay lasts a few days, and recovery requires an additional rest period of about two weeks at home. After this normal moderate activity and sexual intercourse may be resumed. Complete recovery normally takes about six weeks.

See also MINILAPAROTOMY.

laser surgery Surgery performed with a beam of light energy instead of with the traditional scalpel (knife). First used to treat eye disorders, laser sur-gery is being used more and more in gynecological operations, in which it greatly minimizes pain, risk of complications, disability and recovery time. It has been used to stop dysfunctional uterine bleeding (thereby avoiding hysterectomy), correct malformations of the uterus, repair damaged or severed fallopian tubes or perform tubal ligation, treat endometriosis, eradicate genital warts and treat precancerous lesions of the cervix, vulva and vagina. It also is beginning to be used in breast surgery for biopsies, tumor removal and MASTEC-TOMY (see def. 1). A laser is able to destroy only the damaged tissue without injuring surrounding normal tissue. Also, the laser beam seals off small blood and lymph vessels, so the loss of blood and other fluids is much less. Risk of infection is reduced because most laser surgery is done without an incision or direct human contact with the tissue being treated. The disadvantages are that the equipment is very expensive to buy and maintain, and special professional training is required to use it properly.

Leboyer method Also *birth without violence, gentle birth.* An approach intended to ease the trauma of birth for the newborn baby by using a darkened room, eliminating harsh or sudden noises and slowly and gently easing the baby from the mother's body. Frederick Leboyer, the French obstetrician who promoted this approach about 1970, also believed that the baby should not be swaddled in clothes but first be placed in a warm bath resembling its surroundings in the amniotic fluid, and slowly allowed to acclimate itself to a stretched-out position before being dried and wrapped. The general principles of this method have been adopted to some extent in many hospitals.

leiomyoma Another name for FIBROID.

lesbian A woman who is romantically and sexually attracted to other women rather than men. The name comes from Lesbos, an island on which the Greek poet Sappho lived and wrote of her love for other women. Until the latter half of the

20th century lesbians, like homosexual men, were treated as if they were mentally ill. However, more and more authorities began to question this view, and in the 1950s the American Psychiatric Association officially declared that homosexuality is a healthy form of sexual expression. At the same time, in America more and more lesbians had begun to "come out," that is, admit their sexual preference openly and, although they still faced considerable discrimination, ranging from mild curiosity to extreme hostility, from the nonhomosexual ("straight") population, some of the laws discriminating against them began to be overturned. In 2006 Massachusetts became the first state to legalize the marriage of two partners of the same sex (either men or women). While this grants the married couple the same rights and responsibilities as heterosexual couples in Massachusetts, these couples still are denied hundreds of rights and privileges at the federal level. Other states, while slow to go so far, have given legal rights to unmarried partners of the same sex.

Physically lesbians are in no way different from heterosexual women. They undergo puberty, menstruation, childbearing and menopause in exactly the same way. The only difference is that sexually they respond to other women rather than to men. Some lesbians discover this preference early in their lives; others find out much later, sometimes after years of heterosexual marriage.

A number of health care issues particularly affect lesbians, owing to their style of life. If they have exclusively lesbian relationships, they need neither birth control nor obstetric care; therefore they are less likely to seek annual gynecological examinations and may become careless about procedures such as a regular PAP SMEAR. Further, their experiences with conventional clinics and physicians, who often are intolerant of or insensitive to lesbians, may lead them to avoid such contacts whenever possible, and they often lack health insurance because they generally cannot share spousal benefits with their partner. Managed care also may limit their ability to find lesbian-friendly health care providers. Thus, when they contract a serious disease they run a higher risk of its being overlooked in its early, more readily curable stages. Lesbians are less likely than heterosexual women to become infected with syphilis or gonorrhea, but they are just as likely to get some of the common vaginal infections, such as yeast infection, trichomonas and herpes. Also, women can transmit to women herpes, chlamydia and human papilloma virus, which causes genital warts and may increase the risk of cervical cancer. Finally, a lesbian-identified woman is not immune to HIV if she shares needles (for drugs, legally prescribed injectable medicine, tattoo supplies, etc.) or if she has unprotected sex with a menstruating female or a male who has been exposed to HIV.

While many lesbians choose not to parent, many others do have children, some in the context of prior relationships or marriages with men. Others, both single and partnered, choose to adopt children or to bear their own through methods of ARTIFICIAL INSEMINATION or IN VITRO FERTILIZATION, using sperm from a sperm bank or a willing donor. Either procedure may be performed at home or at certain medical clinics. While lingering prejudice in some regions can make it difficult to find in vitro facilities for this procedure, others, mostly in metropolitan areas, welcome lesbian clients. While it is less common, some partners choose a form of surrogate motherhood whereby one partner has her fertilized egg inserted into the other partner's uterus so that their child will have the genetic characteristics of the biological mother and also nine months of in utero bonding with the child-bearing mother. On the other hand, many lesbians do not bear children, which puts them at higher risk for breast and ovarian cancer (the risk is lowered by the normal fluctuations of pregnancy).

Perhaps the most frustrating area for lesbians is that of mental health. Lesbians have the same emotional problems as heterosexual women; in fact, they may have more, simply because they are subject to considerable stress in a society that is, for the most part, different in its preferences and values. Struggles with depression, anxiety and heavy alcohol use are not foreign to either lesbian or BISEXUAL women, especially those who are fearful of coming out, those struggling with "internalized homophobia" and those lacking supportive families or communities.

lesion   Any change in tissue that differentiates it from the same kind of tissue in corresponding areas and that is caused by disease or injury. Examples include wounds such as a cut or burn, a pimple of acne, a chancre of syphilis, a wart or an abscess.

See also PRECANCEROUS LESIONS.

let-down reflex The forcing of milk through the breasts, which may produce a momentary feeling of tightening or tingling. It is caused by the hormone oxytocin, whose production in turn is stimulated by suckling—or a baby's cry or even the mere thought of suckling—in a lactating woman. Oxytocin causes the smooth muscle fibers surrounding the ACINI (milk ducts) to contract, so that they are compressed and the milk secreted is forced into and through the big ducts of the breasts into the nipples. The sensation stops as soon as milk is released. The let-down reflex is strongest during the first few weeks of breast-feeding and usually occurs simultaneously in both breasts. Some women, however, do not notice it at all. If the let-down reflex is triggered while a breast-feeding mother is away from her child, she may be able to prevent milk from leaking by exerting light pressure on the nipple area with the palm of her hand, fingers or arm.

See also BREAST-FEEDING; LACTATION.

leukoplakia, vulvar The formation of white patches on the vulva, which may or may not be forerunners of cancer (see PRECANCEROUS LESIONS). Since they are difficult to distinguish from scar tissue formed after chronic infection in the area and from the thinning and drying of tissue associated with aging, the term is not very exact. The observation of leukoplakia should be followed with tests to determine the cause and what treatment, if any, should be undertaken.

See also PAGET'S DISEASE, def. 2.

leukorrhea See DISCHARGE, VAGINAL.

LH Abbreviation for *luteinizing hormone,* a hormone produced by the pituitary gland. In women it is primarily responsible for OVULATION and for the production of both estrogen and progesterone by the CORPUS LUTEUM after ovulation. (See MENSTRUAL CYCLE for further explanation.) In men LH, also called INTERSTITIAL-CELL STIMULATING HORMONE, stimulates the production of testosterone and sperm.

libido Also *sex drive.* The desire to engage in sexual activity. It varies greatly in intensity and frequency both from one individual to another and within a single person. The range of what is "normal" libido is so broad that it defies definition. The biochemical changes of puberty, particularly the enormous increase in sex hormone production, usually result in a surge of libido during adolescence, especially in boys but also in girls; the difference apparently is due to increased levels of ANDROGEN in boys. However, just as SEXUAL RESPONSE is governed by conscious thought and feeling, so is libido; consequently increases or decreases in sex drive can be caused largely or entirely by psychological or external factors, and not only by the body's chemistry. Seemingly insatiable libido (formerly called *nymphomania* in women) leading to more or less indiscriminate choice of sexual partners (so-called *promiscuity*) nearly always is the result of emotional problems and leads to physical problems only in that it exposes a woman to a much greater risk of SEXUALLY TRANSMITTED DISEASE.

Fatigue and mental preoccupation are major factors in reducing sexual desire in both men and women. So are fear of pregnancy, intense involvement in work, serious personal problems and marital conflict. When reduced libido becomes a chronic problem, it is considered a form of SEXUAL DYSFUNCTION and may be helped by SEX THERAPY. Illness and certain medications, notably numerous psychoactive drugs and some antihypertension drugs, also may diminish sex drive. Some oral contraceptives seem to increase the sex drive (the triphasic ones; see ORAL CONTRACEPTIVE) and others to lessen it; use of an intrauterine device (IUD) has similarly mixed effects. In both cases increased libido may result from removing the fear of pregnancy, but with oral contraceptives changed hormone levels may be responsible as well. Similarly, pregnancy itself makes some women more interested in sexual activity and others markedly less so. After menopause, too, libido may be increased, decreased or unchanged, and some women in their 80s or older—usually those who enjoyed sexual relations when younger—continue to enjoy them in old age. A recent study showed that administering the male hormone testosterone helped postmenopausal women regain libido.

The term *libido* was used by Sigmund Freud and some followers of his theories in a broader sense to mean all physical energy controlled by an unconscious part of the mind that they called the "id."

See also APHRODISIAC.

life expectancy   The length of time an average person is expected to live. Women tend to live longer than men—at present in North America, eight years longer, on the average. With advances in medicine and nutrition, life expectancy for both men and women has been advancing steadily, especially during the 20th century. In 1900 the average woman could expect to reach the age of 49, in 1960 the age of 70, and at this writing it is nearly 80. Consequently more women have become subject to some of the disorders of old age, among them cataracts and other vision problems, hearing loss, osteoporosis and dental problems. However, as more people live long enough to experience these disorders—note that living past menopause was a relative rarity before 1900—it is likely that more preventive measures for them will be discovered as well as more effective treatment.

lightening   Also *dropping.* In a pregnant woman, the descent of the fundus (top) of the uterus from the position it occupies at about 36 weeks of pregnancy to that of the month before (32 weeks), caused by the gradual descent of the baby's head into the pelvic inlet. Most noticeable in a first pregnancy, lightening occurs a few weeks before labor begins. The abdomen changes in shape, the lower portion becoming more pendulous (droopy) and the overall shape less protuberant. The baby's head, which was freely movable until now, becomes fixed in the pelvic inlet. After lightening a woman often finds it easier to breathe, since the enlarged

uterus no longer presses up against the rib cage, but she may find it harder to walk, may suffer from leg cramps and may find she must void more frequently, all owing to pressure on the blood vessels of the legs and on the bladder.

lipoma   A benign (noncancerous) tumor of the breast, made up of fat tissue. If it can be established without a doubt that a growth is actually a lipoma, usually possible only by means of biopsy, it can simply be left alone. If the growth is unusually firm in consistency or has other characteristics making the diagnosis doubtful, it usually is surgically removed.

liposuction   See COSMETIC SURGERY.

lips, inner and outer   See LABIA.

lithotomy   See DORSAL LITHOTOMY.

liver cancer   See CANCER, LIVER.

liver spots   Brown spots on the skin that resemble large freckles, occurring around and after menopause, particularly on the hands, forearms, face and other parts of the body that are frequently exposed to the sun. They are caused by an increase in melanin, the pigment that influences skin color and is itself influenced by hormones such as estrogen, progesterone and melanocyte-forming hormone. It is believed that the formation of liver spots is related to cumulative sunlight exposure over the years, since melanin acts to keep the sun's rays from harming the skin; the hormone imbalance associated with menopause also may be a contributing factor, and some women experience similar skin changes during pregnancy. After menopause, however, even women who formerly were not especially sensitive to sunlight are advised to avoid direct exposure and overexposure from their middle years on. Further, any change in liver spots, such as hardening, thickening or soreness, should be checked with a dermatologist to rule out skin cancer.

See also SKIN CHANGES.

LMP Abbreviation for *last menstrual period,* specifically the first day of the last menstrual period preceding a pregnancy. It is used in estimating the length of gestation.

See also PREGNANCY TEST.

lobular cancer in situ See CANCER IN SITU.

local anesthesia See REGIONAL ANESTHESIA.

lochia A vaginal discharge experienced after childbirth. For the first few days following delivery it consists of blood-stained fluid. After three or four days it becomes paler, and after the tenth day, owing to the presence of additional white blood cells, it becomes yellowish white or whitish. Normal lochia has a peculiar fleshy odor suggesting fresh blood; a foul smell signals postpartum infection.

loop electrosurgical excision procedure Also *LEEP, electrosurgical loop excision.* A technique that combines diagnosis and treatment for cervical abnormalities, such as dysplasia or early-stage cancer. Usually an outpatient procedure, it is both less expensive and less risky than CONIZATION. After local anesthetic is applied to the cervix and guided by a colposcope (a lighted, low-power microscope), a low-voltage, high-frequency radio wave runs through a thin wire loop that is inserted into the vagina and scoops out abnormal tissue in a few seconds. The wound is packed with a medicinal paste that enhances healing, and the tissue is sent out for further analysis. Often all of the abnormal tissue is removed at the same time. There is no pain or discomfort after surgery, infection is negligible and the cervix is completely healed within two or three months.

LTH Abbreviation for *luteotropic hormone,* another name for PROLACTIN.

lubricant Any substance that reduces friction. During sexual arousal the walls of the vagina secrete a lubricant, mucus, to facilitate coitus. Inadequate lubrication can make vaginal intercourse painful and can be a constant problem for some women. A longer period of foreplay for sexual arousal or use of a little saliva to assist penetration may be all that is needed. If these measures do not suffice or if inadequate lubrication is due to hormonal changes, which for some women occur during every menstrual cycle and others only after menopause (so-called VAGINAL ATROPHY) and/or while breast-feeding, the use of a water-soluble lubricant such as K-Y jelly or Lubrifax usually will solve the problem. Some women prefer to use natural vegetable oils, such as safflower or sunflower oil, and others use substances like yogurt. Treatment with hormone creams or pills is also effective, since estrogen promotes vaginal mucus production, but may not be worth its risks or side effects (see ESTROGEN REPLACEMENT THERAPY). Although Vaseline (petroleum jelly) does lubricate, it is not water-soluble and does not wash off readily; further, it damages the rubber of a condom, diaphragm or cervical cap and therefore should not be used together with these birth control devices.

lumpectomy See MASTECTOMY, def. 7.

lung cancer See CANCER, LUNG.

lupus See SYSTEMIC LUPUS ERYTHEMATOSUS.

luteal phase defect See IMPLANTATION.

luteinized unruptured follicle Also *trapped egg syndrome.* A failure in ovulation that occurs when the surface of an ovarian FOLLICLE does not dissolve to release the egg. It tends to occur in women who have been taking fertility drugs to induce ovulation and also in women who have had chronic pelvic inflammatory disease.

luteinizing hormone   See LH.

luteotropic hormone   Also *luteotrophic hormone, luteotrophin, LTH.* Other names for PROLACTIN.

lymph   A pale, yellowish fluid that travels throughout the body by means of the lymphatic system and is derived from tissue fluids. Lymph consists of white blood cells in a plasmalike liquid. It is collected from tissues in all parts of the body and is returned to the blood via the *lymphatic system,* a circulatory network of lymph-carrying vessels, and the *lymphoid organs*—mainly the LYMPH NODES, spleen and thymus—which produce and store infection-fighting white blood cells.

lymphedema   Chronic swelling of the extremities owing to accumulation of fluid that results from obstruction or severance of LYMPH vessels and/or disorders or removal of the LYMPH NODES. It is characterized by puffiness and swelling of the affected arm or leg. Lymphedema is a common aftereffect of lumpectomy and MASTECTOMY when the procedure involves the complete or partial removal of several lymph nodes, thereby impairing lymph drainage. Consequently there may be chronic swelling, ranging from mild to severe, in the arm on that side. Moreover, that arm and hand become more vulnerable to infection, so even a small burn or cut may lead to widespread infection and high fever. Similarly, cancer treatment that requires removal of lymph nodes in the pelvic region or upper thigh and radiation therapy of the chest or groin area sometimes results in lymphedema of the adjacent leg or arm. Other causes are burns, low thyroid levels and infection. In most cases postoperative lymphedema subsides within 6 months, but in 3 to 5% of cases swelling may be noticeable (arm circumference may increase by as much as 2 inches) and persistent. If swelling, redness, hardness or

warmth recur, patients are advised to contact their clinician at once, since the sooner treatment begins, the less swelling will occur. Even when lymphedema disappears, subsequent trauma to the arm or hand may lead to recurrence. The best way for breast cancer patients to avoid lymphedema is to have a SENTINEL NODE BIOPSY instead of axillary node dissection. Some studies indicate that 30 to 40% of breast cancer survivors develop lymphedema, which may occur years after surgery.

There is no effective permanent cure for severe lymphedema, but there are treatments that minimize its extent and avoid its complications. The most effective treatment, long used in Europe but only recently adopted here, is *complete* (or *complex*) *decongestive physiotherapy.* It involves 45-minute massage sessions once or twice a day for a month or until the limb reaches normal (or almost normal) size. It is performed by a certified lymphedema therapist who has completed at least 135 hours of training. (See the Appendix for the directory of such therapists.) Following each treatment the limb is wrapped in a compression bandage to prevent the lymph that was pushed out from re-entering. With the bandage in place, the patient must exercise the muscles and joints of the limb, which results in further outflow of lymph. Each treatment takes three to four hours. Further, the skin and nails of the affected limb must be kept clean and well lubricated (usually with a lanolin-based lotion applied twice a day). When the massage treatments are concluded, a custom-fitted pressure sleeve or stocking is made, which must be worn every day (and bandages applied every night). An alternative to specialized massage, which may not be available, is the use of pneumatic compression sleeves or stockings that rhythmically inflate and deflate; they usually are used in a hospital or clinic.

Precautionary measures to avoid injuring the affected region are to wear gloves when gardening or using strong detergents; wear bathing shoes when swimming in a river, lake or ocean; use a thimble when sewing; avoid touching harsh chemicals and abrasive compounds; take precautions against burns, including sunburn; use an electric razor instead of a manual razor blade for underarm shaving; have all injections, vaccinations and blood pressure tests administered to the unaffected arm; avoid restrictive pressure on that arm and hand; carry antibiotic ointment and bandages to treat unavoidable small injuries, hangnails and scrapes; and avoid tight clothing that can impair circulation. If the legs are affected, patients should not cross them. Also, compression garments are recommended for use during air travel. A serious flareup, with severe pain, fever, and extreme redness requires prompt attention, since it signals a potentially life-threatening infection. It is treated with intravenous antibiotics.

For years doctors advised breast cancer survivors at risk of developing lymphedema to avoid most upper-body exercise or lifting anything heavier than five pounds. However, a study published in 2006 found that slow, progressive weight training did not increase onset of lymphedema nor did it worsen the symptoms of longtime sufferers. The emphasis was on slow and progressive, over a six-month period.

lymph nodes   Small, bean-shaped masses of tissue situated along the vessels of the lymphatic system (see LYMPH). The nodes act as filters, removing bacteria or cancer cells from the lymphatic fluid.

lymphogranuloma venereum   Also *LGV, lympho-granuloma inguinale.* A new SEXUALLY TRANSMITTED DISEASE caused by a strain of CHLAMYDIA organism and transmitted by vaginal, anal and sometimes oral-genital sexual intercourse. It also may be spread by close physical contact other than intercourse. The organisms attack the lymph nodes. Symptoms appear 5 to 21 days (usually 7 to 12 days) after infection, beginning with a tiny painless bump or pimple on the genitals, in men usually on the penis or urethra, in women anywhere on the vulva or in the vagina. The sore usually disappears by itself within a few days and, since it is painless, may not be noticed by the infected person. The organisms then spread from the initial site to nearby lymph vessels and glands, usually those in the groin. The lymph glands in one or both sides

become swollen and tender 10 to 30 days after the original infectious contact. The swollen glands fuse together to form a single, painful, sausage-shaped mass called a *bubo*, which lies in the folds of the groin. The glands swell above and below the groin fold, giving the bubo a grooved appearance. The skin over the bubo becomes a bluish red; some of the glands in the bubo are soft, others hard. In most cases these lymph glands are destroyed and several abscesses form that push to the surface and release pus. In about one-fourth of cases the bubo disappears spontaneously, without treatment.

The formation of a bubo is more common in heterosexual men than in women or homosexual men. In women the original sore is often deep in the vagina, and the organism invades the deeper pelvic lymph glands. In homosexual men the sore may form in the anus and from there also invades the deeper pelvic lymph glands. In these instances visible buboes do not form, and the infected person remains unaware of the disease.

As the lymph glands are invaded, both men and women may have fever, chills, abdominal pain, loss of appetite and joint pain. Backache often occurs when the deep pelvic lymph glands become infected. If treatment is delayed, complications may develop. Among them are anal and rectal problems when the anal area is invaded, especially rectal strictures (narrowing); blockage of fluid in the genital area and consequent swelling, called *elephantiasis* and more common in women than men; and cancerous and precancerous lesions, as a result of excess tissue growth in the rectal and genital areas.

Diagnosis of lymphogranuloma venereum is based on a skin test, involving injection of an antigen, or a blood test, called LGVC-FT, for *LGV complement fixation test;* the latter is more accurate. The treatment of choice is a 21-day course of tetracycline, doxycycline or erythromycin. Buboes on the verge of bursting should be surgically drained. Abscesses often require surgery, but rectal strictures frequently can be dilated. Since LGV can be difficult to eradicate, all patients should receive careful follow-up at least six months.

M

macular degeneration Also *age-related macular degeneration, AMD.* Atrophy of the macula, the central part of the eye's retina, the layer of tissue that registers light. The leading cause of blindness in persons over the age of 55, it is more common in women, especially white women, than in men, and is believed to affect 10 million Americans (one person in four over the age of 75). As the name indicates, age is a major risk factor. Individuals in their 50s have only a 2% chance of developing the disorder, but the risk jumps to 30% in those older than 75. Since women tend to live longer than men, they get the disorder more often, as do those with a family history of the disease. The vast majority (90%) of cases have the *dry* or *atrophic* type, which involves a breakdown or thinning of retinal tissue and loss of photoreceptor cells in the central retina. Small, whitish-yellow deposits called *drusen* often develop underneath the retina. A smaller percentage (10%) of patients have *wet* or *exudative* AMD, in which abnormal blood vessels develop underneath the retina. These new vessels are prone to leaking fluid and blood, which damages cells. The main symptoms of AMD include blurred vision, distorted vision or a blind spot in the central vision.

Because the onset is gradual, a simple test in a doctor's office will detect vision distortions that might be overlooked. It uses an Amsler Grid, a box of cross-hatched lines with a dot in the center. Upon staring at the dot with one eye, if any of the straight lines look wavy it could indicate macular degeneration.

There is no effective treatment for dry AMD, which worsens with age. However, people are usually able to manage quite well in their daily routines with only mild to moderate vision loss. Wet AMD sometimes responds to laser treatment that eliminates some of the new blood vessels; however, some healthy cells are damaged at the same time. Another treatment is photodynamic therapy, in which a drug, verteporfin (Visudyne), is injected intravenously to sensitize the blood vessels to laser light, and then a laser is used to destroy abnormal blood vessels. Another medication recently approved, Lucentis (ranibizumab), blocks abnormal blood vessel growth. It is administered as an injection into the eye and can be repeated if effective. However, it is not without side effects, some of them serious.

Individuals whose parents have wet AMD have a greater risk of developing it themselves. Preventive measures include stopping smoking (a major risk factor). Low antioxidant levels may also be implicated, so a diet rich in leafy green and yellow vegetables may help prevent it. The Age-Related Eye Disease Study of 2001 found that high doses of vitamin E, beta carotene and zinc help protect high-risk individuals from advanced AMD.

magnetic resonance imager Also *MRI;* (formerly) *nuclear magnetic resonance, NMR.* A sophisticated electronic scanner that uses strong magnetic fields up to 30,000 times stronger than the earth's radio wave pulses to provide pictures of, for example, the central nervous system. However, each machine costs several million dollars, and each scan $1,000 or more, so it is not available in every medical center. No radiation is involved in the scanning. The patient is placed in a magnetic field inside a tunnel-like machine and radio pulse waves are bounced off her body. As this occurs, the MRI measures variations in the energy of hydrogen atom nuclei in the cells and a computer records the results. The procedure takes about 45 minutes but occasionally longer. It is painless but extremely noisy (there is a loud, continuous metallic sound), and some individuals feel extremely anxious about being closed in. Earplugs or earphones to listen to music help counter the noise, prism glasses so one can see out of the machine and an explanation of the process help diminish anxiety, but a small percentage of patients require an antianxiety medication. Some centers now have open MRIs, which help claustrophobic patients and also persons too obese to fit into the conventional two-foot-diameter machine. However, open machines have some drawbacks. In closed machines the magnets are wrapped in coils of wire, which create a superconductor of very high magnetic resonance. Most open machines use two non-electrified magnets, generating much less magnetic strength and hence less clear imaging. To compensate, the patient is scanned for a longer time, roughly twice as long. However, improved models of open scanners, called open high-field MRIs, are being developed. MRI is particularly useful in evaluating disorders of the genital and urinary tracts that cannot be seen with other imaging techniques, providing information about fluids that help distinguish between hemorrhage and infection, spotting cancerous lesions and the like. It also can detect tumors in very dense breast tissue that are missed by ultrasound and mammograms but requires the use of an injected dye to evaluate breast cancer.

See also CAT SCAN.

maidenhead   See HYMEN.

makeup   See COSMETICS.

male contraceptive   Interference with the production, storage, chemical constitution or transport of sperm in order to prevent conception. The principal method of male contraception—and a completely reversible one—is the CONDOM, a rubber sheath that collects the ejaculated semen and sperm. It was long widely used in other countries but gained much broader advocacy and distribution in America in the 1980s, owing to fear of HIV transmission. Various chemicals that inhibit sperm production also are being studied. Among them are synthetic hormone compounds, such as TESTOSTERONE, which inhibits the production of FSH (follicle-stimulating hormone), which in turn stimulates sperm production. One study showed that weekly injections of testosterone reduce the sperm count of 98.6% of men to below the threshold needed for conception (specifically, a sperm count of less than 3 million). However, the injections are painful and have unpleasant side effects, such as weight gain, acne and irritability. Another approach has been to administer synthetic progesterone (progestin), which also suppresses FSH and LH (luteinizing hormone) in a daily pill, combined with a slow-release testosterone pellet placed under the skin. The reverse is also being tried, combining testosterone shots with progestin implants. One study reported that injection of these combined hormones proved very effective. An androgen derivative called MENT (an acronym for its chemical formula), delivered through an implant, is 10 times more active than testosterone and is being tested combined with progestin. Still another approach is to take testosterone along with GnRH (gonadotropin-releasing hormone) agonists, which seems to bring the sperm count to zero but requires daily injections. Still other researchers are experimenting with a vaccine that destroys FSH entirely, which would require only a single yearly injection. Also under development is *immunocontraception*, which involves prompting an immune reaction to a protein, eppin, produced in the epididymis and testis, the ducts that carry sperm. Preliminary tests on male monkeys injected every three weeks showed it did not interfere with potency, and fertility was recovered when the injections were stopped. In 1979 the Chinese announced they were testing an oral drug called *gossypol*, a derivative of cottonseed that apparently reduces both sperm count and sperm motility but damages the testes and in some men causes unacceptably low potassium levels and irreversible infertility. Gossypol in vaginal cream form proved an effective contraceptive, but the compound's deep yellow color caused permanent stains on bedding and clothing. Another study, from India, reports an injectable male contraceptive that does not involve hormones and is reversible. It involves injecting a polymer dissolved in dimethyl sulphoxide into the vas deferens, the tubes through which sperm must pass. The injection does not block the tubes but coats their walls and kills sperm as they pass; it can be reversed by flushing out the coating. Allegedly, single injections continued to provide contraception for 10 years. In 2005 researchers announced a way of immobilizing sperm so they cannot swim to the egg; they hope to produce a pill for this purpose, which would be a reversible contraceptive.

Nifedepine, a widely used medication for high blood pressure, has a contraceptive effect by blocking the calcium channels in sperm membranes without affecting hormone production. However, testing on this effect is, at this writing, inconclusive. Another compound, miglustat (Zavesca), used in Gaucher disease, is also being studied, as are materials injected into the vas deferens and plugs preventing sperm motility.

Researchers also are working on a vaccine to inhibit sperm. Other methods of inhibiting sperm production include THERMATIC STERILIZATION and ULTRASOUND (see def. 2). However, none of these methods is currently available in a form as effective as most female contraceptives. The principal means of permanent (nonreversible) male contraception—sterilization—is VASECTOMY.

male menopause Also *male climacteric.* Strictly speaking, the end of male testicular function, meaning greatly reduced production of the principal male hormone, testosterone, and of sperm. As in women, declining production of hormones by the gonads (sex glands) makes the pituitary gland produce more gonadotropic hormones to stimulate testosterone production. Hence the clinical signs of male menopause are low testosterone levels and high levels of gonadotropin; in women the counterpart is high levels of pituitary FSH (follicle-stimulating hormone; see MENOPAUSE). However, unlike the end of ovulation in women, sperm production in men does not end abruptly except when surgery or radiation therapy has damaged the testes. Rather, men undergo a very gradual, long-term decline, which actually begins soon after the age of 20 but usually produces no noticeable symptoms of any kind until after the age of 50 or 55. The first sign is usually diminished potency—decreased ability to have or maintain an erection. Occasion-

ally a man may experience vasomotor symptoms similar to the HOT FLASHES of menopausal women, but the majority of men note no change other than that it takes longer to achieve a full erection and ejaculation and that the time between orgasms (the *refractory period*) lengthens. (See under ORGASM.) Because potency is so intimately related to psychological factors, including boredom, preoccupation with work, fear of aging, mental or physical fatigue and anxiety concerning sexual adequacy, it is not really known how much of the decline is due to lowered hormone production and how much to other factors. (See also IMPOTENCE.) Even clinical tests are not foolproof, because testosterone levels in a single individual vary considerably from month to month, and even from hour to hour, with no known cause or visible effect.

The most common physical problem men encounter after the age of 55 is prostate disorders. It is estimated that more than half of all American men over 60 have some enlargement of the prostate gland, and many encounter more serious disorders, ranging from inflammation and infection to cancer of the prostate, the third most common malignancy in American men. (The prostate is described under PENIS.) A significant number of men find their capacity to enjoy sexual intercourse unchanged in later life, despite decreased hormone levels and less frequent coitus.

malignant Describing a growth or tumor that is cancerous.

See also CANCER.

mammalgia Painful breasts. The pain may be caused by premenstrual edema (fluid retention), poorly fitting brassieres, injury or infection (MASTITIS). After childbirth a common cause of breast pain is the engorgement that occurs when milk is first produced (see LACTATION). Cysts in the breast often cause pain (see FIBROCYSTIC BREAST SYNDROME) but breast cancer rarely does. However, there may be considerable postoperative pain following a MASTECTOMY.

mammaplasty Also *breast augmentation, breast reconstruction, breast reduction.* Plastic surgery performed to increase or decrease the size of one or both breasts, or to restore breast form following surgery for cancer or other breast disease (see MAS-TECTOMY). Breast *reduction* surgery is not always a wholly cosmetic procedure. Extremely heavy breasts can cause chronic backache, breathing problems and skin irritation from brassiere straps and perspiration. However, reducing breast size is a complicated surgical procedure and should not be undertaken lightly. Moreover, if a woman considering breast reduction plans to breast-feed in the future, the surgeon must be particularly careful not to remove too much secretory tissue or cut through the major mammary ducts.

There are two principal techniques for breast reduction surgery. In one, the nipple and areola are removed, and excess tissue is taken from the lower portion of the breast, after which the surgeon replaces the nipple and areola as a skin graft. This procedure greatly reduces nipple sensitivity and also eliminates the possibility of breast-feeding. In the other, the nipple and areola remain attached to the breast by a thin stalk of tissue, the surgeon removes excess breast tissue, and the nipple is then moved to a higher position on the breast. This technique preserves nipple sensitivity and in some cases enough tissue to allow breast-feeding. Reduction surgery takes three to four hours and is performed under general anesthesia in a hospital. The woman remains hospitalized for several days and generally can resume most activities within two to three weeks. Any such surgery is best performed by a board-certified plastic surgeon.

The simplest kind of surgery to *enlarge* breast size or to *replace* tissue lost through disease or mastectomy involves implanting a pouch filled either with silicone gel or with a saline (saltwater) solution. Injecting liquid silicone directly into the breast, a procedure used in the 1950s and 1960s and subsequently outlawed in many places, is extremely dangerous, frequently resulting in infection, poisoning and even the development of cancerous tissue. Silicone gel, an inert material similar in consistency and resilience to normal breast tissue and long considered quite safe, is contained in soft, seamless silicone pouches, to prevent it from migrating into other parts of the breast. The gel-filled pouch is inserted through a small incision at the base fold area of the breast, or breast-to-be,

and positioned under the breast skin. Sometimes, however, it is placed under the major pectoral muscle. In 1988 it was announced that silicone implants had caused cancer in rats, giving rise to concern about their safety in human patients, and subsequently numerous women reported problems with them, including leaks or infection and excessive breast hardness and firmness. In January 1992 the U.S. Food and Drug Administration called for a moratorium on use of silicone gel-filled breast implants, urging manufacturers to stop marketing them and surgeons to stop inserting them. In 1999 an independent panel of scientists concluded that silicone implants do not cause major systemic diseases like lupus or rheumatoid arthritis. But silicone sacs filled with gel or salt water still can rupture or cause local infections or scarring. Late in 2006 the FDA announced its approval of silicone implants, stating that it had reasonable assurance that the devices were safe and effective for cosmetic use in women aged 22 or older and for reconstruction in women of all ages. However the FDA warned that they are prone to rupture, they may contract or they may cause pain and inflammation in the breast, and insisted that doctors advise patients to have biennial MRIs to check for rupture (and remove the implant if rupture occurs). One study found that 69% of recipients experienced a rupture. Moreover, the FDA required the manufacturers to track 80,000 patients for 10 years to make sure no health concerns arise.

In case of rupture, the implant should be removed, along with the capsule of scar tissue surrounding it. Leakage can be detected by surgery or an MRI, but these are costly procedures. In response, a number of laboratories developed diagnostic blood tests to determine if existing implants were leaking. One such test measures antibodies created by the body in reaction to silicone. Symptoms of leakage include pain or hardening of the breast, a rash, extreme fatigue, fever, joint and/or muscle pain, burning or "electric" sensation, skin thickening or skin hardening. Women who experience these are urged to consult their clinicians.

A substitute for silicone implants is a saline implant, involving a two-stage operation. First, a balloon-like expander is placed under the chest wall muscle, and for several months saline (salt water) is injected every few weeks into the expander to stretch the overlying muscles and skin. In a second surgery, the expander is replaced with a permanent saline implant. This kind of implant lasts about 8 to 10 years, after which it is likely to leak and need to be replaced.

The most common complication of implant breast surgery is necrosis (death) of the covering skin. If the flap of skin covering the implant is thin, there may be gradual further thinning or discoloration over a large area of the implant, and occasionally sloughing off of skin, requiring removal of the implant. Other possible complications are blood clots, hemorrhage, infection and edema (fluid retention). Another problem is hardening of the breast into a baseball-like shape, caused by the formation of a capsule of scar tissue around the implant. These contractures, which can occur months or years after surgery (since scar tissue can take a long time to form), can result in abnormalities of breast shape and position, including lumps. They can, however, be treated. Formerly massage and other manipulation from outside, called *closed capsulotomy,* were recommended, but it was discovered this method risked breaking up not only scar tissue but the implant itself. *Open capsulotomy,* a surgical procedure, avoids this problem.

As a result to these and other concerns about implants, more women wishing reconstruction might consider the complex surgery whereby the breast is rebuilt with tissue taken from the abdomen, back or buttocks. A lengthy and expensive operation, it is appropriate only for women who have usable tissue to spare. In the abdominal procedure (called *trans-rectus abdominal muscle flap,* or *TRAM*), an abdominal incision is made, and fat and flesh are tunneled upward under the abdominal skin to the area of the missing breast. This flesh is not detached, so it maintains its own blood supply. Once it is in place, the surgeon shapes the breast. In a later procedure a nipple and areola may be created by skin grafting and tattoo. Although this technique is more complicated, the resulting breast looks and feels more natural, and there is no danger that the body will reject its own tissue. However, it cannot be used in women who smoke or have diabetes or any other condition that could constrict blood flow to the rebuilt breast, and could be problematic for women with back pain, those who are

physically very active and women who want to become pregnant. An alternative uses a portion of the broad back muscle (latissimus dorsi), with its overlying skin and fat; it has fewer complications but also makes a smaller breast. Still another is the *gluteus free flap,* taking tissue from the buttock. The flap must be moved too far to maintain the tissue's blood supply, so the vessels are cut and then reconnected to blood vessels in the chest wall. All these procedures represent major surgery, with its usual potential for complications (mainly infection and uncontrolled bleeding), as well as the danger that the blood supply to the relocated tissue will be compromised by twisting or a clot before it is healed.

Whatever the method of breast reconstruction, a nipple can be formed. In some cases the nipple of a diseased breast can be saved by "banking"; that is, when the breast is removed the nipple is temporarily grafted to another part of the body and is later attached to the reconstructed breast. Or an artificial nipple can be constructed from either part of the remaining nipple or from the vulva or some other part of the body.

Opinion differs as to how long a woman should wait after mastectomy before undergoing reconstructive mammaplasty, but there is increasing evidence that beginning or performing reconstruction at the same time as the mastectomy does not incur medical complications. When performed at the same time, the reconstruction portion of the surgery generally is carried out by a plastic surgeon. Nevertheless, many practitioners prefer to wait three months to a year until the mastectomy wounds have healed completely. If radiation therapy follows mastectomy, most surgeons prefer to wait until it is completed because radiation can cause tissue changes in the breast's skin. There is no maximum time limit for reconstruction following mastectomy, and some women have undergone mammaplasty 10 or even 20 years after their mastectomies.

A woman usually can leave the hospital two to three days after mammaplasty but generally must keep her arm close to her side for a few days longer. Within a month she should have complete use of her arm, although she might not yet be able to undertake vigorous exercise, such as golf, tennis or swimming. Some surgeons ask patients to wear a specially fitted brassiere day and night for the first few months so that the new breast takes on the desired shape.

Mammaplasty is also performed as cosmetic surgery, principally to augment breast size. In 2006 about 330,000 cosmetic breast augmentations were performed in the United States, an increase of more than 10% from the previous year. The procedure can cost from $4,500 to $10,000, including silicone implants (which are more expensive than saline), surgeons' fees and operating room costs. Health insurance generally does not cover cosmetic surgery.

Mammaplasty should not be undertaken lightly. The FDA has published a patient guide that is available online: www.fda.gov/cdrh/breastimplants. The Web site provides considerable information about products, the process and recommendations.

mammary duct ectasia   Dilation of the milk ducts within the breast, which then fill with debris. It usually occurs in numerous ducts and often is associated with the formation of cysts (see FIBROCYSTIC BREAST SYNDROME). If the ducts fill enough to rupture, they may become inflamed and infiltrated by plasma cells and consequently become swollen and painful. This condition, which is relatively uncommon, is called *plasma cell mastitis* and affects mainly older women. Symptoms include one or more hard, poorly defined, immovable masses in the breast (usually both breasts) and a recurrent greenish or brownish nipple discharge. Treatment is palliative—hot compresses and analgesics until the inflammation subsides—but sometimes infection develops, and surgical excision may be required.

mammary duct fistula   A false passage (fistula) or tunnel extending from one of the main milk ducts in the breast out to the surface of the nipple. It usually requires surgical repair.

mammography   An X-ray examination of the breast that is used to detect and diagnose disease, including cancer. It is considered the most reliable mechanical method available for detecting a breast cancer before it can be felt. However, it does overlook some cancers (see below). Nearly half the tumors detected by mammography are too small to be felt on physical examination. For many years the recommendation has been for a baseline mammogram between the ages of 35 and 40, mammograms every other year from 40 to 50, and annually thereafter. In 1997 the National Cancer Institute repeated this recommendation, but the American Cancer Society now recommends an annual mammogram from age 40 on. Since breast cancer tends to develop and grow more rapidly in younger women, annual screening increases the likelihood of finding cancers at an early stage. However, in 2007 the American College of Physicians disagreed with these guidelines, instead urging women in their 40s to consult with their physicians individually about whether to get X-rays. All of these guidelines are for women with *no symptoms* (such as a lump); those with a suspicious mass should be investigated immediately.

Mammography is a valuable diagnostic tool for women who have a palpable lump in the breast or under the arm, in order to help determine whether a biopsy should be performed or the lump is a cyst that should simply be aspirated (drained) and observed. It is similarly useful for women who have noticed changes or abnormalities in the breast skin (dimpling, discoloration, puckering), in the nipples (scaling, discharge, sudden inversion) or in the size or shape of either breast.

The amount of radiation needed to produce a clear mammogram (picture) varies with breast size and density. To avoid undue exposure it is highly desirable to use the lowest possible dose of radiation needed. Mammography should be performed by a radiologist or radiologic technician and preferably at a facility whose equipment and personnel are certified and annually inspected by the Food and Drug Administration (FDA). The maximum radiation dosage per examination per breast should be less than 1 rad (for *radiation-absorbed dose*), and a lead apron should be used to shield the ribs and abdomen from any exposure.

Despite established standards, radiologists who read mammograms can vary considerably in their interpretations of them and in the advice they give women. It would be helpful if there were more specific criteria for radiologists to use both in interpreting the X-rays and in making recommendations as to what course to pursue.

Mammography does not detect all hidden breast cancers, especially in very dense breasts. It misses about 10% of tumors in older women and about 33% in women under 50. One kind of tumor, invasive lobular carcinoma, may not show up at all even if it is large enough to be felt. Also, younger women are more apt to have false positive results. Both false positive and false negative error is probably due to the denser breast tissue of younger women. Some 90% of all screening mammograms find nothing wrong. Should an abnormal area be detected, a special *diagnostic mammogram* might be indicated instead of immediately performing a biopsy. Special views allow the radiologist to see tissues at a different angle or a different area not seen in a routine mammogram. Spot compression and magnification may also allow better visualization.

A newer kind of imaging, *digital mammography,* relies on storing an X-ray image on a computer disk. It offers clearer images, especially of dense breast tissue, and enables comparison of a woman's mammograms from year to year. The digital image enables magnifying an area and adjusting the contrast at a computer workstation, revealing far more detail than film can. Another advantage is that it can be sent electronically to another medical center or doctor for a second opinion. Also, computer-aided detection can be used after digital mammography to help pinpoint suspicious areas. A large clinical study of digital versus traditional mammography, examining the breasts of nearly 50,000 women aged 47 to 62, indicated digital mammography was neither better nor worse than the standard technique. However, in women most likely to have dense breasts, digital mammography did a better job of locating breast cancers. On the other hand, computer-aided mammography was associated with significantly higher false positive rates, recall rates and biopsy rates, and with significantly lower accuracy. Another study published in 2007, however, indicated that human scanners of mammograms, using their eyes and experience, are more accurate. The computer-assisted detection software is more likely to interpret a benign growth as potentially cancerous, and such false positive readings lead to additional scans and needless biopsies. However, a large study published in 2008 indicated that computer-assisted mammography read by one radiologist spotted nearly the same number of cancers as

ordinary mammograms read by two radiologists. The computer-assisted technology is used in 30% of the more than 30 million mammograms performed in the United States each year. Another technique being investigated is *digital tomosynthesis,* which takes X-ray pictures of the breast from 11 different angles, thus providing a series of cross-sections. It eliminates the problem of overlapping structures that can hide a tumor and also cuts down the likelihood of false positive results. At this writing it is being tested only in women already diagnosed with breast abnormalities.

Still another method is *scintimammography,* currently being tested in clinical trials. It involves injecting a radioactive agent into an arm vein which then flows into the breast. An image then taken with a gamma camera shows tumor cells, which take up more of the dye than normal cells do. Expected to be used as a follow-up to conventional mammograms, this method delivers more radiation and also cannot detect tumors smaller than 1 centimeter (⅜ inch).

For dense breast tissue, ultrasound can help determine if a suspicious mass is solid tissue or a fluid-filled cyst, and also evaluate solid breast masses to determine if there actually is a separate tumor or if glandular tissue simply has become more prominent. A newer device approved in 1997, *high-definition imaging ultrasound,* allows viewing of lesions obscured by dense breast tissue. Its readings can spare women unnecessary surgical biopsies, although it, like mammography, yields a high percentage of false positive readings. Ultrasound is a useful addition to mammography but not a substitute for it. Another such addition is magnetic resonance imaging (MRI), which helps locate lesions in dense breasts but cannot determine which are cancerous. In 2007 the American Cancer Society recommended that women at greatest risk for breast cancer also undergo annual MRIs, but not all authorities agree with this advice. A still experimental method to be used for high-risk women who have very dense breasts is *molecular breast imaging.* It involves giving an intravenous dose of a short-acting radioactive tracer that is absorbed more by abnormal cells than healthy ones. Special cameras collect the "glow" these cells emit, revealing more tumors than ordinary mammograms and fewer false alarms. Much less expensive than

MRIs, it requires further testing to compare the results with MRIs. Another technique is thermal imaging, which is based on the fact that heat emitted by blood flow through blood vessels that feed malignancies has a distinctive thermal "footprint." It can detect lesions but is not very specific, since many things besides cancer can increase heat in the breast. Nuclear imaging techniques are also being investigated. One is PET SCAN. Other researchers are examining laser devices to see if the amount of light absorbed and refracted by breast tissue varies with the presence of tumors.

See also MAGNETIC RESONANCE IMAGING; ULTRASOUND.

mammotome See BIOPSY, def. 5.

manic-depressive illness Also *bipolar affective disorder, bipolar depression.* A severe emotional disorder that is equally common in women and men and is characterized by recurrent cycles of mania and depression. Like other kinds of serious DEPRESSION, it is believed to have a biologic basis; it tends to run in families, and possibly it is transmitted by a dominant gene. The mood changes occur for no apparent reason but often can be controlled by medication.

Lithium, which has long been used for the manic phase of the illness, can have toxic effects. Other medications that may be as effective as lithium include such anticonvulsants as carbamazepine (Tegretol) and valproate (Depakote), which also have side effects. The schizophrenia drugs risperidone, quetiapine and olanzapine seem to be effective in treating sudden manic episodes and have fewer side effects. For the depressive stage of the illness, a number of ANTIDEPRESSANTS are used, but since they may cause a swing from depression to mania, they can be used only for short periods and must be closely monitored. Moreover, they appear to be of limited use. Long-term psychotherapy in conjunction with medication does appear to help. A recent study of three kinds—cognitive behavior therapy, interpersonal and social rhythm therapy and family therapy—showed that therapy consisting of 30 50-minute sessions over nine months resulted in greater improvement than short-term treatment, consisting of three sessions over six weeks. There was no significant difference among the three kinds of therapy.

Manic-depressive illness can begin at any time but tends to begin in the early 20s. Untreated, the depressive phase is characterized by extreme despondency, especially early in the morning, and progressive withdrawal from work, social affairs and other human contact. Many patients become suicidal. Typically, after six to nine months of acute depression, a manic phase begins. There is an apparent sense of well-being and heightened self-confidence as well as increased energy. Most patients become hyperactive, uninhibited and extremely talkative. They often exhibit inappropriate behavior, such as spending sprees, bizarre clothing or the like, and sometimes they become very irritable. After three to six months this mood is again replaced by depression. However, the sequence and duration of both mania and depression vary considerably.

In most patients the frequency and duration of these attacks increase with age. Treatment usually requires hospitalization for at least a time and control of symptoms with a variety of drugs, generally over a long term. The disorder may worsen during pregnancy and after delivery, but the use of lithium, the principal drug used to treat manic-depression, must be weighed against possible harm to the fetus and the mother's condition.

mask of pregnancy See CHLOASMA.

massage therapy Various techniques of kneading, stroking, pressure and similar movement of the hands over the skin in order to relax the muscles, sedate pain, improve circulation, and before/during childbirth to help stretch the perineum and ease the pain of contractions. Used since ancient times and in many non-Western cultures, massage in the United States was valued mainly by athletes, dancers and victims of stroke or paralysis until the second half of the 20th century, when it was embraced along with other body therapies by those seeking out alternative healing methods. At this writing 33 states issue licenses to massage therapists, indicating in most cases that they have had 500 hours of training and passed an examination. The American Massage Therapy Association certifies and promotes massage therapy.

There are numerous kinds of massage technique, ranging from light stroking to deep pressure, and most massage therapists use a combination of them. Among the most frequently used techniques are *Swedish,* which uses a set of routine strokes to work over the whole body; *Esalen,* a blend of Eastern and Western techniques, mainly Swedish, *acupressure* and *shiatsu,* the latter two applying pressure to energy points along the same meridians as ACUPUNCTURE; *sports massage,* used as part of athletic training and focusing specifically on muscle recovery rate to relieve aches and pains; *rehabilitation* or *medical massage,* developed after World War II for amputees and other wounded veterans, focusing on relieving pain from neurological problems; *reflexology,* based on applying pressure (stroking, pressing, rotating) to designated areas of the hands and feet that are believed to correspond to specific interior organs. Among the movements used are *effleurage,* light, firm and gentle stroking, used during the first stage of labor to ease the pain of contractions; *kneading,* rhythmic lifting and squeezing of flesh; *tapotement,* light hacking, tapping or clapping over muscles and fleshy parts of the body; *vibration,* rapid shaking and pulsating, done by hand or with a machine; *brushing,* light fingertip contact done slowly and rhythmically; *range of motion,* passive exercise by rotating, flexing and extending the body and limbs to mobilize joints and boost secretion of synovial fluid; and *nerve compression,* exerting firm pressure to relieve pain at nerve points. Various studies have found massage helpful in lessening the pain of hospitalized cancer patients, reducing anxiety in cancer patients, and relieving symptoms of premenstrual syndrome. Massage has also helped alleviate LYMPHEDEMA.

While massage appears to be beneficial in numerous ways, there are definite *contraindications* to its use. Among these are phlebitis, thrombosis (obstructive blood clots), aneurysm (weakness or dilation of an artery) and varicose veins (avoid massaging *both* legs if present in one); skin infections or skin that has thinned due to burns, injury or frostbite. Further, it is advisable to check with one's primary-care physician before receiving deep pressure or soft-tissue manipulation if one has osteoporosis, an arthritic condition, hypertension, kidney disease, diabetes, tumors, is pregnant or has an unhealed fracture or recently torn ligaments, muscles or tendons. Although massage therapy can benefit some of these conditions, it also can be harmful if not correctly applied, so a physician's guidelines may be needed.

mastectomy 1. Surgical removal of the breast. It usually is undertaken as a treatment for cancer, but occasionally a very large benign (noncancerous) tumor cannot be removed without removing the entire breast (as in CYSTOSARCOMA PHYLLODES) or the high risk of cancer warrants surgery (see def. 8 below). There are several kinds of mastectomy, depending on the amount of tissue that is removed. From about 1895 to 1975 some 90% of American breast cancer patients who were operated on underwent the Halsted radical mastectomy (def. 2 below), which removes not only the breast but underlying muscle and adjacent lymph nodes, on the theory that cancer cells spread to other parts of the body through the LYMPH. Since 1975 there has been a growing tendency to regard CANCER as a systemic disease that should be treated locally by removing only the tumor and then systemically by subjecting the patient's body to radiation and/or chemotherapy (anticancer drugs), hormones and other treatment. The revised view of cancer led to the development of various less extensive operations as well as approaches involving nutritional, manipulative and psychological treatment (see CANCER, BREAST). Increasingly, it has been recognized that the patient herself must decide not only whether to undergo surgery but what surgery should be done. Consequently the old *one-step procedure,* in which a patient undergoing breast biopsy allowed the surgeon to decide whether or not the breast should be removed and gave permission for this procedure before being anesthetized, now is rare. Instead, most often there is a *two-step procedure,* in which biopsy and surgery are separated by hours, days or even weeks. With the two-step method the patient has time to make a decision, seek one or more additional medical opinions and exercise some informed control over her own care. Also, the delay allows time for a more careful evaluation of the tissue removed in biopsy as well as tests to determine if a malignant tumor is hormone-dependent (see ESTROGEN-RECEPTOR ASSAY). The type of mastectomy performed must take into account how far the disease has advanced. A recent study indicates that the outcome of mastectomy is improved if surgery is performed during the second half of the menstrual cycle; the reason is not known, and further research is needed to confirm this finding. Whether reconstruction is to be immediate or delayed, it is important to discuss this decision with the surgeon and a plastic surgeon *before* surgery is undertaken, because it can alter the way the surgery is done. Unfortunately a large proportion of breast surgeons do not refer their patients to a plastic surgeon for reconstruction, so it is up to the patient to bring up this issue.

The aftereffects of mastectomy can be as traumatic as the surgery itself, or even more so. Following surgery small drainage tubes are left in place for a few days. It usually takes 10 to 14 days for the scars to heal superficially. The adjacent arm normally is swollen for at least a few days, but simple exercises, such as squeezing a small rubber ball, help control the swelling. Feelings of mutilation, of being "less feminine" and fear of pain and death may be difficult to deal with. Many women lose considerable mobility in the adjacent arm and shoulders, and some suffer more or less permanent LYMPHEDEMA. Also, cut nerves and scar tissue in the breast area may produce a combination of numbness and oversensitivity there, making it painful or unpleasant to be touched. A new surgical technique appears to minimize major scarring. Instead of making the traditional incisions from side to side across the breast, the surgeon places the incision around the edge of the areola, which may yield a better result. Surgery generally must be followed up with RADIATION THERAPY and/or CHEMOTHERAPY, which not only may have unpleasant side effects but also may serve as a constant reminder of life-threatening disease.

At least some of the aftereffects of mastectomy seem to be minimized when the operation is performed using *laser surgery* instead of the conventional scalpel. The CO_2 (carbon dioxide) laser, which emits a light in the infrared spectrum with a wavelength of 10.6 millimeters, vaporizes cancerous tissue with much less damage to the surrounding, healthy tissue. It can be used for any kind of mastectomy (see defs. below). There is less postoperative bleeding, drainage and pain, the hospital stay in reduced to one or two days instead of four or five, and normal activities can be resumed much sooner. However, at this writing laser mastectomy is not nearly as widely available as conventional surgery.

Today there are at least two national programs in the United States to aid the recovery—both physical and emotional—of women who have had mastectomies. ENCORE, a YWCA-sponsored program open to women three weeks after surgery, offers group water and floor exercises to strengthen the affected arm; help in choosing clothing, brassieres and prostheses (devices to replace the missing breast); and the opportunity for women with common concerns to share suggestions and support. Reach to Recovery, sponsored by the American Cancer Society, begins in the hospital, where women who have had mastectomies themselves visit patients on an individual basis, answer questions and provide a kit containing a temporary prosthesis and publications describing exercises and other kinds of rehabilitation. Following mastectomy, a large proportion of women can, if they wish, have breast reconstruction surgery (see MAMMAPLASTY).

2. Halsted radical mastectomy. Also *radical mastectomy.* Surgery involving removal of a cancerous breast and its skin, the underlying muscle of the chest wall (both major and minor), the lymph nodes in the adjacent armpit and fat tissue. The physical results are a flattened and sunken chest wall and the potential for developing more or less permanent LYMPHEDEMA and shoulder stiffness. This kind of surgery, first performed about 1882 by William Stewart Halsted, became the most commonly used procedure for treating breast cancer in the United States. Today it has been largely replaced by less radical techniques.

ASK YOUR SURGEON

1. How many mastectomies do you perform (ideally, 5 or more per month); how many lumpectomies (ideally, 15 or more per month)?

2. Do you perform skin-sparing surgery (removing breast but saving skin for better cosmetic result)?

3. Do you perform nipple-sparing procedures?

4. Do you do sentinel-node biopsies (removing only one or a few lymph nodes)?

5. Do you ever recommend neoadjuvant therapy (chemotherapy before surgery)? If so, when? If not, why?

3. extended radical mastectomy. Also *extended thorough mastectomy, Urban operation.* Surgery identical to the Halsted radical mastectomy (see def. 2) but also removing the lymph nodes of the internal mammary chain, which usually requires removing a section of the rib cage. This procedure was invented in the 1930s, by J. A. Urban and others. It was popular until the early 1960s for patients with tumors between the nipple and sternum (breastbone) but has been largely abandoned.

4. modified radical mastectomy. Also *total mastectomy with axillary node dissection.* Surgery to remove the breast, which removes the nipple and surrounding skin, breast tissue, fat, connective tissue, most of the axillary (underarm) lymph nodes and the lining over the chest muscles, but usually leaving the chest muscles intact. It is the only radical surgery for breast cancer that is still widely performed, mainly for tumors too large to be excised alone, for women who do not want long-term radiation and for women with a precancerous condition who want a guarantee against invasive cancer. It results in a cosmetically more pleasing appearance than the Halsted and preserves normal arm and shoulder strength. This technique was first reported in 1948 by two British surgeons who believed that cancer could not spread through the pectoral (chest) muscles, and results indicate a recurrence-free survival rate comparable to that of the Halsted.

5. simple mastectomy. Also *total mastectomy.* Surgery in which only the breast is removed, leaving intact the axillary nodes and chest muscles. It sometimes is combined with *axillary dissection* (of the lymph nodes nearest the breast), which is performed primarily for the purpose of STAGING, that is, to determine the extent of spread into the lymph nodes and the need for subsequent treatment with radiation and for drugs. It differs from the modified radical mastectomy (def. 4) in that it takes only the axillary lymph nodes closest to the breast. This surgery—total mastectomy with axillary dissection—was recommended by the Consensus Development Panel at the National Institutes of Health in June 1979, to replace the Halsted radical (def. 2) for all women with Stage I cancer (small tumor without spread) and some with Stage II (cancer in some nodes but no spread elsewhere) cancer. If cancer has spread to the nodes, either radiation is used or the affected nodes are removed, or both. If there is no low axillary node involvement, only the breast is removed and the axilla (armpit closely observed following surgery. If cancer later develops in the nodes, they are surgically removed at that time. Traditionally performed under general anesthesia, simple mastectomy sometimes can be performed using only sedation and a long-acting local anesthetic. It apparently reduces postoperative pain and cuts hospital stays from a few days to a few hours.

6. partial mastectomy. Also *segmental mastectomy, quadrantectomy.* Removal of a breast tumor and a small area (2 to 3 centimeters, or 1 inch) of surrounding tissue, including some of the overlying skin and part of the lining of the underlying muscle. A quadrantectomy removes the quarter of the breast with the tumor. The rest of the breast, along with connective tissue, remains intact. Although the breast is partially saved, it still may be markedly disfigured. If appropriate, it can be restored later through plastic surgery, or the other breast may be altered to match the affected one more closely (see MAMMAPLASTY). Opponents of this procedure say it does not take into account the multicentric nature of breast cancer, that is, its tendency to appear in another part of the same breast. About 13% of women undergoing more extensive surgery have been found to have one or more hidden cancers in the same breast, in addition to the one originally detected. To kill any cancer cells that may remain in the breast, partial mastectomy is always followed up with radiation therapy and/or chemotherapy. Also, many surgeons believe that this procedure should be supplemented with removal and examination of at least some adjacent axillary lymph nodes, to gauge the progress of the disease more accurately (see STAGING).

7. lumpectomy. Also *local wide excision, segmental resection, tumor excision, tumorectomy, tylectomy, wedge excision, wide excision.* Removal of only the tumor mass and a small amount of surrounding breast tissue, leaving muscles and skin intact. The least invasive surgery for breast cancer and often requiring only local anesthesia, it may leave the breast looking normal. Most surgeons also perform an axillary node dissection, a small underarm incision to remove a number of lymph nodes (to see if the cancer has spread to them). However, SENTINEL NODE BIOPSY is an alternative to this procedure. Nearly all surgeons performing this operation follow it with radiation therapy lest some cancer cells remain hidden in the breast, and often chemotherapy as well. Long opposed by conservative practitioners, lumpectomy has been found to yield survival rates at least as good as total mastectomy, and it is increasingly used for Stage I and II cancers (see STAGING). Moreover, a recent study indicated that administering chemotherapy before surgery shrinks many tumors originally considered too large for lumpectomy and consequently avoids the more radical surgery. (In this study, one woman in eight with large tumors or malignancy that had spread to nearby lymph nodes experienced complete remission from the presurgical chemotherapy and remained cancer-free for five years.) The new approach is expected to apply eventually to about 45% of early breast cancer cases.

Other research suggests that making a decision between lumpectomy and mastectomy is assisted by an MRI (see MAGNETIC RESONANCE IMAGER).

8. subcutaneous mastectomy. Surgery in which about 95% of the internal breast tissue is removed without disturbing the overlying nipple and surrounding skin, with its fat. It is performed chiefly as a preventive procedure when there is a high risk of malignancy. If, after careful examination of the excised tissue, an invasive cancer is found, both the remaining breast tissue and axillary lymph nodes are removed in a subsequent operation. Sometime after surgery, an implant in inserted into the chest cavity to restore the breast contour.

Subcutaneous mastectomy also has been used as primary treatment for a CANCER IN SITU of the lobe or other noninvasive cancers not close to the nipple. The major objection to this procedure as treatment for invasive cancer is that breast tissue cannot be completely eliminated from the nipple area, so there is a risk of leaving some cancer cells. Subcutaneous mastectomy occasionally is recommended as a preventive measure for women who are at high risk for breast cancer, especially those with any of the following: severe FIBROCYSTIC BREAST SYNDROME; a biopsy that shows moderate to severe noncancerous breast disease; a family history of breast cancer and progressively more nodular (lumpy) breasts; lumps and cysts in one breast and cancer in the other breast.

mastitis An inflammation of the breast, caused by infection, most often by *Staphylococcus aureus* but sometimes by another organism. It is possible to contract mastitis from a bite, as in love play, but most often the organism invades the nipple of a woman who is breast-feeding. The symptoms of mastitis are pain in the affected breast, particularly in one spot, tenderness and swelling. There may be a chill and there nearly always is fever, sometimes quite high. Treated with warm compresses and oral antibiotics, mastitis often subsides within about 48 hours. When it does not, it usually becomes localized (*suppurative mastitis*), forming an ABSCESS that must be opened surgically and drained. Although at one time it was considered mandatory to stop breast-feeding lest the baby become infected, many women with mastitis have found that suckling relieves the pain somewhat by emptying the breast, thereby reducing the opportunity for bacteria to multiply; it does no harm to the child, since the bacteria usually are from its mouth. *Chronic cystic mastitis* is an older name for FIBROCYSTIC BREAST SYNDROME, but it is not accurate because such cysts rarely involve either inflammation or infection. (For *plasma cell mastitis*, see MAMMARY DUCT ECTASIA.)

Some women who prefer HERBAL REMEDIES use local applications of various herbs to ease the pain of caked nipples and mastitis. Among these are poultices made from elderberry blossom (*Sambucus nigra*) and olive oil; grated raw potato; fresh ginger root; and comfrey leaves (*Symphytum officinale*).

masturbation Also *automanipulation*. The practice of sexually stimulating oneself to ORGASM. According to most authorities today, masturbation is quite normal during adolescence, and many feel it is normal at any age. Apparently the orgasms that women experience with masturbation are often more intense, with stronger muscular contractions, than those experienced with a partner, although the clinicians who observed this phenomenon also pointed out that measurable physical intensity is not necessarily identical to a feeling of satisfaction, which may be more profound with a partner. Mutual masturbation of one sexual partner by another, at the same time or in turn, can be a satisfying means of sexual enjoyment. For heterosexual partners it provides an excellent alternative when illness, injury or a fertile period rule out vaginal intercourse. It also is a means for partners to become acquainted with each other's sexual responses and is frequently recommended by sex therapists to help women who have never achieved orgasm (see FRIGIDITY). Women masturbate in a variety of ways, but nearly all involve stimulating the CLITORIS, with their fingers, by crossing their legs and exerting pressure, with a stream of water, an electrical or battery-operated vibrator, a pillow or any other object. Masturbation was frowned on as an unhealthy outlet, especially for women, throughout the 19th and early 20th centuries, at least in Europe and America, and some clinicians actually removed the clitoris (clitoridectomy) or its foreskin to curb the practice. Today, in contrast, some clinicians actually recommend masturbation to postmenopausal women who have infrequent or no sexual relations with a partner, in the belief that frequent lubrication of the vagina through sexual arousal helps prevent excessive drying of the tissues (see VAGINAL ATROPHY).

maternal serum alpha-fetoprotein-3 (MSAFP-3) test See ALPHA-FETOPROTEIN TEST.

maternity home See BIRTH CENTER.

measles Also *rubeola*. An acute, highly contagious disease of childhood marked by fever, cough, inflammation of the eyelids (conjunctivitis) and a spreading rash. It is caused by a virus, lasts about a week and can be prevented entirely by immunization with a live virus vaccine. It usually is not a serious disease in itself, but its complications, such as pneumonia and encephalitis, can be dangerous. It is important that it be differentiated from a similar disease, called German measles or RUBELLA, which can cause birth defects in a baby if the mother becomes infected during pregnancy. Measles is rare in adults but is likely to make a person acutely ill when it does occur.

meconium The stools of the fetus while it is inside the uterus and of the newborn baby during the first few days of life. By the fourth month of development the fetus has developed enough of a gastrointestinal tract to swallow amniotic fluid, absorb much of the water from it and propel what is not absorbed as far as the lower colon, where it remains. By the ninth month the fetus is swallowing as much as 450 milliliters of fluid a day, or about the same amount of breast milk a newborn baby drinks. Before birth meconium consists not only of undigested material from amniotic fluid but various other products secreted, excreted and shed by the baby's gastrointestinal tract. It is dark greenish-black in color. If the fetus suffers from acute lack of oxygen, its muscles relax and it will evacuate meconium from the large bowel into the amniotic fluid. The presence of meconium in the amniotic fluid calls for careful monitoring of the baby's heart rate. If the heart rate is not between 120 and 180 beats per minute or shows certain kinds of slowdown, the baby definitely is being deprived of oxygen; even if the heart rate is normal, there may still be a problem.

Meconium nearly always is expelled into the vagina with a BREECH PRESENTATION, since during labor there is considerable pressure on the baby's abdomen, forcing the meconium out. In a cephalic (head first) presentation, however, the presence of meconium in the vagina signifies that the baby is not getting enough oxygen.

The principal danger of meconium in the amniotic fluid (other than its cause, lack of oxygen) is that the baby may aspirate some into its lungs, where it can cause a severe chemical irritation, *meconium aspiration pneumonitis*. This condition is, after HYALINE MEMBRANE DISEASE, the leading cause of severe respiratory problems in newborn babies and requires vigorous suctioning to clear the lungs as well as specialized intensive aftercare.

After birth the meconium is excreted as a bowel movement. Soft, brownish green and usually odorless, it is made up of bits of tissue shed from the intestinal tract, a few skin and hair cells and bile (the last accounts for the green color). After the third or fourth day, when formula or breast-milk feeding has been established, the meconium disappears and is replaced by light yellow feces with a characteristic smell.

melanoma Also *malignant melanoma.* A malignant (cancerous) tumor that arises out of pigment cells (melanocytes), most often in the skin or mucous membranes but sometimes also in the eye and central nervous system. Some kinds of melanoma spread so rapidly that they are fatal months after they are first detected, making it by far the most dangerous form of skin cancer. Nearly half of all melanomas arise from pigmented moles. There is a definite connection between exposing the skin to intense bursts of ultraviolet light (sunlight) and the development of melanomas. Further, the effect appears to be cumulative; at least one study has found that severe sunburn in childhood carries an increased risk of developing melanoma many years later. The incidence of melanoma in the United States is growing alarmingly fast, and sunscreens apparently do *not* protect against melanoma (as they do against other kinds of skin cancer).

In women melanomas appear most often on the legs, and in men on the torso. Warning signs include any unusual skin condition, but particularly a change in the size or color of a mole or other darkly pigmented growth or spot. Other warning signs are scaliness, oozing, bleeding, the appearance of a bump or nodule and the spread of pigment beyond the border (see also accompanying box). Early treatment, which involves surgical excision of the tumor, adjacent skin and nearby lymph nodes, is nearly 90% successful. Lesions that invade the skin no more than .75 millimeter (mm) have a good prognosis, with 95% of patients surviving five years or more. As the tumors extend deeper, the prognosis worsens, and with lesions thicker than 4 mm, only 50% of patients survive for five years. Once the cancer has spread to distant parts of the body, however, the survival rate is lower still. Consequently, it is wise to check immediately on any suspicious growth or other

ABCD: WARNING SIGNS OF MELANOMA

A **Asymmetry:** One half of the mole does not match the other.
B **Border irregularity:** The mole edges are notched, ragged or blurred (pigment is leaching or streaming from the border).
C **Color:** Mole shows various shades of brown, black or blue, with possibly some red or white areas or tones of pink and gray; pigmentation is not uniform.
D **Diameter:** Mole's diameter is more than 6 millimeters (¼ inch) and/or there is sudden or continuing increase in size.

skin lesions and to undergo a biopsy if melanoma is suspected. When a patient has many suspicious-looking moles, biopsies become time-consuming and costly, as well as leaving numerous scars. A *dermoscope, a* specialized hand-held microscope, may be used to assess the likelihood that a mole or other skin growth is malignant. The technique, called epiluminescence microscopy and amplified surface microscopy, is widely used in Europe but much less often in the United States. Some units have a built-in digital camera and software that analyzes the pictures and assists diagnosis. The dermatologist must be trained in the technology, and there are increasing numbers of training programs in the United States. Adjuvant treatments such as chemotherapy do not seem to be effective. Current research is being directed at a possible vaccine, since melanoma is a cancer that triggers immune system responses in the form of antigens.

melasma Another name for CHLOASMA.

membrane rupture See AMNIOTOMY; DRY LABOR.

menarche The beginning of menstrual periods, which usually occurs any time between the ages of 9 and 16 and, in 5% of girls, between 16 and 18. Menstruation beginning before the age of 9 may be either PRECOCIOUS PUBERTY or a symptom of endocrine disease. In middle-class American girls the average age of menarche is 12.6, showing a steady decline from the average age of 15.5 a century ago. This decline is largely attributed to improved diet, whereby girls attain their CRITICAL WEIGHT earlier. Contrary to a widespread myth, extremes of climate tend to slow down the rate of maturation, so girls in tropical climates do not mature faster than those in temperate ones. Race also is not a factor. However, poor health—physical or mental—can delay menarche.

Menarche usually occurs two to four years after the first signs of PUBERTY appear, when 90% of the rapid weight gain and height growth have taken place. Most girls are close to their mature height by the time of their first menstrual period, thereafter growing only 1 or 2 inches more. The frequency and amount of menstrual flow during the first few years ranges from one period every few months and light staining to full-fledged monthly periods similar to those of adulthood. Early periods usually, but not always, are ANOVULATORY.

See also AMENORRHEA; MENSTRUAL CYCLE.

menopause Also *change of life, climacteric, the change.* Strictly speaking, the ending of menstruation. In common usage, however, the term describes the period immediately preceding the end of menstruation, which in most women lasts from a few months to a few years, although in some it takes only days and in others five or six years; more recently this period has been called PERIMENOPAUSE. It also may refer to castration or *surgical menopause,* that is, menopause induced by bilateral OOPHOREC-TOMY (removal of both ovaries). Although hysterectomy (removal of the uterus) ends menstruation, estrogen production and ovulation continue until the time of natural menopause, provided that at least one ovary is intact. The average age for menopause in America is sometime between 45 and 53, although the normal range is much wider. Menopause occurring before the age of 40 is considered *premature menopause* and calls for careful investigation to make sure no underlying disease is responsible for the symptoms.

Except when it results from surgery, menopause usually is not abrupt. More often the first signs are fluctuations in the menstrual cycle and menstrual flow. Periods may become lighter and/or less frequent, or a period may be skipped altogether; or periods may become heavy and/or more frequent, as often as every 21 days. Sometimes both kinds of change occur in turn in the same woman. Basically menopause is a reversal of puberty. Where in puberty the pituitary gland stimulates the ovaries to increase estrogen production and release eggs, in middle age—usually sometime after the age of 40—estrogen production begins to slacken, ovulation (egg release) becomes irregular and tapers off and eventually menstrual flow ends. Men, who have more abrupt and disturbing symptoms than women at puberty—voice change, more acne and mood swings, strong feelings of aggression—experience a far more gradual decline in sperm and hormone production in their middle years (see MALE MENOPAUSE). When there has been no menstrual flow for 12 months, the reversal is usually, but not always, complete, and thereafter a woman is said to be POSTMENOPAUSAL. Nevertheless, bleeding after 12 months without a period warrants a prompt gynecologic examination to rule out fibroids, polyps, cancer or some other lesion.

Just as increasing hormone production during puberty brings on physical and emotional changes, so menopause is associated with symptoms caused by decreased hormone production. As the ovaries begin to produce less estrogen, the pituitary gland, responding to the feedback system (see MENSTRUAL CYCLE), secretes more and more FSH (follicle-stimulating hormone) to spur on the ovaries. Indeed, the principal clinical sign in a woman undergoing menopause is the presence of higher FSH levels in her blood and urine. Either a test made with a 24-hour urine sample or a blood test is the standard method of diagnosis. Moreover, ovulation is now sporadic, as it was in the year or two following menarche. An increasing number of cycles involve ANOVULATORY BLEEDING, with no egg released from the ovary. Thus, even if FSH makes the ovaries produce enough estrogen to prepare the endometrium (uterine lining) for the first half of the menstrual cycle, without ovulation no progesterone is produced for the second half of the cycle. The endometrium therefore is built up to receive a fertilized egg but does not mature sufficiently to separate and be shed when no egg is implanted. As a result the cycle is thrown out of kilter. Menstrual bleeding may be delayed, or it may commence on time but continue longer than the usual five to seven days of a normal period, or it may be heavier or lighter than usual. Occasionally the endometrium becomes thicker and thicker, and bleeding becomes profuse and prolonged. In this condition either a D and C or hormone therapy (drugs used to treat endometriosis, such as Danazol or GnRH analogs) may be indicated (see ENDOMETRIAL HYPERPLASIA).

Although ovulation after the age of 40 gradually occurs less and less, birth control continues to be necessary until periods have ceased for at least one year. Even then, ovulation sometimes resumes, although the likelihood of becoming pregnant by then has become very small. Intrauterine devices (IUDs) are not advisable during the menopausal period. Oral contraceptives (the Pill) are approved for use until menopause for nonsmoking women without risk factors for heart disease, as is Depo-Provera. Mechanical barriers such as a diaphragm or condom are safest of all. The birth control methods of determining ovulation can be used to check whether a menopausal woman is still ovulating (see NATURAL FAMILY PLANNING) but, given the irregularity of cycles, should not be relied on for birth control.

The most common symptom of menopause is HOT FLASHES. Another change experienced to different degrees by many women, although often only postmenopausally—typically, several years after periods have ended—is thinning, drying and loss of elasticity in the tissues of the vulva and vagina, called VAGINAL ATROPHY. The labia gradually lose some of their fatty layers, making the clitoris appear more prominent, and the vaginal walls become thinner and produce less mucus. Secondary results of this process are painful intercourse (DYSPAREUNIA) and greater susceptibility to vaginal and urinary infections. Like hot flashes, vagina atrophy responds to estrogen therapy, including local applications of estrogen creams and suppositories, which are absorbed by the body. Here, too, the risks must be weighed against the benefits, although in some cases a single application each week may relieve symptoms and may be too small to cause side effects.

Still another symptom associated with menopause and the postmenopausal years is OSTEOPORO-

SIS, a chronic skeletal disorder of aging that affects women sooner and more severely than men. Estrogen replacement therapy definitely slows down this process.

Menopause does not necessarily affect a woman's sex drive, which depends on the production of androgens (male hormones) by the adrenal glands and ovaries and does not seem to diminish. Indeed, many women find their sex life improved when fear of pregnancy is removed. In general, if a woman had satisfactory sexual relations before menopause, it is likely she will continue to have them. Some women find their decline in libido may improve with a small dose of TESTOSTERONE (the male sex hormone), which in women is produced in small amounts by the ovaries and adrenal glands. Postmenopausally, with declined ovarian function and estrogen replacement therapy, a woman's testosterone levels may drop enough to decrease libido.

Most women—an estimated 60 to 80%—experience only minor discomfort during menopause. After a year or two of irregular periods and a number of hot flashes of mild to moderate severity, they simply stop menstruating. About 10 to 20% have virtually no symptoms. For the remaining 10 to 20%, including the majority of those who undergo surgical menopause, symptoms—especially hot flashes—may be a major annoyance and occasionally incapacitating. A striking feature is the great amount of variation found among individuals, no doubt caused by enormous variation in hormone production. Some estrogen continues to be secreted after menopause, by the adrenal glands and probably also by the ovaries (although it is in a different form and is converted into estrogen elsewhere in the body). The amounts produced vary considerably from one woman to another. Postmenopausally, fat women seem to have higher levels of estrogen (in the form of estrone) than thin ones, indicating that fat cells may store it and release it as they are broken down. In any event, there is no doubt that the severity of menopausal symptoms is a physiological phenomenon and is affected only slightly by a woman's emotional adjustment, satisfaction with her life, anxiety or tranquility over aging or similar concerns.

Human beings are the only animal species in which the female long outlives her reproductive capacity; other animals die soon after they stop reproducing. Moreover, until the 19th century few women lived past menopause. Medical knowledge of menopause, therefore, is still relatively new and limited. During the 19th century various attitudes toward—and treatments for—menopausal symptoms developed. Treatments included bleeding (used in London in the 1850s), hysterectomy (invented in 1872), radiation, monkey gland transplants and injections with the cells of unborn lambs. One view that became common, among women as well as physicians, and one that persists to the present day is that menopausal symptoms are to be disregarded, that if one keeps busy and ignores unpleasant symptoms they will disappear. This view continues to be reinforced by some members of the health care professions, whose image of the menopausal woman is that of a childish neurotic, a nuisance to her husband and doctor, casting a pall over family and friends. Menopausal symptoms do have a real basis in physiologic malfunctioning, and some women—fortunately only a minority—do need assistance in getting through the worst of them. Since estrogen replacement therapy carries some risk and tranquilizers and other mood-altering drugs may relieve anxiety but also have undesirable side effects, simpler and safer remedies should be tried first. A well-balanced diet is important, with enough calcium and vitamin D to ward off OSTEOPOROSIS.

Regular physical exercise, especially brisk walking (a 15-minute mile) and swimming, helps keep bones and muscles strong. Weight-bearing exercise of any kind (including walking) counteracts osteoporosis, and swimming helps arthritis (in assisting flexibility). Exercise maintains muscle tone and cardiovascular capacity, and also gives a sense of well-being and burns extra calories.

Extra lubrication, such as K-Y jelly or a plain vegetable oil applied to the vagina, can protect against irritation due to drying tissues.

After menopause, regular physical examinations should be continued, including an annual checkup for blood pressure, height and weight, breast examination (see MAMMOGRAPHY), pelvic examination and a Pap smear. At that time routine blood and urine tests may also be done, and there should be an annual test for glaucoma, a potentially blinding eye disease that usually develops only after the age of 40 and, if detected early, can be controlled. Women should continue to examine their breasts monthly—and probably should, after the age of 50, have an electrocardiogram every five years or so, and more often in the presence of heart disease, high blood pressure or high-risk factors.

menorrhagia See HYPERMENORRHEA; MENSTRUAL FLOW.

menses See MENSTRUATION.

menstrual cramps See DYSMENORRHEA, def. 4.

menstrual cup A soft, plastic, bell-shaped device for collecting menstrual flow. It is inserted just inside the vagina, where it is held in place by suction. Some women prefer to use a DIAPHRAGM to collect menstrual fluid. Like the menstrual cup, it holds far more than a tampon or pad.

See also MENSTRUAL SPONGE; SANITARY NAPKIN; TAMPON.

menstrual cycle The regular, periodic process of preparing the lining of the uterus for the implantation and support of a fertilized egg, which, if no egg is fertilized, ends in menstruation (the shedding of extra uterine tissue in menstrual flow). The cycle, roughly a month in duration, is regulated by the levels and interactions of certain hormones, which govern release of an egg from the ovary (see OVULATION), the preparation of the endometrium (uterine lining) for pregnancy and the shedding of endometrial tissue when no pregnancy is begun (menstruation).

The length of the cycle varies from woman to woman, and in some women it varies considerably from month to month as well. Most cycles are between 23 and 35 days long. The *average* cycle is 28 days long, counting from day 1 of a menstrual period up to (but not including) day 1 of the next period. It is divided into three phases: (1) the *men-*

The Menstrual Cycle

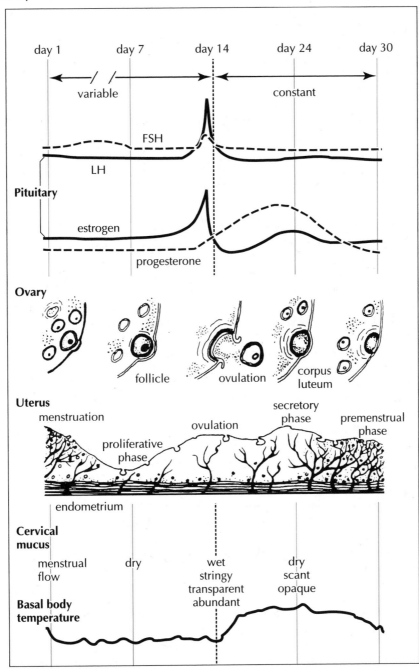

Adapted from *A Book About Birth Control* by Donna Cherniak, Montreal Health Press

strual phase, days 1 to 5; (2) the *proliferative phase* (also called the *preovulatory* or *follicular phase*), days 5 to 13; (3) the *secretory phase* (also called *postovulatory* or *luteal phase*), days 14 to 28. Some authorities do not distinguish between the menstrual and proliferative phases, simply calling days 1 to 13 the proliferative phase.

Between the proliferative and secretory phases, on or about day 13 or 14 (at midcycle), *ovulation*—the release of an egg from the ovary—takes place. In women with menstrual cycles longer or shorter than 28 days, it is nearly always the menstrual and proliferative phases that are longer or shorter; in 90% of women the secretory phase is 13 to 15 days in duration. One can therefore usually determine when ovulation last took place simply by counting back 14 days from the first day of menstrual flow.

The menstrual cycle begins on the first day of menstrual flow. This shedding of endometrial lining results from declining levels of the hormones estrogen and progesterone toward the end of the previous cycle's secretory phase. These low hormone levels also, it is believed, have a positive feedback (or stimulating effect) on the HYPOTHALAMUS, causing it to produce gonadotropin-releasing hormone (GnRH), which in turn acts on the pituitary gland to make it secrete follicle-stimulating hormone (FSH) and luteinizing hormone (LH). FSH stimulates the growth of several follicles (each surrounding one egg) in the ovary, one of which will become the *Graafian follicle*, that is, the one activated to produce a mature egg cell. LH stimulates estrogen secretion by the follicles.

The follicles' secretion of estrogen begins the *proliferative phase*, which starts with the end of menstrual flow and ends with ovulation. During this phase the levels of estrogen increase, all but one of the follicles atrophy while the Graafian follicle continues to develop, and the endometrium thickens in preparation for the implantation of a fertilized egg. As estrogen concentrations rise, FSH levels decline because, it is believed, the higher estrogen level now has a negative effect on the hypothalamus. LH levels remain constant, however. At midcycle, the end of the proliferative phase, the high level of ovarian estrogen causes the pituitary to release a large amount of LH, which in turn stimulates the Graafian follicle to reach

maturity and release an egg (ovulation); the empty follicle is then transformed into the CORPUS LUTEUM, which secretes both progesterone and estrogen.

With ovulation, the proliferative phase, which is dominated by the hormone estrogen, ends. There follows the *secretory phase*, which is dominated by the hormone progesterone, secreted (along with estrogen) by the follicle in its new form, the corpus luteum. During this phase the endometrium thickens still more and the uterine glands begin to produce their secretions of life-supporting substances for the nurture of a fertilized egg. If fertilization does occur, the corpus luteum's secretions are controlled by a different hormone, human chorionic gonadotropin (HCG), manufactured by the placenta. If the egg is not fertilized, the secretions of the corpus luteum are controlled by LH. The higher levels of progesterone and estrogen produced by the corpus luteum now exert negative feedback (an inhibiting influence) on the production of LH and FSH, which begins to decrease. When the level of LH drops, the corpus luteum begins to atrophy and stops producing estrogen and progesterone. The thickening of the endometrium can no longer be maintained and is therefore shed, along with some blood and mucus, in the form of the menstrual flow. The lowered hormone levels again trigger the hypothalamus to produce LRH and FRH, which in turn stimulate pituitary production of LH and FSH, and the entire cycle begins again.

See also the separate entries on each of the hormones mentioned; also AMENORRHEA; ANOVULATORY BLEEDING; FOLLICLE; GRAAFIAN FOLLICLE; OVULATION.

menstrual extraction 1. Also *menstrual regulation, minisuction.* A method of removing menstrual fluid by means of suction or aspiration in order to eliminate the nuisance of menstrual cramps and menstrual flow. A special plastic syringe or cannula is inserted through the cervix at the beginning of a menstrual period. It is small enough so that the cervix need not be dilated first, and it is attached to a small suction machine or foot pump or syringe. By this means the entire menstrual fluid for one period can be sucked out in five minutes. Developed in the 1970s by women who felt that conventional pads, tampons and other ways of dealing with menstrual flow were too troublesome, this method did not gain very wide acceptance and no thorough study has been made of its long-range effects (if any). It definitely carries some risk of infection, since it involves the insertion of a foreign body (the cannula) into the uterus. Otherwise it is similar to VACUUM ASPIRATION except that the cannula is finer and of a smaller caliber, and it is performed at home or in a self-help clinic, usually by nonprofessionals who have been taught the procedure. It *cannot* be done by a woman on herself.

2. Also *preemptive abortion, interception of pregnancy.* The same procedure described in def. 1 but performed for the purpose of ending a possible pregnancy; that is, one that either has not been verified by a positive pregnancy test or that has been verified but is still very early—less than six weeks from the first day of the last menstrual period. Some authorities feel that, since pregnancy can be detected just days after conception (see PREGNANCY TEST), menstrual extraction and vacuum aspiration are one and the same. Also, many believe that there is a greater risk of retaining fragments of fetal and placental tissue with any suction procedure used before the sixth week of pregnancy and therefore recommend waiting until later. This may rule out the very small instrument used in menstrual extraction, since the longer one waits, the more material must be removed. Further, unless pregnancy has been definitely established, menstrual extraction may be totally unnecessary. Nevertheless, its supporters maintain that for a woman whose menstrual period is a few days late and who fears she may be pregnant, menstrual extraction may be a satisfactory alternative. In any case, a thorough pelvic examination and a repeat pregnancy test three weeks after the procedure are recommended.

menstrual flow   Also *menstrual discharge, period.* Vaginal bleeding that occurs on a more or less regular monthly basis from MENARCHE until after MENOPAUSE. The duration of bleeding, called the *menstrual period,* lasts, on the average, from two to seven days. The total amount of discharge varies considerably among different women but 60 to 70 milliliters (3 to 4 ounces) appears to be aver-

age for a single period. The fluid is dark reddish in color but tends to be brighter red if it is very profuse. It consists of blood, degenerated cells from the endometrium (uterine lining; see MENSTRUAL CYCLE for explanation), mucus from the cervical glands and vagina, and bacteria. It usually does not contain clots, nor is the blood component in it capable of clotting. The blood in menstrual flow is actually serum, which already clotted while in the uterus and then was dissolved and reliquefied by enzymes.

In many women menstrual flow is heaviest during the first day or two of their period and thereafter gradually diminishes. This pattern is by no means universal. Some women barely stain for the first two days and then flow more heavily, while others always experience a steady flow (either light or heavy). Some women always have very heavy periods (requiring the use of more than eight sanitary napkins or tampons per day) and some always have quite light ones (only one or two napkins per day). Since the normal range is so wide, a marked *change* in a woman's own pattern is more significant than differences among individuals.

The principal means of dealing with menstrual flow in Western countries are the SANITARY NAPKIN and TAMPON (see also MENSTRUAL CUP; MENSTRUAL EXTRACTION; MENSTRUAL SPONGE). The occurrence of menstrual flow need not prevent vaginal intercourse. In fact, for couples wishing to avoid pregnancy, it may be a satisfactory time since few women ovulate while flowing. Those who find intercourse messy at this time might try using a diaphragm during intercourse to contain the flow.

Scanty flow, or *hypomenorrhea,* sometimes is caused by oral contraceptives and usually is no cause for concern. In contrast, *hypermenorrhea* or *menorrhagia,* meaning very heavy menstrual flow, can result from a number of disorders and should be investigated. One common cause is presence of a FIBROID. Another, often unsuspected, is ectopic pregnancy. Other possible causes include a cervical or endometrial POLYP, PELVIC INFLAMMATORY DISEASE, an ovarian CYST or other tumor and ADENOMYOSIS. Occasionally thyroid disturbances or a platelet deficiency, such as VON WILLEBRAND DISEASE, are responsible. In some women an intrauterine device (IUD) causes such heavy flow that it must be removed and another form of birth control substituted.

Often, however, hypermenorrhea is simply the result of a disruption in hormone balance, which is most likely to occur at menarche and menopause. Such DYSFUNCTIONAL BLEEDING may be corrected either by a D AND C or vacuum aspiration, or by the administration of hormones, either progesterone alone or oral contraceptives containing both progesterone and estrogen.

Hypermenorrhea is both more alarming and potentially more dangerous than scanty flow. It can result in enough blood loss to cause anemia and occasionally even to necessitate a blood transfusion. If heavy bleeding and anemia persist and no other measure proves effective, as a last resort hysterectomy may be performed. A new alternative to hysterectomy is LASER SURGERY, which directs intensely concentrated light beams against the uterine lining and coagulates the blood-filled tissue, creating a thin layer of scar tissue that does not bleed. Performed on an outpatient basis, it usually is preceded by an endometrial biopsy to make sure no cancer is present and by the administration of danazol, which shrinks the endometrium to a thickness of 1 millimeter. The laser beam is carried into the uterus by a flexible fiberoptic device inserted through the vagina and cervix. Some clinicians may try gonadotropin-releasing hormone (GnRH) agonists, which induce a temporary, reversible menopause. A still newer technique is BALLOON ABLATION. (See also BREAKTHROUGH BLEEDING; OLIGOMENORRHEA; POLYMENORRHEA.)

A number of nutritional and HERBAL REMEDIES have been used to deal with hypermenorrhea. Some women find that dolomite, which contains calcium and magnesium, helps both severe cramps and heavy flow; they recommend taking a tablet every few hours during the first day or two of such a period. Vitamin A supplements (but less than 25,000 International Units a day—more is dangerous) also have been so used. Herbal remedies include teas made from yarrow (*Achillea millefolium;* **avoid if pregnant**), red raspberry leaf (*Rubus idaeus*), shepherd's purse (*Capsella bursa pastoris*) or cinnamon bark (stick cinnamon). For painful menstruation and other problems associated with menstrual periods, see DYSMENORRHEA.

menstrual sponge   A small natural sponge inserted into the vagina to absorb menstrual flow. It is used by some women as an alternative to commercially manufactured pads and tampons on the grounds that a sponge is free of bleach and chemicals, less expensive, more convenient and ecologically preferable because it can be reused. A sponge can be cut into whatever size one wishes (for heavier or lighter flow) and holds approximately as much as a pad or tampon. The sponge used should be natural (not the human-made cellulose variety sold for cleaning purposes) and preferably unbleached, meaning it is brown rather than yellow or white. It should first be well rinsed or, if one wishes, boiled, but not for longer than five minutes lest it become tough. It is then dampened and inserted. To make removal easier, one can first tie a piece of strong string or dental floss around it or through one end. A piece of sponge about the size of a small egg is recommended at first. It will expand somewhat when moistened more by the menstrual flow. To remove, one gently pulls on the string or, if none has been attached, on the sponge itself. If the sponge begins to tear, relax, get a firmer hold and resume gentle pulling. Once out, the sponge is rinsed with clear water and reinserted. If rinsing is not possible, it can simply be squeezed out and reinserted. (Some

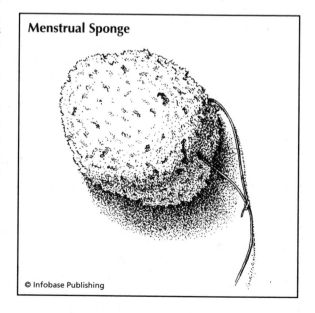

Menstrual Sponge

© Infobase Publishing

women carry an extra sponge in a small plastic bag so as to avoid reinserting a soiled one.) At the end of a monthly period, the sponge can be rinsed several times in water with a little white vinegar (1 tablespoon per 16 ounces of water) to remove any accumulated odor. It is then air-dried and stored until the next period. Some women advocate using soap and water; others believe soap should be avoided. Unbleached sponges last for many months before they deteriorate. Although not widely sold in American drugstores, sponges suitable for this use are available from women's health centers and clinics, direct or by mail order. Although its advocates believe the menstrual sponge is safer than the TAMPON, at least one case of toxic shock syndrome associated with sponge use has been reported.

See also CONTRACEPTIVE SPONGE.

menstruation   Also *menses*. Regular monthly shedding of endometrial tissue and blood through the vagina. The beginning of menstruation is called MENARCHE, the end, MENOPAUSE.

See also MENSTRUAL CYCLE; MENSTRUAL FLOW.

metabolic syndrome   A group of risk factors for heart attack.

See also ARTERIOSCLEROSIS.

metabolic toxemia of pregnancy   See ECLAMPSIA; PREECLAMPSIA.

metabolism   A general term for all the physical and chemical processes whereby the body acquires and uses the foods and energy it requires for life, growth and maturation. It includes the transformation of nutrients into living tissue and the processes whereby complex substances are reduced to simpler ones. *Basal metabolism* is the minimum energy expended by the body while at complete rest for the maintenance of its basic functions: respiration, circulation, muscle tone, body temperature, glandular activity and so on. The rate of basal metabolism, or *basic metabolic rate* (BMR), is measured by a calorimeter and is expressed in *calories* per hour

per square meter of body surface. Disorders of metabolism—that is, inabilities to use nutrients and energy in necessary ways—either are present from birth (genetic or congenital) or are acquired. One congenital defect is phenylketonuria (PKU), the inability to metabolize a particular amino acid, which frequently results in mental retardation. It can, however, be diagnosed immediately after birth by means of a simple test, which in the United States is now mandatory in most states, and with treatment this outcome can be prevented.

metastasis   The spread of disease from one part of the body to another that is not directly connected to it. The term generally is reserved for the spread of CANCER, which is said to *metastasize*. To date there is no sure way to predict when cancers, such as a malignant breast tumor, metastasize, and consequently adjuvant therapy (chemotherapy and radiation) is used almost routinely. However, an increasing number of tests are being devised, most of them performed on cells taken from the original tumor, to find indicators that will predict the chances of spread and so help decisions about further treatment. At this writing they still are considered experimental, but breakthroughs are anticipated in the near future.

metrorrhagia   See BREAKTHROUGH BLEEDING.

microsurgery   Surgery performed with the help of optical instruments, such as loupes or microscopes, to magnify the surgical field. The term also implies the use of particularly fine operating tools, very small nonirritating sutures and special salt solutions (to keep tissues continually moist). Further, the term implies a surgical approach that involves extremely delicate and meticulous handling of tissues. Microsurgery is used in removing pelvic adhesions and scar tissue, repairing damaged fallopian tubes and other procedures.

midcycle   The middle of the MENSTRUAL CYCLE, when ovulation takes place.

See also MITTELSCHMERZ.

midwife 1. A person other than a physician who has some training (formal or informal) to serve as the principal assistant at childbirth. Although there are some male midwives, the majority are women. Midwives have been used since ancient times. In Europe and in America they often were accused of witchcraft, and, indeed, the first witch executed in the Massachusetts Bay Colony, in 1648, was a physician and midwife, Margaret Jones. In Europe midwifery survived the witchcraft craze and midwives were integrated into the health care system. In England and America, however, men were encouraged to enter the field of obstetrics and gradually took it over, eventually as physicians. With the establishment of hospitals and the increase in hospital deliveries, midwifery died out in America except in rural areas, since midwives were not allowed to assist births in hospitals. However, along with the increase in hospital births came growing concern over the very high infant mortality rate—higher than with home births—and in 1931 the first school to train nurses in maternity care was opened in New York. Meanwhile the *granny midwife* of rural areas, especially the American South, continued to function. Such women usually had no formal training but learned from experience, both their own and through apprenticeship to women of the previous generation (often their own mothers) who had practiced midwifery. They attended the majority of American home births until the 1930s. In the late 1930s and early 1940s maternity centers began to open in the rural South. There granny midwives could supplement their experience with formal training in anatomy, nutrition, and other prenatal care, and sterile technique. The modern midwifery movement grew, but slowly, and it faced considerable opposition from both obstetricians and hospitals. Today the majority of states in the United States have licensing and other legal provisions for the practice of midwifery, although some are more restrictive than others.

In Europe, Africa and Asia, midwifery never fell into disrepute, and even in the most advanced European countries midwives continued to account for the majority of deliveries, both in hospitals and at home. Indeed, in addition to the kinds of midwife described in defs. 2 and 3 below, several thousand professional midwives from other countries are now practicing in the United States and Canada. Most are graduates of schools of midwifery in the United Kingdom or Australia and have considerable experience in attending both home and hospital births.

See also BIRTH ATTENDANT.

2. lay midwife. Also *community midwife, independent midwife.* A midwife who, like the granny midwife, may have no formal training or recognized professional education in midwifery but who usually is a younger woman and may have considerable formal education of other kinds. Frequently she begins her career by accompanying doctors or midwives who are attending home births. She gradually takes more and more responsibility for the delivery, until she feels ready to work alone. Lay midwives became very active in the 1970s in the so-called counterculture—in communes on the American West Coast, for example, or at birth centers trying to provide a safe alternative to hospital settings. Today they are the principal attendants at home births. Occasionally they may serve as a birth attendant or labor coach in a hospital birth, but only in an unofficial capacity by private arrangement with the mother-to-be. As a rule lay midwives are opposed to interference with the normal process of labor and delivery (some describe their work as "catching" a baby rather than "delivering" it) and generally concentrate on giving advice and support to the woman in labor as well as dealing with the total health (including the emotional well-being) of the woman and her family. If the lay midwife suspects that a birth may become complicated, she generally takes the woman to a hospital immediately.

The services provided by lay midwives vary widely, since their experience, training and capabilities differ considerably from individual to individual. The best of them provide complete prenatal care, including history, physical examination, pelvic examination and measurements, laboratory tests and discussions of nutrition as well as the standard checkups. They remain with a woman through labor and delivery, provide emergency transport to a hospital should it be needed and give follow-up care after birth. The principal drawback to using a lay midwife, other than that it may be illegal in one's own locality, is that the majority of states permitting them do not regulate them, so there are no set or uniform standards for evaluating their work, and hence no way of determining their competence in advance. However, in recent years they have joined forces with certified nurse-midwives (see def. 3) to create the new Certified Professional Midwife (CPM), with established standards for validating their knowledge and competence.

In some states the practice of lay midwifery is clearly legal, in others it is illegal, and in many others it is legally ambiguous. Even where it is legal, midwifery is often vigorously opposed by physicians on the ground that it constitutes practicing medicine without a license. In some states where no specific law governs lay midwifery, the practice is prohibited by judicial interpretation or attorney general opinion.

3. nurse-midwife. A registered nurse who has taken special postgraduate training in gynecology and obstetrics so that she is qualified to care for women before, during and after childbirth, provided that no complications develop. In the United States she must have fulfilled the requirements for certification by the American College of Nurse-Midwives and is qualified to perform a variety of gynecologic services, including Pap smear, breast and pelvic examination, contraceptive and menopausal counseling, teenage pregnancy prevention, tests for vaginal, pelvic and urinary infections, assistance with breast-feeding and screening for menstrual problems (dysmenorrhea, fertility problems, etc.). She may work in her own private practice, in private physician practices, freestanding birth centers, hospitals and health departments, and occasionally may attend home births. She cares for the mother during a normal pregnancy and stays with her during labor and delivery, most often in a hospital. She also evaluates and provides immediate care for the normal newborn baby and helps the mother care for herself and the infant. She provides prenatal care in conjunction with an obstetrician. Either she or the obstetrician conducts the first examination, including history, pelvic examination and laboratory work. Thereafter it is usually the nurse-midwife who sees the woman in routine checkups, answers questions and perhaps also conducts a childbirth education class.

ASK YOUR POTENTIAL MIDWIFE

- Are you certified by the American College of Nurse-Midwives? May I see your certification?
- Are you covered by my medical insurance? If so, in what settings: hospital? birth center? health maintenance organization clinic? public health department? doctor's office or clinic? for home birth?
- What do you consider a complication requiring backup—breech birth? prolonged labor? bleeding?
- What backup do you use in case of emergency or complications? What physician? Which hospital?
- Are you willing/able to use analgesics if I need them? anesthesia?

The nurse-midwife in effect is a person formally trained to perform duties that were undertaken by informally trained practitioners in the past. Those who are licensed and certified (known as *CNMs*) can practice in all 50 states. Although the American College of Nurse-Midwives was founded in 1955 in order to establish standards for training nurses in maternity care, opposition from physicians continued to keep nurse-midwives from delivering babies in hospitals; they were allowed only to assist physicians. In 1970 the American College of Obstetricians and Gynecologists gave formal recognition to licensed midwives, stating that they may, when working with a physician, assume responsibility for the complete care of uncomplicated maternity patients. However, they must be qualified, that is, have an RN (registered nurse) degree followed by one year of training in obstetrics and gynecology, leading to a degree in midwifery. If, in addition, they take a year of internship, they receive a master's degree along with the nurse-midwifery certificate.

The care provided by nurse-midwives generally is regarded as being of very high quality. Many of them subscribe to the same view as lay midwives—that is, labor should be allowed to progress at its own pace. They tend not to rush patients through delivery, and although they are allowed to administer painkilling medications and oxytoxin (Pitocin), they tend to do so sparingly. Often the midwife meets the mother at the hospital door and remains with her until after the birth, whereas obstetricians are more likely to check the mother periodically rather than staying with her. They do not, however, perform surgery such as a Cesarean section, nor do they use forceps.

There are several drawbacks to using a nurse-midwife. Some physicians refuse to work with them, viewing them as an economic threat, which limits their access to medical backup. The requirements of managed care, limiting the time spent on prenatal visits, may be a constraint. Hospital rules may restrict their activities somewhat, and in some places they may not be allowed to assist a home birth, where "supervision" is less readily available. Also, only 39 or so institutions in the United States offer nurse-midwife training programs, so there are currently about 11,000 certified nurse-midwives in the country.

Although midwife-attended births grew considerably from the 1970s through the 1990s, the number of available midwives, especially nurse-midwives (see def. 3 above), began to decline dramatically from about 2001 on. A principal reason for this decline is the enormous increase in malpractice insurance premiums, ranging from 50% to as much as 400% in some cases, and new limitations placed on midwives' practice by both hospitals and insurers. It has forced the closing of numerous birth centers staffed mainly by midwives, as well as limiting the numbers hired by physicians to work in hospitals. Insurers claim that, with the increase in women having babies later in life and other high-risk patients, the increased premiums are necessary, but opponents hold that it is unfair to penalize midwives, whose care results in fewer Cesareans and other expensive procedures. Furthermore, health insurance tends to cover the full cost of birth in a hospital but awards less for birth in a birth center and still less for birth at home.

The accompanying table lists questions a woman considering using a midwife might ask.

migraine   Also *sick headache*. A recurrent kind of HEADACHE that affects women more frequently than men (some studies say five times as much, others only one and one-half times as much). The headache tends to occur in two stages. In the first, called *premonitory stage* or *aura,* a person has various sensory aberrations or unexplainable mood changes, hyperactivity, or irritability. Common among the sensory distortions are visual disturbances such as seeing flashing lights or zigzag lines or experiencing blind spots. About one of five patients experiences such a distinct aura, usually some hours before head pain develops.

The second stage is characterized by the severe head pain itself. It can affect almost any part of the head except the lower jaw and usually begins on one side (the same side affected during the premonitory stage), in the lower forehead or temple. It tends to move from there to the back of the head, remaining more severe on the side originally affected. The head pain frequently is accompanied by nausea, sometimes with vomiting, and a variety of other symptoms, including increased urination, pallor, abdominal pain, photophobia (intolerance to light), sweating, supersensitivity of the face to heat, cold and touch (called *allodynia*), and/or fever. By the time the nausea passes the headache usually has ended. Typically a migraine lasts 8 to 12 hours, but it may persist for several days.

Migraine can be brought on by such external factors as bright lights, noise, motion and abrupt changes in weather. It also may be precipitated by a change in estrogen levels just before a menstrual period (see below), psychological stress, weather changes, fatigue or sleep disturbances and overuse of over-the-counter pain medications. Although various foods have long been thought to trigger migraine, especially chocolate, red wine, and aged cheese, there is no firm evidence supporting this notion. Migraine tends to run in families. It usually begins between the ages of 10 and 30 and frequently ends after the age of 50.

In at least 60% of women with migraines, their headaches are often or always set off by changing levels of sex hormones, either produced naturally during the menstrual cycle or administered as medication or contraceptives. Typically the headache begins just before menstruation or, more often, at the time of ovulation. Research suggests that the headaches and other symptoms (nausea, mood disturbance, hypersensitivity to light and noise) stem from an abrupt decrease in previously high levels of estrogen. Women afflicted with this so-called *menstrual migraine* also often suffer from fluid retention and breast tenderness in association with menstruation. Fully one-third of such cases begin at the time of the first menstrual period. The headaches generally disappear with pregnancy, during which estrogen levels remain high, and menopause may bring an end to them (although some women get worse postmenopausally). Both oral contraceptives and estrogen replacement therapy aggravate the syndrome, and should be used with caution, if at all.

Migraine was long believed to be brought on by stress leading to the constriction of cerebral arteries, which reduced the blood flow and oxygen supply to the brain. Today migraine is thought to be caused by some disturbance in the function of serotonin, a neurotransmitter (brain chemical) that is also linked to depression and sleep disturbances. While the precise mechanism still is not understood, the most effective medications against migraine act on serotonin.

Mild attacks of migraine may respond to aspirin or ibuprofen taken early, when symptoms are first felt. An over-the-counter medication combining aspirin, acetaminophen and caffeine (Excedrin Migraine) has been approved for migraine relief. Stronger medications are required for a severe attack. They include ergotamine tartrate (dissolved on the tongue, inhaled through the mouth, injected or given by rectal suppository) along with caffeine, which appears to enhance its effect. It too works best when taken early. It should not be taken by a pregnant woman. A newer class of drugs called triptans relieve pain very quickly. The first, sumatriptan, was introduced in 1993 and relieves pain within two hours for about 80% of patients. Marketed as Imitrex, it is available as a subcutaneous self-administered injection, as oral tablets and as a nasal spray. It cannot be used by individuals with heart disease or severe hypertension, because it can constrict coronary arteries, and should be used cautiously if at all by pregnant women. The same cautions apply to zolmitriptan (Zomig), naratriptan (Amerge) and rizatriptan (Maxalt), available in tablet form. The triptans are not ideal, since in 30 to 40% of cases the headache returns within 24 hours. Also, they cannot be used within 24 hours of ergotamine, and they are not advised for women taking serotonin reuptake inhibitors such as Prozac or Zoloft or MAO inhibitors. Another drug for migraine pain, dihydroergotamine mesylate (DHE),

formerly only injected, is available as a nasal spray (marketed as DHE-45 and Migranal). It has a milder effect on arteries than the triptans but should be avoided by women who have poor circulation and diabetes. It takes about three hours to work and must be taken at the first hint of migraine pain. The antihypertensive drug propranolol appears to prevent migraine in some patients or at least reduce the frequency of attacks, but it cannot be used by persons with asthma, severe heart disease and some other disorders. Antinausea medications taken at the onset of a migraine sometimes are helpful; they include prochlorperazine (Compazine), metoclopramide (Reglan) and ondansetron (Zofran). The herb feverfew (*Tanacetum parthenium*) contains a serotonin antagonist and has been found to reduce both the severity and frequency of migraines. Not every feverfew product contains enough of the needed chemical, parthenolide (0.2% is the recommended minimum amount), and further, caution must be exercised, as with other HERBAL REMEDIES.

Two totally different approaches to treatment are now in large trials. One is occipital nerve stimulation (ONS) and the other transcranial magnetic stimulation (TMS). In the former, a pacemaker-like device is connected to electrodes implanted just under the skin at the back of the head. Current delivered through the electrodes aims at relieving or preventing migraine pain. In TMS, a magnetic device is pressed to the back of the head, altering electrical brain activity to halt the progress of a migraine. It is being studied only in patients whose migraines begin with an aura (flashing lights or other visual disturbances).

milk leg   See PHLEGMASIA.

mind visualization   See VISUALIZATION.

minerals   A class of essential nutrients. Those required in large quantities (1 to 2 grams per day) are called macronutrients; those required in small amounts are micronutrients and also are known as trace minerals. The macronutrients include CALCIUM, needed for healthy bones and teeth, as well as blood clotting, muscle function and nerve transmission;

RECOMMENDED DAILY MINERAL INTAKE

Mineral	Amount
Calcium	1,200–1,500 mg ages 11–24 and in pregnancy, during lactation; 1,000 mg ages 25–50; 1,500 mg age 50+
Chloride	750 mg
Copper	900 mcg age 19+; 1,000 mcg during pregnancy; 1,300 mcg during lactation
Fluoride	3 mg for women, 4 mg for men
Iodine	150 mcg age 19+; 220 mcg during pregnancy; 290 mcg during lactation
Iron	18 mg up to age 50; 8 mg age 51+; 27 mg during pregnancy; 9 mg during lactation
Magnesium	320 mg for women; 420 mg for men
Phosphorus	700 mg
Potassium	3,500 mg
Selenium	55 mcg
Sodium	1,500 mg (1,300 after age 50, 1,200 after age 70)
Zinc	15 mg

chloride, which helps balance body fluids and contributes to iron metabolism; magnesium, required for many chemical reactions and to help build bones and teeth; phosphorus, for bone and tooth formation and energy production; and potassium and sodium, both needed for normal nerve and muscle function and to maintain electrolyte balance. The trace minerals include iron, important for hemoglobin and muscle cells; iodine, for forming thyroid hormones; fluoride, to help bone formation and prevent dental caries; copper, to help make red blood cells; selenium, an antioxidant that acts with vitamin E; and zinc, needed for many enzymes and insulin, and healthy skin, wound healing and growth. Iodine deficiency causes goiter; iron deficiency can cause anemia. Most of the necessary minerals are present in a normal diet, but occasionally supplements are needed, particularly calcium for postmenopausal women and fluoride if water supplies are not fluoridated.

See also DIET.

minilaparotomy Also *minilap*. A kind of abdominal TUBAL LIGATION in which the incision is much smaller, only local anesthesia is required and there are fewer unpleasant aftereffects than with tubal ligation performed by LAPAROSCOPY. The clinician inserts a speculum into the vagina, clamps the cervix to hold it steady, and inserts a blunt metal instrument, called an *elevator,* through the cervical canal into the uterus. Next the surgeon makes a 1-inch incision about 1 to 1½ inches (2½ to 3¾ centimeters) above the pubic bone and so manipulates the elevator that the uterus is moved up against the incision. The fallopian tubes are then brought into view, pulled out one at a time through the incision and are cut and tied off with sutures, clips or rings, or closed by means of an electric current or heat (cauterized). The surgeon checks to make sure there is no bleeding and closes the incision with sutures (stitches). There is relatively little discomfort following the operation, which can take as little as 20 minutes, and the woman usually may go home within a few hours and resume all normal activities within a day or two. Because the minilap does not require elaborate surgical equipment and can be performed by trained technicians (rather than surgeons) on an outpatient basis, it is considered a very promising form of permanent birth control in countries where overpopulation poses serious problems. The principal risks are perforation of the uterus by the elevator, difficulty in locating the tubes in obese women, and possible intestinal or bladder injury from the incision.

minipill Also *progestin-only pill.* An ORAL CONTRACEPTIVE that contains only a small dose of progestin (synthetic PROGESTERONE) and no estrogen. Unlike other oral contraceptives, it cannot be relied on to prevent ovulation (it does so in only 50% of cases). Rather, it changes the cervical mucus so that it is no longer hospitable to sperm. It also slows the transport of an egg through the fallopian tube. Since it contains no estrogen, the minipill does not produce many of the side effects of other oral contraceptives. It does, however, give rise to breakthrough bleeding (between periods) and irregular menstrual cycles. Taken daily, it is thought to be about 95% reliable in preventing pregnancy, somewhat less than pills containing estrogen. To enhance its effectiveness, some women use a second method of birth control, such as a diaphragm or condom, at midcycle.

Some women stop having menstrual periods entirely while taking the minipill, meaning they are never sure whether they have missed a period because of pregnancy or the medication. Also, the incidence of ECTOPIC PREGNANCY (outside the uterus, a dangerous condition) is higher in women who become pregnant while taking the minipill, possibly because of the egg's slower transport. **No woman should take the minipill if she is pregnant or has unexplained vaginal bleeding or breast cancer.** Also, it should be used cautiously by those who are breast-feeding or have liver disease (hepatitis, jaundice, cyrrhosis), functional ovarian cysts, cardiovascular disorders or a history of breast cancer. In view of these risks and disadvantages, most clinicians recommend the minipill only when estrogen is contraindicated—in women who have had an estrogen-dependent breast cancer, for example.

minisuction   See MENSTRUAL EXTRACTION, def. 1.

miscarriage   **1.** Also *spontaneous abortion, natural abortion.* The loss of a pregnancy, or expulsion of a fetus before it is sufficiently developed to survive. Such a fetus is defined as one weighing less than 500 grams (1.1 pounds), although some authorities define an infant weighing between 500 and 999 grams (1.1 and 2.2 pounds) as "immature" and others as an "abortion" (see also PREMATURE). The term *miscarriage* is strictly a popular or lay term; physicians use *abortion,* distinguishing only between *spontaneous* or *natural abortion,* which occurs through natural causes, and *induced, elective* or *therapeutic abortion,* which results from artificial intervention. This book follows current popular usage: *abortion* is used only for artificially induced abortion; *miscarriage* is used for natural or spontaneous loss of a pregnancy.

An estimated 15 to 20% of all known pregnancies in North America end in miscarriage; in underdeveloped countries the rate is much higher. Moreover, a much higher percentage of unknown pregnancies (before the woman knows or suspects she is pregnant)—an estimated 50%—end in spontaneous abortion. The majority of miscarriages

occur during the first three months of pregnancy, and in at least half of these the cause lies in the fetus itself, which has some anatomic or genetic abnormality. The woman's activities—jumping, falling, vigorous physical exercise, frequent vaginal intercourse—do not cause miscarriage. Neither does emotional shock or stress. On the other hand, hormonal imbalance, infection or immunologic factors sometimes are responsible (see HABITUAL MISCARRIAGE), although not nearly as often as was formerly believed. However, habits such as cigarette smoking and regular use of certain drugs, such as LSD, do increase the risk of miscarriage. A recent study found that women who took aspirin were 60% more likely to miscarry than those who did not, and users of nonsteroidal anti-inflammatory drugs (NSAIDs) such as ibuprofen were 80% more likely to lose the pregnancy. Other causes for miscarriage in the first trimester are inadequate production of progesterone or some other hormonal lack that either prevents successful IMPLANTATION of the fertilized egg or supplies insufficient nutritional or hormonal support for its growth, or some defect in the endometrium (uterine lining) itself that prevents successful implantation. Fortunately, 90% of women who miscarry once have a healthy pregnancy the next time.

Causes of miscarriage during the second trimester (13 to 24 weeks) include anatomical uterine defects (a double or divided uterus, uterine scar tissue from repeated infection, fibroids, endometrial polyps or a similar problem), an INCOMPETENT CERVIX, infections such as syphilis or genital herpes, or an immunologic reaction causing the woman's body to reject the fetus as if it were a foreign body. Many if not most of these conditions can be corrected by medication or surgery and therefore need not cause miscarriage again.

A single miscarriage usually does not warrant the performance of elaborate tests to determine its cause. However, the risk of miscarriage does rise with a woman's age; one study shows it roughly doubles between the 20s and early 30s, and doubles again between the early and late 30s. For women who have postponed motherhood until their 30s and have had one miscarriage, it therefore may be advisable to determine the cause somewhat sooner, that is, after one miscarriage rather than the three consecutive ones that are considered to constitute habitual miscarriage. Such investigation should include an X-ray of the uterus, an endometrial biopsy timed so as to detect hormonal deficiency following ovulation, blood tests for blood group and type as well as antibody levels of both parents, semen analysis of the father and chromosome analysis of both parents.

The loss of a baby that was planned and eagerly awaited can be emotionally very painful for both mother and father as well as other relatives. Moreover, because miscarriage has a long history of myths and misconceptions, the couple's natural feelings of grief and loss often are complicated by a sense of guilt (What did I do wrong?), anger (It's all his/her fault) and fear (What if I/we can never have a normal baby?). Even persons with rational understanding of the statistics and causes of miscarriage may suffer from nagging doubts and fears. Consequently after any miscarriage it is highly advisable for a woman to ask relevant questions during the follow-up visit with her clinician—with the father also present, if possible—and to discuss the suspected or known causes of this particular miscarriage and the chances of successful future pregnancy.

2. threatened miscarriage. Symptoms indicating that a pregnancy may end prematurely, most often consisting of slight bleeding and mild cramps. Bleeding alone need not be a sign of threatened miscarriage. If the bleeding continues for a time, however, it is advisable to check for a cause other than threatened miscarriage, such as a cervical POLYP. Ultrasound can determine if the fetus is alive, as can a blood test for HCG (human chorionic gonadotropin), whose levels should be increasing. Bleeding and cramps together nearly always constitute a threatened miscarriage, although the cramps are not strong enough to dilate the cervix. When they are, miscarriage usually is inevitable (see def. 3 below).

An early threatened miscarriage, after one or two missed periods, probably cannot be treated effectively, but nearly all clinicians recommend bed rest for at least 24 hours and no vaginal intercourse for a few days. Since it is believed that most such early miscarriages are due to abnormalities in the fetus and are, in effect, nature's way of eliminat-ing a defective fetus, presumably no treatment for the mother would make much difference. For threatened miscarriage later in pregnancy, however, bed rest and avoidance of intercourse are generally recommended (see also under EXERCISE). An asthma medication, terbutaline, occasionally is used to delay premature birth. Hormone treatment of any kind, especially with DIETHYLSTILBESTROL, is to be avoided for threatened miscarriage unless there is a specific hormone deficiency; it may cause birth defects and possibly cancer in the babies that survive.

See also UTERINE MONITORING.

3. inevitable miscarriage. The occurrence of severe vaginal bleeding and/or cramps in a pregnant woman, indicating that no medical treatment can avert a miscarriage. At this point the amniotic membranes have ruptured, the cervix is dilated, and the membranes, fetus and placenta are on their way to being expelled. The woman's clinician should be contacted immediately, and hospitalization may be necessary. If the fetus and other material are expelled at home, they should be placed in a sterile container and brought to the clinician for examination, since they may reveal the reason for the miscarriage. If pain and blood loss are severe and prolonged, further treatment in the hospital may be necessary.

4. incomplete miscarriage. A miscarriage in which not all of the products of conception—membranes, fetus, placenta—are spontaneously expelled. Most often it is part of the placenta that is retained. Incomplete miscarriage usually is marked by continued bleeding, which can be severe enough to constitute a hemorrhage. Sometimes a drug such as oxytocin is administered to stimulate uterine contractions that may expel the remainder, but more often a D AND C or VACUUM ASPIRATION is performed to make sure all the material is out of the uterus, to prevent infection and more blood loss. Incomplete miscarriage tends to occur most often in the second trimester. A recent study indicated that administering misoprostol, used in the induction of labor and to prevent postpartum hemorrhage, is another option.

5. missed miscarriage. The retention of a dead fetus inside the uterus for at least two months. Unlike other kinds of miscarriage (see above), the symptoms often are barely noticeable. There may or may not be vaginal bleeding. Usually the breasts return to prepregnant size and the uterus stops growing; eventually it becomes somewhat smaller, owing to absorption of amniotic fluid. Many women report few or no symptoms, but some complain of lassitude, fatigue, depression and a bad taste in the mouth. Most often uterine contractions eventually begin of their own accord, and the fetus is spontaneously expelled, as in other kinds of miscarriage. When, however, the mother is aware of the fact that the fetus is dead, waiting for spontaneous miscarriage can be emotionally devastating for both her and the family. Consequently many clinicians advise emptying the uterus promptly by inducing labor with oxytocin, by AMNIOINFUSION or by D AND C, the choice depending on the size of the uterus. As with incomplete miscarriage, administering misoprostol may be used to induce contractions and empty the uterus.

See also STILLBIRTH.

6. septic miscarriage. Any miscarriage (see def. 1 to 5 above) that involves infection of the uterus and/or the products of conception. Symptoms include, in addition to the usual vaginal bleeding, marked tenderness of the uterus and lower abdomen, chills, fever and an elevated white blood count.

Septic miscarriage is treated with massive doses of antibiotics for 12 to 24 hours; if labor does not begin by itself, a D and C is performed. Such infections are commonly found following an induced ABORTION performed by an unqualified or sloppy practitioner—they are common where a proper medical abortion is illegal or unavailable—or by women on themselves with instruments ranging from coat hangers to knitting needles. They also may be the result of PELVIC INFLAMMATORY DISEASE or of an INTRAUTERINE DEVICE (IUD) that has failed to prevent pregnancy. Unless treated promptly, such infection may cause enough damage to require removal of the uterus (HYSTERECTOMY).

See also PUERPERAL FEVER.

missed abortion (miscarriage) See MISCARRIAGE, def. 5.

mitochondrial disease See BIRTH DEFECTS.

mitral valve prolapse A ballooning of one or both leaflets of the mitral valve, which lies between the atrium (upper chamber) and the ventricle (lower chamber) on the left side of the heart. This condition occurs in about 5% of Americans, but eight times more often in women than in men. Most often it gives rise to no symptoms whatever, and the condition is discovered only during a routine heart examination with a stethoscope. Occasionally the valve may leak some blood back into the atrium whenever the ventricle pumps blood in the opposite direction. This is known as *mitral valve regurgitation,* and if it is moderate to severe and a fair amount of blood flows back, there may be symptoms such as a shortness of breath. Palpitations or dizziness suggest abnormal heart rhythms. Complications are rare, but patients with structural changes of the valve (which can be detected by an echocardiogram) seem to be at increased risk for endocarditis (infection of the mitral valve). Clinicians may therefore prescribe preventive antibiotics before the woman undergoes dental cleaning, cystoscopy, sigmoidoscopy or any other procedure in which bacteria can be released into the bloodstream. If regurgitation worsens and causes problems, drugs that dilate blood vessels may be prescribed, and if these are not effective, surgery to repair or replace the valve may be in order. For most women, however, the condition presents no problems and calls for no particular changes in lifestyle.

Mittelschmerz A German word, literally meaning "middle pain," used to refer to a cramping pain on one side of the lower abdomen that some women regularly feel at OVULATION. Occasionally the pain is quite severe and mimics the symptoms of acute appendicitis. It may or may not be accompanied by slight bleeding and sometimes even severe bleeding. The reason for these symptoms is not known, especially since many women never feel anything when they ovulate. One theory is that it may be due to irritation of the abdominal lining caused by fluid or blood released from the ruptured egg follicle; another is that follicle growth stretches the surface of the ovary, causing pain (see also GRAAFIAN FOLLICLE). Whatever the cause, *Mit-*

telschmerz usually persists no more than a few hours and rarely more than 24 hours.

mongolism, mongoloid Older names for DOWN SYNDROME.

moniliasis See YEAST INFECTION.

mons veneris Also *mons pubis, pubis, pubic mound.* A cushion of fat that lies over the central portion of the pubic bone, or SYMPHYSIS PUBIS. After puberty it is covered with PUBIC HAIR, usually forming a triangular pattern called the *escutcheon.*

Montgomery's glands See AREOLA.

morning-after pill See EMERGENCY CONTRACEPTION.

morning sickness Popular name for the nausea of early pregnancy, technically called *nausea gravidarum.* It is generally confined to the first three and one-half months of pregnancy, although a small percentage of women continue to experience it either steadily or occasionally until delivery. Although many women find it occurs only in the morning, when they first get out of bed, others experience it at a different time of day, such as late afternoon, and some intermittently throughout the day. Some women feel nauseated, vomit and then are relatively comfortable; others vomit but continue to feel nausea; still others simply feel constantly queasy and never vomit at all. The remedies generally recommended are to eat lightly a number of times throughout the day rather than taking a few big meals, slowly munching dry crackers or toast before arising (nausea is thought to be worse on an empty stomach) and avoiding greasy foods and any particular foods that seem to bring on nausea (many women find meat and other proteins the worst offenders). A variety of both prescription and over-the-counter medications, especially antihistamines and other remedies for motion sick-

ness, have been used over the years. Doxylamine combined with 25 mg of vitamin B_6 four times a day appears to be safe and effective. If these do not work, antinausea medications like Phenergan or Reglan may be prescribed. The condition tends to be worse for women with a history of heartburn or gastric reflux, so antacids like Zantac or Tagamet may help. Women with very severe cases—this condition is called *hyperemesis gravidarum*—usually require hospitalization and find relief only when the fluid-electrolyte balance is corrected by administering intravenous fluids. An herbal remedy that often appears to help considerably is ginger, taken in the form of two to three 500-milligram capsules of powdered ginger root. It should be taken only in gelatin-capsule form because otherwise it can burn the esophagus. However, some women find ginger gives them another kind of indigestion. Still others find they can counter nausea with acupressure (see ACUPUNCTURE) applied to a point (the so-called Neiguan or Nei-Kuan point) approximately three fingers above the wrist joint, between the two central tendons. A remedy long used for motion sickness called Relief-Band may be effective. Approved for morning sickness by the FDA and available by prescription, it is worn on the wrist and turned on whenever the wearer feels nausea.

motility, sperm The ability of sperm to move, which is necessary if they are to travel from the vagina through the cervical canal to the uterus and fallopian tubes to fertilize an egg. For a man to be considered fertile, 60% of the sperm in a sample of his semen must be still moving after four hours (see SPERM for semen analysis). The application of heat to the testes is believed to decrease sperm motility (see THERMATIC STERILIZATION). Hormonal factors, infections and disease of the prostate gland may have a similar effect.

MRI Common abbreviation for MAGNETIC RESONANCE IMAGER.

mucous membrane Also *mucosa.* Glandular tissues that secrete *mucus,* a thick, sticky, lubricating liquid composed of glandular secretions, salts, dead cells and white blood cells. Mucous membranes line practically all of the body cavities with external openings (orifices), including the mouth, nose, rectum and vagina, as well as the internal surfaces of many other organs.

mucus method   See CERVICAL MUCUS METHOD.

mucus plug   A small wad of mucus that fills the cervical canal during pregnancy. Often it is expelled spontaneously as a thick fluid discharge, along with a little blood, as the cervix is slowly dilating. This phenomenon is called the *bloody show,* or *show,* and may occur weeks before the onset of labor, just before labor or during the course of labor.

multigravida   A woman who has been pregnant more than once.

multipara   A woman who has completed one or more pregnancies to the stage of viability (when the baby could live), whether it actually survives or not.

multiple pregnancy   A pregnancy with more than one fetus at the same time, that is, twins, triplets, quadruplets, and so on. There are basically two kinds of multiple pregnancy: *monozygotic,* or *identical,* in which a single fertilized egg divides into two or more individuals; and *dizygotic,* or *fraternal,* in which two or more eggs are fertilized during the same menstrual cycle (possibly but not necessarily during the same act of intercourse). Monozygotic pregnancy involves a single sperm and egg; dizygotic involves two or more eggs and sperm. In both cases more than two individuals (twins) can result. Triplet pregnancy can come from one, two or three eggs. Single-egg triplets are the least common; more often there are two eggs, one of which develops into a single fetus and the other into two. The Dionne quintuplets, born in Canada in 1934—the first set of quintuplets known of whom all five survived—were monozygotic, that is, were derived from the division of a single fertilized egg.

By far the most common kind of multiple pregnancy is twins. Of the twins born in North America, about one-third are identical (monozygotic) and the rest fraternal. Fraternal twins are more like siblings of different ages than twins; they may be of the same or opposite sexes and do not resemble each other more than other, single children of the same parents do, Identical twins are necessarily of the same sex (all the genetic material of the egg divided in two to form them, including the sex chromosomes) and resemble each other closely. Occasionally identical twins do not separate completely but are born conjoined and share some of the same organs; this is the phenomenon known as *Siamese twins* and is caused by failure of the embryo to split entirely in two.

The occurrence of identical twins is, so far as is known, entirely a matter of chance. It is not affected by any identifiable factors and indeed is rare in all other mammals except the nine-banded armadillo, which routinely produces four babies from one egg. In human beings identical twins occur at random in 1 of every 200 pregnancies.

Fraternal twinning, on the other hand, is influenced by the pituitary gland's secretion of FSH (follicle-stimulating hormone) as well as a number of other factors. It occurs far more often in blacks than in whites and far less often in Asians. It is more probable when there is a family history of fraternal twins, presumably because the trait of producing more than one egg at ovulation, called *polyovulation,* or its cause—higher secretion of FSH—is hereditary.

Since the 1960s the incidence of fraternal twins has risen markedly with use of various kinds of FERTILITY DRUG, which stimulates FSH production. Such drugs can result in three or four, or even as many as eight or nine, fetuses. Multiple fetuses also often occur from IN VITRO FERTILIZATION, in which numerous embryos are transferred into a woman's uterus in the hope that at least one will develop into a viable fetus. The chance of bearing fraternal twins also increases with the mother's age and the number of previous pregnancies: At age 20 the chances are 4 for every 1,000; at age 40 they are 16 for every 1,000. After 40, however, they drop again. Fat women are more likely to bear twins than thin women, perhaps owing to higher hormone levels.

With fraternal twins the eggs may be released from one ovary or from both. Each twin has its own amniotic sac and placenta. Identical twins may be formed at various times in the early development of the fertilized egg, but it is presumed that the division usually occurs before the eighth day after fertilization. Some identical twins share a placenta but have separate umbilical cords; these babies often do not survive, because their cords become entangled, cutting off their oxygen supply. More often each twin has its own placenta and cord. Even so, sometimes only one twin is born alive. In such cases the dead twin may be expelled early, in miscarriage, and the live one carried to term. More often, however, the twins will be born at the same time (or at least within one hour), one alive and the other dead, the latter having been carried dead for some months. This tends to happen more with identical twins than fraternal ones and often results from *transfusion syndrome,* in which the twins have an arterial connection whereby one twin in effect bleeds the other to death.

Multiple pregnancy is riskier for both babies and mothers. The rate of miscarriage and stillbirth is much higher than in single births, as is the rate of newborn mortality. The latter is at least partly due to the fact that twins, like all multiple pregnancies, are rarely carried as long as single pregnancies—an average of 37 weeks for twins versus 39 weeks for single births—and PREMATURE babies have a poorer chance of survival. Hence combined perinatal and neonatal mortality is four times higher than with single births. Other complications occurring more often with twins are ABNORMAL PRESENTATION, HYDRAMNIOS, PREECLAMPSIA, PLACENTA PREVIA, PROLONGED LABOR and POSTPARTUM HEMORRHAGE. When treatment for infertility results in a multiple pregnancy considered dangerous to mother or babies, a highly controversial technique called *fetal reduction* may be used. Performed before the 12th week of pregnancy, it consists of injecting a lethal drug into one or more of the fetuses (through the mother's abdomen, guided by ultrasound) in order to give the remaining fetuses (usually two) a better chance of surviving. This procedure has been questioned on ethical grounds. Also, it can lead to miscarriage of all the fetuses.

Often the existence of a multiple pregnancy is not discovered until one baby has been delivered and the size of the mother's uterus indicates it is not yet empty. Some women have even been given oxytocin or another drug to help the uterus continue contracting and return to normal size before it was realized that another baby was still there; this is extremely dangerous to both mother and child and usually can be avoided by palpating the uterus immediately after delivery, so that another fetus would be felt. Occasionally, however, a drug must be administered because the overdistended uterus fails to contract, hemorrhaging begins and labor stops, putting both the second baby and the mother at severe risk.

Multiple pregnancy is suspected when the uterus is much larger than normal for the length of gestation, based on the last menstrual period. Often fetal heartbeats cannot be detected as early, probably because the fetuses are smaller than in a single pregnancy of the same duration. Raised levels of alpha-fetoprotein (see ALPHA-FETOPROTEIN TEST) can indicate the presence of twins by 16 weeks. ULTRASOUND can establish the presence of twins quite early; X-rays usually do not reveal it until the end of the fifth month. By the seventh month abdominal palpation often will reveal the presence of two fetuses.

Especially during the last two months, women carrying twins require extra care to avoid the two major complications likely to occur then: preeclampsia and premature labor. More frequent prenatal visits generally are advisable. Careful review of the mother's diet is important, and she will need extra rest. Some physicians advocate near or complete bed rest from about 28 weeks on to reduce the risk of PREMATURE labor. (See also under EXERCISE.)

Labor usually occurs spontaneously, and the first stage is conducted as it would be for a single birth. Delivery of the first twin usually does not present a problem if it is in vertex (head first) position; ABNORMAL PRESENTATION most often affects the second one, which may present as a breech (feet first) or even lie transversely (sideways). Often a transverse position can be changed to either vertex or breech and then delivered. Such version, or turning, is easier with twins because they tend to be smaller than single babies. Occasionally twins are interlocked so they cannot be safely extracted; unfortunately this may not be discovered until part of the first twin—usually the legs—has already emerged; an emergency Cesarean section then must be performed.

Still another problem encountered with multiple births is that contractions may stop or become very weak after delivery of the first twin. Authorities differ on how long one should wait before extracting the second baby. Some believe the mother should be allowed to resume labor for an hour or more in hopes of a spontaneous delivery, but most feel that so long a delay endangers the unborn baby and favor proceeding with immediate delivery, waiting no longer than 15 minutes between births. If vaginal examination and the position of the second twin permit, the membranes are ruptured and, if necessary, the twin turned to either vertex or breech presentation. Delivery then is hastened by pressing on the fundus (top of the uterus) to engage the presenting part and help propel it down the birth canal. If this is not effective, the baby is extracted with the help of forceps or other instruments.

multiple sclerosis Also *MS*. A recurring autoimmune disease of the central nervous system that attacks the myelin, or covering sheath, of nerve fibers in the brain and spinal cord. These nerve fibers become scarred with hard, sclerotic patches that interrupt message transmission in the nerve pathways of vision, sensation and voluntary movement. As a result, there may be a variety of symptoms, principally ataxia (failure of muscle control, leading to spasm and disturbed coordination), muscular weakness, spasticity and tremor, extreme fatigue, numbness and paralysis in the extremities, difficulty with bladder control, double or blurred vision or other visual disturbances and speech difficulties. Moreover, recent research indicates that the disease also involves the severing of nerves in the brain, presumably by brain chemicals, which accounts for the fact that some patients eventually lose their ability to walk or lose vision in one eye.

Multiple sclerosis affects far more women than men and whites twice as often as blacks. It occurs mostly in colder regions and only rarely in tropical and subtropical areas. It usually strikes between the ages of 20 and 40. The most common symptoms of an attack, which may be mild or severe, brief or long lasting, are changes in vision, muscle weakness and abnormal sensation (numbness, tingling). Its course, however, is so variable that it is virtually unpredictable. A first attack, which usually runs its course in 2 to 6 weeks, may be followed by no symptoms whatever for a period of 10 to 15 years; or the disease may recur in months or even weeks, usually at increasingly shorter intervals. The reason for remission is that the myelin broken down and replaced by scar tissue—demyelinization—can repair itself (remyelinization). There are three main categories of the disease: *relapsing-remitting MS*, with flare-ups followed by recovery; *progressive relapsing-remitting MS*, with flare-ups worsening and leaving the patient more disabled than before; and *progressive MS*, with the condition slowly but steadily worsening.

Multiple sclerosis is difficult to diagnose on the basis of a single attack, or even several attacks, because its symptoms are so varied and often resemble those of cerebral vascular accident (stroke), brain tumors, syphilis, neuritis or other conditions. However, diagnosis almost always can be confirmed by a MAGNETIC RESONANCE IMAGER, which reveals demyelinization. It is considered an AUTOIMMUNE DISEASE. For reasons that are unclear, cells of the immune system turn their potent chemical weapons against the myelin sheath that protects nerve fibers in the brain and spinal cord. Recent research indicates that the Epstein-Barr virus, which causes infectious mononucleosis, may increase the risk of developing multiple sclerosis. No cure is yet known, and research on different treatments has been hampered by the frequent occurrence of spontaneous remission, making it impossible to tell whether a therapy was effective or the disease simply subsided. A genetically engineered form of the immune-system hormone interferon beta-1b (Betaseron) appears to modify the abnormal immune responses associated with MS attacks and won approval for MS treatment in 1993. Soon afterward three other drugs came on the market, interferon beta-1a (Avonex, Rebif), and glarimer acetate (Copaxone). The interferon drugs reduce the number of episodes and may decrease myelin breakdown; Copaxone reduces the number of flare-ups and also improves neurologic symptoms but does not help progressive MS. All these drugs are most effective when they are started as soon as a diagnosis of multiple sclerosis has been established. Corticosteroids such as prednisone also help some patients but have more unpleasant side effects. When nothing else is effective, immune-system suppressants may be tried, but usually they are reserved for patients with rapidly advancing disease. In 2000 a potent cancer-fighting drug, mitoxantrone (Novantrone), was approved for treating advanced multiple sclerosis (progressive relapsing and worsening relapsing-remitting; see above). It is given four times a year by infusion, but is limited to 8 to 12 doses because it may give rise to serious heart problems. Perhaps the most effective drug thus far for preventing relapses, Tysabri (natalizumab) was introduced but then was linked to a rare and often fatal brain disease (progressive multifocal leukoencephalopathy, or PML) as well as impaired immune function. In 2006 the FDA approved its use in a limited number of cases that did not respond to less toxic medications and only as monotherapy (not in conjunction with other treatments) on a carefully monitored basis.

Other treatment is strictly palliative, including medication and physical therapy for spasticity, the avoidance of overfatigue and excessive heat, and prompt attention to urinary infections and similar secondary problems. During a new attack, steroid treatment with oral or injected cortisone and ACTH often relieves specific symptoms.

In women, multiple sclerosis does not affect either menstruation or fertility. Pregnancy is possible. There is some evidence that it worsens the disease's symptoms, but others believe the suppression of the immune system in pregnancy may temporarily improve the condition, and pregnancy has no subsequent effect on disability. The decision to start a family should be based on the woman's disability level at the time, the ability to care for children in later years and the ability to deal with the stress of raising a family. Any kind of birth control device may be used, provided that the woman's

coordination is good enough to insert it. However, IUDs are contraindicated for women with numbness in the pelvic area, since they may not be able to detect slippage of such a device.

The sex drive may be diminished during periods of extreme fatigue, and orgasmic ability is impaired when there is lack of sensation. However, some women who lose sensation in the pelvic area find that other areas of the body become more sensitive to sexual stimulation. During intercourse and masturbation there may be increased urinary incontinence, which sometimes can be prevented by making sure the bladder is quite empty beforehand. During periods of remission, however, many patients are able to lead normal or near-normal lives.

muscular dystrophy   A hereditary chronic disease in which the voluntary muscles become progressively weaker. The most common form, *Duchenne muscular dystrophy,* is a sex-linked recessive-gene disorder (see BIRTH DEFECTS) passed on by mothers to their sons. It usually appears before the age of seven, beginning with difficulties in walking and standing and eventually affecting the shoulders and arms. By puberty most victims are confined to a wheelchair. At present, there is neither a cure nor a specific treatment. However, researchers have uncovered the specific gene defect that is responsible for the disease and have identified a particular protein, dystrophin, that patients lack. It is hoped that these advances will enable the development of treatments to replace dystrophin or compensate for its absence.

myasthenia gravis   A chronic disease characterized by progressive weakness of the voluntary muscles. The cause is not known, but it appears to be an AUTOIMMUNE DISEASE that causes malfunctioning of the enzyme acetylcholine, which normally induces muscles to contract. The onset may be sudden or gradual. The most common symptoms are drooping eyelids and double vision, followed by difficulty in swallowing, speaking and weakness of the limbs. The weakness also can affect the respiratory muscles, which is life-threatening.

Myasthenia gravis most often attacks adolescents and young adults (women far more than men in this age group), newborn babies and adults over the age of 40 (usually with some evidence of a tumor of the thymus). In about one-fourth of the cases, the disease disappears spontaneously. In women, this kind of remission often occurs during pregnancy, and current research is focusing on substances produced by the placenta in the hope of isolating a curative agent. Current treatment consists of either thymectomy—removal of the thymus, which plays a role in the body's immune system—which helps in approximately one-third of cases, or administering various drugs, such as anticholinergic agents that act on the sympathetic nervous system or corticosteroids that suppress immune-system response.

mycoplasma   See VAGINOSIS.

myocardial infarction   Another name for heart attack, during which some of the heart's blood supply is suddenly reduced or cut off, causing the heart muscle (the *myocardium*) to die.

See also ARTERIOSCLEROSIS.

myoma   See FIBROID.

myomectomy   Surgical removal of a FIBROID tumor. When a large fibroid causes significant discomfort and/or extremely heavy bleeding, its removal may be indicated. Traditionally such treatment involved hysterectomy—removal of the entire uterus—on the rationale that fibroids tend to recur, they would probably interfere with a pregnancy, and even if a woman became pregnant she would require a Cesarean section. Also, it was held, myomectomy causes considerable blood loss during surgery and results in the formation of adhesions, which may lead to infertility and chronic pain. Today many authorities agree that often more conservative surgery—removal of the fibroid only—may be tried. It requires general anesthesia, must be done in a hospital and takes one to five hours. Careful examination may enable surgeons to remove early "seed" tumors, thereby avoiding recurrence, and meticulous microsurgical technique often can control bleeding and avoid adhesion formation. For fibroids inside the uterus, some surgeons perform a *hysteroscopic myomectomy,* removing them through the vagina, without opening the abdomen. This procedure not only requires a much shorter hospital stay but also can eliminate the need for Cesarean section in a future pregnancy. Or a *laparoscopic myomectomy* may be possible (see LAPAROSCOPY), done under general or regional anesthesia and leaving a much smaller scar than standard myomectomy.

myositis   A rare muscle disorder characterized by persistent muscle swelling, inflammation and weakness, as well as other complications such as lung disease. The type affecting primarily muscles is also called *polymyositis.* Another form, *dermatomyositis,* tends to be accompanied by a skin rash. An AUTOIMMUNE DISEASE, it affects twice as many women as men. It is diagnosed in just one of every 100,000 patients a year, but authorities suspect that many cases go unidentified. One survey indicated that the average patient sees seven physicians before receiving the correct diagnosis. Dermatomyositis in particular is associated with cancer, a malignancy occurring in about 15% of men patients over age 50 and in a smaller proportion of women, so patients need to be examined and monitored for malignancy. Interestingly, if a tumor is removed, the myositis often goes into remission. The principal treatment for myositis is prednisone, a corticosteroid. If it does not work, immunosuppressants such as methotrexate may be tried, or intravenous immunoglobulins. At this writing clinical trials are going on with a number of anticancer drugs.

Nabothian cyst   See CYST, def. 4.

natural childbirth   See PREPARED CHILDBIRTH; PSY-CHOPROPHYLACTIC METHOD.

natural family planning   Also *biological birth control, calendar method, fertility awareness, periodic abstinence, rhythm method.* A method of both birth control and pregnancy planning that is based on timing sexual intercourse so as to avoid (or seek out) a woman's fertile period, that is, her time of OVULATION. For preventing pregnancy the couple abstains from vaginal intercourse during ovulation and, for more safety, several days before and afterward. Since an egg remains viable for only 24 hours after its release from the ovary, sperm, which can live 48 to 72 hours after ejaculation, must be present in the fallopian tube during that interval if fertilization is to take place.

Natural family planning still is the only means of birth control sanctioned by the Roman Catholic Church. Its success depends entirely on how closely one can estimate the time of ovulation and on avoiding intercourse during this fertile period. The interval between a menstrual period and ovulation is highly variable, both from one woman to the next and in the same woman (see MENSTRUAL CYCLE), but ovulation always occurs approximately 14 days *before* the start of the next menstrual period; thus one can tell when ovulation last took place, but only *after* the fact.

The four main methods of calculating the fertile period are: the calendar method, temperature method, cervical mucus method and combined or sympto-thermic method.

The *calendar method,* also called *rhythm method,* uses the length of past menstrual cycles to calculate the probable time of ovulation. For this purpose a woman must keep track of her cycle for at least six months. A cycle is said to begin on the first day of menstrual flow (day 1) and end on the last day before the next menstrual flow. One subtracts 18 from the shortest cycle to obtain the first fertile day and 11 from the longest cycle to obtain the last fertile day. To prevent pregnancy, one must avoid vaginal intercourse from the first fertile day through the last fertile day. The rest of the month is considered the *safe period.* Another mode of calculation is counting to 15 from day 1 of a period; from that date subtract 6 and also add 6; these 13 days are the possible fertile ones, and the rest are "safe." The calendar method is considered the *least reliable* method of natural family planning and is totally useless for women with very irregular cycles, following abortion or delivery, or during breast-feeding. In Europe a handheld computer, marketed as Persona, has been used to calculate pregnancy risk depending on the day of a woman's menstrual cycle. Studies there suggest that with strict use it is about 94% effective. It is not available in the United States.

The temperature method, also called BASAL BODY TEMPERATURE (BBT), is based on the fact that progesterone, released by the corpus luteum after ovulation, causes a measurable increase in basal body temperature, which remains raised until the next menstrual period. It too is an after-the-fact method of determining ovulation; that is, it provides evidence that ovulation took place, and when. It is somewhat more reliable than the calendar method and can be used by women with irregular menstrual cycles but is inaccurate following abortion or childbirth. Over a period of six to eight months, it may give a good indication of a woman's pattern of ovulation.

The CERVICAL MUCUS METHOD is based on the fact that the cervical mucus in most women changes in consistency during the course of each menstrual cycle. After menstruation and before ovulation, the mucus is thick, sticky, opaque and scant. A few days before ovulation the amount of mucus increases and it becomes clear and more slippery, not unlike raw egg white. A woman checks her mucus manually, for degree of wetness (wettest at ovulation) and appearance, and keeps a record of changes in consistency to establish some kind of pattern for ovulation (she also can use one of several chemical tests on the mucus). This method has not been tested adequately over a long period of time, but it appears to work reasonably well once a woman has become thoroughly familiar with her own body patterns.

The *combined* or *sympto-thermic method* uses both changes in basal body temperature and changes in cervical mucus to estimate the fertile period. Taking the strictest calculation of each, it appears to be the most reliable method of these four. However, none of them is as reliable as oral contraceptives, a diaphragm used with spermicide or intrauterine devices. (See table under CONTRACEPTIVE for a comparison.)

Natural family planning does have certain advantages. For birth control these methods all are totally reversible. They work either for planning a pregnancy or for preventing one. They have no harmful side effects. They are free or require only very inexpensive equipment (but see below), and they involve the male partner's cooperation. Their chief disadvantages are their limited reliability (depending on how regular a woman's cycles are) and the need for self-control exercised by both partners to prevent pregnancy (unless an alternative method of contraception is used during fertile periods). One other risk has been suggested. When natural family planning fails and unplanned pregnancy occurs, there appears to be a much higher than normal rate of miscarriage and birth defects. It is suspected that this is due to fertilization involving an old egg or an old sperm. The best chance for normal pregnancy is fertilization at the time of ovulation. A miscalculation by a couple using natural family planning may lead to fertilization 24 hours after ovulation, with increased risk of defects.

Various devices to measure hormonal changes and thereby predict ovulation have been developed, mainly to help women who wish to become pregnant (see OVULATION), but they are not reliable for birth control.

naturopathy Also *naturopathic medicine, holistic medicine.* An approach to treating illness with diet, exercise and other so-called natural means, instead of drugs or surgery. According to this theory, symptoms are signs that the body is trying to heal itself, and treatment focuses on the underlying cause of illness, especially bad habits of lifestyle that cause the body to accumulate waste products and toxins. The individual is treated as an integrated whole (hence the term *holistic* for this approach). The name *naturopathy* was coined in the late 19th century by a German homeopathic healer, John H. Scheel, to mean treatment of the whole person by natural means. One early naturopathic healer, Sebastian Kneipp, developed a system of *hydrotherapy,* involving walking on wet grass in the morning and running on freshly fallen snow, drinking herbal teas and the like. Followers of Kneipp founded the American school of naturopathy around 1900, and the treatment spread quickly across the United States. In the next five decades various schools and methods of training appeared, but by the early 1960s the movement had nearly died out, at least in part owing to legal problems. In 2000 the North American Board of Naturopathic Examiners began to administer clinical licensing examinations in naturopathic medicine. Today naturopathy is licensed in 13 U.S. states and five Canadian provinces.

Modern naturopaths rely heavily on diet management and herbal remedies. They also use physiotherapy involving light, water, electricity, heat, cold and ultrasound; therapeutic exercise such as yoga; manipulation of joints, soft tissues and spine; acupuncture; diet supplements; massage and acupressure. Most naturopaths do an extensive history for diagnosis, which may include lab tests, X-rays and/or ultrasound. Those considering treatment should ask a naturopath about his or her training and certification and what he or she considers areas of expertise. The principal training schools in

North America are the National College of Naturo-pathic Medicine, Portland, Oregon; Bastyr College, Seattle, Washington; Southwest College of Naturopathic Medicine, Tempe, Arizona; University of Bridgeport College of Naturopathic Medicine, Bridgeport, Connecticut; and Boucher Institute of Naturopathic Medicine, New Westminster, British, Columbia.

nausea   An unpleasant feeling in the upper gastrointestinal tract and abdomen, often associated with vomiting. In addition to being a symptom of gastrointestinal disorders of many kinds, ranging from mild to serious, as well as a side effect of radiation therapy and chemotherapy against cancer, in women nausea is associated with a number of conditions in which hormone levels are temporarily higher than usual. Chief among these is the nausea of early pregnancy, commonly called MORNING SICKNESS. Nausea is sometimes a symptom of spasmodic dysmenorrhea, along with the cramps accompanying the first days of menstrual flow; a side effect of some oral contraceptives, usually those very high in estrogen; and, rarely, a symptom of incomplete miscarriage when some fetal or placental material has remained in the uterus. Nausea also is one of the symptoms of the secondary stage of SYPHILIS and of MIGRAINE attacks.

necrospermia   Absence of live sperm in the seminal fluid, rendering a man sterile.
　　See also STERILITY.

needle aspiration, needle biopsy   See BIOPSY, def. 3.

neonatal jaundice   Also *neonatal icterus, newborn jaundice, physiologic jaundice, hyperbilirubinemia*. Mild jaundice in a newborn baby, manifested in yellowing of the skin and the eyes between the second and fifth days of life. It is caused by a delay in the ability of the baby's liver to deal with bilirubin, a product of the breakdown of hemoglobin (the oxygen-carrying molecule of blood) from fetal red blood cells. Mild jaundice from this source is quite common and rarely lasts more than a week. However, jaundice occurring before the second day of life or after the fifth day is abnormal (it may be a symptom of ERYTHROBLASTOSIS), as is severe jaundice. If the yellow color is particularly deep, a blood bilirubin level test should be performed; levels over 20 milligrams of blood bilirubin per 100 milliliters of blood can cause permanent brain damage in the child. Causes of abnormal jaundice include infection, blood incompatibility or a structural abnormality in the liver, among others. Frequently the cause is never determined. Treatment consists of placing the baby blindfolded (to protect the eyes) under fluorescent lights to lower the blood bilirubin concentration; this phototherapy is continued until levels are within safe limits. In 1988 researchers announced the development of a drug that counters neonatal jaundice. Called Sn-protoporphyrin, it reduces bilirubin levels, either eliminating or reducing the need for light therapy, which has the disadvantage of separating baby and mother for long periods and also is not always available in less developed countries. Because earlier discharge of newborns from the hospital is more prevalent, in 2004 the American Academy of Pediatrics recommended that all infants be examined in the first few days after discharge when bilirubin levels peak.

neoplasm   Another name for TUMOR.

neural tube defects   A class of common, very serious birth defects that involve failure of the baby's spinal cord to close properly. When the tube does not close at the top of the spine, the brain does not develop properly, a condition called *anencephaly*, which is generally fatal within hours after birth. When the failure to close occurs lower down, the condition is called SPINA BIFIDA. The precise cause of such defects is not known, but both genetic and environmental factors appear to play a role. In certain parts of the world (the western United Kingdom, for one) incidence is much higher than elsewhere (1 per 100 births, as opposed to 1.5 per 1,000 in North America). Research has indicated that daily supplements of folic acid before conception and during early pregnancy substantially reduce the recurrence of neural tube defects, and some women may require extra vitamin B_{12} as well. Screening for neural tube defects during pregnancy can be done by means of an ALPHA-FETOPROTEIN TEST; for those parents in a high-risk group (those who have had one baby with a neural tube defect), many practitioners recommend amniocentesis and high-resolution ultrasound to determine if the fetus is normal. Should the fetus have myelomeningocele, in which the spinal cord protrudes from the spine (eventually leading to paralysis and incontinence), it may be possible to perform surgery *before* birth, using a skin graft to patch the spine. This procedure, however, is still experimental.

nidation   Another name for IMPLANTATION.

nipple   The specialized part of the female BREAST through which milk is expressed during lactation. The breast's milk-producing glands, the ACINI, are connected to the nipple by a complex network of ducts that enlarge as they enter the nipple. The enlarged portions are called *lactiferous sinuses,* and their external openings are the numerous pin-sized holes in the nipple. Usually the nipple is cylindrical, protrudes somewhat above the surface of the surrounding AREOLA and is a brownish color somewhat darker than the areola. However, in some women the nipple may be quite flat, almost flush with the areola, or inverted (turned inward), and approximately the same color as the areola. The shape of the normal nipple also varies widely. Usually both nipples are about equal in size and shape, but if one breast is significantly larger the nipple may be larger too. Occasionally a woman has one or more extra (*accessory*) nipples. They usually are located below the breast and are flat, as in a child before puberty.

The nipple is covered with a layer of hairless skin and contains many muscle fibers, through which pass the terminal milk ducts from each lobe of the breast. The contraction of these muscle fibers causes the nipple to become erect during sexual arousal (cold can similarly stimulate erection) and, in lactating women, to expel milk.

An *inverted nipple,* in which the central portion of the nipple appears to turn inward, is also normal, although it may require a little manipulation if a woman is attempting to breast-feed. Surgical repair of this condition is possible but often is only partly successful. Frequently, however, flat or even inverted nipples begin to project somewhat during lactation, and the shape does not interfere with milk production. Using a special plastic shield called a Woolwich Shield during pregnancy and the breast-feeding period helps some women. Also, a nipple-rolling exercise done twice a day may change the shape enough so that the baby can grasp the nipple more easily.

An inverted nipple should be distinguished from a *retracted nipple,* in which the nipple is pulled inward by an underlying tumor or inflammation. Usually in the case of a tumor the nipple becomes larger and flatter as the tumor grows; also, only the nipple of one breast will show this change, giving some warning. Reddening, ulceration or scaling of the nipple, which normally is bumpy and wrinkled in appearance, are also signs of disease.

In the nonlactating woman, discharge from the nipples may be caused by tumors within the breast, either benign or malignant, by disorders of the pituitary or hypothalamus, by infection, as a side effect of some drugs (especially the phenothiazine tranquilizers) or from chronic stimulation of the nipples, as in love play. A thin white discharge is probably milk caused by some endocrine disorder that is producing lactation abnormally. A purulent (pus-laden) discharge is usually the result of an infection, such as MASTITIS. A thick sticky discharge, which may vary in color, is usually a sign of inflammation involving the terminal milk ducts, whereas a serous (thin, clear, yellowish) discharge, with or without some bleeding, usually is caused by either a benign or a malignant lesion, most often a benign DUCTAL PAPILLOMA. The most serious kind of tumor involving the nipple is PAGET'S DISEASE (def. 1).

See also BREAST-FEEDING; BREAST SELF-EXAMINATION; LACTATION.

nit   The egg of a crab louse.
See also PUBIC LICE.

node Also *nodule.* A small mass of tissue resembling a swelling, knot or similar protrusion. It may be normal, as in the case of lymph nodes, which actually are glands, or it may indicate the presence of disease, as when nodes occur on the joints in rheumatic disease.

nongonococcal urethritis (NGU) Also *nonspecific urethritis (NSU).*
  See URETHRITIS.

nonspecific vaginitis Also *NSV.*
  See also VAGINITIS.

non-stress test Also *NST.*
  See also FETAL MONITORING.

Norplant See CONTRACEPTIVE.

NSAID Abbreviation for *nonsteroidal anti-inflammatory drug.*
  See ANALGESIC.

nuchal translucency-biochemical blood test An early test for fetal abnormalities that can be performed between 10 and 13 weeks of pregnancy. The test combines an ultrasound examination of fetal nuchal translucency—that is, it measures skin-fold thickness at the back of the fetus's neck, which is greater in Down syndrome and some other syndromes—with a measure of two biochemical substances in the mother's blood—pregnancy-associated plasma protein, or PAPP-A, and beta human chorionic gonadotropin, or HCG—that can indicate a possible chromosomal abnormality. With a second ultrasound of the fetal nasal bone, these four noninvasive tests increase the accuracy of the detection rate of Down syndrome to 97%. See also under DOWN SYNDROME; PRENATAL TESTS.

nuclear magnetic resonance Older name for MAGNETIC RESONANCE IMAGER.

nucleic acid The genetic substance of all living organisms; that is, the substance whereby the physical characteristics of parents are passed on to their offspring, whether the parents are one-celled organisms or human beings. Chemically nucleic acid consists of large molecules, in turn made up of smaller units called nucleotides. There are two main classes of nucleic acid: *deoxyribonucleic acid,* or DNA, and *ribonucleic acid,* or RNA. In living cells, DNA is the primary genetic material, while RNA helps translate genetic information into protein structures. The *genes,* the basic units of heredity, are molecules of DNA. It is DNA that provides the *genetic code,* which determines the development of cells by controlling the synthesis of RNA. In animal (and human) cells DNA is present in a part of the cell's nucleus called the chromosome.
  See also GENETICS.

nullipara A woman who has never completed a pregnancy to the stage of viability (when the child could live).

nurse A person with considerable training in health care. Formerly lowly assistants to physicians, nurses today may undertake many of the tasks previously done only by doctors and play an increasing role, especially in gynecology and obstetrics. There are, however, numerous kinds of nurse, the most important of which are

- Licensed practical nurse (LPN), also called licensed vocational nurse. Has one year of post-high school education and most often works in a hospital or nursing home, under the supervision of a registered nurse or physician.
- Registered nurse (RN). Has two to four years of nursing school and is licensed by the state to practice nursing.
- Nurse practitioner (NP), also certified nurse practitioner (CNP). Has advanced training beyond two to four years' nursing school, often a master's degree in nursing. Works primarily in ambulatory settings such as clinics, nursing homes, hospitals, or her own office. Provides primary and preventive care, such as managing

common childhood illnesses and working with chronically ill adults. By law must have consulting physicians, but in some states may write all prescriptions.

- Clinical nurse specialist (CNS). Has advanced training beyond nursing school. Works in a hospital or other clinical setting, specializing in a particular area (such as oncology, cardiology, newborn care, etc.); serves as educator/advisor to nursing colleagues and patients.
- Certified registered nurse anesthetist (CRNA). Usually has two to three years' training beyond a bachelor's degree in nursing, all in delivery of anesthesia; administers more than two-thirds of anesthetics given to patients in United States (sole anesthetists in majority of U.S. rural hospitals).
- Certified nurse-midwife (CNS). See MIDWIFE, def. 4.

- Visiting nurse. A registered or licensed practical nurse who works in the home after a patient's hospital discharge or when a patient has chronic or terminal illness. Usually practices through a Visiting Nurse Association or a home-care agency.

nurse-midwife   See MIDWIFE, def. 4.

nursing   See BREAST-FEEDING.

nutrition   See DIET; OBESITY; WEIGHT, BODY.

nymphomania   See LIBIDO.

obesity An excess of body fat. Long defined as weighing 20% or more over what is considered one's ideal weight relative to height and body build, current thinking holds that the *body-mass index (BMI)* is a more accurate indicator of excess body fat. It is calculated by multiplying one's weight in pounds by 703, and then dividing the result by one's height in inches multiplied by itself. For example, a woman who is 64 inches tall and weighs 134 pounds has a BMI of 23 (134 × 703 ÷ [64 × 64]). According to the National Institutes of Health, a woman with a BMI of 25 or more is overweight. Another measure for women is the *waist-to-hip ratio,* calculated by dividing one's waist measure in inches (taken at the smallest area around the waist) by the widest measure around the hips. A waist-to-hip ratio higher than 0.88—a so-called "apple shape," as opposed to a "pear shape"—in women over 40 has been associated with a greater risk of developing heart disease, diabetes and gallbladder disease. Still another measure recently cited as more indicative of problems is a waistline of more than 35 inches, measured at the navel. Even women of normal weight with this measure are at greater risk for cardiovascular disease and other problems associated with obesity.

Although both men and women have a tendency to gain more weight as they grow older, for some reason more women than men are obese, particularly after menopause. Whether such weight gain is due partly to hormonal changes or is simply a matter of eating the same amounts of food while becoming less active physically is not certain. What is known, however, is that obesity is dangerous. During the childbearing years, with its persistent estrogen stimulation, it can interfere with the ovary/pituitary feedback system and thereby impair fertility. After menopause, it makes women more susceptible to a variety of serious and potentially life-threatening disorders, including diabetes, osteoarthritis, heart disease, hypertension and cerebral vascular accident (stroke), gallbladder disease, and breast and endometrial cancer. It is also linked to numerous other kinds of cancer, including colorectal, esophageal, pancreatic, kidney, gallbladder, ovarian, cervical, liver, prostate, multiple myeloma and Hodgkin's lymphoma. Moreover, a recent study showed that the higher the BMI, the greater the risk of cancer death.

There is no easy way to convert an obese woman into a slender one. It is estimated that 3,500 calories of food produce a single pound of fat. The woman who is 50 pounds heavier than she should be must therefore reduce her usual food intake over a period of time by a total of 175,000 calories. In theory, at least, one can lose a pound of fat per week by reducing one's food intake by only 500 calories a day. Unfortunately, the weight loss on such a diet is rarely constant, owing to fluid retention and metabolic factors that are not completely understood. Nevertheless, to avoid malnutrition—and even obese persons can be malnourished if they eat mainly junk food and get inadequate vitamins and minerals—the best diet for weight reduction for an adult woman in otherwise good health provides 1,000 to 1,200 calories per day and consists of small servings of a large variety of foods that meet the necessary vitamin and mineral requirements, with 20 to 25% of the calories from protein, 15 to 30% from fats and the remainder from carbohydrates. Any such diet should be accompanied by regular and gradually increased physical exercise, preferably by making a conscious effort to change one's daily habits to include more physical exertion. Before undertaking a more vigorous exercise program, cardiovascular and respiratory status should be evaluated first (see also EXERCISE). Fad diets that emphasize eating one or a few foods and eliminating most others should be avoided. In general, even if fad diets and medication help a person lose weight, that weight generally is gained back very quickly when diet or medication is discontinued. Many persons find group plans or behavior modification groups, which aim at reeducating eating habits, helpful as a long-term solution.

In 2007 the FDA approved an over-the-counter version of the weight-loss drug Xenical to be sold without a prescription. Sold as Alli, it blocks the breakdown and absorption of fat in the intestine and at the same time blocks absorption of calories from fat, as well as creating an aversion to eating excessive fat. However, it has some unpleasant side effects, notably diarrhea and oily stools, and is effective only when combined with exercise and a low-fat, reduced-calorie diet. Individuals with diabetes and those using blood thinners are told to consult a physician before taking the drug. Other weight-loss drugs are available by prescription. Sibutramine (Meridia) is considered effective and safe for up to two years, although it can increase blood pressure and therefore requires careful monitoring. Orlistat, the prescription version of Xenical, which inhibits fat absorption, can interfere with the absorption of fat-soluble vitamins (A, D, E and K) and should not be used for more than two years. Not everyone responds to these medications. Indeed, clinical experience indicates that an individual who has not lost at least a pound a week during the first month on a weight-loss drug is not likely to benefit from it.

Another route taken is liposuction, COSMETIC SURGERY to reduce fat deposits in the abdomen, thighs and elsewhere. It requires general anesthesia, several days of hospitalization, and considerable subsequent pain and discomfort. Moreover, the procedure is relatively risky, with considerable danger of complications.

In some women obesity is the result of *compulsive overeating*, a psychological disorder in which food is used to cope with stress, emotional problems or even simple day-to-day problems. It takes the form of episodic binges of uncontrollable eating, followed by a sense of profound guilt and shame for indulging in this behavior (see BULIMIA). Unless it is accompanied by periods of rigid dieting (as it sometimes is), bingeing can cause obesity. Psychological counseling of the kind used for other eating disorders, such as ANOREXIA NERVOSA, is the only known treatment.

For a time grossly obese persons, who weigh twice as much or more than they should, sometimes were treated with a surgical procedure called an *intestinal bypass operation*. It involved bypassing a section of the small intestine from the normal flow, reducing its effective length and thereby diminishing the total absorptive surface for nutrients. However, the side effects from it were so severe that it has been abandoned. A different procedure, called *gastric bypass*, which bypasses part of the stomach, is increasingly being performed, but only as a last resort for those who are morbidly obese (exceeding ideal weight by at least 100 pounds). The number of such surgeries quadrupled between 1992 and 2002 and continues to grow. Called *bariatric surgery*, it is attracting more and more practitioners and is often covered by health insurance. The procedure involves dividing the stomach into two parts and reattaching the smaller upper stomach to the small intestine, creating a tiny pouch. A narrow connection between the pouch and the intestine slows the flow of food to the rest of the digestive tract, so one feels full after eating only a little food. Bariatric surgery is not without risk. About 1% of patients die from complications of surgery, mainly infections and blood clots, and about 8% develop serious problems, such as ulcers and bowel obstruction. Anyone considering the procedure is advised to find a highly qualified surgeon, preferably a member of the American Society of Bariatric Surgery. During the past decade surgical treatment for the severely obese has increased exponentially. See BARIATRIC SURGERY. Also see DIET; WEIGHT, BODY; WEIGHT GAIN.

obstetrician   A physician who specializes in *obstetrics*, that is, childbirth, including prenatal care, delivery (both vaginal and surgical) and postpartum care.

See also BIRTH ATTENDANT; GYNECOLOGIST; MIDWIFE.

off-label drug use Using a medication in ways or for a purpose other than those approved by the U.S. Food and Drug Administration (FDA). Once a drug is FDA-approved, it may legally be prescribed for any condition or at any dosage or in conjunction with other medications. Off-label prescribing is common in medicine, accounting for about 20% of all prescriptions written in the United States each year. In many instances such use is a judgment call by the prescribing clinician, and it may even eventually become the standard of care. For example, estrogen was long ago approved to relieve hot flashes and other menopausal symptoms, and progestins to treat endometriosis and abnormal bleeding. In the 1980s the two were combined to offset endometrial hyperplasia caused by giving estrogen alone, but this use was not officially approved for another decade. In other cases, however, a combination may prove dangerous, as it did with the weight-loss drug fen/phen (fenfluramine and phentermine)—giving rise to heart problems—and had to be withdrawn. Sometimes unexpected reactions to a previously approved drug are reported, and the FDA will then require a change in the drug's labeling. This occurred with the osteoporosis drug alendronate (Fosamax), which caused esophageal irritation, and the label was revised to indicate that one must take it with 8 ounces of water. Many cardiologists today prescribe taking a daily aspirin, to prevent heart attack, and even this use of such a well-known analgesic constitutes off-label drug use. No medication is entirely without risk, so consumers are advised to inform themselves of a drug's use, its possible side effects, and any interaction with other medications (both prescription and over-the-counter) they might be taking.

oligomenorrhea Infrequent menstruation, with intervals of 38 or more days between menstrual periods. It is particularly common at MENARCHE, when intervals of two or three months between periods often occur in girls during the first few years of menstrual periods. It also is common during PERIMENOPAUSE, from the age of 45 on. In both instances it usually constitutes ANOVULATORY BLEEDING, that is, menstruation in the absence of ovulation, which is caused by hormone imbalance. Some women, however, regularly have a longer than normal cycle, and if they menstruate fairly regularly every two months instead of monthly, that alone should not be a cause for alarm or require treatment. Occasionally emotional problems, crash diets and obesity can upset the hormone balance enough to cause oligomenorrhea.

See also MENSTRUAL CYCLE.

oligospermia Also *subfertility*. A relatively small number of SPERM in a semen sample, usually defined as 20 to 40 million sperm per milliliter of seminal fluid. Most clinicians believe that at least two analyses of seminal fluid must be performed for any evaluation of sperm. Currently there are over-the-counter tests available to test male fertility. One, marketed as Baby Start, evaluates the concentration of sperm in semen to see if 20 million per milliliter are present. Oligospermia may result from nutritional problems, acute or chronic illness, general metabolic disease, specific poisoning or occupational hazards such as exposure to radiation, excessive use of alcohol or marijuana, central defects in the pituitary or hypothalamus, specific disease in the genital tract (such as gonorrhea or chlamydia) causing blockage to the vas deferens and scarring of the tubes, varicose veins in the testes (see VARICOCELE), congenital defects such as Klinefelter syndrome or a tiny defect in the Y chromosome. In addition, a number of medications lower sperm count, among them chemotherapy for cancer, cimetidine for ulcers, spironololactone for high blood pressure, testosterone and anabolic steroids used by athletes to bulk up muscles and phenytoin to prevent seizures. Even with all these possibilities, in some men the cause can never be determined.

Among the principal remedies recommended initially are attention to a proper diet and adequate rest, severe restriction of smoking and alcoholic drinks and avoidance of heat in the genital area (no tight underwear or prolonged tub baths; see THERMATIC STERILIZATION for explanation). Clomiphene nitrate (see FERTILITY DRUG) in low doses over a long period (three months to a year) sometimes effects an increase in sperm count; so may a daily vitamin supplement high in vitamin C (300 milligrams), the B vitamins and zinc, and the decongestant pseudoephedrine (30 milligrams twice a day). Also, advances in microsurgery have enabled correcting some anatomical problems.

In cases where the volume of the ejaculate is large (more than 5 million milliliters) but the sperm count low, a technique called *split ejaculation* may be effective. The man deposits only the first portion of his ejaculate in the woman's vagina; since this portion often contains the majority of the sperm, this technique in effect concentrates it. For some men with oligospermia, however, ARTIFICIAL INSEMINATION may be the only way to fatherhood.

See also STERILITY.

omega-3 fatty acid   See CHOLESTEROL; DIET.

oophorectomy   Also *ovariectomy*. Surgical removal of one or both ovaries. The former is called *unilateral oophorectomy;* the latter is *bilateral oophorectomy* and usually is performed in conjunction with removal of the fallopian tubes and uterus as well. Removal of both ovaries constitutes both *sterilization* and *castration,* since these organs are the source of both ova (eggs) and most of the body's estrogen. Following bilateral oophorectomy a premenopausal woman will experience all the symptoms of MENOPAUSE, often in quite severe form owing to the suddenness of change in hormone levels. A postmenopausal woman should have much less of a problem, or none at all. Many clinicians prescribe ESTROGEN REPLACEMENT THERAPY to ease these symptoms but it is not without risk. Removal of one ovary reduces a woman's chances of becoming pregnant but does not make her infertile, since eggs continue to be released from the remaining ovary, which also still produces estrogen.

Because of the radical nature of bilateral oophorectomy, in women of reproductive age it should be performed only when careful diagnosis pinpoints ovarian disease and more conservative treatment is ineffective. The principal indications for bilateral oophorectomy are cancer of the ovaries and severe infection secondary to a condition such as pelvic inflammatory disease. Also, many clinicians believe that it should be performed, along with salpingectomy (removal of the fallopian tubes),

in all women over 40 who must have a HYSTERECTOMY, on the grounds that their ovaries will cease functioning in a few years with menopause and the surgery will eliminate all risk of ovarian cancer. Others maintain that this reasoning is open to question, that the ovaries continue to produce some hormones after menopause and that each woman should make her own decision, based on full knowledge of the various alternatives. Further, some clinicians feel that even a malignant (cancerous) tumor, if it is small and confined to one ovary, does not necessitate removal of the other ovary, although they do recommend that such patients be observed and checked with extra care and frequency for the rest of their lives lest cancer develop in the remaining ovary (see also CANCER, OVARIAN). The main other indication for unilateral oophorectomy (besides infection and cancer) is a benign (noncancerous) ovarian tumor that is too large to be removed without excising the ovary.

Oophorectomy is major surgery. It usually requires several days of hospitalization and three to six weeks for full recovery. The procedure is performed either abdominally, involving either a vertical or a transverse (bikini) incision of about 5 inches, or laparoscopically (see LAPAROSCOPY). Oophorectomy changes the hormonal balance both before and after menopause (the ovaries continue to produce some hormones postmenopausally). Not only does removal of both ovaries result in a sudden menopause, but it also ends the production of ovarian androgens (male hormones), which affect both sexual desire and sexual response. Testosterone, the principal male sex hormone, can also be replaced, but when administered orally or by injection it tends to give rise to masculinizing effects, such as facial hair, acne and lowered voice. These effects can be avoided by administering the hormone through a slow-release pellet inserted under the skin in the hip area; it must be replaced every six months. However, this procedure, although well known in Britain, is not familiar to most American physicians.

Formerly performed almost routinely with hysterectomy, oophorectomy, while perhaps performed more often than necessary, is usually confined to women with serious ovarian disease or cancer in the pelvic area.

See also CYST, def. 6; PELVIC INFLAMMATORY DIS-
EASE; POLYCYSTIC OVARY SYNDROME.

oral contraceptive Also *the Pill, birth control pill.* A
hormone preparation taken by mouth that interferes with ovulation, fertilization or the implantation of a fertilized egg and therefore prevents
pregnancy. Available since 1960, it was the first
method of birth control that was nearly 100%
effective (provided a woman *never* forgot to take
her pill), and it is estimated that today some 80 to
100 million women in the world are using birth
control pills. However, disillusionment with the
Pill began as soon as women experienced its side
effects, and many women abandoned it because
they found them so unpleasant. One oral contraceptive, the sequential pill, was found dangerous
enough to be taken off the market. Once associated with increased risk for certain potentially
life-threatening disorders, such as heart attack and
cerebral vascular accident (stroke), the Pill today
contains much smaller amounts of estrogen and is
considered much safer than before. In fact, recent
studies have shown it associated with *lower* risk of
heart disease and stroke, and its association with
a greater risk for breast cancer also has been discounted. It currently is the most frequently used
reversible method of contraception in the United
States.

There are two main kinds of pill used today: the
combination pill and the minipill. The first contains both synthetic estrogen and progesterone; the
second contains only progesterone (see MINIPILL).
The rest of this entry applies only to the first, combination Pill. By keeping body levels of these two
basic hormones of the MENSTRUAL CYCLE constant,
the pill blocks the feedback mechanism whereby
rising and falling levels of the hormones trigger
ovulation. The combination pill usually is taken
once a day for 21 days and then is discontinued for
7 days. (Some brands come in a 28-day package,
in which 7 tablets containing no hormones and
distinguishable by their color are taken from day
22 to 28 of the cycle.) During the no-pill week,
hormone levels drop, causing bleeding similar to
menstruation but usually lighter, shorter and with
few or no cramps. The Pill provides a very regular
cycle; a woman who takes it at the same time each
day can accurately predict exactly when her period
will begin. To change that day, she can omit one
or more days of the Pill at the end of the cycle or
add one or more days. She should not delay starting a new package of pills for more than seven
days following the previous one, or her cycle may
become very irregular. Sometimes there is staining or breakthrough bleeding between periods; if
it occurs in the *first* half of the cycle, it usually is
caused by not enough estrogen; in the second half,
it usually is caused by not enough progesterone.
Spotting that occurs during the first three cycles
of the Pill may have no significance; if it continues
beyond that time, a different formulation, with a
different combination of progesterone and estrogen, often will eliminate the bleeding. In 2003 a
product called Seasonale was approved. It contains
the same hormones as the original Pill but works
on a 91-day cycle, reducing the number of periods
a woman has from 13 to 4 a year. The pill is taken
every day for 84 days, and then a placebo is taken
for the final week. One side effect of this regime
is nearly two weeks of bleeding or spotting during
the first cycle. However, excess bleeding or spotting
tends to diminish with continued use.

Some women have no periods when taking the
Pill. A woman who misses more than one period
should have a pregnancy test; if she is not pregnant
and continues to miss periods after three months
on the Pill, she may need a kind with less progesterone. Similarly, some kinds of pill have androgenic effects, causing the growth of facial hair, oily
skin and acne; women already susceptible to these
characteristics should switch to another kind of pill.
However, a pill should be tried for three months
before switching to another kind, since side effects
often disappear.

The principal advantages of oral contraceptives
are their high rate of effectiveness, simple method
of use, ease of discontinuing use and beneficial
effects on the menstrual cycle, mainly regulariz-
ing the cycle and reducing premenstrual tension,
menstrual flow and cramps. In addition, the newest forms of the Pill also cause a slight drop in LDL
cholesterol and a rise in HDL cholesterol, both of
which tend to lower the risk of heart disease. (See
CHOLESTEROL for further explanation.) The Pill also

is associated with reduced rates of ovarian and endometrial cancer, and possibly with decreased rates of benign tumors of the breast and uterus. Further, it may slow bone loss (osteoporosis) in women approaching menopause. The greatest disadvantage of the Pill is slightly increased risk of blood clots. Also balanced against the advantages are commonly experienced unpleasant side effects and certain absolute contraindications, meaning that *no* woman with these conditions should even consider oral contraceptives. **No woman should use the Pill if she has any of the following conditions:**

Pregnancy, suspicion of pregnancy or pregnancy ended within the previous three weeks
Breast-feeding and less than six weeks after delivery
Known or suspected breast cancer or endometrial cancer or any estrogen-dependent tumor
Untreated high blood pressure
Any circulatory disorder associated with blood clots (phlebitis or embolisms, severe varicose veins) or a past history of these disorders
Disease of the blood vessels supplying the brain or heart (stroke, heart disease, arteriosclerosis)
Kidney disease
Cystic fibrosis
Jaundice during previous pregnancy or Pill use
Sickle-cell disease
Diabetes with vascular changes (blocked arteries)
Active liver disease (hepatitis, liver tumors or cancer)
Moderate to severe hypertension (high blood pressure)
Severe migraine
Cigarette smoking over age 35
Obesity (BMI, or body-mass index, of 30 or more)
High triglyceride levels (250 mg or higher)

Some authorities feel this list of contraindications also should include a family history of serious circulatory disorders (hypertension, heart disease), especially if close relatives became ill at a young age, as well as oligomenorrhea, undiagnosed amenorrhea and heavy cigarette smoking at any age. Further, epilepsy and other seizure disorders, migraine, asthma and kidney disease all

may become worse as a result of fluid retention caused by the Pill, and anyone taking oral contraceptives who has these conditions requires careful monitoring.

The greatest risk of oral contraceptives is their association with the increased occurrence of blood vessel and clotting disorders, which include superficial or deep-vein thrombosis (formation of a THROMBUS, or blood clot), pulmonary EMBOLISM (a blood clot blocking the lungs) and the blocking of an artery (as in heart attacks and stroke). These risks, higher in all women taking oral contraceptives, are still higher in women who also smoke (especially smokers over 30 who use 15 or more cigarettes a day) and in all women over the age of 35. Also, those pills containing synthetic progesterones, especially desogestrel or gestodene, appear to double the risk of venous blood clots as compared to the older kinds of pill. Other risks associated with the Pill are increased incidence of a rare liver tumor and increased risk of developing high blood pressure. Further, a number of studies have tied use of the Pill to increased risk of breast cancer. However, the results are considered somewhat ambiguous, and critics point out that the lower dosage of estrogen in most brands of the present-day Pill—20 to 35 micrograms—avoids this risk.

Minor but unpleasant side effects are common. Sometimes they pass after a few months of medication, and at other times they can be minimized or eliminated by changing to a different kind of pill. They include edema (water retention), with associated nausea, leg cramps, bloating, weight gain, headache, vision changes, irritability and breast tenderness (early in the cycle they may be due to excess estrogen and during the no-pill week they may be due to excess progesterone); skin changes, especially darkening of the skin around the eyes and mouth (CHLOASMA, due to excess estrogen); androgenic changes, such as oily skin and hair, acne, increased body hair (due to excess androgens); loss of hair (due to excess progesterone); changes in normal vaginal discharge (too much or too little estrogen); depression (excess progesterone); and repeated yeast infections (excess progesterone). Some women experience changes in appetite and sex drive as well as mood changes. Pill users take twice as long to eliminate caffeine from their bodies as nonusers and therefore may develop insomnia, anxiety and tremors from what for others would be moderate amounts of coffee, tea, soft drinks and other caffeine-containing substances. Several dozen brands of Pill are available, and changing brands sometimes relieves discomfort.

The results of numerous laboratory tests can be altered by oral contraceptives, so it is important that a Pill user reports this fact when being tested for thyroid function, liver chemistry, iron level, blood cholesterol and fat levels, glucose tolerance, blood sugar, white cell count and tuberculin skin test. The Pill also interacts with other drugs, sometimes causing adverse drug effects or becoming less effective for birth control. Among these are tetracycline and ampicillin, barbiturates, epilepsy drugs and arthritis drugs, so any doctor prescribing medication should be told if a woman is taking the Pill.

If a woman decides she wants a child, she stops the Pill but is advised to wait until she has at least one period so as to calculate the dates of the pregnancy. Some women do not ovulate for several cycles after stopping the Pill and either have no periods or very irregular ones. In most cases this corrects itself within six months; for the 2 or 3% of cases in which it does not and in which there also is secretion from one or both breasts, other medication may be needed after disease has been ruled out (see POST-PILL AMENORRHEA).

A woman should not begin to use oral contraceptives until she has menstruated for at least six months lest the estrogen in the Pill prematurely stop her bone growth (see PUBERTY). Before taking the Pill, which is available by prescription only, she should have a complete checkup, including weight, blood pressure, breast examination, pelvic examination, a blood test for cholesterol and sugar levels, and a history that will rule out health factors contraindicating its use. In addition to the usual tests (see GYNECOLOGIC EXAMINATION), black women should be tested for SICKLE-CELL DISEASE. Tests for liver function and glucose tolerance also may be indicated.

In starting the Pill, a woman waits for her period, counts the first day of flow as day 1 and takes the first pill on day 5. She continues taking one pill a day for 21 days, takes no pill for seven days and then starts a new package. She continues the pattern of 21 days on, seven days off, which enables her always to start on the same day of the week. Her period usually will begin several days after the last hormone pill of a cycle is taken. She starts the new round of pills seven days later, whether her period has actually come or not. The Pill should be taken at nearly the same time every day to keep hormone levels in the blood as constant as possible.

If a woman forgets a pill she should take it as soon as she remembers, even if that means taking two pills in one day. The chance of pregnancy is still very small. The risk of pregnancy increases, however, if she forgets more than one pill in a single cycle. In this case she should take the pill as soon as she remembers, but should not take more than two in a day and must use a second, backup method of birth control through the remainder of that cycle. Some clinicians say if three pills in a row are missed, the woman should stop the Pill until the next period and then start a new round; if her period does not come, a pregnancy test should be made.

Women who become nauseated sometimes find that taking the pill with a meal or just before bedtime helps. If repeated vomiting persists for more than a day, a backup method of birth control should be used for the rest of the cycle because the pill may not have been absorbed in the stomach.

Certain signs of serious complication warrant seeking *immediate* medical attention, even if it entails going to the emergency room of the nearest hospital. They are:

Severe leg pain or swelling (in calf or thigh)
Severe abdominal pain
Severe headache
Severe chest pain
Shortness of breath
Dizziness, weakness or numbing
Changes in vision (blurring), flashing lights,
  blindness
Jaundice (yellowing of skin)

All women on oral contraceptives should return to their doctor or clinic three months following the first prescription for a thorough checkup and review. If all is well, checkups thereafter may be yearly. A woman who becomes pregnant while taking the Pill should stop taking it immediately. Also, women scheduled for surgery of any kind should stop taking the Pill at least one month before entering the hospital in order to avoid increased risk of circulatory complications. For women who like the method of oral contraceptives but cannot tolerate estrogen, an alternative is the minipill, which contains only progesterone but is slightly less effective in preventing pregnancy.

In 1999 the Food and Drug Administration approved marketing of a generic (non-brand name) pill. It contains desogestrel and ethinylestradiol and is usually less expensive than brand name equivalents.

In addition to their use for birth control, oral contraceptives have been used to treat ENDOMETRIOSIS, POLYCYSTIC OVARY SYNDROME, ovarian CYST, extremely heavy menstrual bleeding, and as a form of EMERGENCY CONTRACEPTIVE.

See also ESTROGEN.

oral sex Also *oral-genital intercourse*. A form of sexual intercourse in which one or both partners use their mouths (lips, tongue) to stimulate their partner's genitals. Oral sex may be performed in addition to or instead of other kinds of sexual intercourse (anal, vaginal). There is no medical reason for a couple who wish to engage in oral sex not to do so except in the presence of venereal disease. AIDS, SYPHILIS and GONORRHEA all can be transmitted by oral-genital contact, and HERPES INFECTION is thought to be transmitted in this way too. The two principal forms of oral sex are CUNNILINGUS and FELLATIO.

See also ANUS; COITUS; SEXUAL RESPONSE.

orgasm Also *climax, coming* (slang). A sudden release of congestion and muscle tension, accompanied by a feeling of intense pleasure, that is the peak of physical gratification in a sexual experience. In women the lower vagina and surrounding tissues as well as the uterus contract rhythmically. In men rhythmic contractions of the pelvic muscles cause EJACULATION, the forcible release of seminal fluid. In men orgasm is usually sudden and quite

brief. In women there is more variation, both among individuals and in one woman at different times; orgasm may be sudden and brief, or it may be long and slow. Also, with continued sexual stimulation, women are able to experience multiple orgasms, that is, a series of orgasms separated by only a few minutes or less. However, women tend to take longer than men to reach orgasm, on the average 15 minutes as opposed to three minutes for men. (Individuals vary widely, however.)

A woman's ability to experience orgasm does not alter with age. In men, however, the time between potential orgasms, called the *refractory period*, definitely increases with age, beginning with 30 to 60 seconds in an adolescent boy and becoming, on the average, 12 hours in a 50-year-old man; there is considerable variation among individuals and in the same individual at different times. To some extent a woman's ability to reach orgasm increases with practice; some women, however, have great difficulty reaching it or never do so at all and are said to suffer from FRIGIDITY. Orgasm in women is most easily achieved through stimulating the CLITORIS, which can be done manually by a woman herself (see MASTURBATION) or by her partner, as well as during vaginal, oral or anal intercourse. Many women find that the penile thrusting of vaginal intercourse does not stimulate their clitoris sufficiently to bring them to orgasm and find that additional stimulation, manual or other, is necessary. A woman can enjoy sex without orgasm, and women who have no sensation in the pelvic area due to disease or injury may find other parts of their body capable of considerable response to sexual stimulation.

Although a person experiencing orgasm is nearly always aware of it, his or her partner often is not and may need to be told when it occurs or has occurred. Regular sexual stimulation without orgasm (that is, stopping short of orgasm) can lead to pelvic discomfort and even to chronic congestion of the pelvic tissues when the engorged blood vessels in that area do not empty promptly. Indeed, for many women orgasm is an effective way of relieving pelvic congestion associated with menstrual cramps (see DYSMENORRHEA, def. 4). A small number of women experience an intense throbbing headache that begins during intercourse and peaks at orgasm, subsiding shortly thereafter. The cause of such an *orgasmic headache* is not known, but it is suspected that it results from the dilation of blood vessels in the brain (caused by increased blood pressure and heart rate). It may be similar to the cause of MIGRAINE, and indeed migraine sufferers are more apt to experience it.

For more information about the physiology of orgasm, see SEXUAL RESPONSE.

os   See CERVIX.

osteoarthritis   Also *degenerative joint disease*. A gradual breakdown of the cartilage that faces the body's joints. The most common form of ARTHRITIS, it strikes nearly everyone sooner or later to some degree but rarely begins before the age of 45. The onset is gradual and restricted to one or a few joints, which feel painful after being exercised and stiff after a period of inactivity. Eventually the affected joints become enlarged. Almost any joint may be affected, but the principal ones are in the spine, hips and legs, and, in women particularly, the fingers. Osteoarthritis of the hand is far more common in women than in men. Characterized by morning stiffness in the hands or thumb and loss of range of motion, it may be followed by bony nodules on the joints, especially the joint at the base of the thumb and joints closest to the palm. It is generally treated with hot or cold packs, special exercises and sometimes splints for use during the day or at night. Involvement of the knee and hip, more common after the age of 60, can become increasingly troublesome and occasionally disabling. Osteoarthritis of the spine may be quite severe without many symptoms.

The cause of osteoarthritis is not known, and treatment is largely palliative. Overweight creates further strain on weakened joints, so weight loss often is recommended. (A recent study showed that eliminating obesity in women over 50 could prevent 25 to 50% of all cases of osteoarthritis in the knee and 25% of cases in the hip.) Frequent rest of the involved joints may help, and canes or crutches may help take the strain off affected weight-bearing joints. Heat helps relieve pain and

muscle spasm, and isometric exercises help maintain muscle tone (appropriate exercises should be prescribed by a physician or physical therapist, because some kinds that help maintain motion also further damage the joints). Many patients find swimming and water exercises helpful. Aspirin, ibuprofen, other nonsteroidal anti-inflammatory drugs (NSAIDs) and the newer COX-2 inhibitors (see ANALGESIC) relieve pain and reduce inflammation, and a stronger anti-inflammatory agent, indomethacin, available only by prescription, also may be effective in those who can tolerate these medications (the principal adverse reactions are gastrointestinal upsets and rashes which can be offset by protective medications). Some patients have found relief from a substance long used in veterinary medicine: combined glucosamine and chondroitin sulfate. Sold as a dietary supplement rather than a drug, it may have a role in cartilage formation, but the evidence for its effectiveness is still mainly anecdotal. It may take three months to be effective, and if no improvement occurs by then it should be discontinued. Further, glucosamine should be avoided by pregnant women, patients with Type II diabetes and the very elderly, and chondroitin by patients taking blood-thinners such as heparin or coumarin, because it could lead to excessive bleeding. A new approach to treating osteoarthritis of the knee involves a series of three or five weekly injections into the joint of hyaluronic acid. Marketed as Synvisc, Orthovisc and Suplasyn, they are believed to help restore the normal consistency of the joint's synovial fluid, a viscous liquid that lubricates it and that breaks down as arthritis progresses. In about two-thirds of patients knee pain is reduced, mobility increased and the need for surgery may be delayed. There are few side effects but to date long-term use has not been studied. For advanced joint degeneration, orthopedic surgery, ranging from simple joint debridement (removal of dead tissue) to replacement of the joint with a prosthesis (artificial joint, especially successful in the case of hip and knee joints), may be required. In 2006 the FDA approved an alternative to total hip replacement. Called the Birmingham Hip Resurfacing System, it machines away the rough, damaged surface of the hip joint bones and covers them with high-carbide cobalt chrome. This procedure is done mostly in active women under the age of 55, with severe pain, no signs of bone loss and normal kidney function. Presumably it could also be done in older women who are not sedentary or overweight.

See also RHEUMATOID ARTHRITIS.

osteopenia   Low bone mass, a potential forerunner of OSTEOPOROSIS. A diagnosis of osteopenia, based on a bone density scan, indicates the need for preventive measures, specifically quitting smoking, adequate calcium and vitamin D intake, and weight-bearing exercise.

osteoporosis   A general decrease in bone mass that appears to be part of the aging process but that occurs more severely and far earlier in women than in men. At any age bone tissue is constantly being worn out, resorbed (absorbed into the bloodstream and eventually excreted) and replaced by newly formed bone. Both men and women are believed to attain their peak bone mass at approximately 35, although one study showed the beginning of bone loss as early as age 25 in 10 to 15% of the individuals studied. Thereafter bone mass either remains constant or more bone tissue is lost than replaced. As bone mass decreases, the bones become more brittle and more fragile, breaking easily (osteoporosis means "porous bones"). The rate of loss in women is for a time considerably greater than that in men, though by the age of 80 men have caught up. Part of the reason is that women's bones are less dense to begin with than men's. Also, women tend to be less active physically than men, and exercise appears to slow down bone loss. Further, bone loss in women speeds up after menopause, apparently because the decline in estrogen makes the body less able to absorb calcium from the diet and incorporate it into bone.

About one-fourth of American women suffer from osteoporosis of varying severity—as opposed to only one-eighth of American men—most of them past middle age and postmenopausal; nearly 90% are affected by the time they reach 75. Spinal osteoporosis is four times more common in women than in men (see COMPRESSION FRACTURE), hip frac-

WHO SHOULD HAVE A BONE DENSITY SCAN*

- All women aged 65 and over
- Postmenopausal women under 65 with one or more osteoporosis risk factors
- Postmenopausal women who have broken a bone
- Women who have been on long-term estrogen replacement therapy
- Women considering osteoporosis treatment if the test would help make a decision
- Women who have taken glucorticoids for two months or longer
- Women with a medical condition placing them at risk for osteoporotic fractures
- Women who have lost an inch or more in height
- Women with a body mass index (BMI) below 18

*Recommended by National Osteoporosis Foundation or National Institutes of Health or World Health Organization

tures two and one-half times more common—they often are the start of permanent invalidism in the elderly and may even precipitate death—and forearm and wrist fractures 10 times more common. Black women, very tall women and obese women are less susceptible than Asian and Caucasian women. Cigarette smoking, heavy use of alcohol (more than two drinks a day), use of steroid medication, anticonvulsants and the anticoagulant heparin, inflammatory bowel disease (Crohn's disease and ulcerative colitis) and a sedentary lifestyle also increase the risk. Thin women with small frames are at greater risk, as are women whose mothers had vertebrae fractures. Other, less crippling symptoms of osteoporosis are backache and loss of height (due to collapse of vertebrae in the spine, with as much as 1 to 1½ inches lost during each decade after MENOPAUSE), abdominal distention and DOWAGER'S HUMP.

A loss in height of an inch or more may be the first sign of an osteoporosis-related spinal fracture and should be checked with one's doctor. Several kinds of *bone density scan* techniques currently are available to measure bone density in women, a procedure now recommended not only for those who are at high risk or already have symptoms but preferably for all women beginning at menopause (or age 50). *Single-energy X-ray absorptiometry* and *peripheral dual-energy X-ray absorptiometry* assess the mineral content in the bones of the forearm, finger and sometimes the heel; *radiographic absorptiometry* measures the mineral content of the bones of the hand; *quantitative computerized tomography (QCT)* can measure trabecular bones of the lower spine; and *dual-energy X-ray absorptiometry (DEXA)* measures the total bone content of hips and spine (it is the quickest and most precise test and delivers the lowest dose of radiation). The machines for performing these tests are expensive and not every insurance plan covers the procedure. Medicare covers a DEXA every two years after age 65. However, a simpler and less costly means, *ultrasound densitometry,* which uses ultrasound (high-frequency sound waves) to measure the density of a woman's heel, knee or other peripheral sites, although less precise, may be adequate. Occasionally a more detailed picture of bone quality is needed. For this purpose a new type of CAT scanner, the Scanco X-Treme CT, is currently being tested. It can image the smallest aspects of bone microarchitecture and help distinguish women with low bone density who actually have strong bones from those who do not and are at risk for fracture and need medication. However, it is not yet widely available.

All these tests compare the condition of a woman's bones to the density of a normal 35-year-old woman. The results are given in standard deviations (SDs); 1 SD below normal is equivalent to a 10 to 12% decrease in bone density. Within 1 SD, bones are considered healthy; between 1 and 2.5 SDs, bone mass is at serious risk for osteoporosis; and at 2.5 SDs or higher, osteoporosis is diagnosed.

The ultimate cause of primary osteoporosis is still unknown. (Occasionally the condition is secondary to kidney disease or specific endocrine disorders and then is treated by eliminating the underlying problem.) Since heredity plays a role, researchers are looking into genetic markers. One has already been found that accounts for about one-third of a person's overall risk; it shows how dense bones will be in early adulthood, an important indicator of future risk.

After significant bone loss has occurred, no treatment currently known can restore normal density. Physical discomfort can be relieved with painkillers such as aspirin, heat, massage and orthopedic supports when needed. A recent study shows that spinal compression fractures, which can be quite painful and disabling, may be treated by minimally invasive surgery. One kind is *vertebroplasty,* in which a needle inserted into the broken bone injects cement. Another kind is *kyphoplasty,* in which a tiny balloon expands the disk back to its original height before cement is injected. Symptoms are relieved within hours or days, and the benefits of the procedure may last for at least two years.

There are preventive measures. It is known that physical stress stimulates an increase in bone mass, while bed rest leads to a decrease. Exercise, especially weight-bearing kinds (walking, jogging, dancing) increases bone mass. Also, insufficient CALCIUM in the diet—which is thought to be true for practically all American adults—accelerates bone loss, while too much phosphorus (found in meats, poultry, fish, cola drinks and many processed foods) seems to impair the body's ability to use what calcium it does get. Therefore regular exercise and a well-balanced diet high in calcium (with milk and other dairy products the best source; calcium supplements are far less effective) will at least strengthen connective tissue (muscles, ligaments, tendons) and thus slow down the osteoporotic process. Before menopause, 1,000 mg of calcium a day, and, afterward, 1,500 mg are recommended, along with 400 I.U. of vitamin D (and 600 I.U. after age 70; some authorities recommend 800 to 1,000 I.U.), and 30 to 45 minutes of weight-bearing exercise (such as walking) on most days. Avoiding smoking and excessive alcohol are also recommended.

ESTROGEN REPLACEMENT THERAPY slows down bone resorption but, owing to numerous risks it presents, is not recommended for simply avoiding bone loss. Oral medications called bisphosphonates, taken daily, are widely recommended for slowing bone loss. Among them are alendronate (Fosamax), risedronate (Actonel) and ibandronate (Boniva). Also effective for slowing bone loss is the SELECTIVE ESTROGEN–RECEPTOR MODULATOR raloxifene (Evista). Fosamax may also be taken once a week or once a month, in higher dosages, and Boniva may be taken once a month as well. Studies show that Fosamax is effective when taken for five years, and its effects continue for about five years after it is discontinued. In 2006 an unusual side effect of the bisphosphonates (Fosamax, Actonel and Boniva) appeared. Some patients developed osteonecrosis of the jaw, that is, destruction of parts of the jawbone. However, the number of cases reported was tiny, and the link is still uncertain. Evista is somewhat less effective but apparently quite risk-free. A different drug that appears to stimulate bone growth is teriparatide (Forteo), based on parathyroid hormone. Approved by the Food and Drug Administration in 2002, it is taken in daily self-administered injections and is recommended mainly for individuals with significantly low bone density and at high risk for fractures. It has such side effects as nausea, headache, leg cramps and dizziness, but results in marked increase of bone density. Taken for three months or so and then stopped, it needs to be replaced by one of the bisphosphonates or raloxifene to maintain the increase in bone formation. If taken for more than two years, it may increase risk of a bone cancer (osteosarcoma), but its effects persist after it is stopped. Research is currently underway on variants of the drug that can be taken in pill form, as a nasal spray or as a cream. A synthetic steroid, tibolone (Livial), is currently available in 70 countries in Europe, South America, Mexico and Asia. It appears to grant bone protection, relieve hot flashes and vaginal dryness, and does not stimulate breast growth; at this writing there are questions about its cardiovascular effects and it has not yet been approved in the United States. The FDA also has approved zoledronic acid (Zometa) and pamidronate (Aredia), which are given intravenously for cancerous bone tumors, to combat osteoporosis. They are administered once a year via an intravenous infusion taking about 15 to 20 minutes, and have been found to decrease the risk of vertebral fractures by 70% and hip fractures by 41%, as well as other bone fractures. A recent study showed that another brand of zoledronic acid, Reclast, reduced the risk of death following hip fracture by 28%. It is given intravenously once a year. Another intravenous bisphosphonate, ibandronate (Boniva), which comes as a monthly pill, may be given intravenously every three months but its results have not been adequately documented. Calcitonin (Calcimar, Miacalcin) is taken as a nasal spray or is injected. The nasal spray can cause a runny, irritated nose; the injection can cause nausea, rash, and flushing of the face and hands. It slows bone loss and increases bone density in the spine in women who are at least five years past menopause. Another medication currently being tested is denosumab, a monoclonal antibody that appears to build bone density and is expected also to reduce bone fractures; it is given by injection once every six months. Like all medications, these are not without side effects. The best means of assessing the effects of treatment is a blood or urine test (not a repeat bone scan) to measure the proteins and enzymes released as bone is resorbed and new bone replaces it. These biochemical markers may show, at the beginning of treatment and three to six months later, the body's response to medication.

ostomy   A surgical opening in the abdomen through which waste material is discharged when the normal function of bowel or bladder is lost. There are three principal kinds of ostomy: COLOSTOMY, ILEOSTOMY and UROSTOMY. The ostomy is fashioned by bringing the opened portion of the remaining intestine or urinary vessel through the abdominal wall. The technical name for the opening is *stoma*. Elimination through the stoma cannot be controlled voluntarily. In most cases it is collected in a plastic or rubber pouch, called an *appliance*, which is attached to the abdomen at all times and is emptied periodically through a bottom opening. Some colostomies, however, are controlled by irrigation (enema) and require only a small gauze pad or plastic stick-on pouch to cover the stoma between irrigations.

Ostomy surgery of and by itself need not interfere with sexual relations or childbearing. In men, however, it may impair sexual functioning, at least for a time. About 10 to 20% of men with ileostomies suffer some impairment of sexual function and potency. Such impairment may be temporary, but in some cases recovery takes as long as two years. For men with urostomies and colostomies, impairment tends to be more severe. Those who have had urinary surgery early in childhood usually can sustain an erection but may be sterile; men who have such surgery as adults usually become impotent. Men with colostomies vary anywhere from full potency to complete impotence. Often potency is retained but the man becomes sterile; in some cases surgery is so extensive that potency is lost permanently.

Ileostomy is the most common kind of such surgery in women of childbearing age. (Urinary ostomy is performed mostly in the very young and in those over 50 for cancer; most colostomies are performed in women over 40.) Ostomy surgery does not alter the physical structure of the vagina or uterus. Immediately following surgery there may be local sensitivity and pain, but once the abdominal incision has healed normal sexual relations can be resumed. When the rectum has been removed, the perineal area may be sore for some months—in some cases much longer—but this varies with individuals.

So far as pregnancy is concerned, it was formerly feared that an enlarging uterus might compress the stoma or that a woman's muscles, nerves and digestive system might be damaged. Today most authorities agree that although bowel or bladder surgery may have been extensive and any pregnancy may be physically taxing, an ostomy need not limit the number of children a woman bears unless other complications are present. Nor need there be a particular waiting period before pregnancy; some births have occurred within a few days of ostomy surgery, although more conservative physicians advise a wait of two years after surgery before conception, and most advise a limit of two pregnancies.

The most common problem during pregnancy is swelling of the stoma, which tends to become tender and protrude during midpregnancy whether the abdomen is much distended or not. Usually the stoma returns to normal size soon after delivery. Because of this change, however, the ostomate who wears a reusable appliance must make sure the opening fits the enlarged stoma properly to avoid exerting damaging pressure on it. Although ostomates may be advised that delivery may have to be by Cesarean section, in most cases a normal vaginal delivery is possible.

Apart from the physical problems of such major surgery, ostomy can be emotionally devastating.

For this reason, support groups have been formed in which former patients help counsel individuals before and after surgery. The United Ostomy Association (see the Appendix), publishes lists of local support groups and extensive explanatory literature.

outpatient   A person who receives treatment at a hospital or other health care facility without being admitted as a resident, or *inpatient.* Many surgical and medical procedures can be performed on an outpatient basis, at a considerable saving of time and money. However, health insurance plans vary, and a procedure that may be covered completely by insurance when a person is hospitalized may be accorded less or even no coverage if performed on an outpatient basis.

See also CLINIC; SURGERY, OUTPATIENT.

ova   The plural of OVUM, or egg.

ovarian cancer   See CANCER, OVARIAN.

ovarian cyst   See CYST, def. 6.

ovarian dysgenesis   See TURNER'S SYNDROME.

ovariectomy   Another name for OOPHORECTOMY.

ovary   The female gonad, or sex gland, primarily responsible for secreting the female sex hormones, estrogen and progesterone, and for producing female germ cells (ova, or eggs). There are two ovaries, located at the back of the broad ligament on either side of the uterus, just below the fallopian tubes, whose outer ends curve over them. In mature women each ovary is about 3½ by 1½ by 2 centimeters (1½ by ½ by ¾ inches) and is shaped like a flattened egg, covered by a grayish-white membrane. Each of the ovaries is attached to its side of the uterus by a special ligament about 4 centimeters (1 to 2 inches) long, but they are suspended by other ligaments as well, and they can shift position somewhat.

At birth the ovaries contain several hundred thousand primordial egg follicles. After puberty, during every menstrual cycle, some 20 of these follicles begin to ripen, but only one (sometimes two) mature completely and release an egg (ovulation). After the egg is extruded from the ovary and drawn into the adjacent fallopian tubes, the empty follicle is transformed into the CORPUS LUTEUM, which secretes progesterone for the next two weeks and then disintegrates. If the egg was fertilized by a sperm (while in the tube) and was implanted in the uterus, the placenta takes over progesterone production. If it was not fertilized, the lowered levels of hormones trigger the cycle to begin again (see MENSTRUAL CYCLE for further explanation). After menopause the remaining egg follicles disintegrate and the ovary shrinks to about one-third its size during the reproductive years.

Palpating (feeling) the ovaries is an important part of every gynecological examination. A difference in size between the two ovaries can be significant, as is enlargement of both ovaries beyond a certain size. The most common disorders affecting the ovaries are cysts (see CYST, def. 6) and cancer (see CANCER, OVARIAN). The ovaries also can be infected in PELVIC INFLAMMATORY DISEASE and the various SEXUALLY TRANSMITTED DISEASES or develop multiple cysts (see POLYCYSTIC OVARY SYNDROME). Surgical removal of the ovaries, which brings on MENOPAUSE if both are removed, is called OOPHO-RECTOMY and should be undertaken only if more conservative treatment is useless.

See also OVUM.

oviducts See FALLOPIAN TUBES.

ovulation The regular release of an egg, or ovum, from the ovaries, which takes place more or less monthly, except during pregnancy, from soon after menarche until after menopause, or roughly from the ages of 14 to 54. At puberty the production of sex hormones is greatly increased, and the pituitary gland begins to produce FSH (follicle-stimulating hormone), which stimulates the growth and development of a number of follicles in the ovary. Each follicle contains an egg cell. As the follicles develop, they produce estrogen, which in turn stimulates the pituitary to produce LH (luteinizing hormone). LH, together with estrogen, suppresses the growth of the numerous follicles stimulated during this cycle except for one, or occasionally two. This follicle, the GRAAFIAN FOLLICLE, grows to maturity and moves toward the ovarian wall. As it moves, that portion of the wall thins and bulges outward. In response to LH, the follicle ruptures, bursting through the ovarian wall and allowing the egg it contains to move out through the opening. Fingerlike ends of the nearby fallopian tube—the fimbriae—move toward the opening in the ovarian wall to catch the egg as it emerges and draw it into and through the tube. It takes an egg about four days to travel the length of the tube, but unless it is fertilized by sperm that has traveled up the tube to meet it within 24 hours of its release from the ovary. The egg will no longer be viable. Sometimes two eggs are released during a single cycle; such *double ovulation*, if both eggs are fertilized, results in the birth of fraternal twins (see MULTIPLE PREGNANCY).

In some women ovulation is marked by pain and/or vaginal bleeding, which may range from slight to severe but usually will last only a few hours (see MITTELSCHMERZ). Many women, however, have no symptoms. Because an egg is viable for such a short time, women who wish to become pregnant, as well as those trying to avoid pregnancy, may want to know when they ovulate. The length of a woman's menstrual cycle is no indication until after the fact: Ovulation tends to occur 14 days (give or take two days) before the next menstrual flow. In a 23-day cycle this would be on or about day 9; in a 40-day cycle it would be on or about day 26. Since many women have highly irregular menstrual cycles, other means are needed to time an attempted conception. The principal methods used for determining the time of ovulation are by taking BASAL BODY TEMPERATURE, which rises at ovulation and stays up until menstruation, and by testing or examining the cervical mucus, which changes in color and consistency just before ovulation. The former method is used mostly by women wishing to conceive, and the latter as a method of preventing conception (see also NATURAL FAMILY PLANNING; CERVICAL MUCUS METHOD). In addition, a number of home ovulation test kits on the market predict ovulation by measuring a sudden monthly surge in the concentration of LH (luteinizing hormone) in the urine (ovulation usually takes place within a day after this surge). To identify the start of the surge, a woman must test urine samples each morning for several days around the middle of her cycle. The device will then indicate the presence of LH with a colored line, dot or test area, whose intensity must be compared against a reference. Lack of a positive result may mean that the woman did not ovulate that month or that her LH surge was too low to be detected by a home test or that her surge was too brief (less than 10 hours) and so was missed by the daily test. Not all these tests have been fully evaluated, but the most sensitive of them appear to be reliable for about 85% of women. Nevertheless, they are most appropriate for women wishing to conceive and are not considered reliable for contraception. Still other over-the-counter preparations are saliva tests. During ovulation, the amount of salt in the saliva rises. Placed on a microscope slide, the crystallized salts in dried saliva produce a fern-leaf appearance if a woman has begun to ovulate. Hand-held microscopes are available for relatively low prices ($25 and up). Their advantage over urine-stick tests is that they can be used over and over for as long as a year. They indicate ovulation as many as four days in advance and can be used at different times during the day. If none of these methods indicates that a woman is ovulating, a clinician may perform an endometrial biopsy, usually by VACUUM ASPIRATION, and examine the endometrial (uterine lining) tissue, which can indicate conclusively whether ovulation has taken place, but not when.

See also ANOVULATORY BLEEDING.

ovulation method   See CERVICAL MUCUS METHOD; NATURAL FAMILY PLANNING.

ovum   Also *ova* (pl.). The Latin word for "egg," the female reproductive cell in all animals that reproduce sexually, including human beings. Unlike sperm—the male reproductive cells that are produced by the testes after puberty—the ova already are present in the ovaries at birth but begin to mature and be released only after puberty. The human ovum is very tiny, about $1/200$ inch in diameter (perhaps $1/5$ the size of a printed dot). At birth a baby girl's ovaries contain 1 million ova; by puberty, at age 11 or 12, there are only 300,000. Despite the degeneration of so many ova, there are always far more than can mature during a woman's lifetime. The average ovum survives outside the ovary for about 24 hours before it degenerates; ideally fertilization (the union of ovum and sperm to form a fertilized egg) takes place within 12 hours after the release of an ovum from the ovary, the release being called OVULATION. In 2004 researchers reported that female mice continue producing eggs throughout their lives, overturning a long-held belief that the number of ova at birth can only decrease. Specifically, they discovered active germ-line stem cells in both young and adult females, from which new ova develop. This finding, if proved to be true in human females, could have huge implications for fertility treatments, for dealing with menopause, and similar issues.

oxygen in childbirth   The administration of oxygen to the mother during labor. It is used to saturate the blood with oxygen when there is fetal distress or the mother experiences hyperventilation, nausea or other discomfort. Oxygen may be administered to a baby after birth, especially a PREMATURE baby and/or one suffering from respiratory distress, as in HYALINE MEMBRANE DISEASE. However, if too much oxygen is given to a newborn baby, there is danger that the retinas of its eyes will be damaged, possibly resulting in blindness (see RETROLENTAL FIBROPLASIA), so the levels administered must be carefully monitored.

oxytocin   A hormone stored and released by the pituitary gland in response to stimulation by the

HYPOTHALAMUS. Its main functions are to stimulate uterine contractions during labor and to contract the cells of the breast's milk ducts, causing the expulsion of milk (see LET-DOWN REFLEX). It was first isolated by Vincent du Vigneaud in the 1930s and was synthesized (made in a laboratory) in 1953. In its synthetic form, for which common brand names are Pitocin and Syntocinon, oxytocin is used both to induce labor and to strengthen uterine contractions during labor. However, indiscriminate use of the drug can cause too violent contractions, threatening the baby's oxygen supply or causing other damage, and the U.S. Food and Drug Administration has ruled that it may not be used in elective induction (see INDUCTION OF LABOR). For *oxytocin challenge test*, see FETAL MONITORING.

Paget's disease **1.** A form of breast cancer in which the NIPPLE and AREOLA become encrusted and look inflamed. The underlying cause is a cancerous growth between the milk ducts deep in the breast, from which malignant cells have spread upward along the ducts that end at the nipple. Paget's disease tends to occur in middle-aged women. Treatment usually consists of a simple mastectomy and removal of affected lymph nodes. Sometimes only the nipple and surrounding tissue are removed.

2. A CANCER IN SITU of the VULVA that is characterized by a reddish lesion interspersed with white epithelial "islands," which under the microscope are revealed to be large, pale "Paget" cells. Usually it is not associated with an underlying cancer, although in 5% of patients it is associated with cancer elsewhere in the body. Treatment consists of extensive local excision.

3. A progressive bone disease of unknown cause that affects more men than women and that eventually causes distortion, thickening and overgrowth of various bones. The bones most often affected are those of the pelvis, hips and skull. The disease usually does not begin until middle age and progresses quite slowly. No cure is known, and treatment is directed principally at relieving discomfort from the distortions.

pain See CHRONIC PAIN; PELVIC PAIN.

palpate To press lightly on the surface of the body with the fingers to determine the size and position of an underlying structure, such as the uterus or ovaries (see GYNECOLOGIC EXAMINATION) or to locate abnormalities such as lumps, as in BREAST SELF-EXAMINATION. Palpation is a basic technique in physical examination.

palpitations The unpleasant sensation of one's own heartbeat, perceived as abnormally fast or unusually violent or somehow irregular. It may indicate actual *tachycardia,* that is, a rapid heart rate, or a structural change (see MITRAL VALVE PROLAPSE), but often it does not and there are no demonstrable signs of any kind. Palpitations frequently accompany an ANXIETY attack and also are associated with MENOPAUSE.

pancreas An ENDOCRINE gland situated behind the stomach, between the spleen and duodenum, whose principal functions are to secrete digestive fluids into the intestine and to secrete the hormone insulin (see DIABETES). It occasionally becomes inflamed, a very painful condition called pancreatitis, which may be caused by gallbladder problems or exposure to certain drugs or alcohol abuse. Acute pancreatitis is characterized by sudden severe abdominal pain, which becomes worse when one lies down. Because it can be life-threatening, it requires immediate medical attention. There is also a chronic form of the disease that develops from long-term use of various drugs, alcohol abuse or unknown causes. The pancreas then gradually loses its ability to secrete digestive enzymes, and the patient begins to lose weight (since food cannot be absorbed) and can even develop diabetes. Pancreatitis is treated with drugs or surgery, depending on the cause and extent of damage.

Pancreatic cancer, a disease occurring mostly after the age of 50 and twice as often in men as in women, is frequently not diagnosed until it is far advanced and is a leading cause of death. The average survival rate five years after diagnosis is only 5%. Because there is a strong familial factor, some individuals take the extreme route of having their pancreas removed, which has the inevitable consequence that they will become diabetic.

panic disorder   See ANXIETY.

papilloma, ductal (intraductal)   See DUCTAL PAPILLOMA.

Pap smear   Also *Papanicolaou smear, Pap test.* A valuable test for cervical cancer named for its inventor, Dr. George Papanicolaou, that should be performed on a regular basis. The test itself consists of scraping away a thin layer of cells from the surface of the cervix, using a wooden or plastic spatula. The cells are placed on a slide, sprayed with fixative, stained and examined under the microscope by a pathologist or specially trained technician. The test is quite sensitive, detecting the presence of abnormal cells on the cervix and reliably revealing early, precancerous or potentially cancerous changes. It also helps evaluate estrogen production and determines the presence of common vaginal infections. It does not, however, reliably detect cancer of the vagina, uterus or ovaries. If a Pap test picks up suspicious premalignant changes, it usually is followed up with a biopsy to remove cervical and endocervical tissue for further examination (see BIOPSY, def. 7).

There are several ways of classifying the type and degree of abnormalities detected by a Pap smear. The most commonly used current system of staging for cervical cancer (the Bethesda system) ranges from normal cells to probable malignancy:

Negative: all cells normal.
ASCUS (atypical squamous cells of undetermined significance): some atypical cells; HPV (Human papilloma virus) testing warranted; if positive, COLPOSCOPY indicated.
LSIL (low-grade squamous intraepithelial lesions): More abnormal cells and more severe abnor-malities; questionable or suspicious; colpos-copy indicated.
HSIL (high-grade squamous intraepithelial lesions): Possible malignancy; colposcopy indicated; if negative, repeat Pap smear in a few months.
Positive: probable malignancy, biopsy indicated.

Other names for these designations are benign for ASCUS, mild to moderate dysplasia for LSIL, severe dysplasia for HSIL, and carcinoma in situ or invasive cancer for positive. (See also CANCER, CERVICAL.)

Most Pap tests result in negative findings, meaning the cells are normal, but anywhere from 1 to 6% are positive. In rare instances a woman will receive a "false negative" report, which can be identified only in retrospect, after a malignancy is diagnosed through a biopsy or positive reading and earlier Pap test results are reviewed. To help ensure proper treatment, a patient should ask whether the laboratory to which her clinician sends the smear is certified by the American Society of Cytology or the American Society of Clinical Pathologists. Researchers also have developed a technique involving infrared spectroscopy of cervical cells, which they hope will lead to a quicker method that will replace the Pap test. Although taking a Pap smear takes little time, doctors usually send the cell samples to outside laboratories and results are not available for a week or two; spectroscopy would yield results almost immediately, but the test is not yet available at this writing. However, a liquid test, called ThinPrep, has been approved to replace the conventional Pap smear. Instead of smearing collected cells onto a slide, with ThinPrep the cells are rinsed off the collecting tool into a vial of preservative solution. The sealed vial is sent to a laboratory, where a processor filters out blood and mucus and deposits a single thin layer of cells on a slide. It offers a clearer picture of cells and therefore is more accurate in detecting low-grade lesions. Two other new techniques, PapNet and Auto Net, use computers to re-image conventional Pap smears and make it easier to identify abnormalities missed the first time.

An annual Pap smear is advised for all women, starting within three years of the onset of sexual activity, or by age 21. Thereafter screening should be done annually until age 30. If a woman aged 30 or older has had three normal test results in a row, the interval can increase to two or three years, provided she has none of the following risk factors: cigarette smoking, infection with a cancer-causing form of human papilloma virus (HPV; see below), HIV, herpes, virus, or chlamydia; poor diet; exposure to DES in utero; treatment with immune-suppressing medication; or a personal or family history of cervical cancer. In these cases annual screening is recommended. Most women aged 70 and older who have had three or more normal Pap tests in a row and no abnormal test in the previous 10 years and those who have had a total hysterectomy can stop cervical cancer screening. However, in cases of abdominal hysterectomy where the cervix was preserved, Pap tests should be continued on a schedule determined by the woman's age and risk for cervical cancer. But if the cervix was removed during a hysterectomy for cervical, ovarian or endometrial cancer, Pap tests still should be continued to monitor for changes in vaginal tissues.

Because human papilloma virus (HPV) is thought to be implicated in 90% of cervical cancers, a new procedure, called Hybrid Capture HPV DNA Assay, adds another step to the Pap smear process for ASCUS and LSIL tissue samples. They are tested for the presence of the virus, and if it is found, a microscopic examination of the cervix (see COLPOSCOPY) and removal of the lesion are indicated. If no infected cells are found, a follow-up Pap smear in a few months is suggested. A large study showed that this test identified 100% of cancers (as opposed to 92% with an ordinary Pap smear) and 90% of precancerous lesions (as opposed to 78%), so it appears to warrant the extra cost incurred. For women who have been vaccinated against HPV (see HUMAN PAPILLOMA VIRUS), this advanced test may not be necessary.

How to proceed when Pap smear findings are other than negative (completely normal) is usually a matter of the clinician's judgment, based partly on the patient's risk factors. If the latter are low, a single abnormal finding may warrant a wait-and-see approach with a follow-up Pap test in four to six months. Many ASCUS and LSIL abnormalities do disappear spontaneously, but if they show up

in a second test, COLPOSCOPY should follow. Nevertheless some clinicians proceed with colposcopy after even one abnormal smear, and that course of action is recommended for patients with previous abnormal Pap findings, those with risk factors for cervical cancer and those who are unlikely or unwilling to return for follow-up Pap screening. Long a mainstay at detecting cervical cancer, the new vaccine against human papilloma virus along with a newer genetic test that detects the DNA of 13 of the virus's cancer-causing strains and 90% of precancerous lesions are beginning to play a larger role in screening and may eventually make the Pap test obsolete.

paracervical anesthesia   Also *paracervical block*. A kind of local ANESTHESIA that is administered chiefly for a D AND C or for an abortion. It involves injecting a local anesthetic through the vagina into the area around the cervix, that is, the ligaments and walls of the lower part of the uterus.

Formerly used in labor, paracervical anesthesia is now considered unsafe in childbirth because it lowers the mother's blood pressure, which may impair the baby's oxygen supply.

paraplegia   Partial or total paralysis of the lower extremities, with severe impairment or complete loss of sensitivity to touch, pain and temperature in that area. It usually results from an injury to the spinal cord, most often one caused by a traffic, industrial or sports accident; such damage from tumors, infections, abscesses and congenital defects is less common. The complications and sexual implications of paraplegia are similar to those of quadriplegia, in which all four limbs are impaired, except that autonomic hyperreflexia (see QUADRIPLEGIA) occurs less frequently and, since the patient has use of his or her arms, masturbation is possible.

parathyroid   Four small ENDOCRINE glands located behind the thyroid gland. They secrete a hormone that, in conjunction with vitamin D, regulates the body's metabolism of calcium and phosphorus.

parturition Another name for childbirth. See also LABOR.

patients' rights A general term that describes a person's just claims on health care services. Health care institutions such as hospitals, especially large ones, often have a built-in tendency to overlook the concerns of the individual patient. Further, the long-standing traditional attitude of health care professionals is that their knowledge and expertise should override such considerations as the patient's understanding of his or her illness, treatment and prognosis. These tendencies became even more exaggerated with increasing professional specialization and technological advances in medicine. Beginning in the 1960s, however, there was a growing reaction in the United States, and patients, individually and in groups, began to assert their rights. For example, when a young child required hospitalization, formerly it was taken for granted that the hospital's normal rules limiting visiting hours should be obeyed. As a result, many young patients were so frightened by being separated from their parents that hospitalization represented a far more traumatic experience than their illness. Increasingly, parents began to fight these rules, and today it is not unusual for a hospital to provide sleep-in accommodations for a young child's parent or, at the very least, to allow very liberal visiting hours. The same is true for fathers of newborn babies. Similarly, it was traditional for a patient to sign very broad consent forms when admitted to a hospital, in effect letting the physician and/or the hospital staff make all the decisions concerning treatment, including surgery. The patients' rights movement, in contrast, stressed the principle of *informed consent*, whereby before consenting to any treatment a person is given the maximum available information, in everyday language rather than in special medical terms, about his or her condition, the alternative treatments available and all their consequences (positive and negative), the effects of treatment compared to no treatment at all, and similar facts.

While patients' rights apply equally to both sexes, this concern necessarily affects women more than men simply because women use health care facilities and personnel far more often. Women seek medical care when they are not ill or injured: for birth control, pregnancy, childbirth, abortion, routine cancer tests. Moreover, this greater dependency on the medical profession has fostered the very attitude the patients' rights movement is combating, the traditional doctor-patient relationship in which the physician is an authority figure who tells the patient what is best. The dependent and passive status of patients also has led to their abuse, especially when they lack funds and/or education or have a poor command of English. Such patients may find themselves undergoing unnecessary surgery, being given experimental drugs or being otherwise exploited.

To combat this situation and at the same time improve the quality of health care, the patients' rights movement directed its efforts in two major directions: (1) informing everyone of his or her rights as a health care consumer; and (2) urging the use of a patient advocate. Lists of patients' rights have been developed by the American Hospital Association, medical committees for human rights and similar bodies as well as by women's health collectives and self-help centers. While they vary in minor details, they cover the same basic ground: the right to know the identity and professional status of the caregiver; the right to know the nature of the illness and its prognosis (including all test results); what treatments are possible and their pros and cons (including benefits, side effects and risks), their costs and coverage by medical insurance and the necessity for hospitalization; the right to know the contents of one's own medical records and to privacy of one's person and records; the right to refuse to take part in experiments, research or procedures performed for educational purposes, and to refuse any drug, test or treatment; the right to get a second medical opinion concerning one's condition or any proposed treatment, to leave the health facility at any time regardless of physical or financial status and to refuse to be transferred to another facility. Today many larger teaching hospitals give patients a printed list of their rights when they are admitted, and many other hospitals and clinics post such lists on bulletin boards or make them available on request.

To ensure that these rights are honored, it may be helpful to have a *patient advocate*, a friend or relative who accompanies the patient to a clinic or doctor's office and stays with the patient in the examining room, to give both general support and to uphold the patient's demands for his or her rights. A few hospitals now assign every patient to an advocate on the staff who is available to answer questions, uphold the patient's rights, assist in clarifying the nature of decisions the patient must make and otherwise support the patient. In recent decades the growth of *managed care,* a system of health care financing and delivery that gives health insurers considerable power over the practice of medicine, has had new impact on patients' rights. In order to cut burgeoning costs, insurers may, for example, decide whether or not a patient should see a specialist, limit the time of a hospital stay or even deny needed medical care altogether. Moreover, although managed care began as a non-profit physician-managed system, in the 1990s for-profit managed care firms increasingly prevailed in the market, making for increased pressure to make larger profits by offering lower quality and fewer services.

See also PREGNANT PATIENTS' RIGHTS; SURGERY, UNNECESSARY.

pediculosis pubis   See PUBIC LICE.

pelvic cavity   See PELVIS.

pelvic examination   See GYNECOLOGIC EXAMINATION.

pelvic exenteration   Radical surgery formerly performed for very advanced cancer of the cervix. It involved the removal not only of cervix, uterus, fallopian tubes and ovaries, but also of rectum and bladder, which were replaced by special openings in the abdomen (see OSTOMY). Today chemotherapy and radiation therapy have largely replaced this procedure.

pelvic inflammatory disease   Also *pelvic infection, PID, salpingitis.* Inflammation and/or infection of the fallopian tubes, which often involves the ovaries and uterus as well. Strictly speaking, inflammation of the tubes is *salpingitis,* of the uterus *endometritis* and of the ovary *oophoritis.* Some authorities use the term *pelvic inflammatory disease* as another name for salpingitis because it primarily involves the tubes; others use it more broadly, for any pelvic inflammation or infection, sometimes even including CERVICITIS.

Pelvic inflammatory disease can range from a mild to a very serious, even life-threatening disorder. It may be *acute* (a sudden, severe infection), *subacute* (less severe) or *chronic* (with persistent inflammation and low-grade infection). In its acute form it is characterized by severe lower abdominal pain and tenderness, felt especially on movement of the cervix. Other symptoms include high fever, chills, a purulent (pus-filled) cervical discharge, vaginal bleeding and a raised white blood cell count, signaling an active infection. A frequent finding is the rapid development of adhesions (scar tissue) between any of the adjoining pelvic structures (ovaries, tubes, uterus) or between them and the small intestine, colon or rectum. The pain felt on palpating these adhesions is similar to that felt with appendicitis and pyelonephritis (kidney infection), which therefore must be ruled out.

Diagnosis includes a pelvic examination (to locate pain and swelling) and laboratory analysis of the cervical discharge. If there is doubt, an exploratory LAPAROSCOPY may be needed, and, should an ABSCESS be suspected, ULTRASOUND may be used to locate it. An *abscess* is a serious complication; if it ruptures, the infection can spread through the tubes into the entire pelvic and abdominal cavity, causing peritonitis (the peritoneum is the lining of the abdomen), a medical emergency; it can cause death in as little as an hour. Because such an abscess often does not respond to antibiotic treatment, it may require surgical incision and drainage. Another serious complication of acute pelvic inflammatory disease is massive enlargement of a fallopian tube with fluid (*hydrosalpinx*) or pus (*pyosalpinx*), which may cause it to rupture. Still another is *septicemia* (blood poisoning), which usually occurs only when the disease is a sequel to childbirth, abortion or miscarriage; the infection then spreads into the bloodstream through open blood vessels in the uterus. Fortunately, the severe discomfort of acute pelvic inflammation usually prompts a woman to seek medical attention before these serious complications can develop.

Pelvic inflammatory disease is a bacterial infection. Usually the organisms responsible enter the body through the vagina and work their way up into the pelvic cavity. The gonococcus, which causes GONORRHEA, and *Chlamydia trachomatis,* which causes CHLAMYDIA INFECTION, are thought to be responsible for one-third to one-half of cases. The rest are caused by other bacteria, principally *Escherichia coli,* which may enter through the cervix during childbirth, abortion, miscarriage or by means of an intrauterine device (IUD), either during insertion or, some authorities believe, up the device's string. A recent study indicated that gram-negative and anaerobic gram-positive bacteria also are often involved. Because these are strongly associated with ENDOMETRITIS, it is recommended that all women with PID be treated with medications that include the broad-spectrum antibiotic metronidazole. Occasionally, although quite rarely, the disease is caused by tubercle bacilli (which cause tuberculosis) that have spread into the pelvis or by some tropical infectious organism.

Once the diagnosis has been made, treatment with broad-spectrum oral antibiotics usually is begun at once and continued for about two weeks. In a severe acute case the patient may be hospitalized and antibiotics given intravenously. At home, bed rest is generally recommended, at least until the temperature returns to normal, to help prevent jarring of the uterus and tubes, which may increase inflammation and slow down healing. Certainly all vigorous activities, especially any that jostle the pelvis, such as sexual intercourse, should be avoided. Heat often is beneficial in the form of a hot bath, lasting 15 to 20 minutes, taken four times a day. If the condition improves within two weeks, treatment usually is continued for another week to ward off a recurrence. If there is no improvement or the condition worsens, a new antibiotic probably will be tried. If three different courses of treatment fail to effect improvement, the disease may be termed a case of *chronic* PID (provided the original diagnosis was correct).

Chronic pelvic inflammatory disease is a low-grade infection that may persist from several weeks to many months. Symptoms may include more or less constant abdominal pain or discomfort, weakness, fatigue and very heavy menstrual periods, often with severe cramps. A mild case, however, may give rise to few or no noticeable symptoms. Nevertheless, persistent pelvic discomfort should be checked, because even a subclinical (almost symptom-free) infection can give rise to the most common aftermath of pelvic inflammatory disease: partial or total INFERTILITY. The disease, even in a mild form, can permanently scar the delicate tissues of the fallopian tubes, so that bands of scar tissue (*adhesions*) distort the shape of the tubes or seal their open ends (near the ovaries). As a result eggs are blocked from passing into and through the tubes, and fertilization cannot take place. Also, partial obstruction of a tube can lead to an ECTOPIC PREGNANCY, because the fertilized egg, unable to pass down into the uterus, instead becomes implanted in the tube or elsewhere. Finally, the presence of scar tissue increases the risk of recurrent infection and, depending on its location and abundance, can cause severe pain during sexual intercourse and during menstrual periods. Early treatment, however, minimizes these complications.

Chronic pelvic inflammatory disease that does not respond to bed rest and oral antibiotics is treated in a number of ways. Hospitalization and intravenous antibiotics may be tried first. Sometimes the patient may decide to live with the disease and its potential risks. Some women have found relief through a variety of HERBAL REMEDIES, usually in conjunction with antibiotics. Among these are heat treatment with a poultice of fresh ginger root or yucca plaster, made from coarsely grated yucca (a tuber; if not available, substitute red-skinned Irish potato). Herbal teas used include one made from goldenseal root (*Hydrastis canadensis*) and myrrh (*Commiphora myrrha*), and another from red raspberry leaf (*Rubus idaeus*), ginseng (*Panax quinquefolium*) and cinnamon bark (*Cinnamonum zeylanicum*).

For severe, crippling chronic infection that responds to no other treatment, surgery may be the only resort. One conservative surgical procedure that may help involves releasing some of the adhesions. Sometimes, however, only removal of the infected organs—one or both tubes, the uterus and sometimes one or both ovaries—will eradicate the disease.

Prevention and early treatment of pelvic inflammatory disease are much simpler than a cure. One of the easiest preventive measures is always wiping from front to back after a bowel movement, to prevent rectal bacteria from entering the vagina. After abortion, D and C, miscarriage or childbirth, the cervix remains somewhat dilated and more open to infection for several weeks. During this time women should avoid inserting anything into the vagina—fingers, tampon, diaphragm, penis. Also, showers are probably safer than tub baths during this period. Women susceptible to infection—especially to vaginal infections—should use a form of birth control other than an IUD. Women who do use IUDs should pay prompt attention to any symptoms of pelvic infection and have a routine check of their IUD once a year. Women who may have been exposed to gonorrhea should have a gonorrhea culture at once because 80% of those infected will have no symptoms of the disease; the symptoms of gonorrheal pelvic inflammatory disease usually appear a week to 10 days after exposure. Even if the gonococci that have invaded the pelvis are killed or die off, they may be followed by other infection-causing bacteria. Condoms, spermicide and diaphragms all discourage the transmission of gonorrhea but should not be considered protection against it. Further, although women rarely pass on gonorrhea to one another, it is not impossible, so sexually active lesbians also should have routine gonorrhea cultures.

pelvic pain Discomfort, ranging from mild and intermittent to severe and unremitting pain, in the general area of the genital tract (ovaries, uterus, vagina). The pain may be felt principally in the lower back or, more often, in the lower abdomen. The site usually depends on the cause, but sometimes the discomfort is very generalized (widespread).

Sudden severe pain in the lower abdominal area may be caused by acute PELVIC INFLAMMATORY DISEASE (especially if an abscess forms), ECTOPIC PREGNANCY, the twisting on its stem of either an ovarian cyst (see CYST, def. 6) or a uterine FIBROID, or ovula-

tion (see MITTELSCHMERZ). Any sudden severe pain in the pelvic area should be considered a medical emergency and warrants prompt attention, especially if it is accompanied by nausea, vomiting, rapid pulse, pallor and faintness. Sensations of painful pressure in the vaginal, urinary or rectal areas may be caused by pelvic relaxation, that is, prolapse of the uterus, urethra, bladder or rectum (see CYSTOCELE; PROLAPSED UTERUS; RECTOCELE; URETHROCELE) or by a pelvic tumor. Deep abdominal or vaginal pain felt during vaginal intercourse (DYSPAREUNIA) may come after surgery resulting in a shortened vagina (such as vaginal HYSTERECTOMY) or may be a symptom of either pelvic inflammatory disease or ENDOMETRIOSIS. Endometriosis causes pain and tenderness in various places, depending on where the endometrial tissue is growing, but characteristically it is most apparent in the days just before menstruation and in the early days of menstrual flow. Painful menstruation (see DYSMENORRHEA, def. 4) may begin just before or during menstrual periods and may persist for a few hours or throughout the entire period; it may focus in the abdominal area, the lower back or both. Another source of pelvic pain is ENDOMETRITIS.

Not all pelvic pain is caused by disorders of the reproductive organs. Nongenital sources of pain usually involve the urinary tract (kidney, ureters, bladder), the gastrointestinal tract or the skeletal system and supporting tissues. Pelvic pain thus may be caused by cystitis, a renal calculus (kidney stone), diverticulitis (inflammation of the large bowel), appendicitis, cholecystitis (gallbladder disease), colitis (inflammation of the large intestine), osteoarthritis or osteoporosis affecting the lower spine, a ruptured disk, poor posture, scoliosis or a bone tumor. Another possible source of pelvic pain is a small bundle of nerves at the base of the spinal cord, called *superior hypogastric plexus*. It relays pain sensations from the pelvic cavity to the brain. With chronic stimulation of the nerves, the pathway may be reversed, with pain signals traveling from brain to pelvis. In time, normally healthy pelvic areas then become sources of pain, or trigger points, which in turn may tense pelvic floor muscles and cause spasms, called *pelvic floor tension myalgia*.

In some cases virtually all sources of pelvic pain—both genital and nongenital—are ruled out

Side View of Female Pelvic Organs

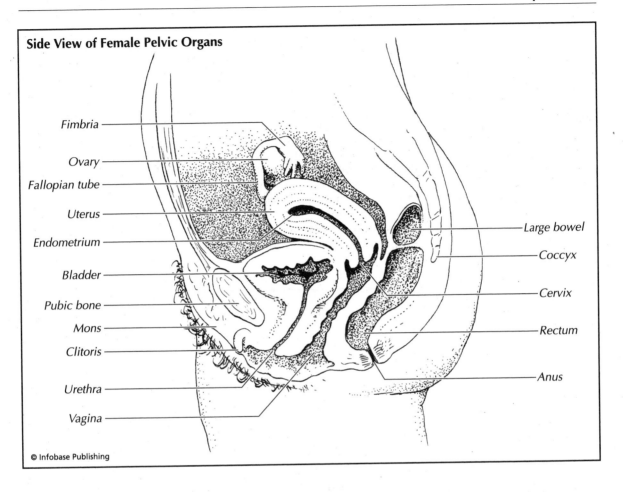

Fimbria

Ovary

Fallopian tube

Uterus

Endometrium

Bladder

Pubic bone

Mons

Clitoris

Urethra

Vagina

Large bowel

Coccyx

Cervix

Rectum

Anus

© Infobase Publishing

and no organic disorder can be found. Some clinicians may then suggest that the pain is psychogenic in origin and advise the patient to seek counseling or some form of psychotherapy. Combination therapy, including anti-inflammatory medications such as ibuprofen, oral contraceptives, low doses of tricyclic antidepressants, muscle relaxants, anticonvulsive medications, acupuncture, physical therapy and nutritional and psychological counseling, may be helpful. Special pain units established at some hospitals have been successfully dealing with CHRONIC PAIN by such means as physical therapy, heat, massage, low-voltage electrical stimulation and biofeedback. Trigger point therapy involves injecting the anesthetic lidocaine into tender pelvic or abdominal muscles; it often provides immediate relief but may have to be done periodically. In cases where the condition stems from nerve pain, nerve blocks may be achieved by injecting an alcohol solution to destroy pain-causing nerve fibers. Surgical options include removal of scar tissue and cutting certain nerves in the lower back, or implanting a pacemaker-type device that stimulates the nerves with electrical current. For pain that continues to be chronic and severe, a clinician may suggest surgery to remove one or more (or all) of the pelvic organs. However, if the cause of pain cannot be identified, it hardly seems reasonable to suppose that radical surgery will succeed in eliminating it, and it often does not.

pelvis The bony girdle located at the bottom of the spinal column just above the bones of the thighs. It encloses the *pelvic cavity*, the lowermost portion of the abdominal cavity, which contains the internal reproductive organs (uterus, fallopian tubes, ovaries) as well as the bladder and rectum.

penis   Also *phallus; dick, cock* (slang). The male organ of urination and copulation (sexual intercourse). It is made up of three sections of spongy erectile tissue. Two of them lie side by side, forming the upper part of the *shaft* of the penis; near the top they separate and anchor the penis to the underlying pubic bones. The central section runs between the other two and then forms the lower part of the shaft; it contains the urethra. At the tip it widens to form the *glans*, the dome-shaped, highly sensitive end of the penis. The outside of the penis is covered with loose skin that is attached to the circumference of the glans, or *corona*. A fold of this skin, called the *prepuce* or *foreskin*, loosely covers the glans. It is this fold only that is removed in CIRCUMCISION. Uncircumcised men must regularly pull the prepuce back to clean the glans of *smegma*, a waxy secretion produced by glands under the prepuce. At the tip of the glans is the urethral opening, through which both urine and sperm are transported to the outside.

The average penis is 3½ to 4 inches (8½ to 10 centimeters) long when not erect. During sexual arousal the spongy sections of the penis, which are

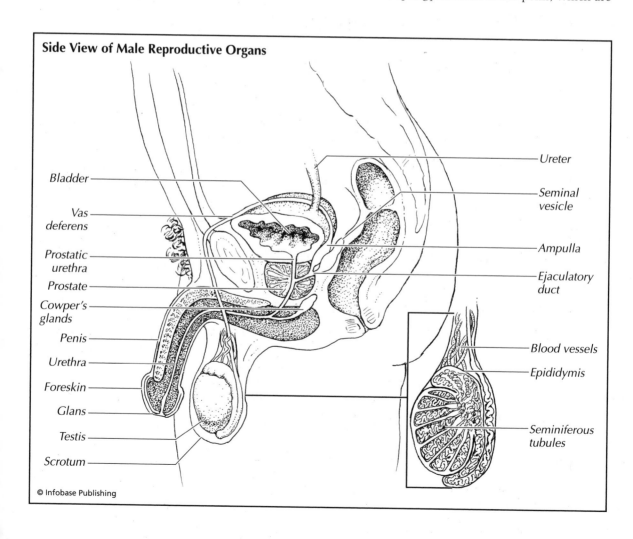

Side View of Male Reproductive Organs

Bladder

Vas deferens

Prostatic urethra

Prostate

Cowper's glands

Penis

Urethra

Foreskin

Glans

Testis

Scrotum

Ureter

Seminal vesicle

Ampulla

Ejaculatory duct

Blood vessels

Epididymis

Seminiferous tubules

© Infobase Publishing

rich in blood vessels, become engorged with blood, causing the penis, which normally hangs down, to become hard, erect (upright) and enlarged, on the average 6 to 7½ inches (15 to 19 centimeters) long and about 1½ inches (4 centimeters) wide. This phenomenon, called *erection,* enables the penis to be inserted into the female vagina. When the peak of sexual excitement and release, or ORGASM, is reached, the sperm and other secretions, together called *semen* or *seminal fluid,* are ejaculated through the urethral opening.

SPERM, which begin to be manufactured at puberty by the two testes in tiny adjacent tubes (the *seminiferous tubules*), pass up from each testis to a coiled tube behind it called the *epididymis.* From there they pass up through a second tube on each side, the *vas deferens,* each about 18 inches (45 centimeters) long. The vasa deferentia run from the groin up to the bladder, behind which each vas widens into an *ampulla,* where the sperm are stored. Muscular contractions of the vasa deferentia push the sperm up to the ampulla. On the outer side of each ampulla lies a 2-inch-long gland called the *seminal vesicle,* which produces secretions important to the survival of the sperm. The duct of the seminal vesicle joins that of the ampulla to form the *ejaculatory duct.* It is here that gland secretions and sperm are mixed together into seminal fluid just before ejaculation occurs. The ejaculatory ducts from each side join the urethra within the *prostate gland.* This gland, made up of gland and muscle tissue and located under the bladder, also produces an alkaline fluid that helps the sperm to propel themselves. The urethra runs from the bladder through the prostate, whose secretions enter it through many tiny ducts and mix with the sperm only seconds before ejaculation. One other structure, *Cowper's glands,* which join the urethra as it leaves the prostate, contributes lubricating fluid during sexual arousal.

A common problem in men from about age 55 on is enlargement of the prostate, which often is benign but sometimes is cancerous. Because it can be severe enough to block the flow of urine, sometimes suddenly and completely, standard treatment long was surgery (usually a transurethral resection of the prostate), which cured the problem but often left the man impotent. Recent research has shown

that a particular hormone, dihydrotestosterone, stimulates prostate growth, and current efforts are directed at finding a medication that blocks its formation. At the same time, surgeons worked to develop different techniques and operations that would preserve sexual function, even in men whose tumors were cancerous. While their success rate is not yet 100% (and may never be), there has been definite improvement in the outcome of many cases. An alternative to surgery is radiation therapy, which often yields good results. Prostate cancer, which frequently progresses very slowly, occurs mostly after the age of 50 and the risk increases with each decade of life.

peptides Hormonal proteins that currently are being manufactured in synthetic form for a variety of uses in both men and women. The first peptide to undergo intensive study was an analog of gonadotropin-releasing hormone (see GNRH).

percutaneous umbilical blood sampling Also *PUBS, funipuncture.* A method of prenatal testing for birth defects by testing the fetus's blood. Guided by ultrasound, a needle is guided through the mother's abdomen and uterus into the umbilical vein, and the blood withdrawn is tested for most of the same conditions detected by AMNIOCENTESIS, but results are available in as little as 24 hours. However, the technique is considered riskier and therefore should not be substituted unless absolutely necessary. The test is performed between 18 and 36 weeks of pregnancy.

perforated uterus See D AND C.

Pergonal Brand name for HUMAN MENOPAUSAL GONADOTROPIN.

perimenopause The two to six years or so preceding the end of menstruation (see MENOPAUSE), characterized by the beginning of irregular menstrual periods and such symptoms as mood swings, loss of concentration and HOT FLASHES. Estrogen levels begin to drop from about age 35, and it is hormonal imbalance that accounts for irregular periods. Irregularities themselves are normal, but certain symptoms can signal the possibility of serious disease. Extremely heavy bleeding (faster and heavier flow than a heavy period, often with clots), bleeding at intervals shorter than 21 days, lengthy staining outside menstrual periods (for three to four weeks) and bleeding after there have been no periods for 12 months all warrant a prompt gynecologic examination to rule out fibroids, polyps, cancer or some other lesion. In addition to menstrual irregularities, hot flashes are the symptom most closely associated with perimenopause. They are experienced to some degree—ranging from very slight and infrequent to very severe and frequent—by about three-fourths of women and can persist for years. Particularly annoying at night (so-called night sweats), they are believed to result from a disturbance of the HYPOTHALAMUS, which regulates body temperature, caused either by lower estrogen levels or by higher follicle-stimulating hormone (FSH) levels. The exact mechanism is still not understood, but hot flashes can be relieved by estrogen, indicating that their cause is hormone imbalance. Just when ESTROGEN REPLACEMENT THERAPY should begin, if at all, is controversial. Taking estrogen before menopause might cause ovulation and irregular bleeding.

Besides the menstrual irregularity and hot flashes directly attributable to changing hormone levels, perimenopause is associated with other symptoms, some of them by-products of hormone imbalance and others the result of general aging. As ovarian function declines, the proportion of muscle to fat decreases, and gradual thickening around waist and abdomen are common. Some women experience symptoms identical to those of premenstrual tension (DYSMENORRHEA, def. 5), with edema, headache, abdominal bloating, constipation and breast changes; they probably are due to the secretion of estrogen in the absence of progesterone. Others are afflicted with dizziness and/or PALPITATIONS, thought to be caused by disturbances of the vasomotor system, similar to those that cause hot flashes. In still others, frequent hot flashes and night sweats give rise to nervousness and irrita-

bility as well as profound fatigue, brought on by constantly interrupted sleep. For severe discomfort, some authorities believe low-dosage oral contraceptives might be the answer, since they override the pituitary gland by supplying a regular dose of estrogen and a progestin to regulate the cycle.

Continued discomfort of this kind, as well as hormonal imbalance itself, can bring on mood changes not unlike those of puberty, including anxiety and depression. Moreover, the mixed feelings of an adolescent girl approaching womanhood and the accompanying new responsibilities have a counterpart in the middle-aged woman who may be experiencing other life changes and must face the prospect of aging, with its largely negative connotations in a society that equates attractiveness with youth. New drugs for depression, such as Prozac, have become popular because they have fewer side effects than older drugs; they begin to work only after several weeks of treatment.

There are less risky alternatives to alleviate symptoms and moodiness. Among those widely recommended are changes in diet. Reducing salt intake may help relieve edema (fluid retention) and other symptoms resembling premenstrual tension. Avoiding foods high in tyramine, a chemical that raises blood pressure and is present in red wine, chocolate, canned and dried fish, avocado, raisins, soy sauce, aged cheeses and certain other foods, as well as increasing the intake of naturally DIURETIC foods (cucumbers, celery, parsley) also may help. A well-balanced diet is always important, and the addition of certain vitamins appears to be particularly helpful during menopause. The B-complex vitamins combat stress (and B$_6$ particularly helps the premenstrual syndrome); brewer's yeast, whole grains and seeds are good natural sources. Some women have found that vitamin E relieves hot flashes (it is found in wheat germ, whole grains, vegetable oils, peanuts, navy beans and salmon, but women who have diabetes, rheumatic heart disease or high blood pressure are advised to *limit* their intake of vitamin E to 125 International Units per day or less. Vitamin C helps the absorption of vitamin E and may help prevent vaginal infection. The mineral CALCIUM, the need for which increases with age, helps combat osteoporosis; it is best taken from natural sources such as milk, yogurt and cheese and requires adequate intake of vitamin D, which assists calcium absorption. If menstrual flow is long and profuse, additional iron may be needed to prevent anemia. Since individual nutritional requirements vary greatly, vitamin supplements (in pill form) should be used with caution. Regular EXERCISE is important, and ideally it should include aerobic, muscle-building and flexibility-enhancing activities.

Women have long used various homeopathic and HERBAL REMEDIES to relieve menopausal symptoms. For the premenstrual tension symptoms, the same herbs used for congestive dysmenorrhea may give relief. Licorice root (*Glycyrrhiza lepidota*) contains a substance chemically similar to estrogen, and sarsaparilla (*Smilax officinalis*) contains one similar to progesterone; a tea brewed from these is used to relieve hot flashes. GINSENG root (*Panax quinquefolium*), long used in China, is used by some women for hot flashes, as is dong kwai (or tang kuei; *Angelica sinensis*), a Chinese herb that can be chewed, boiled into a tea or taken in powdered form. Long profuse periods have been treated with a tea made from either shepherd's purse (*Capsella bursa pastoris*) or bearberry (*Arctostaphylos uva-ursi*).

perinatology   The medical specialty of caring for sick babies before, during and after birth. With a HIGH-RISK PREGNANCY it is advisable for the mother to be near a medical center with a perinatologist, if at all possible.

perineal massage   Also *prenatal perineal massage.* A technique for slowly and gently stretching the skin and tissues around the vagina and perineum so as to ease the passage of a baby during childbirth and help reduce the risk of tearing and the need for EPISIOTOMY. Using a lubricant such as K-Y jelly or vegetable oil (or natural vaginal secretion), the woman places her thumbs 1 to 1½ inches inside her vagina, presses downward and outward at the same time, and gently but firmly keeps stretching until she feels a slight burning, tingling or stinging sensation. At that point she holds the pressure steady with her thumbs for about two minutes, until the area becomes a little numb and the tingling is less acute. Still pressing, she slowly and gently massages back and forth over the lower portion of the vagina, working the lubricant into the tissues for three to four minutes, and gently pulling outward (forward) to help stretch the skin. Performing this massage daily from about the 34th week of pregnancy is recommended. Increased flexibility and stretchiness should begin to be felt after a week or so. The massage also may be performed by the woman's partner, using either index fingers or thumbs. However, one must be careful to avoid the urethra (urinary opening). Further, massage must be *avoided* if the woman has active herpes lesions, lest they be spread to other areas.

perineum   Technically, the muscles and fascia (fibrous tissue) of the entire region underlying the urethral and vaginal openings and the anus as well as the pelvic floor. In common usage, however, the term is used for the area between the scrotum and anus in men, and in women for the section of fibrous tissue between the anus and vagina, which during childbirth may be stretched considerably and often tears. To prevent tearing, obstetricians may enlarge the vaginal opening surgically (see EPISIOTOMY). Some authorities believe that PERINEAL MASSAGE of the area between anus and vagina during late pregnancy decreases the risk of tearing and the need for episiotomy.

persistent sexual arousal syndrome   A rare condition in which a woman feels constant spontaneous and intense genital arousal, with or without orgasm or genital engorgement. It is not accompanied by feelings of sexual desire and is not relieved by orgasm, which sometimes cannot be reached. It was not diagnosed until 2002, probably because women were too embarrassed and ashamed to report it to their clinicians. The feelings of arousal are very strong and persist for extended periods of time—hours, days or weeks. Orgasm, if achieved, sometimes provides temporary relief but symptoms soon return. The condition is extremely disruptive, impairing concentration and causing great physical discomfort. To date no one cause has been identified. In some women it begins after brain or bladder surgery, or seizures; in others it is triggered by an antidepressant medication, Trazodone, which causes priapism, an equivalent condition in men. Treatment may involve psychological counseling, or medications such as antidepressants, antiandrogenic agents or anesthetizing gels.

pessary A hard rubber or plastic device that is inserted into the vagina to support a PROLAPSED UTERUS and weakened vaginal walls. It should be checked a few days after being inserted to ensure that it is not damaging vaginal tissue or causing urinary problems. It must be removed regularly for meticulous cleaning, either by the clinician every six to eight weeks or by the woman herself. It has several other drawbacks as well: It may cause an irritating and smelly discharge, which then requires regular douching and the use of vaginal creams; it can abrade the delicate tissues inside the vagina; and it can interfere with vaginal intercourse, shortening the vagina and thus limiting penetration. (Some of these drawbacks are lessened if the woman removes the pessary every night, both to avoid irritation and make intercourse easier.) For these reasons it is used mainly in women for whom surgery to repair a prolapsed uterus represents too great a risk. Occasionally a pessary is used to keep a repositioned RETROVERTED UTERUS in place. Pessaries have been in use since the 19th century. By 1868 some 120 different kinds were available in the United States, of various sizes and shapes, ranging from a simple plug to a complicated device that had to be worn under a large hoop skirt.

PET scan Common name for *positron emission tomography*, a kind of diagnostic radioactive imaging used to detect abnormal function in various organs. In the case of heart and cardiovascular disorders, a substance needed for heart function, such as sugar, is labeled with a radioactive substance that gives off positrons and is injected into a vein so that it quickly reaches the heart. PET then determines how much blood is reaching different parts of the heart muscle. PET scans sometimes are helpful in determining whether a breast cancer has spread to the lymph nodes, and also in monitoring response to chemotherapy.

Pfannenstiel incision A horizontal incision into the lower abdomen, about 5 inches (12½ centimeters) long, over the pubis, near the top of the pubic hair, which is used for hysterectomy, Cesarean section or abdominal tubal ligation. It leaves a less noticeable scar than the midline vertical incision formerly used exclusively.

phallus See PENIS.

phenylketonuria Also *PKU*. A hereditary disorder thought to result from lack of a gene needed to produce an enzyme that converts the amino acid phenylalanine to a similar acid, tyrosine. As a result of this chemical block, phenylalanine is converted to phenylpyruvic acid, which builds up in the body fluids and, frequently, causes severe mental retardation. PKU occurs in 1 of every 10,000 births and is detectable by means of a simple urine and blood test as soon as a baby begins digesting food. It also can be detected prenatally through CHORIONIC VILLUS SAMPLING. Practically all babies born in American and Canadian hospitals today are tested routinely for PKU. If treated at once, with a diet low in phenylalanine until the child is five years old, retardation is prevented. Moreover, some authorities maintain that treatment must be continued for life, since a number of studies report subsequent mental and behavior problems if therapy is terminated at this age. In any event, the child still carries the inborn defect responsible for the condition and hence can transmit it to his or her children. Also, there now is growing concern about women with PKU whose treatment ended at age five or six and who are now experiencing a very high rate of miscarriage or delivering babies with numerous defects, including mental retardation. Many of these women did not know (or remember) that they had PKU early in life and recognize the consequent hazards to their children. The problem is a new one, since until the early 1960s newborns were not tested or treated for PKU and consequently most PKU women were severely retarded and rarely bore children. Among the solutions under consideration is establishing routine premarital blood tests for PKU and, if a pregnancy is planned by a PKU woman, returning immediately to a low-phenylalanine diet, even before conception, to prevent buildup of phenylpyruvic acid that would be transmitted to the baby via the placenta. Experience with such a solution is too limited at this writing to draw any conclusions.

In 2007 the FDA approved the first drug to treat phenylketonuria, which is thought to be effective in 20 to 50% of patients. Called Kuvan and known generically as sapropterin dihydrochloride, it reduced levels of phenylalanine by about 30%. Patients need to try the drug for a month or two before abandoning their special diet, since there is no way to predict whether it will be effective.

phlebitis   Also *venous thrombosis, thromboembolic disease, thrombophlebitis.* An acute inflammation of the veins—most often the deep veins—characterized by the formation of small blood clots, or thrombi (see THROMBUS), in them. Depending on the severity of the inflammation, there may be no symptoms or there may be tenderness, pain, swelling, warmth and redness of the overlying skin and/or prominence of the superficial veins in the area involved. Phlebitis most often affects leg veins and pelvic veins. Pain usually is felt when standing and walking but is relieved by sitting or lying down with the affected leg elevated. Even when there are no symptoms, if phlebitis is suspected it is important that it be diagnosed correctly, particularly if deep veins are involved. Usually a *venogram* is made, which involves injecting a dye into the veins and then taking an X-ray. Although the disease may be self-limiting, simply subsiding in a few weeks, there is danger that one of the clots formed might move to the lungs and create a potentially fatal blockage (a pulmonary EMBOLISM). Phlebitis in the pelvic veins is a possible complication of pregnancy and childbirth, gynecologic or urinary tract surgery and serious pelvic infections (pelvic inflammatory disease, puerperal fever). Treatment consists of bed rest with the legs elevated, anticoagulant drugs (which help prevent clot formation) and, after release from bed, the use of elastic supports and frequent leg elevation (no prolonged

standing or sitting) in order to prevent edema (swelling due to fluid retention). Because estrogen is somehow associated with increased formation of blood clots, a woman who has (or has ever had) phlebitis should avoid medications containing estrogen, such as oral contraceptives and estrogen replacement therapy.

phlegmasia   Also *milk leg, white leg.* Inflammation of the femoral vein in one or both legs after childbirth (see also PHLEBITIS). The leg becomes swollen, tender and usually bluish white in color owing to constricted blood vessels. Formerly very common, especially after a difficult labor, phlegmasia today is relatively rare. Treatment consists of bed rest with the leg elevated, elastic supports, pain relievers and, if deep veins are affected, anticoagulants to prevent clot formation.

physical examination   Also *physical.* See under GYNECOLOGIC EXAMINATION.

pica   A craving for ingesting unusual substances that are not normally considered food. Traditionally associated with pregnancy, such cravings frequently are for lump laundry starch, flour, baking powder, baking soda, clay or chopped ice, and some authorities believe they may reflect genuine dietary deficiency, specifically of iron. Others believe that eating these substances, practiced more among the poor and the poorly educated, reflects a folk tradition or social custom rather than true need. Eating clay—even iron-rich red clay—is not beneficial because clay forms a filter in the digestive system that actually blocks iron absorption, causing severe ANEMIA. Whatever its source, the practice can damage both mother and baby. Another form of pica is the consumption of paper and other inedible materials by young children; eating paint chips can lead to lead poisoning and irreversible brain damage.

PID   Abbreviation for PELVIC INFLAMMATORY DISEASE.

pigmentation   See CHLOASMA; LIVER SPOTS; MELA-NOMA; SKIN CHANGES.

piles   See HEMORRHOIDS.

Pill, the   See ORAL CONTRACEPTIVE.

pineal body   Also *pineal gland.* A tiny, egg-shaped body located in the midline of the brain that secretes at least one hormone, *melatonin,* which is believed to inhibit (suppress) the function of the sex glands (testes, ovaries). Its relation to the reproductive system was first described in 1896 by a German physician who found a tumor of the pineal gland in a small boy with PRECOCIOUS PUBERTY. Melatonin was not isolated until 1950, from a cow, and its action in human beings still is not totally understood. However, in animals it is known to be affected by prolonged light or dark-ness, which in turn affects reproductive activity, and therefore it is believed to act as some kind of regulator between environmental stimuli, such as light, and the reproductive system. Experimental use of prolonged light at night in order to suppress the vasomotor instability causing HOT FLASHES in menopause suggests that the pineal may exert an effect on the hypothalamus, which controls body temperature. Exposure to sunlight for prolonged periods, as in countries near the North Pole dur-ing June and July, inhibits melatonin production and may increase fertility and combat DEPRESSION (def. 3).

piriformis syndrome   A condition in which the piriformis muscle in the buttock irritates the sciatic nerve. It may involve pain in the buttocks, lower back and down the back of the thigh, in other words, along the entire course of the sciatic nerve. Piriformis syndrome is much more common in women than men, and is more likely to occur in the 15% of individuals whose sciatic nerve goes through the piriformis muscle rather than passing under it. Diagnosis is based on the symptoms and a physical examination of the back, hip and legs.

Hip motion tends to produce the pain. Treatment involves stretching exercises. Also, applying ice or heat to the mid-buttock and using anti-inflamma-tory medication (an NSAID) may be helpful. Physi-cal therapy may be recommended; in stubborn cases a local anesthetic and steroid may be injected into the area. To prevent the condition, which can be caused by any sport that tightens the hamstrings and buttock muscles, it is important to do appropri-ate stretching exercises.

To help relieve the condition, a particular stretch-ing exercise is recommended. Sitting on the floor, cross the leg on the affected side over the other leg, placing the foot alongside the knee. Using the opposite hand, pull the upright knee across the midline of the body, and hold for 10 to 30 seconds. The stretch should be felt in the affected buttock and outer thigh.

Pitocin   Also *pit* (slang). A brand name for synthetic OXYTOCIN, used to strengthen uterine contractions.

pituitary gland   Also *hypophysis.* One of the ENDO-CRINE glands, located below the base of the brain, to which it is attached by a stalk. An oval structure about 1½ centimeters (½ inch) long and less than 1½ centimeters wide, it consists of two parts. The *adenohypophysis* or *anterior pituitary,* which consti-tutes three-fourths of the total gland, produces protein hormones that are tropic hormones—that is, they regulate the growth and hormone pro-duction of other endocrine glands—as well as hormones that directly influence body growth, metabolism and lactation. The anterior pituitary was once believed to be the "master gland" of the endocrine system, until it was discovered that most of its functions in turn are controlled by the hypo-thalamus. The principal hormones it produces are somatotropin, or growth hormone, corticotropin, FSH, LH, thyrotropin, PROLACTIN and melanocyte-stimulating hormone; their functions are described in the accompanying chart. The *neurohypophysis* or *posterior pituitary* is the storage site of two important hypothalamic hormones: OXYTOCIN, which stimu-lates milk let-down and uterine contractions, and

PITUITARY HORMONES

Hormone	Function	Regulated by
Somatotropic hormone (STH) (Growth hormone)	Causes protein synthesis, growth of epiphyseal cartilage, mobilization of fat; opposes insulin	Increased by amino acids, lowered blood sugar
Adrenocorticotropic hormone (ACTH) (Corticotropin)	Stimulates adrenal growth and secretion of cortisol	Increased by lower cortisol levels, stress; decreased by higher cortisol levels
Follicle-stimulating hormone (FSH)	Stimulates growth of ovarian follicles; causes sperm formation	Decreased by higher estrogen levels
Luteinizing hormone (LH)	Causes follicle growth, stimulates estrogen production, causes ovulation; stimulates testosterone production	Stimulated by low doses of estrogen and progesterone; decreased by high steroid levels
Prolactin	Causes lactation and breast growth; inhibits FSH and LH production	Released by suckling, brain stimulation
Melanocyte-stimulating hormone	Stimulates melanocytes and skin pigmentation	Increased by absence of cortisol (in Addison's disease)
Thyroid-stimulating hormone (TSH) (Thyrotropin)	Stimulates growth of thyroid and production of thyroxin	Increased by low thyroxin, decreased by high thyroxin

vasopressin, which affects the blood vessels, uterus and kidneys (see HYPOTHALAMUS). Sometimes the pituitary gland must be excised to treat breast or other cancers. See HYPOPHYSECTOMY.

Problems caused by the failure of the pituitary gland to produce adequate amounts of certain hormones sometimes can be treated by administering the needed hormone. For example, inadequate production of growth hormone can result in extremely short stature. For some years growth hormone was extracted from pituitary glands obtained at autopsies, but the supply was much smaller than the need. Today, however, synthetic human growth hormone has been produced using genetically engineered bacteria. This synthetic hormone can be administered to abnormally short children to trigger a growth spurt.

PKU See PHENYLKETONURIA.

placebo Treatment that is not directly related to relieving the condition for which it is given. Placebos often are used in research to determine whether a medication being tested actually is effective. In a *double-blind* study, neither the clinicians nor the patients (researchers nor subjects) know who is getting a medication and who is being given a placebo; often the placebo is a pill that looks real but contains sugar or some other harmless substance. Clinicians also use placebos in general practice in order to obtain the *placebo effect*, that is, improvement that results from any therapeutic intervention (some patients get better simply because they believe a particular treatment or doctor will help them). A placebo most often takes the form of medication (powder, pill, capsule, liquid), but strictly speaking the term can be used for any treatment, including hypnosis, manipulation, surgery or simply the presence and attitude of a clinician. Studies have shown that placebos not only can cure conditions but, like drugs, can cause side effects such as nausea, diarrhea or a rash. How and why placebos work is not yet known. Among the theories proposed are that a placebo reduces stress, allowing the body to heal itself; that special molecules act in the brain to carry out response to a placebo; and that placebos work because the brain is organized to act on what is expected to happen next (that is, improvement). This last hypothesis, called *expectancy theory*, is currently being studied by neuropsychologists.

placenta Also *afterbirth*. A highly specialized organ that connects a fetus to its mother and enables the exchange of soluble, bloodborne nutrients and secretions, including oxygen. The placenta usually lies at the top of the uterus and is connected to the fetus by the UMBILICAL CORD. Part of it, called the *fetal placenta*, develops from the CHORION, the outermost membrane that covers the fertilized egg and nourishes it until the placenta is fully developed. The rest of it, called the *maternal placenta*, develops from the part of the endometrium, or uterine lining, to which the fertilized egg is attached (see IMPLANTATION). The development of the placenta is stimulated by the hormone progesterone, which is secreted by the CORPUS LUTEUM. After the placenta has developed, it secretes estrogen and progesterone, which are needed to sustain the pregnancy.

In addition to estrogen and progesterone, the placenta produces at least two other hormones, HUMAN CHORIONIC GONADOTROPIN (HCG) and chorionic somatomammotropin, associated with fetal growth. Estrogen promotes the growth of the uterine muscles and blood vessels that supply oxygen to those muscles; progesterone delays uterine contractions, so that the baby is not pushed out prematurely. In addition to its hormonal and nutritional functions, the placenta also serves as a barrier to some infections (but not to some viruses or to typhoid fever and syphilis).

Without an intact, functioning placenta, a fetus cannot survive. In ABRUPTIO PLACENTAE and PLACENTA PREVIA, in which the placenta becomes detached from the endometrium, the fetus's oxygen and food supply are threatened. Once the placenta has separated completely, no oxygen can be transferred through it. Toxic wastes build up in the baby's tissues, and its brain, which can survive only eight minutes of oxygen deprivation, begins to suffer irreversible damage.

At term, after nine months' gestation, the human placenta is a disk-shaped mass measuring about 15 to 20 centimeters (8 inches) in diameter and 2 to 3 centimeters (1 inch) in thickness. It weighs about 500 grams (1.1 pounds) and is located in the upper two-thirds of the uterus. The fetal side is covered by a transparent membrane (the amnion). Fetal blood flows to the placenta through the two umbilical arteries, which carry deoxygenated (venous) blood. Maternal blood with a significantly higher oxygen content returns to the fetus from the placenta through the single umbilical vein.

During childbirth the placenta becomes detached in the course of labor and is expelled after the delivery of the baby, still attached to it by the umbilical cord. Contractions of the uterine muscles close the openings of the uterine blood vessels where it is torn from the endometrium; this is why the uterus must continue to contract after delivery and, if it does not, hemorrhage may occur. The delivery of the placenta is called the third stage of LABOR. Occasionally it is not completely detached during labor and must be removed, either manually, by pushing down on the mother's abdomen near the top of the uterus to help expel it, or with instruments. The clinician, midwife or other birth attendant should always examine the placenta after delivery to make sure it is intact; retention of part of the placenta can cause hemorrhage in the mother.

For *placental insufficiency,* see POSTMATURE.

placenta previa Location of the PLACENTA over or near the internal cervical os (opening), that is, where the cervix widens into the body of the uterus, instead of near the top of the uterus. Placenta previa is, along with ABRUPTIO PLACENTAE, one of the two main causes of hemorrhage in the latter part of pregnancy. The placenta may cover the os completely (*total previa*) or partly (*partial previa*), or it may simply encroach on it (*low-lying* or *marginal placenta previa*), so that dilation of the cervix during labor may cause it to be detached. The degree of placenta previa depends in part on how much the cervix is dilated. A low-lying placenta previa at 2 centimeters of dilation can become a partial placenta previa at 8 centimeters, simply because the wider opening of the cervix uncovers more of the placenta. In both total and partial placenta previa, the placenta partly separates from the uterine wall and consequently disrupts the blood vessels there; this is what causes hemorrhage. With a low-lying placenta previa, separation does not occur until the cervix is dilated considerably—that is, well along in labor—so bleeding usually does not occur until that point.

Placenta previa is not very common—it occurs in about 1 of every 200 pregnancies. Both age and parity (number of previous children) play a role: Women over 35 and women with numerous children are three or four times more likely to develop placenta previa than younger women and women who have had no children. Also, once it has occurred, it is quite likely to recur in subsequent pregnancies.

The chief sign of placenta previa is painless bleeding (usually heavy but sometimes light) during the eighth month of pregnancy. The initial hemorrhage usually stops by itself and is rarely (if ever) fatal, but it may recur at any time. Sometimes, however, there is a continuous discharge of smaller amounts of blood. With low-lying placenta previa, the bleeding usually does not occur until the onset of labor and then may be light or very profuse.

Whenever there is bleeding late in pregnancy, placenta previa or abruptio placentae is suspected. Diagnosis is easiest by means of ULTRASOUND (def. 1). Manual examination (in either vagina or rectum) should *never* be performed except in a well-equipped operating room (prepared for Cesarean delivery and blood transfusion) because it may precipitate a life-threatening hemorrhage.

The major danger of placenta previa to the fetus is premature labor and birth before it is sufficiently developed. Consequently, the safest treatment for both mother and child is hospitalization. If ultrasound or X-ray shows that the baby is still too small for safe survival and the mother is not threatened by massive hemorrhage, most clinicians advise waiting as long as possible before delivery. If the baby is sufficiently large and developed there is no need to wait.

With total placenta previa delivery *must* be by Cesarean section, which also is indicated for any kind of placenta previa with massive bleeding or fetal distress. Cesarean section results in less blood loss because delivery is so much faster, and therefore it may be indicated even if the baby has died before delivery. However, for women who have had children previously, have a low-lying placenta and are already well into labor, with the cervix dilated to at least 4 centimeters—conditions that apply to about half of the cases—a simple vaginal delivery may be possible provided that bleeding is not too severe, delivery is imminent and the baby is in no distress.

plasma cell mastitis   See MAMMARY DUCT ECTASIA.

PMS   Abbreviation for *premenstrual syndrome*. See DYSMENORRHEA, def. 5.

polycystic ovary syndrome   Also *PCOS;* formerly, *Stein-Leventhal syndrome.* A condition in which both ovaries are studded with numerous small cysts, which actually are egg follicles from which the eggs cannot, for some reason, be extruded. The eggs therefore collect under the follicle capsules, making them look like small cysts. Women with this condition do not ovulate, since no eggs are released, and hence are infertile. They also menstruate irregularly or not at all, show mild or marked hirsutism (excess body and facial hair), and often are obese. The syndrome is suspected if these symptoms are present and both ovaries are enlarged.

The syndrome, originally named for Irving Stein and Michael Leventhal, the physicians who first described it in 1935, is believed to affect as many as 10% of women. It is caused by a hormone imbalance, specifically an excess of male hormones. This accounts for such cosmetic symptoms as acne that does not respond well to treatment, dark and coarse facial hair, hair on abdomen and chest and male-pattern balding. The ovaries continue to produce estrogen and LH (luteinizing hormone) but, in the absence of ovulation, they produce almost no progesterone; hence the endometrium (uterine lining) continues to grow, creating an increased risk of endometrial cancer. The condition is also associated with high levels of cholesterol and triglycerides, creating increased risk of heart disease and stroke, and high levels of insulin, which can be a forerunner of Type II diabetes.

Owing to these symptoms, diagnosis should involve a full work-up by an endocrinologist familiar with hormone disturbances. It should involve blood tests for LH, prolactin, thyroid-stimulating hormone, progesterone, testosterone, blood lipids (cholesterol and triglycerides), a blood glucose tolerance test and, sometimes, ultrasound to view the ovaries. The syndrome's cause is not known but it does tend to run in families, so upon diagnosis it may be wise to test other family members.

Treatment depends on the severity of symptoms and the woman's goals. Diet and weight loss are the first approach, and sometimes reverse the symptoms. A diet low in carbohydrates helps reduce the level of insulin the body produces to process glucose. Oral contraceptives can regulate periods, whereas infertility is often treated with clomiphene citrate (Clomid or Serophene) to induce ovulation. For women who don't want to take birth control pills but are concerned about the risk for endometrial cancer in the absence of menstruation, a progesterone drug such as Prometrium taken every few months will induce a period. For those who are insulin-resistant, insulin sensitizers such as metformin (Glucophage), pioglitazone (Actos) and rosiglitazone (Avandia) may be helpful, although the last is associated with increased risk of heart failure. Spironolactone (Aldactone) blocks male hormones and may help hirsutism, as does the topical cream Vaniqa, which slows down hair growth. If these drugs are not effective, a surgical procedure called *bilateral wedge resection,* in which a wedge of the affected tissue is cut from each ovary, can be performed. Done laparoscopically (through tiny abdominal incisions), it creates little scar tissue but does not restore fertility. Some women find help in support groups through chapters of the Polycystic Ovarian Syndrome Association (see Appendix).

polygalactia Excess secretion of breast milk. It usually occurs before breast-feeding is well established (immediately after birth), before the supply has been regulated by the infant's demand for milk, and during weaning, especially if there is some reason for weaning very quickly (rather than gradually reducing the number of feedings per day over a period of several weeks).

See also BREAST-FEEDING; LACTATION.

polyhydramnios Another name for HYDRAMNIOS.

polymenorrhea Frequent menstrual periods, with intervals of fewer than 20 days between menstrual flows. It usually signifies a hormone imbalance, that is, too much estrogen in the absence of progester-

one (or relative to progesterone), a condition found mostly in young girls who are not yet ovulating and in women approaching menopause (see ANOVULATORY BLEEDING). It also may be caused by a uterine FIBROID. For young girls threatened with anemia from too frequent periods, progesterone alone or sometimes an oral contraceptive containing both estrogen and progesterone may establish a more normal cycle. In older women fibroids and other growths, benign or malignant, should be ruled out before giving any medication. Some women routinely menstruate every 19 or 20 days and, in the absence of anemia or other problems, such a short MENSTRUAL CYCLE is no cause for alarm or for treatment.

polymyalgia rheumatica Also *PMR.* A form of rheumatic disease that involves the tendons, muscles, ligaments and other tissues around the joints. Characterized by severe pain, aching and morning stiffness in the neck, shoulders, lower back and hips, it sometimes is the first sign of GIANT CELL ARTERITIS. The onset may be gradual or occur over just a few days, and the cause is unknown, but some researchers suspect a hereditary tendency toward the disease. Although occurring in both men and women of all races, it is twice as likely to occur in women and is more common in white women over the age of 60. It often occurs in association with GIANT CELL ARTERITIS. Polymyalgia may take months to diagnose because it resembles so many other disorders, such as rheumatoid arthritis, that affect muscles and joints. Diagnosis is based on a history, physical examination and laboratory tests. A strong indicator is a high erythrocyte sedimentation rate (ESR). Treatment consists of anti-inflammatory drugs, including corticosteroids, rest and mild exercise to relieve pain and stiffness. Untreated, the disease progresses, with fatigue, long-term low fever and significant weight loss. In some cases it eventually runs its course, typically lasting three to five years and then gradually disappearing. However, some patients may have lost vision in one or both eyes, owing to arterial inflammation affecting the optic nerve. Corticosteroid therapy, usually with prednisone, makes the symptoms disappear within a few days, but continuing the drug in low doses over a long period—18 months to three years or longer—is recommended, along with careful monitoring for side effects.

polyp   **1.** A soft, fleshy, easily crumbled, non-cancerous tumor, usually attached to normal tissue by a stem or pedicle. Common sites for such growths are the nasal passages, vocal cords (larynx), gastrointestinal tract and pelvis.

2. cervical polyp. A polyp that develops high up in the cervical canal, near the entrance to the body of the uterus. It may occur singly or multiply and is an overgrowth of normal tissue from the lining of the cervix or uterus. It may give rise to no symptoms at all, or it may cause bleeding between periods or staining in postmenopausal women. Very large polyps sometimes cause cramping as they push down through the cervical canal. Diagnosis is relatively easy, because such polyps usually protrude into the vagina and so can be seen on pelvic examination. Normally they can simply be removed under local anesthesia in the clinician's office or in a clinic or hospital on an outpatient basis, but occasionally a D AND C may be needed to remove them completely.

3. endometrial polyp. Also *intrauterine polyp, uterine polyp.* A polyp that develops inside the body of the uterus and can grow into and through the cervix. A long endometrial polyp may protrude all the way into the vagina. Like cervical polyps (see def. 2 above), it represents an overgrowth of normal endometrial tissue and may be either symptomless or cause bleeding between periods or after menopause, as well as cramping pain as it pushes down through the cervix. Also like cervical polyps, endometrial polyps may occur singly or in numbers. Most endometrial polyps occur before the age of 50 and their rate of appearance declines after menopause. Often they are symptomless, but they can cause vaginal bleeding, sometimes cause pain and can interfere with becoming pregnant. They usually are identified during a pelvic or transvaginal ultrasound, or by a more accurate technique, *hysterosonography,* in which saline is used to distend the uterus before an ultrasound probe is placed in the vagina. The vast majority of endometrial polyps are benign, but if they are troublesome or suspicious they should be removed. To remove them, a D and C or hysteros-

copy must be performed, and sometimes a second D and C is required to locate an additional polyp that was missed the first time. Occasionally, if polyps continue to recur and/or if they persistently cause postmenopausal bleeding, a hysterectomy is performed to eliminate them entirely.

See also ENDOMETRIAL HYPERPLASIA.

4. colorectal polyp. A growth of tissue from the intestinal or rectal wall that protrudes into the large intestine or rectum. It may be cancerous, precancerous or benign. Because there is considerable risk that even benign polyps may become cancerous, they should be removed. Because most polyps cause no symptoms, they usually are detected during flexible sigmoidoscopy. If polyps are found, the entire large intestine is further examined via colonoscopy, which allows both biopsy and removal, using a cutting instrument or electrified wire loop. After polyps are removed, colonoscopy is repeated a year later and then at other intervals.

See also CANCER, COLORECTAL.

positron emission tomography   See PET SCAN.

postcoital test   See SIMS-HUHNER TEST.

posterior presentation   Also *posterior position.* In childbirth, the position of the baby, head first but with its face up, toward the mother's belly (instead of her back) as it comes down the birth canal. It is the most common form of abnormal position, the norm being *anterior,* or face down. In about 94% of cases the baby eventually rotates by itself into the much easier anterior position, although often it may not do so until the head has reached the pelvic floor. Generally labor is somewhat prolonged with a posterior position, especially with a first baby, and frequently back discomfort is felt. If the baby does not rotate spontaneously and the clinician is unable to turn it manually or with forceps, a forceps delivery in posterior position may be necessary. Since the use of forceps nearly always requires enlarging the vaginal opening with a considerable EPISIOTOMY, it is preferable to turn the baby to an anterior position if at all possible.

postmature The condition of an infant born more than two weeks beyond full term, that is, 42 or more weeks following the last menstrual period. Approximately 4% of all pregnancies are prolonged for more than two weeks. The effects vary. In some cases the fetus continues to grow at a significant rate and suffers no harm. In others, its growth stops as the pregnancy continues, and the fetus may show evidence of starvation, with loss of soft tissue and low birth weight at the time of delivery. In such cases, in which the PLACENTA has become insufficient—that is, it functions inadequately in transporting nutrients and oxygen to the baby—the baby's needs may not be met and the pregnancy usually must be terminated, either by INDUCTION OF LABOR or by Cesarean section. *Placental insufficiency* is readily measured by the amount of estriol (an estrogen produced by the placenta) in the mother's urine or blood. A steady level of estriol, as determined by tests once or twice a week, shows that the placenta is continuing to function as before and there is no problem for the baby. If this test, combined with a weekly non-stress test (see FETAL MONITORING), attests to the baby's well-being, no action need be taken. If the results of either test are poor, induction of labor or a Cesarean section should be done immediately.

Most postmature infants lack lanugo (soft downy hair covering the shoulders of most newborns) and have long nails, abundant scalp hair, pale skin with some evidence of drying, and apparent increase of alertness. There may be little amniotic fluid, and it may be stained with MECONIUM.

The reasons for postmaturity are not understood except in those cases in which the infant is born severely damaged, when it is thought to be due to long-term malfunctioning of the placenta.

A recent study showed that infant and maternal risks begin to rise as early as at 40 weeks of gestation. Among them are increased rates of prolonged labor, Cesarean delivery, postpartum hemorrhage, cephalopelvic disproportion (infant's head too large for mother's pelvis) and abnormal fetal heart rate. These findings suggest that the definition of postterm pregnancy should be earlier than 42 weeks.

postmenopausal bleeding Any staining or bleeding that occurs in a woman aged 45 or older 12 or more months after her last menstrual period. Such bleeding should be investigated promptly, even if it consists of only a little staining or spotting, because it can be a sign of cancer or some other serious disorder. An endometrial biopsy may need to be performed to rule out endometrial cancer; sometimes a D and C will be required. Some menopausal women do resume menstrual periods after an interruption of 12 months or so, usually on a quite irregular basis, until they finally stop menstruating. Consequently some authorities define menopause as the cessation of menstrual periods for two years. Nevertheless, to be on the safe side, any bleeding after a full year's interruption calls for a prompt gynecologic checkup.

See also MENOPAUSE.

postnatal care See POSTPARTUM.

postpartum Pertaining to the period after childbirth, also called the PUERPERIUM or postnatal period. Routine hospital care during the first 48 hours after delivery involves taking the mother's pulse, temperature, blood pressure and respiratory rate every six hours. In most hospitals a woman may get up and use the bathroom within a few hours, depending on the mode of delivery (vaginal or Cesarean) and anesthesia (none, local, regional or general); in birth centers or at home it may be even sooner. A few women have trouble urinating after delivery, especially if the labor was difficult or forceps were used, and they may require catheterization intermittently until the bladder resumes normal function. BREAST ENGORGEMENT normally occurs within two days after delivery; for women who decide not to breast-feed, the engorgement may take several days to subside. Uterine contractions (AFTERPAINS) continue for some days and often are triggered by breast-feeding. Vaginal bleeding called LOCHIA, subsiding to a moderate discharge, usually persists for three to six weeks. Menstrual periods generally resume in seven to nine weeks in non-breast-feeding women but not for many months in nursing mothers (occasionally not until nursing is stopped).

After a Cesarean section the woman usually may get up within a day; a catheter is nearly always used for the first 24 to 48 hours, and possibly also intravenous feeding. Stitches or clips are usually removed after four days (unless they are the kind that resorb), and until then the incision site should be kept dry. There usually is pain at the incision site, relieved by administration of analgesics (sometimes narcotics like morphine). Intestinal gas pressing against the incision site also may cause pain, which may be relieved by walking or lying with the knees drawn up. Sometimes an enema is needed to help the gas escape.

If all goes well, most hospitals discharge a woman after two days (four days following Cesarean section). Thereafter she usually may resume a fairly normal life, but should allow for more rest, take warm sitz baths if hemorrhoids from pushing or the stitches from episiotomy are uncomfortable and drink extra fluids if she is breast-feeding. (Some doctors warn against tub baths, however, because of the danger of infection through the still-dilated cervix.) Most clinicians advise avoiding vaginal intercourse for three to four weeks, or until the woman feels comfortable, indicating that the uterus has healed; however, some women prefer to engage in it sooner and others to delay even longer. The biggest risks of having sex too soon are tears in the incisions (if any) or infections in the uterus caused by bacteria carried by sperm. In rare cases, a woman having sex within a week or so of giving birth may die of an air embolism (air bubbles in the major arteries to heart and brain). Apparently, soon after childbirth women are more vulnerable to this complication because air forced into the uterus during sex can enter the bloodstream through blood vessels damaged during delivery.

The *postpartum examination,* usually performed four to six weeks after delivery, involves weight, blood pressure and hemoglobin measurements, checking the breasts and a pelvic examination. This is the time for discussing current and future methods of birth control, perhaps being fitted for a diaphragm since size may change after childbirth, and discussing future pregnancies if any are being considered.

Persistent pain of any kind during the postpartum period, both before and after hospital discharge, a smelly vaginal discharge or a fever above 100.4 degrees Fahrenheit (38 degrees Celsius)

should be reported at once, since they may signal an infection. Other symptoms calling for prompt medical attention are nausea and vomiting, painful or urgent urination, pain or swelling in the legs, chest pain or cough, and hot, tender breasts. The principal medical complications following childbirth are bleeding and infection.

See also DEPRESSION (def. 2); POSTPARTUM HEMORRHAGE; PUERPERAL FEVER.

postpartum depression   See DEPRESSION, def. 2.

postpartum hemorrhage   Heavy bleeding during the postpartum period, that is, following childbirth. Such bleeding occurs most often when the uterus does not contract sufficiently after delivery of the PLACENTA. Other causes are failure to expel all of the placenta from the uterus; occasionally such retained pieces of placenta form growths similar to POLYPS in the uterine wall, causing menstrual irregularity, abdominal pain and heavy bleeding.

Unlike other kinds of massive bleeding, postpartum hemorrhage usually involves no sudden gush of blood but rather constant moderate bleeding over a period of hours. A blood loss of 500 milliliters or more during the first 24 hours after delivery is defined as a hemorrhage, since it is enough to be life-threatening at this stage. The principal danger to the mother occurs in situations where no blood transfusion is quickly available, as in a home birth.

To prevent hemorrhage, after delivery of the placenta the fundus (top of the uterus) should always be palpated to make sure it is well contracted. If it is not firm, it should be massaged firmly with the fingertips until it is. Many clinicians routinely inject ergonovine (a drug to induce or strengthen contractions) after every delivery; others prefer to use oxytocin but only when bleeding persists despite massage of the uterus. If bleeding continues, most authorities recommend beginning a transfusion immediately and employing *bimanual uterine compression* (with one hand inside the vagina and the other outside the abdomen, pressing the two hands together to compress the uterus). If bleeding still continues, the uterine cavity should be inspected for retained fragments of the placenta or severe lacerations; the former then may have to be removed, and the latter repaired.

post-Pill amenorrhea   Also *post-oral contraceptive amenorrhea*. Failure to resume menstrual periods within six months after stopping the use of ORAL CONTRACEPTIVES, in the absence of pregnancy or menopause. Sometimes accompanied by galactorrhea (inappropriate production of breast milk), it is generally a sign that the HYPOTHALAMUS is failing to produce gonadotropin-releasing hormone (GnRH), which would stimulate the pituitary to produce the FSH (follicle-stimulating hormone) and LH (luteinizing hormone) needed for a normal menstrual cycle, and prolactin-inhibiting factor (to stop lactation). Since the same symptoms can be caused by a tumor of the pituitary gland, this condition must first be ruled out. However, some studies hold that if ovulation is resumed within a year, there is no cause for concern.

Menstruation normally begins within three months after stopping the Pill, but a small number of women have post-Pill amenorrhea. It is most common in younger women who had irregular and anovulatory menstrual cycles before starting to take oral contraceptives, suggesting that the problem may have existed before pill use began. Treatment depends on the individual. In women who want to become pregnant as soon as possible, ovulation and menstruation often can be restored with hormone therapy: first progesterone to stimulate withdrawal bleeding; if not effective, combined estrogen and progesterone; after bleeding is established, clomiphene citrate to induce ovulation. If all these fail, the administration of synthetic pituitary gonadotropins may succeed. When there is no particular reason to restore menstruation quickly, the condition may be allowed to clear up of its own accord, which often happens in one or two years.

potency   See IMPOTENCE.

poultice   See HERBAL REMEDIES.

precancerous lesions   Growths or other changes in tissue that may, under certain conditions, become malignant (cancerous). In the uterine area such lesions can be eliminated totally by hysterectomy (removal of uterus and cervix), but so radical a procedure may not be necessary. CANCER IN SITU of the cervix and uterus, often with no symptoms other than mild staining between menstrual periods or after intercourse, is confined to the surface cells. An even earlier precancerous condition is DYSPLASIA of the uterus and cervix, which may disappear spontaneously but sometimes develops into cancer (see also ADENOCARCINOMA, def. 2). Authorities do not always agree as to whether a lesion is precancerous or not. In the case of ENDO-METRIAL HYPERPLASIA—thickening of the normally thin uterine lining—some clinicians believe that, in postmenopausal women, this condition readily develops into cancer and therefore recommend hysterectomy, whereas others prefer more conservative treatment, such as a D AND C.

See also LEUKOPLAKIA, VULVAR; PAGET'S DISEASE. def. 2.

precocious puberty   The occurrence of sexual development and menstrual bleeding in girls before the age of eight or nine (and sexual maturity in boys before the age of 10). It is at least twice (some say three to five times) as common in girls as in boys, and 80 to 90% of cases in girls are idiopathic, that is, no underlying cause can be found. However, a major study of American girls from 3 to 12 years old, published in 1997, revealed that by the age of 8, 15% of white girls and 48% of African-American girls had some breast development, pubic hair or both. These figures and more recent studies indicate American girls are maturing faster than previously. The cause is not known, but hormones in food, pesticides and other chemicals, and leptin, a protein secreted by fat cells, may be implicated. One cause may be accidental drug exposures from products that are used incorrectly in the household, such as testosterone skin cream, estrogen-containing shampoos and the like. The average age for MENARCHE, however, between ages 12 and 13, remains unchanged. In about half of cases the early growth stops by itself and no treatment is needed. If, however, it is progressive and various tests do not show an organic cause, treatment with GnRH (gonadotropin-releasing hormone) may be indicated.

Precocious puberty results from premature signals from the hypothalamus, pituitary and adrenal glands, which trigger the growth of pubic and axillary hair, breast development and menarche. Because these signals can be stimulated by a tumor of the brain, ovaries or some other organ, these conditions should first be ruled out by means of X-ray, blood and urine tests and electroencephalography (EEG). If there is no underlying disease calling for specific therapy, administering a GnRH (gonadotropin-releasing hormone) analog, marketed as Lupron, appears to slow down precocious pubertal changes. Administered in monthly injections, it is quite expensive, its long-term effects are not known and in some girls it has the side effect of terrible mood swings resembling those of menopause. Both careful explanation and emotional support should be given to the physically precocious girl and her family, since most such children have the psychological maturity appropriate for their actual age. Her breast development should be described as "early"—not "abnormal"—and the process of menstruation should be thoroughly explained, preferably before menstrual flow actually begins. After menses begins, explicit sex education is important, since she could become pregnant.

preconception care Medical care for a woman who is planning pregnancy *before* she becomes pregnant. It focuses on the conditions and risk factors that could affect a woman if she becomes pregnant, as well as factors that can affect a fetus or infant. Preconception care should begin at least three months before a planned pregnancy. Among the issues involved are taking prenatal vitamins and folic acid supplements to prevent neural tube defects, rubella vaccination to prevent congenital rubella syndrome, stopping smoking and alcohol consumption and detecting and treating existing health conditions to prevent complications in the mother and reduce the risk of birth defects. These conditions include diabetes, hypothyroidism, HIV/AIDS, hepatitis B, PKU (phenylketonuria),

hypertension (high blood pressure), blood diseases and eating disorders. The physician should review medications that can affect the fetus or mother, such as epilepsy medicine (see also DRUG USE AND PREGNANCY), reviewing pregnancy history (has she lost a baby before?), family planning and counseling to avoid unwanted pregnancies and counseling to promote healthy behavior (nutrition, exercise, oral health). Preconception care can be provided by a gynecologist or primary-care physician.

See also PRENATAL CARE.

preeclampsia Also *pregnancy-induced hypertension, PIH, metabolic toxemia of late pregnancy, toxemia*. The development, in the last trimester of pregnancy, of hypertension (high blood pressure), proteinuria (protein in the urine) and edema (fluid retention) associated with a rapid weight gain. If not treated, this condition can progress to ECLAMPSIA and possibly death. Moreover, the progression from preeclampsia to eclampsia can be very rapid (a matter of hours), and therefore preeclampsia requires very prompt treatment.

The precise cause of preeclampsia is not known, but recent research indicates it is caused by an imbalance between two kinds of factor, those that turn on and those that shut down new blood vessel growth. Early in pregnancy more blood vessels are needed to supply the fetus; later this process must be reversed lest the woman bleed heavily. In preeclampsia the shutdown occurs too early. Why the condition develops in approximately 5 to 8% of all pregnancies is not known. It occurs most often in first pregnancies and in women who already have hypertension or vascular disease. Indeed, some authorities lump together preeclampsia, eclampsia and hypertension that develops in late pregnancy, calling them "hypertensive disorders of late pregnancy," but one cannot exclude already hypertensive women who become pregnant. The hypertension of preeclampsia is caused by vasospasm, that is, constriction of the blood vessels that inhibits the flow of blood, especially to the liver, uterus and kidneys. Older women have a greater risk of preeclampsia, as do women carrying more than one fetus. Also, the risk rises if either the woman's mother or her husband's mother had preeclampsia.

Since the symptoms of preeclampsia occur with varying severity, and some, such as edema and weight gain, are characteristic of just about all women in late pregnancy, specific standards have been established. In true preeclampsia hypertension must be present along with either proteinuria or edema. Hypertension is defined as a rise of at least 30 mm (millimeters) Hg over the usual systolic blood pressure or an absolute systolic pressure of 140 or more; a rise of at least 15 mm Hg over usual diastolic pressure, or an absolute diastolic level of 90 or more; and these high levels must be observed on two or more occasions at least six hours apart with the patient resting on her left side (see under HYPERTENSION for explanation of these measurements). Proteinuria is defined as urinary protein in concentrations greater than 0.3 grams per liter in a 24-hour collection (all urine passed is collected over a 24-hour period), or 1 gram per liter or more in a random clean sample on two occasions at least six hours apart. Edema is defined as generalized fluid accumulation in the tissues (not just swollen feet or ankles), especially if it is associated with rapid weight gain (at least 1 kilo, or 2.2 pounds, per week). *Severe preeclampsia* is defined as a blood pressure of 160/110 or higher, proteinuria of 5 grams or more in 24 hours and diminished urine output (400 ml or less in 24 hours), with cerebral or visual disturbance, pulmonary edema or cyanosis, liver capsule tenderness and hyperreflexia (exaggerated reflexes).

The only specific treatment for severe preeclampsia is terminating the pregnancy; delivery alone can prevent convulsions and the death of the baby. Because the baby usually will be premature, there may be a temptation to delay until its chances of survival increase, but severe preeclampsia itself may kill the baby, and it is much safer for the mother not to wait.

Preeclampsia probably cannot be wholly prevented. In earlier times, some clinicians tried to do so by strictly limiting a pregnant woman's weight gain and sodium (salt) intake, and by almost routinely prescribing diuretics to prevent fluid retention. However, it was found that these measures themselves can be dangerous, leading to protein deficiency, sodium-electrolyte imbalance and other problems. More recently studies indicated that aspirin can forestall high blood pressure during pregnancy among those already at high risk for preeclampsia, but it does not confer any benefits to women who are at moderate or low risk. Early detection, on the other hand, may prevent development of life-threatening eclampsia. It is for this reason that good PRENATAL CARE calls for increasingly frequent checkups in the last trimester and routinely includes checking weight gain, blood pressure and testing the urine for albumin (protein). One promising development is the discovery of a marker for the disease in pregnant women's blood that appears about five weeks before its onset. It is a gene, sFlt1, that blocks growth factors, but it can be counteracted by growth-stimulating drugs. Also being worked on is a urine test for a protein, placental growth factor, low in women at high risk.

Once symptoms appear, most physicians believe the woman should have complete bed rest on her left side, at home or in the hospital. Weight, blood pressure and urine must be checked frequently. A protein-rich diet is used, and at least one authority believes that such a diet throughout pregnancy will prevent the development of preeclampsia. If the condition cannot be controlled with these measures or hypertension is present before pregnancy, small amounts of medication to reduce blood pressure are considered safe. If these do not work, strong sedation and anticonvulsant drugs may be given to prevent eclampsia. The principal drug used is magnesium sulfate, which may lessen symptoms and prevent convulsions. Because the condition may persist after delivery, the drug is often continued for 24 hours after birth. If high blood pressure persists as well, beta-blockers or other medication may be used until blood pressure returns to normal.

Research indicates that women who have had preeclampsia are at higher risk for cardiovascular problems later in life. It is not clear whether women who get preeclampsia were already at risk for these problems or whether preeclampsia predisposes them toward them.

pregnancy The condition of a woman who is carrying a fertilized egg (ZYGOTE) or embryo or fetus.

She also is said to have *conceived*. An uninterrupted normal pregnancy, called a *full-term pregnancy,* continues for approximately nine months or 39 to 40 weeks, which for the sake of convenience is divided into roughly equal three-month periods called *trimesters.* It is dated from the beginning of the last menstrual period (LMP), from which the time of birth is calculated. (The easiest way of calculating is to subtract 3 months from LMP and add 7; for example, if the LMP began on January 10, delivery would be due October 17.)

Pregnancy is characterized by complex physiologic changes, which begin almost immediately after conception. (The changes undergone by egg, embryo and fetus are described under GESTATION.) The earliest signs of pregnancy usually are a skipped menstrual period, somewhat swollen and tender breasts, nausea (so-called MORNING SICKNESS), sleepiness and fatigue, urinary frequency, increased vaginal discharge and slight cramping in the area just above the pubis. The presence and intensity of these signs vary greatly from woman to woman, and also from pregnancy to pregnancy. Some women experience few or no symptoms during the first trimester other than absence of menstruation. Some even continue to have slight monthly bleeding resembling periods for two or three months after conceiving, although this is rare. Or pregnancy may occur in a woman who has never menstruated but has ovulated.

These signs and symptoms all reflect hormonal changes in the body. Within five to seven days of conception, chorionic gonadotropins appear in the woman's blood and urine. Their presence or absence is the basis of every PREGNANCY TEST. Progesterone and estrogen levels gradually rise. The blood supply to the pelvis becomes greatly increased, resulting in such early clinical changes as CHADWICK'S SIGN and HEGAR'S SIGN. However, none of this evidence is conclusive. Until recently pregnancy could be definitively established by clinical signs only during the second trimester, when the baby's heartbeat can be heard as distinct from that of the mother (today use of a doptone or ultrasound can detect heartbeat at 11 weeks or earlier), the baby's movements can be felt by the examining clinician and the fetus can be "seen" by X-ray. Now ultrasound can detect pregnancy as early as three

or four weeks after conception, and a PREGNANCY TEST much earlier yet.

By the second trimester the abdomen is enlarged, and the shape, size and consistency of the uterus have changed enormously. In many women there are pigment changes, especially darkening of the skin around the nipples and sometimes on the face (see CHLOASMA); also, a dark line from the navel to the pubic region (called *linea nigra*) may become evident. The skin over the enlarging abdomen is stretched, sometimes leaving pink stretch marks, or STRIAE. Some women, about midway through the second trimester, begin to leak a little fluid from their breasts (see LACTATION). There may be gastrointestinal discomfort from the enlarging abdomen, principally constipation and heartburn. As a result of pressure, VARICOSE VEINS may become troublesome in the legs, vulva and/or rectum (HEMORRHOIDS). The blood volume increases—by 30 to 50% over the nine months of pregnancy—and the heart beats faster to pump the increased amount, causing some women to experience palpitations. There may be leg cramps and/or nosebleeds, the latter from congestion of the mucous membranes. Some women perspire and salivate more during pregnancy. Also, there is a growing tendency toward EDEMA, especially swollen ankles, feet, hands and wrists toward the end of the day. In general these discomforts are intermittent and not too severe; many (perhaps most) women regard the second trimester as the most comfortable period of pregnancy.

In the third trimester considerable enlargement of the uterus and abdomen begin to cause increasing discomfort. More striae appear. The fetus is larger and its movements are more evident, sometimes enough to cause night waking. Pressure from the growing uterus on other organs may cause shortness of breath, increased indigestion (especially heartburn, sometimes after every meal), constipation, urinary frequency and more discomfort from varicose veins and edema. Even without any of these symptoms, practically all pregnant women experience increased fatigue in the last trimester simply from carrying 15 or more extra pounds.

Good PRENATAL CARE is important from the moment pregnancy is verified, with special attention to DIET and EXERCISE. Except in unusual circumstances, most women are able to continue all of their usual activities (including sexual relations) throughout the pregnancy, provided they get the extra rest they need. Even with good care and the absence of foreseeable special complications (see HIGH-RISK PREGNANCY), problems can arise. They include vaginal bleeding early or late in pregnancy, severe or persistent abdominal pain, urinary infection, premature rupture of the membranes, fetal death (see STILLBIRTH), PREMATURE LABOR, ABNORMAL PRESENTATION and PREECLAMPSIA. These situations rarely develop without some warning, so most clinicians advise a woman to **seek emergency medical care at once if any of the following danger signals occurs:** severe persistent abdominal pain (no matter where in the abdomen, or in what stage of pregnancy); vaginal bleeding at any time during pregnancy (light staining in the first half of pregnancy can wait till morning; if it occurs during the second half, it is considered an emergency, even if the amount is slight, except for bloody show; see MUCUS PLUG); dimness or blurring of vision, especially in the second half of pregnancy; puffiness or swelling of the face, eyelids or fingers, especially if sudden; fever and chills; severe persistent headache (especially during the last trimester); absence of fetal movement for 24 hours after the fifth month; membrane rupture (breaking of the waters; see AMNIOTIC SAC).

See also DIET; DRUG USE AND PREGNANCY; LABOR; PREGNANCY COUNSELING; PREGNANT PATIENTS' RIGHTS; PRENATAL CARE.

pregnancy, mask of   See CHLOASMA.

pregnancy counseling   Assistance in deciding whether to continue an unplanned pregnancy, or whether to become pregnant (sometimes called *preconception counseling*), involving a careful review of the options available and their effect on the woman and her partner. In theory there are three basic options for a pregnant woman: continuing the pregnancy and keeping the child; continuing the pregnancy and giving the child up for adoption; and terminating the pregnancy by ABORTION. In practice, however, not every woman has all three

options. Keeping a child fathered by a man other than the woman's husband (the result of rape, for example) might not be emotionally acceptable to both partners. Nor might continuing a pregnancy be an option when it is equally certain that the child will be brain-damaged or have some serious birth defect (see GENETIC COUNSELING). Similarly, abortion might not be possible for a woman opposed to it on religious grounds or for a woman who lives where it is not legal or not available and cannot afford to travel elsewhere. A trained counselor can help a woman (or couple) determine her (their) priorities and alternatives as well as refer her to appropriate agencies (an adoption agency, abortion facility, etc.) to help carry out her decision.

Because BIRTH CONTROL and legalized abortion have made parenthood an optional matter for many couples, an increasing number of women (and couples) seek advice *before* planning a pregnancy. They need to consider if having and raising a child fits in with their desired style of life (including professional and educational plans), whether their motives for childbearing are valid ones, how parenthood will affect their partner and their relationship, and similar questions. Increasingly, professional counselors and therapists are helping to find answers to these questions, so that the field of pregnancy counseling has been broadened to include pregnancy planning.

See also GENETIC COUNSELING.

pregnancy-induced hypertension   Also *PIH*.
See also PREECLAMPSIA.

pregnancy test   A test to determine whether or not a woman is pregnant. There are two basic kinds of pregnancy test: a blood test and a urine test. Both are based on the presence of HUMAN CHORIONIC GONADOTROPHIN (HCG), a hormone secreted by the fertilized egg during its journey from the fallopian tube to the uterus, and later by the placenta. HCG is detectable in the woman's bloodstream as early as six to eight days after conception and in the urine 21 to 28 days following conception. Its production reaches a peak 50 to 60 days later and then steadily declines.

pregnant patient's rights 351

The urine and blood tests used all indicate how HCG inhibits a chemical reaction. Some work in as little as two minutes, and others take two hours or so. They vary principally in their sensitivity, that is, the level of HCG to which they respond. The two blood tests (see RADIORECEPTOR ASSAY) are more sensitive (respond to lower levels of HCG) and more accurate than any urine test. They are particularly useful if ECTOPIC PREGNANCY (outside the uterus) is suspected, because in this life-threatening condition HCG levels usually are too low to be detected by any urine test. However, blood tests are available only through hospitals and specialized laboratories and also are more expensive than urine tests.

Urine tests are widely available and usually adequate for most women's needs. There are two principal kinds: tube tests (two-hour) and slide tests (two-minute). The former supposedly are accurate as early as 37 days after the last menstrual period (LMP; the first day of flow is day 1) or about 14 days after the first missed period was due, whereas slide tests rarely are accurate before 41 days after the last menstrual period. Both are more accurate if they are performed somewhat later—ideally, two weeks later, when HCG in the urine has reached its peak. All urine tests require use of the first urine voided in the morning after a night's sleep because it is more concentrated and so increases the chance of detecting HCG. (For pregnancy tests one can perform at home, all based on urine testing, see EARLY PREGNANCY TEST.)

Blood tests for pregnancy can be positive *before* a period has even been missed in more than 90% of pregnant women, when only 1 to 5 International Units per liter of HCG are present in the bloodstream. However, at that early stage they can yield a *false negative* result—that is, indicate that a woman is not pregnant when she really is—simply for lack of sufficient HCG levels. They also may give a *false positive* result caused by a surge of LH (luteinizing hormone), which is chemically similar to HCG; at such low levels the results are not definitive, and the test may have to be repeated one week later. Urine tests yield positive results for 80% of pregnant women by 42 days after the last menstrual period and for 95% of pregnant women by 56 days after the last period. However, the

incidence of false negative results is even higher than with blood tests, since higher HCG levels are needed for accuracy.

For all pregnancy tests, a *positive result* most often means a woman is pregnant unless the test is performed very early; only rarely does a tumor, infection or medication cause false positive readings. As noted, however, a negative result is less certain, because HCG levels may be too low. The earlier the test is made, the less likely that a negative reading is accurate, and some clinicians feel that every negative result calls for a repeat test one week later.

The first satisfactory pregnancy test was devised by Ascheim and Zondeck in 1928 and took three to five days to give results. It involved the injection of urine into an immature female mouse or rat that was killed after three to five days; if blood spots or hemorrhagic follicles appeared in her ovaries, the result was positive. A similar test induced ovulation in rabbits in 24 to 48 hours (the *rabbit test*); however, use of rabbits was quickly abandoned because they were too expensive. With another early test, urine was injected under the skin of a toad; if the test was positive, the animal laid eggs within 12 to 24 hours (if negative, no eggs were laid). These animal tests, called *bioassay* (for *biological assays of HCG*) were 95% accurate when positive a few days after the missed period, but they also yielded many false negative results.

pregnant patient's rights A general term that describes pregnant women's just claims on health care services. Since about 1930 there has been increasing medical care (detractors call it medical "intervention") in childbirth, at least in the United States and Canada. From the 1950s on, however, when the so-called natural childbirth movement gained momentum in these countries, there was growing skepticism about traditional hospital practices during labor and delivery, which involve various drugs and procedures (some of them not always necessary) that may be potentially damaging to the baby, the mother or both. It was feared that increasingly widespread use of both anesthesia and forceps damaged babies, sometimes inflicting permanent brain damage. Some of the drugs used also could harm the mother. Consequently a number of groups, including women's health centers, consumer groups, self-help clinics and organizations devoted to maternal and child health, devised lists that spell out a woman's right to participate in decisions involving her own welfare and that of her unborn child.

These rights include the right to know about the direct or indirect effects, risks or hazards to herself or to her child that may result from the use of a drug or procedure prescribed for or administered to her during pregnancy, labor, birth or lactation; and the right to be fully informed of any proposed treatment and its alternatives, including childbirth education classes that can help prepare her for labor and delivery and thereby reduce or eliminate the need for drugs and other intervention. Many of these practices have become the norm in numerous, but by no means all, hospitals. Some advocates go further, insisting that a woman has the right to have medical assistance no matter where she intends to give birth (at home, in a clinic, etc.); to refuse any drugs; to ask the health worker to avoid an episiotomy if possible; to labor at her own rate of speed, without intervention, and to give birth in whatever position she chooses; to keep the baby (if healthy) with her from birth on, nursing it immediately and whenever she wishes to; and to have her partner and/or friends with her throughout labor, delivery and the hospital stay. (See also PATIENTS' RIGHTS.)

Owing to the rapidly rising cost of health care and hospitalization, health plans in the 1980s began to cut back coverage for childbirth hospitalization. By 1988 the majority of U.S. health plans covered only a 48-hour hospital stay for normal labor and delivery and three to four days for Cesarean delivery. Some institutions cut this period even shorter. In 1998 the U.S. Department of Labor made clear that new laws covering health insurance say a woman is entitled to 48 hours in a hospital, beginning *after* delivery, and after a Cesarean section she is entitled to four days in a hospital. Critics point out that this arbitrary rule could harm some new mothers, contributing to complications during the postpartum period. Feeding problems, some congenital abnormalities and NEONATAL JAUNDICE often do not show up until the third or fourth day after delivery. Further, early discharge can be extremely hard on inexperienced first-time, single, or very young mothers, as well as on women with several young children at home and no household help. Supporters hold that the hospital is a costly and not very restful environment for recuperation. Some suggest that the best solution is to use a BIRTH CENTER for a longer period after delivery for those women who are likely to need it or who find they need more time to convalesce, and that an experienced home health care aide visit for several weeks after hospital discharge.

premature Also *preemie* (slang). Describing any infant born before 38 weeks of GESTATION, so its chances of survival may be impaired. Infants born after 35 weeks of gestation usually do quite well. Some authorities believe that a birth weight of less than 2,500 grams (about 5.5 pounds) serves as a good definition of prematurity. Infants weighing more than this generally have as good a chance of surviving as any that are larger; infants weighing less may not. There are, of course, many exceptions, and indeed this definition can be applied only to white infants. Black infants on the average weigh 100 grams less than white ones, and full-term Asian babies are smaller still. At the lower end of the scale the definition is even less clear. Generally speaking, however, a birth weight under 500 grams (1.1 pounds) indicates no chance whatever of survival; 500 to 999 grams (1.1 pounds to 2.2 pounds, sometimes called *immature*) indicates a poor chance of survival; and premature infants, ranging from 1,000 to 2,499 grams (2.2 to 5.5 pounds), have a chance ranging from poor to good, depending on their weight (the higher, the better) and the care they receive. Size alone, however, is not an adequate criterion. Babies of diabetic mothers often are large but may not be well developed (see DIABETES). Further, prematurity cannot always be defined by *obstetric gestational age*, that is, completed weeks of pregnancy counting from day 1 of the mother's last menstrual period. Since fetuses develop at different rates, *pediatric gestational age*, indicated by the physical characteristics of the baby at birth and a neurological examination of maturity, also must be taken into account. (See also APGAR SCORE; GESTATION.)

In North America prematurity is the principal cause of death in newborn babies, accounting for about one-half of such deaths. (Of these, 80% occur within 24 hours of delivery.) Improved pediatric care and public health programs have done little to change this statistic. The best means would seem to be prevention, but in more than half the cases prematurity is idiopathic (the cause is not known).

Not all babies weighing less than 2,500 grams are premature in terms of development. Some suffer from intrauterine growth retardation, others from congenital malformation and still others from intrauterine infection. Malnutrition before birth may be caused by inadequate blood flow or by placental insufficiency; that is, the nutrients from the mother do not reach the baby. Congenital defects such as DOWN SYNDROME also are associated with low birth weight, as are maternal infections such as RUBELLA. Conditions in the mother that seem to slow down the baby's weight gain include poor nutrition, hypertension (high blood pressure) and cardiovascular disease, preeclampsia, placenta previa and habitual cigarette smoking. Women whose mothers were given diethylstilbestrol during their pregnancies may be more likely to give birth to premature infants than unexposed women. MULTIPLE PREGNANCY usually involves premature labor and small babies.

The principal danger to the premature infant is respiratory distress (see HYALINE MEMBRANE DISEASE). The use of steroids 24 hours prior to delivery can help mature the lungs and reduce the incidence of bleeding in the infant's brain. Other problems frequently occurring are inability to suck strongly and inability to maintain body temperature (hence the frequent use of warmers). Further, premature infants are more apt to suffer from respiratory and gastrointestinal infections and, if they require high levels of oxygen, risk developing RETROLENTAL FIBROPLASIA. On the positive side, today about 93% of babies born in the 28th week—almost three months premature—survive, the vast majority with no major disability. But for babies born sooner and smaller, the shorter their time in utero and the less they weigh, the poorer their chances for a good long-term prognosis. (See also MISCARRIAGE.)

Since the 1990s a number of different medications have been used to stop premature labor, but

SYMPTOMS OF PRETERM LABOR
(OCCURRING 3 OR MORE WEEKS BEFORE DUE DATE)

- Contractions occurring four or more times an hour
- Pelvic pressure, a feeling that baby is pushing down or is going to fall out
- Increase or change in vaginal discharge
- Breaking of waters, a sudden gush of clear watery fluid

none has delayed it for more than a couple of days, and they also have been associated with serious side effects. The only effective treatment found to date is the hormone progesterone, administered in weekly injections beginning between weeks 16 and 20 and stopped at week 36.

The number of premature births has been reaching record highs, increasing by 35% in a decade. A major cause is an increase in multiple pregnancies, many of them resulting from infertility treatment; about half of twin pregnancies and nearly all pregnancies of triplets or more end before 37 weeks of gestation. Other risk factors are maternal infections, which may account for the higher rate of prematurity among African Americans and the poor; women over age 35; cigarette smoking; too little or too great a weight gain during pregnancy; health problems such as diabetes or high blood pressure; and chronic stress, which can trigger early labor. If experiencing symptoms of preterm labor (see accompanying table), the woman is advised to call her clinician; if the symptoms persist for an hour and she is unable to reach the clinician, she is advised to go to the nearest hospital. Even if she did not plan to be hospitalized, a premature baby is best off in a hospital with a neonatal intensive care center.

A technique for identifying premature labor promptly is UTERINE MONITORING. In addition, researchers are studying various ways to predict premature labor. One that won approval in 1998 is a saliva test called SalEst (for saliva and estrogen) that measures levels of the hormone estriol, which helps prepare the uterus for labor and delivery and peaks three weeks before childbirth. The test correctly predicts 57% of premature births. Women with risk factors, such as a history of premature birth, could be tested several times near the end of pregnancy to assess the likelihood of early delivery. If prematurity can be predicted, drugs to prolong pregnancy or corticosteroids might be prescribed. Another marker for prematurity is presence of infection in the amniotic fluid. Testing for and treating infection may greatly reduce the number of premature births.

A new test for screening for premature labor checks for fetal fibronectin, or fFN, in the vaginal tract. Its presence during weeks 24 to 34 indicates an increased risk of preterm labor. Its absence, on the other hand, indicates that the pregnancy will most likely continue for another two weeks. A positive result for the test, which involves simply a swab of vaginal fluid and 24-hour laboratory analysis, enables attempts to postpone labor. The screening is recommended only for women considered at high risk for premature labor.

The standard venue for premature babies is a neonatal intensive care unit, or NICU, where they are placed in an isolette. Because the unit houses numerous babies in what can be a chaotic atmosphere, with monitors going off and ventilators running, there has been a growing movement to design private rooms in NICUs that mimic some of the qualities of the mother's womb, dark and relatively quiet, with close contact with the parents. They are sometimes called *womb rooms*. By mid-2007, only about 20 of the 800 or so NICUs in the United States have completed womb rooms and about 40 others were planning to build them.

premature ejaculation   See EJACULATION, def. 2.

premenstrual dysphoric disorder   Also *PDD*. A mood disorder that resembles an exaggerated version of premenstrual tension (see DYSMENORRHEA, def. 5). It features at least five of the following symptoms: anxiety, sadness, mood swings, persistent irritability, withdrawal, difficulty concentrating, fatigue, marked changes in appetite and sleep patterns, a feeling of being overwhelmed, and physical symptoms such as headache, joint and muscle pain, weight gain and bloating. More severe than premenstrual tension, the condition can significantly interfere with daily living—work,

social activities and relationships. Similar to the symptoms of major depression, PDD disappears after the menstrual period begins. It is treated with antidepressants, specifically fluoxetine (Sarafem) and sertraline (Zoloft). Like any medication, these can trigger side effects, such as upset stomach, fatigue and agitation.

premenstrual tension   Also *premenstrual syndrome, PMS.* Another name for congestive dysmenorrhea. See also DYSMENORRHEA, def. 5.

prenatal care   Medical care for a woman from the time she suspects that she may be pregnant until the birth of the baby. In large measure, prenatal care is preventive, its chief purpose being to assure the delivery of a healthy baby without danger or harm to the mother. It is designed to detect at their onset conditions that may, if unchecked, adversely affect mother and/or child. Many such conditions can, if recognized early, be corrected or controlled. Among them are signs or symptoms of urinary infection, genital HERPES INFECTION and other kinds of infection, ECTOPIC PREGNANCY, PREECLAMPSIA and abnormal uterine growth, all conditions requiring treatment to prevent serious damage. Some authorities, including the Centers for Disease Control and Prevention, believe that waiting to see a physician until one is pregnant is too late to avoid possible problems and recommend that care begin at least three months before becoming pregnant (see PRECONCEPTION CARE).

Prenatal care is available from private physicians (general practitioners, family practitioners, obstetricians), nurse-midwives, birth centers and clinics. Since a pregnant woman will be seeing her health care provider for nearly a year, it is advisable to select one (or a facility) with some care. Among the factors to be considered in this choice are location (can the person/place be reached readily? are the hours convenient?); qualifications (see also CLINIC; MIDWIFE; OBSTETRICIAN); cost (the total cost of pregnancy and delivery should be clarified at the outset); general orientation (approve of PREPARED CHILDBIRTH? willing to consider and/or attend HOME BIRTH? qualified to perform surgery if needed or backed up by qualified person?); and personality (willing to answer questions? give adequate individual attention?).

The initial visit usually takes place at the time when pregnancy is confirmed, or soon after, and ordinarily takes longer than subsequent ones. It should include a complete medical history with special attention to previous obstetric history (for example, complications in previous pregnancies, birth defects in the family, etc.); a complete physical examination, including pelvic examination, breast examination, height and weight, blood pressure; and a number of laboratory tests. Chief among the tests are a complete blood count (including hemoglobin and hematocrit) and blood tests for syphilis, blood type (should transfusion be needed), RH FACTOR and possible antibody levels (including RUBELLA); a PAP SMEAR; tests for sexually transmitted diseases (STDs), including hepatitis B and HIV; and a urine test (for protein and sugar) and urine culture. Further, black women should routinely be tested for SICKLE-CELL DISEASE and Jewish women for TAY-SACHS DISEASE. Following the examination the clinician should advise the woman concerning diet, exercise, general hygiene and sexual activity, and answer any questions she may have. Either then or later in the pregnancy, suggestions may be made concerning childbirth education of one kind or another.

Many pregnant women require medications to manage previously diagnosed conditions such as asthma or hypertension. However, some medications should be avoided because they can harm the fetus. Among those the FDA considers risky are progesterone, tetracycline, aspirin, cortisone, tretinoin (Accutane), lithium, estrogens, simvastatin (a cholesterol-lowering drug), trazolam and warfarin (Coumadin). See also DRUG USE AND PREGNANCY.

After the initial visit, most women require monthly visits through 28 weeks, every two weeks until 36 weeks and weekly thereafter. These visits generally involve only a check for blood pressure (a rise may warn of possible preeclampsia), weight and urine, along with external examination of the abdomen, listening for the fetal heartbeat and measuring the uterus to check on the growth of the fetus. In addition, at 30 weeks a glucose test is routinely done for gestational DIABETES.

See also DIET; HIGH-RISK PREGNANCY; PREGNANT PATIENTS' RIGHTS; PRENATAL TESTS; WEIGHT GAIN, def. 2.

prenatal tests Any of a number of tests performed before or during pregnancy to detect possible BIRTH DEFECTS or disorders in the fetus. Some tests can be performed *before* pregnancy is established. When IN VITRO FERTILIZATION is done (fertilization of egg and sperm in the laboratory), the resulting embryo can be tested for some genetic disorders, such as TAY-SACHS DISEASE and CYSTIC FIBROSIS, before being implanted in the woman's uterus. This procedure is also called *preimplantation genetic diagnosis,* or PGD. (In 1994 the first baby that had been so tested—for Tay-Sachs disease when she was an eight-cell embryo—was born free of the disease.) Today even more exhaustive testing of embryos, including an intense DNA analysis, can be done. It also may be performed to discover genetic traits that raise the risk of developing diseases like cancer later in life. Most such tests are done for infertile couples or older women who suffer repeated miscarriages, a condition often due to chromosomal errors easily identified in an embryo. However, such screening is still very expensive, running into tens of thousands of dollars. Moreover, a recent study showed that preimplantation genetic screening based simply on a woman's age—in this study 35 to 41—actually reduced the rate of pregnancy and number of live births. Another procedure involves removing a single cell from a three-day-old embryo, which consists of eight cells. Although designed for discovering specific genetic defects, it began to be more and more widely used for older women having difficulty conceiving in the belief that weeding out embryos with abnormalities would enhance their rate of successful implantation.

A few congenital conditions, such as spina bifida, are being treated in the womb by surgery at about seven months, but such treatment is still highly experimental. However, further development is expected to enable treating and eliminating many more problems at early stages of fetal development.

Tests performed *during* pregnancy to detect genetic disorders include AMNIOCENTESIS, CHORI-

ONIC VILLUS SAMPLING (CVS), ALPHA-FETOPROTEIN TEST (AFP), and PERCUTANEOUS UMBILICAL BLOOD SAMPLING (PUBS). (Also see NUCHAL TRANSLUCENCY-BIOCHEMICAL BLOOD TEST.) One center screens for Down syndrome in the second trimester of pregnancy, using a detailed sonogram and maternal blood levels of alpha-fetoprotein plus human chorionic gonadotropin and estriol and combining those levels with the woman's age to obtain a risk estimate. Two blood tests plus a sonogram also may be performed during the first trimester; they can indicate whether the fetus has the extra 21st chromosome that causes Down syndrome with a high degree of accuracy and without endangering the pregnancy. Another new technique enables sifting fetal blood cells from the mother's blood to detect chromosomal defects such as Down syndrome. It is performed at the end of the first trimester and yields results in 72 hours. In *fluorescent in situ hybridization,* individual chromosomes can be tagged with material that glows when fluorescently lighted under a microscope. See also under DOWN SYNDROME.

New techniques such as *embryoscopy* now permit viewing a six-week-old embryo. Although FETOSCOPY had for some time enabled such viewing during the second and third trimesters, it is much riskier. Embryoscopy involves inserting a tiny viewing scope into the mother's abdomen through an ultra-thin needle (guided by ultrasound); an endoscope attached to a camera is then passed through the needle, enabling the practitioner to see neural tube defects and other abnormalities.

prepared childbirth Also *natural childbirth, childbirth education.* A system of preparing a woman (sometimes also her partner) for labor and delivery through education concerning the process of birth, exercises to be used prenatally and during labor and other means. A number of different methods are in current use, but their overall objective is essentially the same: to eliminate a woman's fear of childbirth by replacing it with knowledge of what to expect, and to prepare her mentally and physically for the sensations she will encounter during labor and delivery in order to avoid, as much as

possible, the use of pain relievers, anesthesia, forceps delivery and other medical intervention that could possibly harm her or the baby.

The earliest method of prepared childbirth to become popular was devised by an English physician, Grantly Dick-Read; the DICK-READ METHOD was used in North America from the late 1950s on. During the next decade a method devised by a French doctor, Fernand Lamaze, the PSYCHOPROPHYLACTIC METHOD, virtually replaced the Dick-Read method. Still another method, devised by an American obstetrician, is called *husband-coached childbirth* or the BRADLEY METHOD, after its inventor. Each of these methods not only has its advocates but has attracted teachers who have invented variations of their own. There also is a version of yoga devised by a Danish-trained teacher called *prenatal yoga* or *Euronie method of yoga,* which involves exercises alone (no education concerning birth). Still other childbirth educators urge parents to find their own way through labor and delivery without relying on any set system, allowing the mother's body to function as naturally as possible.

prepartum Before childbirth.
See also PRENATAL CARE.

prepuce Also *foreskin.* A sheath of skin, partly retractable, that covers the penis in men and the clitoris in women. The operation called CIRCUMCISION, performed for hygienic or religious purposes, surgically removes part of the prepuce.

primigravida A woman who is pregnant for the first time.
See also PRIMIPARA.

primipara A woman who has delivered one child.
See also MULTIPARA.

probiotics Live microorganisms administered as dietary supplements aiming to confer a beneficial health effect. Most probiotic products contain bacteria (one-celled organisms) from the genus *Lactobacillus, Bifidobacterium* or yeasts. Basically they supplement organisms already found in the body's intestinal tract. They are available in the form of capsules, tablets or powders, and in certain foods where they either occur naturally or are added (for example, milk, yogurt, miso, tempeh, some juices, soy beverages). Although extensive scientific evidence is not yet available, probiotics appear to help the symptoms of irritable bowel syndrome, antibiotic-resistant diarrhea in children, respiratory and urologic infections and other conditions. Side effects appear to be mild and digestive, such as gas or bloating. Probiotics are considered a form of ALTERNATIVE MEDICINE and should not be used in place of conventional medical care. Moreover, one's health care provider should be informed if they are used. Probiotics are sold over the counter and the labeling can be confusing. The bacteria are measured in colony-forming units (CFUs), and 1 billion CFUs is the minimum per day thought to be effective. However, some labels claim a larger amount of CFUs than they actually contain. Some yogurt products display the National Yogurt Association's Live & Active Cultures seal, which indicates that when manufactured they contained at least 100 million CFUs of live bacteria per gram.

progesterone   A hormone produced after ovulation by the CORPUS LUTEUM that builds up the uterine lining, or endometrium, for the reception and nurture of a fertilized egg and helps maintain a pregnancy. It also is released in tiny amounts by the adrenal glands in both men and women, in men by the testes and in pregnant women in very large amounts by the placenta, which takes over progesterone production after the corpus luteum disintegrates. It was first discovered and isolated in 1934, but it took several years before its role in the MENSTRUAL CYCLE was understood. Progesterone production is triggered midway through the cycle by the pituitary hormone LH (luteinizing hormone). In the absence of fertilization, the built-up endometrial tissue is shed during menstruation, and the lowered levels of progesterone and estrogen stimulate the cycle to begin again. Progester-

one causes the body temperature to rise about 1 degree Fahrenheit, making it possible to tell when ovulation occurs (see BASAL BODY TEMPERATURE). In pregnancy progesterone inhibits movements of uterine muscle, stops ovulation and stimulates breast development. Infertility specialists may use the *progesterone withdrawal test* to determine if a woman is capable of menstruating. It is given orally or by injection; her period will then usually begin 14 to 20 days later. Progesterone may play a role in premenstrual syndrome (PMS; see DYSMENORRHEA, def. 5) but that role has not been definitively established.

Synthetic progesterone, called *progestogen,* includes micronized, plant-derived progesterone, which is chemically identical to the body's hormone, and laboratory-synthetized *progestin,* which differs somewhat from natural progesterone and therefore may have slightly different effects. Consequently the correct compound must be carefully selected for each patient when it is used as a medication. Progestogens are used to control anovulatory bleeding (when estrogen has stimulated endometrial buildup for too long and bleeding is therefore heavy). They are used along with estrogen in oral contraceptives and in ESTROGEN REPLACEMENT THERAPY, as well as to treat secondary amenorrhea (AMENORRHEA, def. 3), endometriosis and some cases of endometrial cancer. In estrogen-replacement therapy, progestogen is believed to help prevent endometrial buildup that may eventually lead to malignancy. Progestin is the only active ingredient in the MINIPILL, developed for women who could not tolerate the estrogen in combined estrogen-progestin oral contraceptives. A progestin medroxyprogesterone acetate, DEPO-PROVERA, is used as a contraceptive given by injection (a single intramuscular injection affords 99% protection against pregnancy for three months). Another form, levonorgestrel, is used in Norplant, a contraceptive implant. Progestogen also is used in an INTRAUTERINE DEVICE (IUD) impregnated with the hormone, which it releases in small amounts in the uterus to help increase its effectiveness.

Progestogens have relatively few side effects, though some women taking them have reported the development of acne, breast tenderness, premenstrual depression and greasy hair. Used in oral contraceptives they may cause weight gain, abdominal and leg cramps, fluid retention, mood changes, reduced menstrual flow and breakthrough bleeding. They should be avoided during pregnancy and by women with jaundice or other liver disease, kidney disorders or Addison's disease. The micronized progestogens are said to have fewer side effects (such as bloating and fluid retention) than the progestins but also can increase the risk of blood clots and should not be taken by women who have severe liver disease, breast cancer or allergies to the plants from which they are derived.

Current research is directed at developing selective progesterone receptor modules, which activate the hormone in some parts of the body and block it in others, in effect acting on progesterone much as a SELECTIVE ESTROGEN-RECEPTOR MODULATOR does on estrogen.

progestin Also *progestogen*. Synthetic (human-made) PROGESTERONE, used in oral contraceptives, estrogen replacement therapy and other medications.

prognosis A forecast as to the probable outcome of a disease. A favorable prognosis means recovery is likely; a poor prognosis means it is not.

prolactin Also *luteotrophin, luteotropic hormone, LTH*. A HORMONE secreted by the pituitary gland that stimulates the breasts to secrete milk and also inhibits the production of the pituitary hormones LH (luteinizing hormone) and FSH (follicle-stimulating hormone), which stimulate ovulation. Women who lactate without having given birth are said to have *galactorrhea* and lack a substance called the *prolactin-inhibiting factor* (PIF), produced by the HYPOTHALAMUS. Since galactorrhea can be a symptom of serious disease, such as a pituitary tumor, it always should be investigated (see also AMENORRHEA-GALACTORRHEA SYNDROME). Such tumors tend to be benign (non-malignant) and respond to drug therapy. Another hypothalamic substance, *thyrotropic release hormone (TRH)*, also stimulates prolactin production.

See LACTATION.

prolapse Also *pelvic organ prolapse*. The protrusion into the vagina of the uterus, bladder, urethrum or rectum. Pressure, pain, difficulty urinating or defecating and sexual problems may result. Long believed to result from muscle and tissue damage from multiple vaginal births, recent research indicates that some women may have a genetic predisposition to these conditions that also may affect women who have never given birth. For prolapsed bladder, see CYSTOCELE; for prolapsed rectum, RECTOCELE; for uterine prolapse, PROLAPSED UTERUS.

prolapsed cord In childbirth, the condition existing when the umbilical cord lies ahead of or beside the presenting part of the baby (head, shoulders, buttocks) in the vagina. This phenomenon is extremely dangerous for the baby, whose oxygen supply and circulation can be impaired with any compression of the cord. It rarely occurs with vertex (head-first) presentation when the head is engaged by the time the membranes rupture, because the head normally presses against the cervix, allowing no room for the cord. If for some reason the head is not engaged, the baby is very small or the pelvis is too small, or if some other part, particularly a shoulder or foot, presents (leads the way), the cord can prolapse when the membranes rupture. Treatment depends on how much the cervix is dilated and on the position of the baby. If the cervix is fully dilated, the baby's life usually can be saved if it can be delivered immediately. If the cervix is only partly dilated and the baby is mature, an immediate Cesarean section may save it. (Even if the cervix is fully dilated a Cesarean section may be performed lest there be too long a period of compression before delivery, during which the baby would be deprived of oxygen.) Even with prompt measures, however, the probability of the baby's death is fairly high (about 17%).

prolapsed uterus Also *fallen uterus, uterine decensus, uterine prolapse*. Partial descent of the uterus into the vagina, owing to pelvic relaxation, that is, weakening of the pelvic floor muscles that normally hold the uterus in place. The condition usually results from childbirth (a long labor, large babies, many pregnancies) and tends to get worse after menopause. In severe cases the uterus drops completely out of the vagina, causing considerable irritation to the delicate cervix, which then rubs against clothing, and producing discharge and bleeding.

A prolapsed uterus may give rise to no symptoms at all, but usually there is a sensation of heaviness or pressure in the vagina. There also may be urinary incontinence (especially when coughing, laughing or sneezing; see URINARY INCONTINENCE) and backache. The condition, which often is found in conjunction with a prolapsed bladder or rectum (see CYSTOCELE; RECTOCELE), can be diagnosed readily during a pelvic examination. In mild cases no treatment may be needed, or the prolapse may be partly corrected by trying to strengthen the pelvic floor muscles with KEGEL EXERCISES; for overweight women, losing weight may also help. In severe cases, the insertion of a PESSARY can alleviate the symptoms, and its use is advisable in women for whom surgery represents too great a risk. Otherwise, surgery to repair the support structures, usually performed vaginally but sometimes abdominally, may be the answer. Another possibility is a vaginal HYSTERECTOMY (removal of the uterus through the vagina) along with any needed repair to the bladder or rectum. The vagina may be smaller after surgery but not necessarily shorter. Problems may recur if the factors causing prolapse are not corrected. After surgery patients are advised to forego smoking, control their weight, avoid constipation and avoid activities, such as heavy lifting, that put pressure on the pelvic muscles.

proliferative phase The first portion of the normal MENSTRUAL CYCLE—usually days 1 to 14—when estrogen secreted by the ovarian follicles causes the endometrium (lining of the uterus) to grow in preparation for the implantation of a fertilized egg.

See also SECRETORY PHASE.

prolonged labor Any portion of childbirth that lasts longer than the generally accepted established norm. The technical term for any difficult labor,

whatever the cause, is *dystocia*. The causes fall into three general categories: ABNORMAL PRESENTATION, with the baby in a position from which it cannot be pushed out; *pelvic contraction* or *cephalopelvic disproportion*, in which a part of the mother's pelvis is not large enough to permit the baby's passage; and, most often, *uterine dysfunction* or *uterine inertia*, meaning insufficiently strong or insufficiently regular contractions of the uterine muscles to dilate the cervix and expel the baby.

The duration of labor varies greatly. A first baby nearly always takes longer than subsequent ones, but even then there are exceptions. The first stage of LABOR, which is by far the longest and involves dilating the cervix to a diameter of about 10 centimeters, lasts in an average first labor about 12 hours (seven hours in subsequent deliveries). This first stage is often subdivided into a *latent phase (early labor)*, characterized by weak, irregularly spaced contractions as the cervix is slowly dilated to about 3 or 4 centimeters, and an *active phase (hard labor)*, in which contractions are stronger, more regular and dilation proceeds more rapidly, until it reaches 8 centimeters. The latent phase may last six to nine hours, but the active phase rarely lasts more than three to six. In the final portion of active labor, called the *transition*, dilation proceeds to 10 centimeters, usually within one hour. It is followed by the second stage, the expulsion of the baby, which lasts one to three hours, and the third stage, delivery of the placenta, which takes 15 to 60 minutes. (All these times refer to a first baby.) (See also the chart for "normal labor" under LABOR.)

Given these average times, *prolonged latent labor* is defined as 20 hours for a first baby, 14 hours for subsequent babies; *prolonged active labor* is marked by cervical dilation of less than 1.2 centimeters per hour with a first baby and less than 1.5 centimeters per hour for subsequent babies. Also, labor is considered prolonged if progress comes to a halt at any point. Prolonged labor tends to occur in older women (35 or older for a first baby), with large babies in a first pregnancy, with POSTERIOR PRESENTATION, the most common abnormal position, and with BREECH PRESENTATION.

Uterine dysfunction (inefficient muscular action) may be caused by excessive use of analgesics (pain relievers) before the onset of active labor, minor degrees of cephalopelvic disproportion, malposition of the baby to even a slight degree (such as extension of the head) or, most often, by some combination of these factors. A slow labor, while unpleasant for the mother, rarely is dangerous for her, but it poses a much increased risk of injury, infection and (rarely) death to the baby. The longer the labor, the greater the risk. If, therefore, progress in dilation of the cervix ceases, especially during active labor, the clinician generally checks first to make sure it is not caused by a malposition. If the cervix stops dilating, amniotomy (membrane rupture) may be done to speed up the labor, and if this cannot be performed safely or is not effective, the administration of oxytocin (to strengthen contractions) may be begun. Since oxytocin is a very powerful drug, constant careful monitoring of both mother and baby must accompany its use (see also under INDUCTION OF LABOR). If oxytocin fails to increase cervical dilation, often an intrauterine pressure catheter is inserted into the uterus. A soft, flexible cord, it lies next to the baby and will accurately measure the strength of contractions. If contractions are found to be strong but there is no change over the next two hours, it is presumed there is cephalopelvic disproportion (the baby's head is too large for the mother's pelvis) and a Cesarean section is necessary.

promiscuous   See LIBIDO.

prophylactic   1. The medical term for "preventive." For example, penicillin or another antibiotic often is used following abortion to prevent the risk of possible infection; in this example giving penicillin is a prophylactic therapy, since no infection is present when it is given.
2. Another name for CONDOM, which prevents conception.

prostaglandins   A group of fatty acids found in human and animal tissue that act on almost every organ system of the body. They play an especially important role in the reproductive, gastrointestinal and cardiovascular systems that is not yet completely understood. Some of them are capable of stimulating uterine contractions and therefore have been used for abortion, principally by injection into the uterus (see AMNIOINFUSION) and in conjunction with the ABORTIFACIENT RU-486. They also have been used in the form of vaginal suppositories, but though they work faster in this way they may cause violent nausea, intense uterine contractions, diarrhea and sometimes fever. Prostaglandins also are suspected of being responsible for severe menstrual cramps (see DYSMENORRHEA, def. 4), causing contractions of uterine muscle and blood vessels that are perceived as pain. Several NSAIDs (nonsteroidal anti-inflammatory drugs) used for arthritis that also have antiprostaglandin properties appear to be effective in reducing severe menstrual discomfort.

prostate gland   See PENIS.

pruritis   See ITCHING.

pseudocyesis   See FALSE PREGNANCY.

psychogenic   Describing a symptom or set of symptoms caused by emotional or psychologic factors that has no objective manifestations. For example, a person may complain of a headache or stomachache, or pain on urinating, and careful medical examination will uncover no physical reason for the pain. These symptoms may be a response to short-lived emotional distress or the expression of a severe emotional disorder, such as depression or anxiety. For an extreme example, see HYSTERIA, CONVERSION.
See also PSYCHOSOMATIC.

psychoprophylactic method   Also *Lamaze method.* A method of PREPARED CHILDBIRTH that concentrates on teaching women about the physiology of reproduction and chilbirth and that instructs them in exercises to be used before and during labor and delivery, including special kinds of breathing (slow

LAMAZE CHILDBIRTH EDUCATION

Phase of Labor	What You Might Feel	What You Can Do
State I Early Phase 0–2 fingers 0–4 cm	Backache Diarrhea or constipation Abdominal cramps Show Ruptured membranes Excitement, anticipation Regular contractions	No Food Time contractions Call nurse and doctor Pelvic rock for backache Slow deep breathing Get accustomed to contractions Conscious relaxation
Mid-phase 2–4 fingers 4–8 cm	Stronger, more frequent contractions More serious concentration Dependent on companionship Discouragement, doubts Restlessness Back and/or leg pain Weepy	Out breathing or rapid shallow breathing Effleurage (bring powder or corn starch) Ice chips Relax Vary position of bed and pillows Mild medication Back rub Concentrate on one contraction at a time Husband: give encouragement
Transition 4–5 fingers 8–10 cm	Leg cramps and shaking Nausea and vomiting Heavy show Hot and perspiring "Sleeping" between contractions Total involvement and detachment Apprehension Inability to concentrate Dizziness Increased pressure Desire to push	Rapid-shallow with "hoo-ha" breathing Remember time is short Wet cloth or face Husbands urges wife to concentrate *Specific* instructions Lots of encouragement Hand over mouth for tingling in hands and feet—or hold breath between contractions Slump and blow DON'T PANIC!
Stage II Expulsion of baby	Contractions may slow down Urge to push Pressure to rectum and perineum Total involvement May experience exhaustion and difficulty concentrating harder	Specific instruction for each contraction Relax perineal muscles 3 pushes per contraction Don't be afraid to push hard Husband: support shoulders and urge to push Be ready to stop pushing
Stage III Expulsion of placenta	May feel slight contraction	Follow instructions

Courtesy of Lamaze Childbirth Education, Inc., Watertown, MA.

chest breathing, panting, blowing) to be used at various stages of labor. It was originally devised by a French physician, Fernand Lamaze, who based it on the work of Russian practitioners, particularly the Pavlovian school of conditioned reflexes (learning to respond in a particular way to a given stimulus). In childbirth, it is applied by blocking out painful sensations with counterstimuli. Thus the occurrence of a contraction (labor pain) serves as a stimulus to relax certain muscles, a process assisted by using a particular breathing pattern. The name *psychoprophylactic* was created from words meaning "mind" and "preventive" and refers to the ability of the mind to prevent or minimize painful sensations.

The psychoprophylactic method is taught in a series of six weekly classes attended by the woman and, if possible, her husband or partner, beginning in the seventh month of pregnancy. The partner, or *labor coach,* assists her during labor by timing the length and frequency of contractions, massaging her back, wiping her face, reminding her of the responses she learned and generally providing support and encouragement. The earliest and principal proponent of the psychoprophylactic method in America was Elisabeth Bing, who began teaching it about 1960 and over the years devised variations and refinements on it. In England Erna Wright based her method on it as did Sheila Kitzinger (who called her method *psychosexual preparation*); both introduced somewhat different breathing techniques, and Kitzinger a different method for bearing down during the second stage of labor. Since then, numerous minor variations on the method have been devised, from altering the number and timing of classes to changing techniques to lessen pain during labor, but its basis continues to be the most popular method of so-called natural childbirth.

Critics of the psychoprophylactic method hold that it concentrates on blocking out pain instead of going along with body rhythms and "riding with" the pain. Also, they say the light panting method of breathing may deprive the baby of needed oxygen, and some criticize the technique of holding one's breath while bearing down during the pushing stage.

See also BRADLEY METHOD; DICK-READ METHOD.

psychosomatic A broad term used to describe a physical symptom or disorder in which psychological or emotional factors play an important but not clearly understood role. The symptom or illness is physically present and demonstrable, but it is either precipitated by or aggravated by psychic factors. Among the disorders in which emotional factors are believed to play an important role are hypertension (high blood pressure), coronary artery disease, diabetes, rheumatoid arthritis, peptic ulcers and asthma. However, the relative importance of psychological factors in such disorders varies greatly among different individuals; besides, they are difficult to separate from other factors, such as hereditary predisposition, allergy, individual personality, and individual responses to drugs and social pressures.

See also PSYCHOGENIC.

psychotherapy Also *counseling, therapy.* A general term for the treatment of mental and emotional disorders that is based primarily on verbal communication between patient and therapist. Psychotherapy is conducted by psychiatrists and other physicians specially trained in this area as well as by psychologists, social workers, psychoanalysts, lay analysts, nurses, pastoral counselors and others with professional training of various kinds in the technique. Psychotherapy may be conducted on a one-to-one basis (individual approach) or in a group with other clients (*group therapy*) and one or more therapists. Families and couples also may be treated together. In addition, some groups—self-help or *support* groups—function on their own, their members acting as therapists for one another.

Psychotherapy is performed most often in an office setting and on an outpatient basis, but seriously disturbed persons may require hospitalization, or they may use a day hospital (returning home every night) or residential program in a halfway house or other supervised facility. Psychotherapy can be carried on alone or in conjunction with psychotropic drugs (principally TRANQUILIZERS, ANTIDEPRESSANTS, antimanic drugs and antipsychotics) and/or electroconvulsive (shock) therapy, the latter usually performed only in a hospital or clinic setting.

There are many different psychotherapeutic approaches, ranging from classical psychoanalysis, developed by Sigmund Freud, and numerous therapies based on it (existential analysis, Jungian analysis, will therapy, etc.) to behaviorist therapy (and others based on it, including rational-emotive therapy, cognitive therapy, sex therapy, psychobiology, etc.) to purely group approaches, such as family therapy and psychodrama.

See also FEMINIST THERAPY; SEX THERAPY.

puberty The period during which sexual maturity is attained. In girls it begins several years earlier than in boys (at about the age of 9 or 10) and lasts for about 5 years. (In boys the average age for onset of puberty is between 12 and 14, but a much wider range—10 to 18—is considered normal.) During this time girls experience a period of rapid growth in height and weight gain—the so-called *growth spurt*. Most women reach their mature height soon after the onset of menstruation, or MENARCHE, which occurs three or four years after puberty has begun (at an average age of 12.6 in North America today). At this time increased levels of estrogen cause closure of the growth centers at the ends of bones, thus ending their growth. (Male sex hormones have a similar effect in boys, but much later.) Estrogen also causes the deposit of increased amounts of fat in the subcutaneous tissue of the breasts, upper arms, buttocks, hips and thighs, producing the characteristic shape of the female body. Influenced by estrogen, the uterus enlarges and the vagina lengthens; the inner lips of the vulva, the labia minora, begin to grow until they may protrude somewhat between the thick outer lips, or labia majora. The relative proportion of lean body mass (muscle and bone) to total body weight lessens, so that muscles look less prominent, masked by the higher proportion of fat. In boys, on the other hand, increased androgen levels produce both greater muscularity and more prominent muscle definition, seen especially in the shoulders and chest. For these reasons women can rarely, if ever, develop the same upper body strength as men, though they are able to develop as much leg strength. Their larger proportion of fat, on the other hand, makes women better able to retain body heat in cold temperatures and also makes them more buoyant. (See also ATHLETIC ABILITY, WOMEN'S.)

Puberty is the time of developing *secondary sex characteristics*. In both boys and girls there is growth of pubic and axillary (underarm) hair, and the enlargement of axillary sweat glands, producing increased perspiration and also perspiration odor. In girls BREAST size increases gradually, one breast often growing markedly faster than the other for a time; in boys the penis and testes grow, chest hair and facial hair appear and the voice deepens. These changes take place gradually, and at various rates in different individuals. Many adolescents worry

about changing too soon (precocious puberty) or, more often, too late (delayed puberty). For most, little more is needed than frequent reassurance that their progress is "normal." *Delayed puberty* caused by later hormone production, although worrisome to children and parents, is in itself no cause for alarm, but when little or no pubertal change of any kind is apparent in girls by the age of 16 (or in boys by the age of 18), medical investigation is warranted to rule out a tumor or serious disease. Total *pubertal failure*, which is more common in boys than in girls, is due nearly always to a deficiency either in the sex glands (testes or ovaries) or in the pituitary stimulation of those glands, and usually responds to treatment with androgens or estrogens.

See also AMENORRHEA, def. 2; PRECOCIOUS PUBERTY.

pubic hair   Hair that grows over the skin of the genital area during PUBERTY. In women it grows over the MONS VENERIS, or pubis, in a roughly triangular pattern (with the base of the triangle at the top), called the *escutcheon*. In men the pattern is less well defined and the hair tends to extend farther up toward the navel and down on the inner thighs, roughly diamond-shaped, as it is in some women, too. The pubic hair may be sparse or profuse, and straight or curly. Its function, like that of axillary (underarm) hair, is to absorb moisture and to trap the scent secreted by the APOCRINE GLANDS. In girls it usually begins to grow about one year before menarche (the first menstrual period). If no pubic hair is evident by the age of 16 (in boys, 18), it may be wise to investigate the cause of delay. Pubic hair sometimes becomes infested with tiny parasites (see PUBIC LICE).

pubic lice   Also *crabs, pediculosis pubis*. A parasitic infection that can be transmitted by sexual contact but also by infested bedding or clothing. The pubic louse (*Phthirus pubis*) is a tiny, yellowish gray creature, about 1 millimeter long, with three pairs of claws and four pairs of legs, giving it a crab-like appearance. It moves by swinging from hair to hair and then inserts its mouth into the skin, where it feeds on tiny blood vessels. If separated from human skin, it can survive only 24 hours at the most. During their 30-day life span the adult lice mate frequently, the female daily laying about three oval white eggs called *nits,* which she cements to one side of a hair. They hatch in seven to nine days. Symptoms of infection vary from none (rare) to intense itching (usual). Scratching brings no relief and helps spread the lice via the fingers to other hairy parts of the body (thighs, underarms, scalp). Diagnosis is made by finding the lice or their nits attached to pubic hairs. Treatment is with any of several over-the-counter drugs available as creams, shampoos and lotions. The safest and most effective of them is permethrin (Nix), sold as a cream rinse. Others are pyrethrin with piperonyl butoxide (R.I.D.) and lindane (Kwell); the latter should be avoided by pregnant women and children. Both may require repeat treatments. None should be used around the eyes (if crabs are in the eyebrows). After treatment, clothing and bedding should be changed and washed (though after 24 hours any remaining lice will have died), and non-washable items such as upholstery and mattresses should be sprayed with an appropriate pesticide to prevent reinfestation.

pubis   Another name for MONS VENERIS.

pubococcygeous   One of the important muscles of the pelvic floor that support the bladder, rectum and uterus. It is the muscle used when one wishes to stop the flow of urine. It and the other pelvic floor muscles often become over-relaxed after childbearing, leading to problems such as URINARY INCONTINENCE, RECTOCELE, CYSTOCELE and PROLAPSED UTERUS. One way to strengthen the pubococcygeous is with KEGEL EXERCISES.

pudenda   Another name for VULVA.

pudendal anesthesia   Also PUDENDAL NERVE BLOCK. A kind of REGIONAL ANESTHESIA administered during childbirth, when delivery is imminent (late in

the second stage of LABOR). The pudendal nerves around the vagina and vulva are injected through both sides of the vagina with a local anesthetic that blocks their transmission of pain messages to the brain. These nerves are hard to locate and are placed differently in some women. Hence it takes considerable skill to block them, and as a rule the anesthetic is only about 80% effective. About the only risk of such anesthesia, other than the slight one of an allergic reaction in the mother, is injection of the anesthetic into the pudendal artery which can cause shock and (rarely) death. Pudendal anesthesia does not block the sensations of labor, only of delivery, and therefore is useful for low FORCEPS deliveries and the performance of a large EPISIOTOMY. It does not interfere with uterine contractions, and the effects of the anesthetic are not transmitted to the baby.

puerperal fever   Also *childbed fever, postpartum infection, puerperal sepsis.* Infection of the genital tract, usually of the endometrium (uterine lining), following childbirth. Its name comes from the fact that it nearly always is marked by a rise in body temperature (fever), and, indeed, the presence of fever after delivery is almost invariably a sign of infection. In this context, fever is interpreted as a temperature of 38 degrees Celsius (100.4 degrees Fahrenheit) or higher on any two of the first 10 days following delivery.

Puerperal fever was the leading cause of maternal death until fairly recently. It was first described in ancient times by Hippocrates and Galen, but its cause—wound infection—was determined only in 1847 by an Austrian physician, Ignaz Semmelweis, who believed that infection was introduced by the examining fingers of physicians, midwives and students. He ordered all persons who examined women in labor to disinfect their hands with chlorine solution, and the mortality rate in his Vienna Lying-In Hospital dropped from 10 to 1% almost immediately. Nevertheless, his ideas were not widely accepted for many years. Epidemics of puerperal fever continued to occur in hospitals for another century—as late as 1968 in the United States—although in the course of time aseptic techniques, antibiotic therapy, a reduction in traumatic deliveries and very long labors, and better general maternal health markedly reduced the death rate.

Puerperal infection can be caused by various organisms, but by far the most common source is the streptococcus. Infection usually occurs during the course of labor. Fortunately most such infections respond well to prompt antibiotic treatment, the choice of drug being based on the organism isolated by laboratory test. More recently, a sudden severe, potentially fatal infection in women who have given birth has been associated with *Staphylococcus aureus.*

See also TAMPON.

puerperium The period immediately following childbirth. A *puerpera* is a woman who has just given birth.

See also POSTPARTUM.

pulse See ARTERY.

purulent Also *suppurating.* Filled with or exuding PUS.

pus A thick, yellowish liquid that forms in infected tissue. It consists chiefly of dead cells and white blood cells and contains the bacteria causing the infection.

See also INFECTION.

pustule See ACNE.

pyelonephritis Also *kidney infection.* An acute infection of one or both kidneys, usually caused by bacteria that enter the body through the urethra and work their way up through the bladder and ureters to the kidneys. It is especially common in young girls and in pregnant women as well as in both men and women who have diabetes or who have undergone catheterization or some other procedure in which an instrument is introduced into the urinary tract. The most common cause is *Escherichia coli,* an organism that normally resides in the gastrointestinal tract. Typically, pyelonephritis comes on quite rapidly and is marked by fever, chills and back pain on one or both sides near the waistline. There also may be nausea and vomiting. Bladder irritation from the infected urine may cause frequency and urgency of urination, which also may be painful, and hematuria (blood in the urine). Treatment should be promptly sought, because pyelonephritis can cause permanent kidney damage. The causative agent can be identified by testing the urine, but antibiotic treatment is usually begun before urine culture results are available. As with other urinary tract infections, drinking a great deal of water—at least six to eight glasses a day, and preferably more—helps by diluting the urine and so making it less hospitable to bacterial growth. Urinating frequently and completely emptying the bladder help to keep the bacteria from multiplying, and eliminating coffee, tea and alcoholic beverages, which all contain kidney irritants, also may help relieve the symptoms.

quadriplegia Partial or total paralysis of all four limbs (both arms and both legs), usually resulting from injury to the spinal cord in the cervical (neck) segments. Such injury may occur in a traffic, industrial or sports accident, or in wartime; less often it results from tumors, infections, abscesses and congenital defects. Once the spinal cord is injured, its nerve cells and fibers are unable to regenerate and the damage is irreversible, with a permanent lesion now obstructing the paths of sensation and motor control. The extent of disability is determined by the extent and level of the lesion in the spinal cord. Quadriplegics suffer serious impairment or complete loss of sensitivity to touch, pain and temperature in all the areas affected. Other problems are disturbances in blood circulation, loss of skin and muscle tone, and loss of voluntary bowel and bladder control. As a result, quadriplegics are apt to suffer from certain secondary complications, especially urinary infections and kidney and bladder stones, pressure sores (decubitus ulcer), muscle contractures of paralyzed joints (hips, knees, elbows) and fractures of weight-bearing bones. Another common complication is *automatic hyperreflexia:* Because the spinal cord, although cut off from the brain by injury, is still living tissue, when stimulated it generates a massive response that cannot be checked by the brain. Symptoms of hyperreflexia, which may occur alone or in combination, include throbbing headache, flushing of the face, neck and upper body, sweating, seizures, nasal obstruction, chills and hypertension. The most common precipitating cause of such violent reactions is retention of urine. Quadriplegics who have lost conscious urinary control normally live with an indwelling catheter (tube), which must be checked periodically for blockage.

In quadriplegic women, menstruation, fertility and pregnancy are not affected. Oral contraceptives and intrauterine devices (IUDs) for birth control are generally contraindicated because circulatory problems are very likely to develop in paralyzed limbs and could go undetected because of lack of sensation, as could a pelvic infection. Sexual intercourse may be difficult in certain positions owing to hip and leg spasms, and there is an increased risk of autonomic hyperreflexia during sexual arousal (and also during labor and delivery). There also is an increased risk of urinary and bowel incontinence during masturbation and intercourse. Masturbation is difficult or impossible without assistance and, depending on the exact location of the spinal cord lesion, there may be no sensation of orgasm or no reflex sexual response with genital stimulation. However, other parts of the body (usually above the site of the lesion) may become highly sensitive to sexual stimulation, and some women report feelings identical to orgasm when these are stimulated.

See also PARAPLEGIA.

quickening The perception of the movements of the fetus by a pregnant woman. It usually occurs sometime between the 16th and 20th weeks of pregnancy, and it may be perceived initially as a very faint flutter or, especially later in pregnancy, as quite vigorous "kicks." The fetal movements also can be felt by placing one's hand over the lower abdomen. The movements of the fetus depend on the presence of the amniotic fluid, in which it floats. During the fourth and fifth months the fetus is small in relation to the amount of fluid. A sudden tap or simply pressure on the abdomen causes the fetus to sink in the fluid; it then rebounds to its original position, as if tapping back at the examining hand. This passive movement of the fetus is called *ballottement*. Both it and the more active movements can sometimes be felt upon vaginal examination to test for ENGAGE-MENT; after engagement the fetus is fixed in the pelvis and cannot be ballotted. From the 30th week of pregnancy on, complete absence of fetal movements for a period of 24 hours or longer is a sign of possible fetal distress and should be investigated.

rabbit test   See PREGNANCY TEST.

radiation therapy   Also *irradiation, radiotherapy.* Treatment of cancer by directing X-rays, cobalt or other sources of ionizing radiation at specific parts of the body. If administered just as a cancer cell is ready to reproduce (divide in two), radiation will stop cell division and the cell will eventually die. Because cancer cells multiply faster than normal cells, they are more susceptible to radiation.

Radiation therapy is effective as a primary treatment—that is, used alone, without surgery—for many cancers, such as skin cancer, Hodgkin's disease, some non-Hodgkin's lymphomas, cancer of the cervix, early cancers of the prostate, larynx, esophagus, lung and nasal passages. Some specialists believe it can be used in this way for breast cancer as well, along with only minimal surgery (see MASTECTOMY, def. 6, 7), but others disagree. Radiation therapy is the principal primary treatment for inflammatory breast cancer (see CANCER, INFLAMMATORY BREAST), for local control of inoperable breast cancers (in women who cannot or will not undergo surgery, or whose cancer is very advanced); as an adjunct to mastectomy or lumpectomy; to shrink a large tumor to operable size; and to alleviate pain, especially bone pain caused by distant METASTASIS, and in multiple myeloma, advanced lung and esophagopharyngeal cancer, gastric cancer, sarcomas and brain metastases. Implanting a radiation source temporarily at the site of a tumor can supplement external radiation in destroying cancer cells (also see below).

Like CHEMOTHERAPY (anticancer drugs), radiation also affects some healthy cells, particularly those subject to rapid growth, such as hair roots and gastrointestinal mucosa. Consequently it causes similar unpleasant side effects, the most common being hair loss, skin irritation, nausea, vomiting and sores in the mouth. Loss of libido also is common, and although it usually returns after treatment is completed, treatment for prostate, testicular or cervical cancer may result in permanent hormonal or structural changes that affect sexuality. These sometimes can be aided by hormone therapy.

Radiation usually is less disfiguring than surgery. In the case of breast cancer, treatment may cause a temporary sunburnlike blistering, but the final appearance of the skin is not much scarred in about 75% of patients. Others have quite extensive scarring, however. Radiation occasionally leads to other complications. In breast cancer these include radiation-induced rib fractures, damage to the underlying lung and bone marrow, short-term lung inflammation and, more rarely, scarring of the pericardium (the sac surrounding the heart).

Newer techniques being explored are called *partial-breast irradiation,* which exposes less tissue to radiation and cuts treatment time from five to seven weeks to a few days. It limits treatment to where the tumor had been and a few centimeters around it. *Accelerated partial-breast radiation* involves 10 treatments lasting about 15 minutes each and given twice a day for five days. One approach, also called BRACHYTHERAPY, delivers radioactive "seeds" through catheters inserted into the breast, either a series of 10 to 20 or a single balloon catheter. Another approach is a single dose of radiation to the lumpectomy site at the time of surgery; it is called *intra-operative radiotherapy.* The probe so inserted into the tumor bed stays in place for about 25 minutes and then is removed. Still another technique uses an external beam of radiation, after three-dimensional scans plot and shape the delivery from the outside. At this writing it is not known if partial-breast radiation is as safe or effective as standard care following lumpectomy, in which the entire breast is irradiated. It is advised only for women over 50, with ductal cancer either invasive or confined to the ducts, a tumor 2 centimeters or less in size, negative surgical margins at least 2 millimeters in all directions and no lymph node involvement. It should be performed only by a surgeon or radiation oncologist who has appropriate training in the technique. Another new technique is proton radiation, very expensive and not widely available. Its chief advantages are that it targets the tumor precisely and has fewer side effects than conventional X-ray therapy. On the horizon is therapy using beams of carbon ions, thought to be even more powerful in killing tumors. Several medical centers are planning to install combined proton and carbon therapy centers.

With cervical cancer, a slender metal instrument containing radium or cesium may be inserted through the vagina and left in place for several days. Cancers of the tongue and uterus also may be treated with implants containing radioactive elements such as cesium, iridium and certain forms of iodine. They are inserted under general or local anesthesia and remain in place for about a week. While they are in place, the patient must remain fairly still so as to assure proper positioning, and remain in the hospital because she emits a small amount of low-level radiation. Another kind, *radiofrequency ablation*, has been successful on liver cancer and is being tested in breast cancer with tumors of 1.5 centimeters or smaller. Guided by ultrasound, a needle-thin probe is inserted into the tumor, and the probe opens like an umbrella with alternating current sent up the spokes. Heating the tumor cells above 212 degrees Fahrenheit, the current kills them. *Laser ablation* works similarly but uses laser energy to heat and kill the tumor.

It is highly advisable to use a radiologist who specializes in breast imaging to look at all of one's imaging studies—mammograms, breast ultrasounds, breast MRIs—on a daily basis. Occasionally a radiologist is so focused on the main cancer that a tiny tumor elsewhere in the breast or even in the other breast is overlooked.

See also CANCER.

radical hysterectomy   Also *Wertheim procedure.* Surgical removal of the uterus, cervix, pelvic lymph nodes and ligaments, and the upper portion of the vagina, and sometimes also the ovaries and follicle-stimulating hormone.

See HYSTERECTOMY.

radical mastectomy   See MASTECTOMY, def. 2, 3, 4.

radioimmunoassay   See RADIORECEPTOR ASSAY.

radionuclide imaging   Also *scanning*. The administration of radionuclides (radioactive isotopes) to a person whose body is then subjected to special visualizing equipment for the purpose of diagnosis. The radionuclides are administered orally, by injection or directly into the part of the body being investigated. The particular one used depends on the tissue being examined, because different organs incorporate (take up) specific substances differently. Thus, different elements are used for liver scans, pancreas scans, spleen scans, central nervous system (brain) scans, bone scans and so on. Radioactive iodine is used in thyroid scans to detect cancer and other disorders, because the thyroid gland takes up iodine. Polyphosphate is used for bone scans, which often can detect minute cancerous invasions of bony tissue and thus pinpoint the spread of breast or other cancers to bone very early.

The radionuclides used for scanning are produced artificially. They emit ionizing radiation in the form of gamma rays, which are detectable outside the body by various kinds of scintillation detector. Because modern instruments permit detection of very small amounts of gamma rays produced by a tiny tracer dose of radionuclide, there is no danger in their use, and they can be employed even in very young children. However, because scanning introduces radioactive substances into the bloodstream, it should be avoided, if possible, during pregnancy and breast-feeding, since the effects on a fetus or a very young infant (through breast milk) are not known.

radioreceptor assay   A PREGNANCY TEST developed in the mid-1970s that is so sensitive it can give a positive result in more than 99% of pregnant women before a period has been missed. Like other pregnancy tests, however, it also can yield false negative results. A blood test, it is sensitive to only 200 International Units per liter of HCG (pregnancy hormone) in the bloodstream, whereas other tests require a level five times as high. Another blood test that is almost as sensitive is a serum *radioimmunoassay*, which can detect pregnancy as early as the sixth to eighth day after ovulation. Both these tests rely on the competition of the HCG to be measured with radioactively labeled HCG for sites on an antibody. Very low levels can, however, be mistaken for a pregnancy; they actually are not HCG but LH (luteinizing hormone), which rises drastically at ovulation. Therefore, to be sure, all such tests should be repeated a week later when, if levels are higher, the woman is presumed to be pregnant.

radiotherapy See RADIATION THERAPY.

raloxifene See SELECTIVE ESTROGEN-RECEPTOR MODULATOR.

rape Any sexual assault, up to and including undesired sexual intercourse (anal, vaginal, oral), on a man, woman or child. Except in special situations (such as prison), women and children are by far the most common victims. In the United States each state has its own laws governing rape, which in legal terms is classed as a felony, but in all 50 states it is defined as obtaining sexual intercourse through physical force or the *threat* of physical force. From the mid-1970s on the number of rapes reported yearly in the United States was increasing faster than any other crime of violence (murder, assault, robbery), and even then reported figures were believed to be but a fraction (an estimated one-tenth) of the reality because so many victims are reluctant to report the crime.

In the 1950s, when rape began to be brought to public attention, a large number of myths concerning it were widely believed. As a result women's groups and other organizations dedicated to fighting rape directed their efforts toward publicizing the true facts about rape. Rape is a crime of violence, not of sex. About half of all reported rapes are committed by someone known to the victim, and the actual number is thought to be much higher because women are more reluctant to report a rape involving a relative or friend. Half take place in the victim's home, which is usually entered by force. Rapists tend to choose their victims because they appear to be vulnerable and alone. Most rapes (70%) are planned in advance, and most rapists (85 to 90%) use physical force or the threat of force (such as displaying a weapon). Victims range in age from infancy (as young as six months) to old age (80 and older). Most rapists are married or have a regular sexual partner, making it clear that they are not motivated by sexual frustration. Most rapists, when tested, are not psychologically abnormal and tend to admit that their crime was motivated by a desire to dominate, humiliate and hurt. They rarely kill their victims.

Because rape was long viewed as a sexual crime, women who reported it were frequently made to feel that they had somehow provoked it and perhaps even enjoyed it. Therefore another area addressed by antirape groups is the treatment of victims by hospitals, law enforcement authorities and the courts. Recognizing that rape hurts a woman both physically and psychologically, they have urged the establishment of rape crisis centers staffed with counselors who help rape victims go through the procedures necessary to protect themselves medically and to enable them to prosecute attackers. Rape victims are urged to take the following steps:

1. If possible, the woman should call a local rape crisis center promptly for counseling on medical care, police procedures, prosecution and help through the court process, and emotional problems resulting from the attack.
2. The woman should promptly get a medical examination from a physician trained in handling rape evidence. (All physical evidence must be dealt with in accordance with local laws concerning evidence.) The clinician should first treat any injuries sustained, even minor ones (all of which should be recorded in detail), and then give a standard pelvic examination

(see GYNECOLOGIC EXAMINATION) during which he or she should perform a Pap smear and ask the pathologist to examine it for sperm cells, as well as test the cervix and vaginal walls for acid phosphatase, produced by the male prostate gland (and therefore present in ejaculated seminal fluid). For this test a small amount of saline solution is introduced into the vagina and then withdrawn with a syringe, and the fluid withdrawn is tested for both acid phosphatase and sperm. The clinician should record both the number of sperm seen and whether they were moving. (Evidence of sperm may disappear in eight hours, so promptness is important.)

3. Tests for GONORRHEA, SYPHILIS and AIDS should be performed. Since none of these venereal diseases produces symptoms in the early stages, a second test for gonorrhea should be done two weeks later, a second blood test for syphilis three months later, and a test for HIV antibodies six months later. If the rape was oral or anal, specimens from the woman's mouth or rectum should be taken as well.

4. The woman's body and clothing should be checked for substances that could be used as evidence, such as blood or grass stains on clothes, scrapings from under the fingernails (especially if she resisted), pubic or scalp hair different from hers, and so on.

5. If the risk of pregnancy appears to be considerable—if the rape occurred at midcycle and the woman was not protected by a contraceptive—use of the MORNING-AFTER PILL within 72 hours of rape, or performing MENSTRUAL EXTRACTION when the next period is due, might be considered. Another morning-after alternative, inserting an INTRAUTERINE DEVICE, is not advisable, because if the rapist was harboring an infection this insertion could carry bacteria into the uterus.

6. The rape should be reported to the police immediately (a decision as to whether to prosecute can be made later). Some localities have provisions for reporting to the police anonymously. The report should include a full account of what happened and the attacker's appearance, if possible; women who do decide to prosecute, so that the police will try to arrest the rapist and

he can be tried on the woman's charges, often discover that a prompt report to the police is a point in their favor in court.

7. After these immediate measures are taken, a woman should seek some kind of postrape counseling. Such counseling is available in some hospital psychiatric departments, through local rape crisis centers, through women's self-help clinics and other community resource organizations. Most women find that they have at least temporary emotional problems in the aftermath of a rape and some develop long-term ones, especially in the area of sexual relations. Denial and depression often mask their initial fear and anger, and it is easiest for them if these feelings are expressed honestly and worked out. Sometimes a professional therapist is needed. Even supportive friends, family and lovers may not be able to help enough. Children and teenagers particularly may need special care and counseling to understand what happened and to resolve their own feelings. It is now recognized that rape can sometimes lead to post-traumatic stress disorder, which may require treatment with antianxiety and antidepressant medication and psychotherapy (or behavior therapy).

Like many areas affecting women's health, rape is one in which prevention is far preferable to treatment. Among the suggestions made by antirape groups are:

- Prepare yourself beforehand. Imagine what you might do (for example, fight, run, scream, talk to the attacker, disgust him by pretending to vomit). Prepare to resist, although yelling may not make sense if no one is nearby, or running if there is nowhere to run to.

- If you live in a place with other vulnerable women (apartment house, college dormitory, etc.), set up a rape squad to patrol, as a deterrent, and/or a special call-for-help signal, such as a police whistle.

- At home, use deadbolt locks on outside doors, keep windows locked, especially at night, put iron grids on first-floor windows, keep shades drawn at night, do not hide your key near the door or in some other obvious place.

- If you live alone, list only your first initials in the phone book and on the mailbox.

- Do not let strangers into the house; if you suspect that someone has broken in while you were out, do not enter the house alone.

- Acquire some self-defense skills; even if you cannot use judo against an armed man, your knowledge will give you more confidence and also make you appear less vulnerable.

Raynaud's phenomenon A circulatory disorder characterized by spasms of the peripheral blood vessels, especially in the fingers and toes, which are triggered by exposure to cold. Named for the French doctor who first described it, it may be secondary to other conditions, such as SCLERODERMA, RHEUMATOID ARTHRITIS, SYSTEMIC LUPUS, or to trauma such as repetitive stress injury (as from extended typing). However, about two-thirds of cases are idiopathic (without known cause), a form called *Raynaud's disease*. Raynaud's affects mainly women, in whom it appears 20 times more often than in men and usually begins between the ages of 15 and 40. The spasms may last a few minutes or several hours, turning the digits bluish or purplish and sometimes numb; they usually are not painful. They can be relieved by warming the affected areas. Since the spasms cut off blood supply to the fingers and toes, they leave them vulnerable to damage, particularly in secondary Raynaud's phenomenon. Over time the skin of the fingers becomes smooth and shiny, the blood vessels become smaller in diameter and lessen blood flow, and small painful ulcers may appear, which, left untreated, may progress to gangrene. Treatment consists of protecting the body (especially the extremities) from cold and using mild sedatives. Smoking is harmful, since nicotine constricts blood vessels, and therefore must be avoided. When these measures do not control the disorder, other medications may be indicated, such as the calcium-channel blocker nifedipine or the antihypertensive drug prazosin. Some patients have learned to control symptoms by BIOFEEDBACK. Women who experience the symptoms of Raynaud's should see their clinician, since these traits may be the first signs of an underlying disorder such as scleroderma.

rectocele A bulging of the wall of the rectum into the vagina, owing to pelvic relaxation, that is, weakening of the muscles that ordinarily hold the rectum in place. It may occur alone or in conjunction with a PROLAPSED UTERUS and/or CYSTOCELE (fallen bladder), and like them usually results from childbirth (long labor, large babies, many pregnancies). Rectocele usually causes discomfort during a bowel movement, when pressure is felt. Some women must actually put a finger inside their vagina when they defecate in order to hold back the rectal wall. The condition can be corrected by minor surgery, in which the surgeon makes an incision along the back wall of the vagina, pushes the rectum back and up and sews it into place.

recurrence The return of symptoms or signs of a disease. In the case of CANCER, the return of symptoms in the same general area as the primary tumor.

reflex sympathetic dystrophy Also, *complex regional pain syndrome, RSD*. A form of chronic pain in which nerves send incessant pain signals to the brain. About 60 to 80% of patients are women. The condition usually follows trauma, such as an accident or surgery. The pain, most often involving the arms, hands, legs or feet, can be constant and very severe, affecting daily activities. The condition is difficult to diagnose, and it may be confused with Lyme disease or lupus. It is thought to be caused by nerve injuries that are too small to detect in standard examinations, which measure the flow of electrical impulses along specific nerve pathways. It is also difficult to treat. One therapy involves injecting large doses of ketamine, an anesthetic, which induce a coma. This is thought to block the transmission of pain signals. The treatment is risky, and, even if it relieves pain, in about half of the patients the pain returns. A surgical treatment involves implanting an electrical stimulator in the affected limb or near the spinal cord to send benign impulses at regular intervals along the injured nerve. The patient can turn the stimulator on or off by holding a special magnet over the skin. This treatment, too, may have complications, mainly from infection or electrode malfunction.

regional anesthesia Also *conduction anesthesia, local anesthesia.* Administering an anesthetic that causes a loss of feeling in a particular part of the body by blocking the conduction of pain sensations from that part to the brain. The principal kinds of regional anesthesia used to relieve the pain of childbirth and surgery in the pelvic area are CAUDAL, EPIDURAL, PARACERVICAL, PUDENDAL and SPINAL.

remission The decrease or disappearance of the symptoms and signs of a disease, either spontaneously or in response to medication or other treatment. Also, the period during which this change occurs. The term *remission* ordinarily is reserved for serious illnesses that have a tendency to recur or flare up, such as cancer or multiple sclerosis. Acute temporary ailments are usually said to be "cured."

respiratory distress syndrome See HYALINE MEMBRANE DISEASE.

restless legs syndrome Also, *anxietas tibialis, Ekbom syndrome, hereditary acromelagia, leg jitters.* A neurological disorder in which a person feels intense crawling sensations in the legs and an irresistible urge to move them. Though movement relieves discomfort, symptoms return upon sitting or lying down. Typically occurring after the age of 50 and at night, the syndrome interferes with sleep, sometimes causing severe sleep deprivation, as well as with any prolonged sedentary activity, such as sitting on an airplane. The condition's cause is unknown, but it tends to run in families. It may be due to iron deficiency, which can be detected by blood tests. Even if blood iron levels are normal, there can be iron deficiency in the brain. Individuals with a mild case of restless legs syndrome may find relief through moderate exercise, massage of the legs, hot or cold packs and eliminating intake of caffeine and alcohol. For more severe cases, medi-

cation may be indicated. The best response usually is to medications that act like the neurotransmitter dopamine, principally ropinirole (Requip), pramipexole (Mirapex) or pergolide (Permax). These also are used in Parkinson's disease, but restless legs syndrome is not a form of or precursor to Parkinson's. However, both Permax and another Parkinson's drug, cabergoline (Cabaser, Dostinex), have been linked to heart valve damage ranging from moderate to severe, indicating they probably should not be used. In any event, no one drug seems to work for all cases. Others that may be tried are opioids (painkillers) like codeine, benzodiazepines (tranquilizers) or anticonvulsants.

retarded ejaculation See EJACULATION, def. 3.

Retin-A See ACNE; SKIN CHANGES.

retroflexed uterus A uterus that is doubled back on itself.
See also RETROVERTED UTERUS.

retrograde ejaculation See EJACULATION, def. 4.

retrolental fibroplasia A potentially serious eye condition in PREMATURE infants who are exposed to high concentrations of oxygen during the first few days of life. The premature retina develops abnormally, the extent of abnormality depending on the oxygen concentration and length of exposure. At first the retinal blood vessels proliferate and later fibrosis may develop. In extreme cases the retina becomes detached and partial or total blindness may result. The disease is almost entirely preventable by keeping oxygen concentration below about 30%. When 100% oxygen is needed to resuscitate the baby, which sometimes happens, it should be given for the briefest possible time. Infants with chronic hypoxia (oxygen deprivation) because of HYALINE MEMBRANE DISEASE or some other condition limiting the extraction of oxygen from the air they breathe may need high concentrations of oxygen for several days in order to survive. In such instances their arterial oxygen must be monitored carefully in order to prevent this toxic effect on the retina. A recent study indicates that high doses of vitamin E given to babies who need oxygen within 24 hours of birth greatly reduced the severity of retrolental fibroplasias that did develop, but it is still considered experimental. Dimming the intense lighting used in intensive-care nurseries also may help prevent retinal damage.

retroverted uterus   Also *tipped uterus, tipped womb.* A condition in which the uterus, which usually tilts forward slightly at almost a right angle to the vagina, is instead tilted backward (see UTERUS). It occurs in 25 to 30% of women, most of whom are not even aware of it and require no treatment. Symptoms, when they do occur, usually consist of a vague backache or, in extreme cases, pain during vaginal intercourse (because the uterus is tipped so far that it lies adjacent to the vagina). Often a tipped uterus is congenital, but sometimes it occurs after pregnancy, owing to stretching of ligaments that normally keep it tilted forward, or after multiple infections create scar tissue (adhesions) that in effect pull the uterus back. Endometriosis also can make it adhere to the back. It was formerly believed that a retroverted uterus hindered conception; today women with a retroverted uterus who have trouble becoming pregnant usually are told to try positions for intercourse other than the conventional "missionary" position (with the woman on her back and her partner on top), since in that position the cervix is not bathed in the pool of semen. Pregnancy generally causes the uterus to move forward, although it then returns to its retroverted position after delivery. If it does not move forward, occasionally the cervix locks into the pubic bone and blocks the outlet to the bladder. This problem, called an *incarcerated uterus,* usually occurs during the the third or fourth month of pregnancy and causes considerable difficulty in urinating. It may be corrected by having the clinician press on the back of the uterus through the vagina. If that does not work, a catheter is put through the urethra into the bladder to drain it and remains in place until advancing pregnancy corrects the condition as the uterus grows out of the pelvis. Other than that, treatment is needed only if there is extensive infection or a large FIBROID is distorting the uterus unduly. Often the treatment consists of inserting a PESSARY (ring) into the vagina that, in effect, holds the uterus in a better position. Formerly a retroverted uterus was repaired surgically in an operation called *uterine suspension,* in which the surgeon made an abdominal incision, cut any adhesions and sutured (sewed) the stretched ligaments to the abdominal wall so they could again support the uterus in a forward tilt. Today such surgery is rarely performed.

Rett syndrome   Also *Rett's disorder.* A rare genetic disorder related to autism that affects mainly girls—one in 10,000—and can leave them unable to walk, talk, use their hands and have breathing and other difficulties. After seemingly normal development, the disorder appears some time between the ages of five months and four years. Head growth slows and language and social skills deteriorate. Eventually mental retardation develops, usually severe, and the patient will require full-time care. There is no cure at present, but in 2007 researchers announced that they had been able to reverse the condition in mice by means of genetic engineering, and it is hoped that one day this work will be effective in humans.

rheumatoid arthritis   Also *rheumatism* (pop.). A chronic, progressive, systemic disease, the principal manifestation of which is inflammation of the joints, often accompanied by anemia. It affects approximately 6.5 million Americans and occurs three times as often in women as in men (some studies say eight times). Although it can strike at any age, its onset typically is between the ages of 20 and 45. Progressive joint destruction, pain and decreased mobility can lead to severe crippling and deformity.

Rheumatoid arthritis is the most common form of *synovitis,* that is, inflammation of the synovial membrane lining a joint. Cells in the membrane divide and grow, until the joint appears red, swollen and feels puffy or boggy to the touch. Increased

Rheumatoid Arthritis Damage

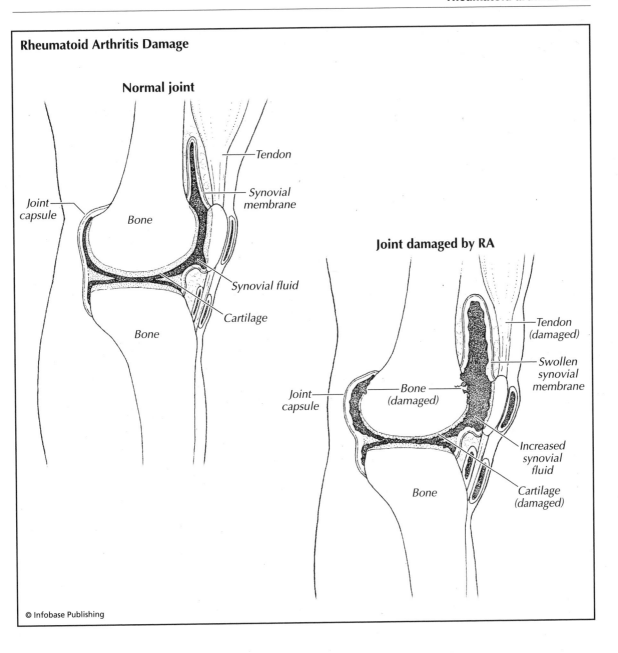

Normal joint

Tendon

Synovial membrane

Joint capsule

Bone

Bone

Synovial fluid

Cartilage

Joint damaged by RA

Tendon (damaged)

Swollen synovial membrane

Joint capsule

Bone (damaged)

Increased synovial fluid

Cartilage (damaged)

Bone

blood flow that is part of the inflammatory process makes the area feel warm. Cells release enzymes into the joint space, and these cause further irritation and pain. If the process continues for years, as it sometimes does, the enzymes gradually may digest the cartilage and bone of the joint, which becomes virtually immobile. Synovial inflamma-

tion also increases the risk for cardiovascular problems; recent research indicates a significantly increased incidence of atherosclerosis and heart attack in rheumatoid arthritis patients.

The earliest symptoms of rheumatoid arthritis are swelling and pain in one or more joints that persist for at least six weeks. The wrists and knuckles are the joints most often afflicted, but the knees and metatarsals (ball of the foot) often are involved as well, and indeed any joint may be affected. Diagnosis is made through two blood tests. One measures high-sensitivity cardiac-specific *C-reactive protein*, which also indicates the risk for cardiovascular disease. The other measures the *erythrocyte sedimentation rate*, which indicates the degree of inflammation. Diagnosis is further aided by measuring the presence and amount of a protein called the *rheumatoid factor*. X-rays are not very useful for diagnosis at the outset, although they can reveal damage to the bone and cartilage and reveal the progress of the disease over time. Other symptoms, in addition to pain in the affected joints, are general muscle aches and fatigue (similar to those of flu or another virus infection, but longer-lasting), muscle stiffness (especially first thing in the morning) and sometimes low fever.

The disease usually takes one of three courses. It may be a single brief illness, lasting a few months at the most and not leading to permanent disability; it may involve several episodes of extreme symptoms, or *flare-ups*, separated by periods of total remission, with little or no physical impairment remaining; or it may become chronic and constant, lasting several years or for life. The last is the most common course of rheumatoid arthritis.

The cause of rheumatoid arthritis is not known, but it is almost certainly an AUTOIMMUNE DISEASE, in which the body's immune system goes awry and it begins to make antibodies against some of its own normal tissues. Since there is no specific cure for rheumatoid arthritis, the patient usually must learn to live with it. Both overexertion and too much rest worsen joint stiffness, so a middle road between enough rest and sufficient exercise must be found. Work with a professional physical therapist to find the right exercise program sometimes is of great benefit. Other treatment consists of administering high doses of aspirin (under medical supervision), which helps both the pain and the inflammation. Other anti-inflammatory agents, such as ibuprofen and indomethacin, also may be used. Their chief side effect is gastrointestinal disturbances, which, if severe enough or if bleeding occurs, means the drug must be stopped. The COX-2 inhibitors avoid this risk but have other side effects (see ANALGESIC), and are currently undergoing further investigation for safety following the 2004 removal of Vioxx from the market.

Two main kinds of medication are used for rheumatoid arthritis. They reduce joint swelling and relieve pain. The first kind are called disease-modifying antirheumatic drugs, or DMARDS; they slow or stop changes in the joints. Some come in oral form (pills), and others are injected. Both kinds suppress the immune system, that is, slowing down the body's attack on itself, leaving one a prey to serious infections. Also, they can take weeks or months to start working, and a pain reliever may be needed until they do. Since some of them can

PRINCIPAL DMARDS			
Generic name	Brand name	Form given	Notes
Hydroxychloroquine	Plaquenil	Pill	
Leflunomide	Arava	Pill	Can cause serious birth defects
Methotrexate	Rheumatrex, Trexall	Pill	Serious birth defects; possible liver, kidney problems; low red blood cell counts; painful mouth sores; avoid during breast-feeding.
Sulfasalazine	Azulfidine, Sulfazine	Pill	
Adalimumab	Humira	Injection	
Anakinra	Kineret	Injection	Does not work as well as other injected DMARDS
Etanercept	Enbrel	Injection	
Abatacept	Orencia	Intravenous	
Infliximab	Remicade	Intravenous	
Rituximab	Rituxan	Intravenous	

cause serious birth defects, it is important to use two kinds of birth control (such as the Pill and a condom) while taking DMARDS.

The second kind are steroids, which help with joint pain and swelling, but it is not known if they can slow down the disease. The steroid most often used is prednisone. It can weaken bones, raise blood sugar, and cause weight gain. Therefore steroids are often prescribed in low doses and for a short time.

The accompanying table lists the principal DMARDS, how they are administered, and their side effects. If one DMARD does not work, switching to another may help, or adding a second kind, or adding prednisone.

Sometimes damaged joints can be restored by orthopedic surgery, such as hip or knee replacement, synovectomy (removal of the diseased synovial membrane) of the knee or knuckles, or resection of the metatarsis (foot). Although such surgery is a major undertaking, in severe cases it may be preferable to some of the stronger experimental drugs or a life of invalidism.

In women, rheumatoid arthritis affects neither the menstrual cycle nor fertility; in fact, pregnancy sometimes brings on a remission or an exacerbation. Delivery may be complicated if the hips or spine are deformed. Oral contraceptives must be used with caution, since rheumatoid arthritis patients have circulatory problems. Intrauterine devices (IUDs) may be inadvisable if a woman is at all anemic, since they may cause heavier menstrual flow. Though sexual response is unaffected, the sex drive may be diminished owing to both pain and fatigue, and deformities and pain may interfere with intercourse in certain positions (as well as with masturbation).

See also OSTEOARTHRITIS.

Rh factor   An ANTIGEN that is present in the red blood cells of most men and women, whose blood is then said to be *Rh-positive*. When it is absent, the blood is said to be *Rh-negative*. If a woman with Rh-negative blood carries an Rh-positive fetus (because the father's blood is Rh-positive), her body may become sensitized and develop antibodies to attack the Rh-positive blood cells in the fetus. This condition is called *Rh incompatibility*. In some cases it occurs when the fetal blood enters the mother's bloodstream via the placenta. More often, however, it occurs during delivery. Either AMNIOCENTESIS or CHORIONIC VILLUS SAMPLING can be used to determine whether a fetus suffers from Rh incompatibility. A promising newer test that carries less risk and yields faster results uses some of the mother's blood to see if the Rh factor in the fetal blood is compatible with the mother's (as early as 14 weeks into pregnancy the mother's blood carries enough of the fetus's DNA for this determination). However, this test is not yet available for general use.

Rh incompatibility occurs in about 0.5% of pregnancies and can result in the death of the fetus from erythroblastosis, a kind of anemia, as early as four months along in the pregnancy. The only way to save a fetus so threatened is to give an exchange transfusion, that is, replace its blood supply with Rh-negative blood that will not react to the mother's antibodies. Formerly such babies were given exchange transfusions immediately after birth, but for many this was too late. In 1963 a New Zealand physician, A. William Liley, developed a way of transfusing the fetus with Rh-negative blood by injecting it directly into the mother's abdomen, a technique so successful that mortality from Rh incompatibility was greatly reduced. More recently another technique of *intrauterine transfusion* was developed in France, whereby blood is administered through the umbilical cord as early as the 18th week of pregnancy. Less risky is the preventive administration of *Rhogam*, an anti-Rh gamma globulin, or vaccine. When injected into an unsensitized Rh-negative mother who has just given birth or who has had a miscarriage or abortion, it prevents her body from forming Rh antibodies that might harm future babies. The vaccine must be given within 72 hours of delivery or abortion in order to be effective.

All pregnant women should be tested for Rh factor, even if they plan to terminate the pregnancy. If a woman is Rh-negative and the father also is Rh-negative, no problem of incompatibility arises; if the father is Rh-positive or paternity is unknown, however, the mother's blood must be tested to see if she has developed any Rh-antibodies. Even if she has never been pregnant before, she may have been sensitized through a blood transfusion using Rh-positive blood. If no antibodies are present, the test should be repeated monthly between the 28th week of pregnancy and delivery to see if antibodies have developed. Should they be present, she then must receive special care through the remainder of the pregnancy. Antibody levels must be checked every month; if they rise significantly an intrauterine fetal transfusion may be performed. AMNIOCENTESIS is performed first to assess the extent of damage to the fetus, which can be evaluated from the level of bilirubin in the amniotic fluid. If the fetus is sufficiently well developed, premature delivery by induction may be considered.

The majority of Rh-negative women have no difficulty in a first pregnancy, but about 10 to 15% become sensitized after one or more pregnancies. For about 90% of those potentially sensitized, injection of Rhogam eliminates all risk in the next pregnancy; however, it must be administered again after every pregnancy, whether ending in delivery, miscarriage or abortion.

rhythm method   See NATURAL FAMILY PLANNING.

rimming   See ANUS.

ripe cervix   The softening of the cervix that occurs near the end of a full-term pregnancy. It may be somewhat dilated (1 to 2 centimeters), show some EFFACEMENT and is usually anterior in position. This condition usually indicates that the cervix would respond favorably to INDUCTION OF LABOR should it be necessary.

rooming-in   The practice of allowing a newborn baby to stay in the same hospital room as its mother instead of in the hospital nursery. Supporters of rooming-in say this practice helps establish successful breast-feeding from the very beginning of life as well as a close bond between mother and baby (see BONDING). Opponents say the mother should have maximum rest after delivery and

therefore should not have to care for the baby so soon. Some favor a compromise, called *modified rooming-in*, in which the baby remains in the mother's room during the day but sleeps in the nursery at night, so the mother can have an uninterrupted eight hours' sleep.

rosacea   A skin disorder that produces persistent redness, bumps or pimples and tiny spidery surface blood vessels, mostly on the central part of the face. It usually appears after age 30, more often in women than men. There are four subtypes of rosacea: (1) characterized by flushing and persistent redness on the face, sometimes accompanied by visible blood vessels (this type does not necessarily progress to more severe forms); (2) resembling acne, with pimples and pustules, often accompanied by persistent redness but without blocked pores; (3) thickened skin, especially at the nose (more common in men); (4) eye irritation, potentially severe enough to threaten sight.

Neither the cause nor a cure for rosacea is known, but treatment is available, best begun as early as possible. Initially a topical antibiotic may be used; for more difficult cases an oral antibiotic such as tetracycline may be used. Laser surgery can eliminate or improve the spidery blood vessels (called *telangiectases*). Eye irritation is usually treated with cleansing and tearing agents, and if necessary, antibiotics and medicated eyedrops. To prevent flare-ups, patients are advised to use sun protection (sunscreen, a hat, sunglasses), and avoid spicy foods, alcohol, caffeine and hot, humid environments.

rubella   Also *German measles, three-day measles.* An infectious disease of childhood that, when contracted by a pregnant woman, can lead to miscarriage, stillbirth or serious birth defects in the baby. The earlier in pregnancy the disease is contracted, the more serious the effects. During the first 12 weeks of gestation the fetus lacks the ability to create antibodies against the rubella virus. Therefore, if the virus is transmitted from the mother's bloodstream to the fetus, it continues to multiply at a much greater rate there. As a result, if the fetus survives early pregnancy at all, it may be born with any or all of the following defects: deafness and other ear abnormalities; cataracts and other eye disorders; brain damage; heart malformations; abnormalities of other internal organs. The danger to the fetus is greatest during the first four weeks, of pregnancy, when some 60% will suffer irreversible damage; 35% will be affected during the second four weeks and only about 10% during the third four weeks. Because of the high risk for the fetus, a woman who contracts rubella during early pregnancy may be advised to seek an abortion, if possible. If legal, religious or medical reasons rule out abortion, she may be given large doses of gamma globulin, though many authorities believe it to be ineffective.

The connection between rubella and birth defects was first observed in 1914, and since 1969 an effective vaccine against rubella has been available. Women who intend to bear children and have not had rubella during childhood (or think they might not have) should definitely be vaccinated at least four months before conception is planned and be sure that all of their older children (if any) have been vaccinated. They also should use a reliable method of birth control during that four-month period. Rubella vaccine is given to babies by itself at the age of 12 months or together with measles and mumps vaccine at 15 months. A simple blood test can determine whether one has antibodies to the virus, resulting from earlier vaccination or infection. The four-month waiting period after vaccination is necessary before conceiving because the vaccine is made from attenuated (weakened) live virus; it is therefore not advisable to vaccinate a woman already pregnant. A woman already pregnant who has neither had rubella nor been vaccinated should make every effort to avoid infection.

Rubella is found everywhere and is endemic in larger cities. Typically the symptoms appear 16 to 18 days following exposure, though the incubation period is anywhere from two to three weeks. In children a rash consisting of pinkish raised spots, lighter than those of regular measles, often is the first sign of illness. They form on the face first and then move rapidly down the body, but since they often fade in a day or so the facial rash may be gone by the time the last of the body rash appears. Slight cold symptoms may accompany the rash. In adolescents and adults the illness is usually more severe. However, unlike measles in adults, rubella usually runs its course in a few days. Most cases are so mild that no treatment (other than aspirin, perhaps) is needed.

Newborn babies with rubella, who acquired it before delivery, may be severely ill. The worst problems are those of infants with extensive red patches caused by bleeding inside the skin, which may be symptomatic of generalized internal bleeding; more than one-third of these babies die within the first year of life. With less severe infection, there may be marked improvement after about six months, when the body finally gets rid of the virus and the child begins to gain weight and grow normally.

Rubin test Also *carbon dioxide test, tubal insufflation.* A procedure long used to detect an obstruction in the fallopian tubes that prevents a woman from becoming pregnant. Carbon dioxide gas is blown into the cervix under pressure carefully monitored with a mercury manometer, which can indicate if the tubes are partly or wholly blocked. The Rubin test is performed in an office or clinic and takes only a few minutes. After the gas has passed through the tubes, it escapes into the surrounding cavity, causing some shoulder pain when the woman sits up. If it cannot pass through because of blockage, it is simply expelled through the vagina. Sometimes the test itself will get rid of an obstruction, clearing the tubes of small bits of scar tissue or mucus. The test cannot, however, define the nature of a tubal problem or provide enough other information, so many clinicians prefer the more accurate findings of HYSTEROSALPINGOGRAPHY.

RU-486 See CONTRAGESTIVE.

S

saddle block anesthesia See SPINAL ANESTHESIA.

safe period See NATURAL FAMILY PLANNING.

safe sex See AIDS.

saline abortion See AMNIOINFUSION.

salpingectomy Surgical removal of one or both fallopian tubes, a procedure usually performed in conjunction with OOPHORECTOMY and/or HYSTERECTOMY. *Unilateral salpingectomy* means removal of one tube, *bilateral salpingectomy* of both. The principal indication for unilateral salpingectomy is the removal of a fetus that has become implanted in the tube rather than the uterus (see ECTOPIC PREGNANCY). In such a case, diagnosis can be confirmed by CULDOCENTESIS or LAPAROSCOPY, and the surgeon then usually removes the affected tube. Sometimes, if the other tube already has been removed because of earlier ectopic pregnancy, the surgeon may try to save the remaining tube by repairing it, but such a procedure often leaves scar tissue or other damage, increasing the risk of yet another tubal pregnancy.

salpingitis Inflammation and/or infection of the fallopian tubes, most often caused either by GONORRHEA or as a sequel of childbirth or abortion. See PELVIC INFLAMMATORY DISEASE.

sanitary napkin Also *sanitary pad, Kotex.* An externally worn pad of absorbent material, designed to soak up menstrual flow. Such napkins were developed during World War I by Kimberly Clark, an American manufacturer of surgical dressings that was looking for a way to use up its surplus cellucotton and marketed it as a sanitary napkin under the brand name Kotex (which has since become a popular name for all such napkins, regardless of brand). Prior to that—and even today, in many parts of the world—women used rags or other pieces of cloth or paper for this purpose.

See also MENSTRUAL CUP; MENSTRUAL SPONGE; TAMPON.

sarcoma A malignant (cancerous) TUMOR made up of closely packed cells embedded in a homogeneous tissue. Sarcomas often are found in connective tissue, such as bone. Though in the pelvic area they are less common than other kinds of malignancy, they can affect the endometrium, ovaries and vagina.

scabies A parasitic skin infection caused by the tiny itch mite *Sarcoptes scabei,* which can be transmitted by sexual contact. The principal symptom is extreme itching, particularly at night, after bathing and after exercise. The most common sites of infection are the hands and arms, feet and ankles, genitals, buttocks and armpits. The female mite burrows into the skin to lay eggs for a week and then dies; sometimes the mites' burrows, fine wavy lines, can be seen, especially on the hands. The eggs hatch into larvae and mature in about 10 days. Scabies is transmitted by skin-to-skin contact, as among members of the same household or during sexual contact. The incubation period is about five weeks. The symptoms are due to an allergic reaction to the mite, so individuals who have been infected before get symptoms sooner. Treatment consists of a single application of permethrin cream (Nix) over the entire body, which should remain in place for at least 12 hours. Lindane cream or lotion (Kwell) also is effective but should be avoided for treating infants or pregnant or breastfeeding women. Itching may persist for some days or even weeks but constitutes the aftermath of allergy; the treatment need not be repeated. Applying calamine or aloe vera lotion may help, as may an antihistamine. Towels, clothing and bed linens used for the previous two weeks should be washed or dry-cleaned to kill any residual mites or larvae.

scan, scanning See CAT SCAN; MAGNETIC RESONANCE IMAGER; RADIONUCLIDE IMAGING.

scanty flow Exceptionally light bleeding during regular menstrual periods.

See also MENSTRUAL FLOW.

Schiller test A diagnostic test for vaginal or cervical cancer. The cervix and vaginal walls are coated with an iodine solution (Schiller's stain or Lugol's solution), which stains normal cells brown but is not absorbed by abnormal cells, which remain pink (or sometimes yellow or white). If abnormal tissue is revealed in this way, it is usually further examined by COLPOSCOPY, and some is removed for biopsy to determine its nature. The solution stains clothing, so a sanitary pad should be worn after this test.

schizophrenia A group of serious emotional disorders of unknown cause that are characterized by disturbances of thought, mood and behavior. Typically the schizophrenic patient seems withdrawn and isolated, emotionally detached from other people. His or her fundamental perceptions of reality are fragmented and distorted. Hallucinations, especially auditory (hearing imaginary voices), are common, as are delusions of persecution. Behavior varies. It may be torpid, silent and apathetic, or very agitated. Moreover, symptoms vary in severity, from mild to very severe.

There is considerable disagreement about all aspects of schizophrenia, including its causes, classification, treatment and outcome. However, most authorities today agree that it involves both biochemical and genetic factors. Some cases seem to cure themselves spontaneously; most, however, become chronic and may be crippling. Treatment includes a variety of drugs, principally potent antipsychotic agents, as well as various forms of psychotherapy, counseling and social management.

scleroderma Also *systemic sclerosis*. A disease involving the connective tissue and blood vessels that may cause widespread hardness of the skin and other organs. Four times more common in women than in men, it typically strikes between the ages of 20 and 50, although children also can be affected. Scleroderma appears to be an AUTOIMMUNE DISEASE involving dysfunction of the vascular system, although the cause is still unknown. Exposure to certain chemicals can cause conditions similar to scleroderma, and leakage from silicone breast implants may have this effect, although evidence is far from conclusive. There are two forms of scleroderma: localized, which affects mostly the skin, and systemic, which includes scarring and blood vessel damage in the skin, lungs, esophagus, heart and kidneys. It also can slow motility in the gastrointestinal tract and cause arthritis, muscle inflammation, dry eyes and dry mouth. Patients with systemic scleroderma eventually suffocate or starve to death. Most patients have cold-induced spasms of small blood vessels in their hands and feet, known as RAYNAUD'S PHENOMENON. Diagnosis is based on clinical symptoms and findings, which can be confirmed by a skin biopsy. At present there is no cure, and treatment is directed most at relieving symptoms. Physical therapy can help joint disability; corticosteroids can as well but have been found to worsen kidney problems and high blood pressure. Cancer drugs such as methotrexate often combat scarring in the lungs, and the cancer drug cyclophosphamide (Cytoxan) has been shown to slow skin thickening and lung function deterioration, but to a limited extent. ACE inhibitors (high blood pressure medications) can reverse kidney damage and THALIDOMIDE may retard scarring. Nifedipine, a calcium channel blocker, may help control Raynaud's phenomenon. A genetically engineered hormone called Relaxin allows the skin to stretch by boosting collagenase and decreasing collagen. Among the avenues being explored is the use of stem cell transplants, a variant of bone marrow transplants.

Research is also looking into causes. Because the disorder affects more women than men, and mostly women who have borne children, some speculate that cells from a woman's fetus may continue to circulate in her bloodstream and somehow affect her immune system, and indeed scleroderma patients do have higher levels of such cells. Other research is focusing on finding a scleroderma gene.

sclerosing adenosis A benign (noncancerous) lesion, often found in the breasts of relatively young women (during the childbearing years), that consists of distorted tissue of the ACINI. It is perfectly harmless but sometimes is difficult to distinguish from a malignant tumor, so to rule out cancer with certainty it usually is excised (cut out) for biopsy.

sclerotherapy   See VARICOSE VEIN.

scoliosis A progressive lateral curvature of the spine that is four or five times more common in women than in men and most often begins at puberty, between the ages of 11 and 15. As the condition progresses, it contracts the ribs and compresses the lungs and heart, restricting breathing and circulation. It also may cause degenerative disease of the spine, leading to osteoarthritis, disk problems and sciatica. Eventually, without treatment, it is possible for scoliosis to cause total invalidism and death.

About 10% of American adolescents have scoliosis. Of these, about one-fourth require medical attention of some kind, ranging from observation for future progression of the curvature to the use of a brace or surgery, depending on how advanced the curvature is at the time it is first detected. The earliest detectable symptoms are the protrusion of one shoulder blade, one hip looking higher or more prominent than the other, clothing hanging unevenly, an odd gait and a slight thickening on one side of the neck.

There are many causes for the development of scoliosis, including various nerve and muscle disorders, diseases such as poliomyelitis and abnormal development of the vertebrae. However, 80 to 90% of the cases are idiopathic—that is, no cause can be determined. Scoliosis tends to run in families and so may be genetic, but it is not known what triggers the development of the curvature or why some curves progress more than others. Scoliosis occurs in otherwise perfectly healthy individuals. Because it may appear at any time during the growing years and is painless in its early stages, it is important to check a child's spine regularly until growth is complete, especially during the rapid growth spurt of the early teen years. The easiest way to check is to have the child stand and bend forward, with the arms hanging down loosely and palms touching at about knee level. In this position, either one shoulder higher than the other *or* a curve of the vertebrae, which are very prominent, is cause for suspicion. Lordosis (swayback) and kyphosis (humpback), in which the spine curves abnormally toward the front or the back, also are indications for further checking. Some cases of scoliosis are mild enough to require no treatment. For adolescents whose curves range beyond 25 to 30%, some kind of treatment is indicated, most often a spinal brace that keeps the curve from progressing. The brace is worn 23 hours a day for two to three years, and daily exercises generally are advised. More drastic treatment involves spinal fusion or other surgery. Because early detection is so helpful, school-based screening programs, which can be carried out by school nurses, physical education instructors and volunteers who have some training, are highly recommended and have become mandatory in some localities.

scopolamine A hypnotic drug that induces amnesia and for years was given during LABOR

Common Kinds of Scoliosis

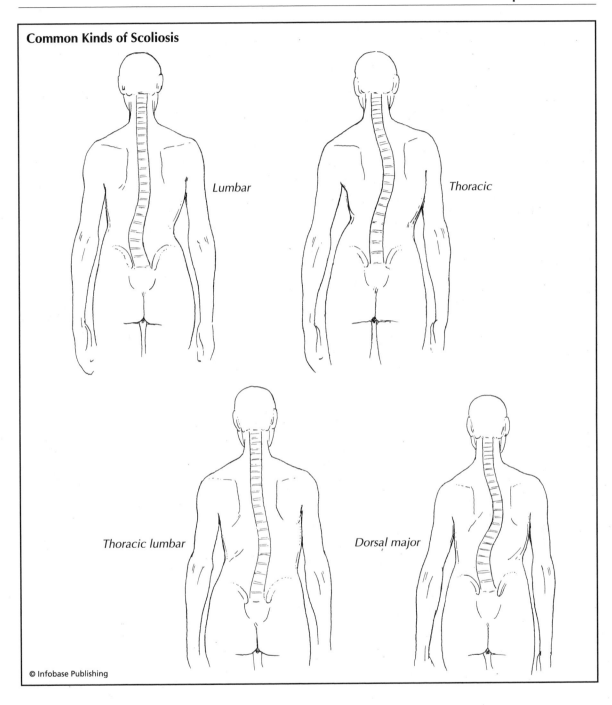

Lumbar

Thoracic

Thoracic lumbar

Dorsal major

to make a woman forget its pain afterward. Usually it was administered together with various narcotic drugs for their analgesic (pain-relieving) and euphoric effects, and sometimes also with barbiturates. Scopolamine induces a kind of "twilight sleep." However, it causes some restlessness as well and sometimes even hallucinations and delirium. Therefore, a woman given scopolamine requires constant observation by a trained attendant, and she cannot cooperate in her labor or use any relaxation techniques. Its effect on babies has never been evaluated satisfactorily, and today it has been largely replaced by narcotics, especially meperidine (Demerol), sometimes combined with tranquilizers to produce analgesia and sedation. A newer use of scopolamine, administered in low doses to be absorbed through the skin, is to combat severe motion sickness in adults.

scrotum   A two-chambered sac of thin, wrinkled skin that hangs between and slightly in front of a man's thighs, behind the PENIS. After puberty it is covered with pubic hair. Inside the scrotum are the testes (see TESTIS). The scrotum itself is sensitive to sexual stimulation and to temperature change. In cold weather muscles in the scrotal wall contract to bring the testes closer to the body (for warmth).

seasonal affective disorder   Also *SAD*.
See DEPRESSION, def. 3.

sebaceous cyst   See CYST, def. 2.

secondary sex characteristics   The external physical characteristics that distinguish women from men, which are the result of increased levels of different sex hormones (estrogen in women, androgens in men).
See also PUBERTY.

secretory phase   The latter portion of the normal MENSTRUAL CYCLE, when estrogen and progesterone stimulate the uterine glands to secrete life-supporting substances in preparation for the implantation and nurture of a fertilized egg (pregnancy). If an egg actually is implanted, the secretions continue to be produced. If conception does not occur, progesterone and estrogen levels drop sharply and the endometrium (uterine lining), unable to support

the growth that took place in preparation for pregnancy, breaks down and is shed as menstrual flow.
See also PROLIFERATIVE PHASE.

selective estrogen-receptor modulator   Also *designer estrogen; SERM.* A synthetic compound that stimulates certain of the body's estrogen receptors, duplicating estrogen's activity in some tissues but not in others. Among them are tamoxifen, a compound that blocks estrogen's effects on the breast and breast cancer but acts like estrogen in increasing bone density and raising HDL (high-density lipoproteins, the good cholesterol). It is used to treat estrogen-dependent breast cancer. Another is raloxifene (Evista), used post-menopausally to counter vaginal dryness and hot flashes, and help prevent osteoporosis; it lowers LDL (low-density lipoproteins, the bad cholesterol) but does not raise HDL, and it appears to reduce the risk of endometrial and breast cancers. Numerous other such compounds are being developed and tested in the hope of finding one that will have all of the good effects of natural estrogen (preventing bone loss) and none of the bad ones (triggering cancers).
See also ESTROGEN.

self-help   Routine gynecologic care, involving breast and pelvic examination, simple laboratory tests, fitting and insertion of birth control devices and similar procedures, carried on in a group setting where women are encouraged to participate in their own health care. The development of the self-help movement in North America began in the late 1960s, when a small but growing number of women rebelled against the male-dominated profession of gynecology. Gynecologists, they felt, tended to regard routine care in the same way as acute illness, that is, with the authoritative professional making all basic decisions for a passive, dependent, uninformed woman patient. In contrast, women involved in the self-help movement wanted to take charge of their own routine care themselves, exchanging knowledge and expertise with one another in a group setting, usually taking the form of a *self-help clinic,* in which health care providers—physicians, nurse-practitioners, nurses—encourage them to share in observing, advising, treating and being treated. In such a setting women met in groups to discuss their common health concerns and learn to know their bodies better. With the guidance of professionals they learned to perform pelvic examinations on themselves and each other, using a speculum, hand mirror and lamp, and to recognize early signs of vaginal infection, venereal disease and pregnancy as well as to check the position of diaphragm or IUD. They also learned breast self-examination, and some undertook pregnancy testing and other simple laboratory work.

As self-help groups and clinics grew in number, they varied somewhat in their approach. Most clinics recognized the need to integrate the self-help approach with technical expertise and established their own gynecology and obstetrics services.

Self-help is not a new concept. Up to the early 1800s most women cared for themselves and their families with little or no professional advice, using herbs and household remedies passed down to them from mothers and grandmothers. Those women who proved to be particularly skillful often helped their neighbors as well. In 1790 in America there was approximately one trained physician for every 10 such "domestic practitioners." Only during the next century did medicine—especially gynecology and obstetrics—become a formal profession. By the late 19th century there were several hundred medical schools in America. Most of them were proprietary, meaning any man could take a course of lectures by paying a fee; no women were admitted. Then licensing laws began to be enacted and stricter standards for training and practice were established. These brought to an end the practice of domestic medicine and the role of women as healers, at least outside their own immediate families, and early in the 20th century they also brought to an end the proprietary medical schools, which were replaced with medical schools on the European model. During the next two decades the rapidly growing medical profession cracked down on patent medicines and quackery of various kinds, which competed with their services. Simple home remedies and patent medicines alike were replaced with newly developed drugs and treatments, available only by prescription from licensed physicians.

The feminist movement in the 1960s, with its consciousness-raising groups, soon gave rise to discussions of women's health problems and health care. As women talked together about their innermost concerns, they often discovered a common ground of experience with health care. Using the services of physicians when they were not actually ill—seeking routine checkups, contraceptives, abortions and obstetrical care—they still were treated as "patients" and often were kept in ignorance of their condition, or treated patronizingly or condescendingly. It was this aspect of their experience that led some of them to seek alternative kinds of care, giving birth to the modern self-help movement. About 1970, self-help clinics for women's health care began to be formed, and in the next few years hundreds of them were established. By the following decade the self-help movement, although still small and involving principally white, middle-class American women, had through its educational role alone exerted some influence on the American health care system, which gradually seemed to be becoming more sensitive to women's needs. Today self-help clinics are also known as *women's* or *feminist health centers/clinics*. In most the emphasis is more on a caring environment in which information is shared, but the clinical work is in the hands of trained nurses and practitioners. The independent self-help groups are now largely *support groups* in which women share their experiences with various disorders, therapies (including alternative therapies), mental health and lifestyle problems such as those experienced by parents of schizophrenics, new mothers and the like.

See also CANCER SUPPORT GROUP. For resources for women with specific problems, see the Appendix.

semen   Also *seminal fluid*. The fluid discharged when a man reaches orgasm and ejaculates. It consists of gland secretions and sperm. For semen analysis, see under SPERM.

See also EJACULATION; PENIS.

senile vaginitis   See VAGINAL ATROPHY; also VAGINITIS.

sentinel node biopsy A technique for staging breast cancer, that is, seeing how far it has spread (see STAGING). Instead of removing a number of lymph nodes, which tend to be the first place to which breast cancer spreads, radioactive and blue dyes are injected at the site of the tumor. By following their path, the sentinel lymph node—the one that first receives drainage from a tumor—is located. If this node contains no cancer cells, it is assumed that the remaining nodes also do not. (Some practitioners remove any node that absorbs the dye.) A less invasive procedure that eliminates the pain and other postoperative complications of standard lymph node dissection, sentinel node biopsy appears to be just as reliable.

See also CANCER, BREAST.

septic abortion **1.** A miscarriage caused by infection in the pelvis, resulting from pelvic inflammatory disease, an intrauterine device or some other cause. See MISCARRIAGE, def. 6.

2. An elective abortion that was improperly performed, resulting in infection, hemorrhage or both. See ABORTION.

SERM Abbreviation for SELECTIVE ESTROGEN-RECEPTOR MODULATOR.

serologic test, serum See BLOOD TEST.

serotonin poisoning Also *serotonin syndrome.* A toxic reaction to a combination of drugs or to an overdose of some drugs that raise the amount of the neurotransmitter serotonin to life-threatening levels. Symptoms include confusion, disorientation, agitation, irritability, unresponsiveness, anxiety, muscle spasms and rigidity, loss of coordination, tremors, shivering, fever, profuse sweating, rapid heart rate, raised blood pressure and dilated pupils. These signs occur in any number of other diseases, making the condition difficult to diagnose. Moreover, a huge number of drugs can trigger the syndrome. A frequent trigger is the combination of a powerful ANTIDEPRESSANT such as an SSRI with another serotonin-raising substance, especially an antipsychotic drug. The condition can occur at any age and can occur even weeks after a serotonin-raising drug has been stopped (since some of these drugs remain active in the body for weeks). The most important form of prevention is notifying one's doctor of all drugs one regularly takes, both prescription and over-the-counter. Once the syndrome occurs, it is crucial to stop drugs immediately and seek emergency care. In most cases treatment of such symptoms as fever and increased blood pressure will suffice. More severe cases call for sedation and medication that inhibits serotonin.

sex, determination of The establishment of a baby's sex, which depends on whether the particular sperm responsible for fertilization carried, after dividing, an X (girl) or Y (boy) sex chromosome (see GENETICS). In 1987 researchers announced they had found the particular gene responsible, which they called *testis determining factor* and which resides on the Y chromosome. The chances for either sex are believed to be about equal (50%). Over the years numerous theories and techniques have been developed concerning possibilities of increasing the chances of conceiving a child of the desired sex. (Some couples try to choose their child's sex for medical reasons, mainly to avoid the risk of an inherited sex-linked disorder.) According to one recent system that claims an 80 to 85% chance of success, to conceive a boy intercourse should take place a few hours before or just at the time of OVULATION; before intercourse the woman should use an alkaline douche (2 to 3 tablespoons of baking soda per quart of water); the penis should penetrate deep into the vagina at ejaculation; and the woman should experience orgasm. For a girl baby, the last intercourse should take place 2 to 3 days before ovulation, preceded by an acid douche (2 tablespoons vinegar per quart of water); the penis should not penetrate too deeply at ejaculation; and the woman should not try to achieve orgasm. A technique offered by a number of fertility clinics in the United States and Canada, as well by some private practitioners, involves filtering the semen so as to remove most of the X chromosomes, thereby increasing the chances of producing a male to about 75%. The filtered semen is then introduced by artificial insemination. Invented by Ronald Ericsson, a physiologist, it relies on the principle that sperm carrying Y chromosomes move faster through a viscous liquid than those carrying X chromosomes. However, the procedure is not officially endorsed, has never undergone controlled clinical trials and is considered of questionable validity by some researchers. The most recent methods of sex selection require in vitro fertilization. With one kind, the embryos are tested for sex before being placed in the uterus and the parents may decide if they want only those of one sex or the other. Pregnancy is not guaranteed, and the entire procedure can cost $20,000 or more. Another method, used before the eggs are fertilized, involves sorting sperm by means of a system called MicroSort. Semen usually has equal numbers of female- and male-producing sperm cells, but the system can shift the ratio to either 88% female or 73% male. Not widely available, it costs $4,000 to $6,000 for the sorting alone and accepts only parents who have a genetic disorder or request family balancing. It is not available for a first baby. Couples who undergo IN VITRO FERTILIZATION and are at risk for passing on certain sex-linked genetic disorders may consider preimplantation genetic diagnosis, in which embryos are tested for the disease gene before being implanted. Even though such testing is done very early, when the embryos consist of just eight cells, it is opposed by those who feel rejecting embryos is equivalent to throwing away potential babies. Most professional groups oppose sex selection, but one, the American Society for Reproductive Medicine, does not oppose sperm sorting, which does not involve discarding embryos of the "wrong" sex.

sex therapy   A form of short-term therapy dealing with male and female sexual problems that usually are solely psychological but sometimes occur in conjunction with organic disorders. The main medical problems that may contribute to SEXUAL DYSFUNCTION are diabetes, hypertension, hormonal prob-

lems, alcoholism, side effects of medication, and the aftermath of treatment for various kinds of cancer.

Sex therapy is behaviorist in approach, that is, it focuses principally on changing behavior rather than delving into its underlying causes. A therapist may treat an individual or, more often, a couple. The treatment includes taking a detailed history of the individual's or couple's sex life, a thorough explanation of the anatomy and physiology of the sex organs and of sexual response and, often, a series of exercises for the couple to perform at home in order to change their behavior. These exercises help a couple to concentrate on gentle forms of touching and caressing in order to discover what they enjoy and find arousing (what pioneer sex therapists William Masters and Virginia Johnson called "sensate focus exercises"; see also SEXUAL RESPONSE). Their goal is to reduce anxiety and increase pleasure, in place of feeling that one must live up to some mythical standard of "performance." This approach appears to work well both for women unable to achieve orgasm and for men who cannot achieve or sustain an erection (see FRIGIDITY; IMPOTENCE) or who ejaculate prematurely. For sexual problems that have deeper emotional origins, therapists tend to use a psychosexual approach, which combines behavioral tasks with psychodynamic exploration. Survivors of cancer therapies often have a diminished sense of self-worth as well as some physiological problems resulting from their treatment. Sex therapists can guide them and their partners, helping them overcome both physical and emotional obstacles to sexual intimacy and enjoyment.

Until about 1960 a couple who had difficulty with sex could seek counsel from a family doctor, gynecologist or psychotherapist. Sex therapy as such is still a relatively new field, and as the work of Masters and Johnson, Helen Singer Kaplan and other researchers became known, numerous individuals, some well qualified and others totally unqualified, set themselves up in practice. Its very nature makes sex therapy readily open to abuse by unscrupulous and/or unqualified practitioners. Also, standards for licensing are not well established. The best way to find a reputable practitioner is through the American Association of Sex Education Counselors and Therapists, a national association that has established requirements for certification and publishes a national register (available from it or in many libraries; see Appendix). Suggestions for surgery of some kind on the genital area (such as opening the HYMEN) should never be accepted without seeking at least two other medical opinions. Further, reputable therapists *never* engage in sexual relations or exercises of any kind *with* their clients, nor do they urge clients to engage in practices that might seem morally questionable (for example, observing sex acts, partner swapping, group sex, surrogate therapy or indiscriminate choice of many partners).

sexual dysfunction   A disturbance or disorder that frequently or always prevents an individual from engaging in satisfactory sexual intercourse. Such dysfunctions may arise anywhere in the cycle of desire-arousal-orgasm (see also SEXUAL RESPONSE). A disorder of the desire phase is often described as a man's or woman's low LIBIDO, that is, lack of interest in or desire to experience sexual relations. Disturbances of the arousal phase in a man result in difficulty in achieving and/or maintaining an erection (see also IMPOTENCE); in women it results in difficulty in becoming excited and achieving vaginal lubrication during sexual activity. Disorders of the orgasm phase in men include premature or retarded ejaculation (see EJACULATION) and in women failure to reach ORGASM. Another female sexual dysfunction is VAGINISMUS, making penile penetration difficult and painful, but this condition is much rarer than the other dysfunctions. The most common condition, experienced by an estimated 30 to 60% of women—understandably statistics in this area are not very accurate—is failure to reach orgasm during vaginal intercourse, although they can experience orgasm with a partner by other means. The second most common problem is failure to reach orgasm with a partner, although they can achieve it with masturbation. Only about 9% of adult women are preorgastic, that is, have never experienced orgasm (see also FRIGIDITY). The most common dysfunction in men is premature ejaculation, experienced by about 25%.

An often overlooked cause of sexual dysfunction is a side effect of psychoactive drugs, especially with long-term use, which can involve decreased or lost sexual desire, inability to achieve an erection or ejaculation and delayed or blocked orgasm. Tricyclic ANTIDEPRESSANTS and selective serotonin reuptake inhibitors like Prozac are often implicated. Blood pressure medication (diuretics, beta-blockers, etc.) can cause reduced libido and difficulty in reaching orgasm. Cancer therapy can cause vaginal dryness, reduced libido, and difficulty reaching orgasm. Numerous physical conditions also may be at fault, among them estrogen insufficiency; diabetes; thyroid, adrenal, and pituitary disorders; sickle-cell anemia; spinal cord damage, stroke and Parkinson's; endometriosis; arthritis; and Sjögren's syndrome. Although Viagra (sildenafil citrate) has been very helpful to men, it has proved to be less so for women. Small doses of TESTOSTERONE do enhance libido.

See also SEX THERAPY.

sexually transmitted disease   Also *STD, venereal disease, VD.* An infection that is, for the most part, transmitted by sexual contact between two persons. Recent studies show that women are twice as likely as men to contract an STD. Despite the development of powerful new antibacterial agents during the second half of the 20th century, the incidence of certain STDs—especially gonorrhea and chlamydia infection—has been increasing in the United States and Canada at an alarming rate. Most attack the genital-urinary tract, with which the infecting organisms originally come in contact, but some, notably gonorrhea and syphilis, can attack and damage other organs, such as the heart. The principal venereal diseases are AIDS, GONORRHEA, SYPHILIS HERPES INFECTION, CHANCROID, PUBIC LICE, HEPATITIS B, CHLAMYDIA INFECTION, LYMPHOGRANULOMA VENEREUM, GRANULOMA INGUINALE and CONDYLOMA ACUMINATA. It is possible to be infected with more than one of them (for example, gonorrhea and syphilis) at the same time. In addition, SCABIES, TRICHOMONAS, UREAPLASMA, nonspecific URETHRITIS, nonspecific VAGINITIS, bacterial VAGINOSIS and CYSTITIS all may be transmitted by sexual contact, as may various intestinal infections (viral, parasitic and bacterial), principally through anal sex.

Because sexually transmitted disease is associated with sexual promiscuity (relations with many different partners), a sense of shame, embarrassment and other feelings resulting from religious and cultural taboos often prevent its early detection and treatment. Further, some of the sexually transmitted diseases, notably gonorrhea and chlamydia, can be virtually without symptoms in one or both partners, who then unwittingly pass on the infection. Pregnant women also can infect their babies. As with most infectious diseases, prevention is the best control. Measures that may reduce the chances of infection, especially if used in combination, are

For men: 1. Use of a condom during vaginal and anal intercourse. 2. Washing the genitals before and, even more important, right after sex, with soap and water.

For women: Use of a diaphragm or female condom with spermicidal jelly, cream or foam, and use of these spermicides in the anus for anal intercourse. The cervical cap and use of spermicides alone also afford some protection.

For both sexes, selectivity of choice in sex partners is a preventive measure; the more different partners one has, the higher the risk of infection. If one is sexually active with several partners and has any reason to suspect exposure to infection, an STD test is recommended every three to six months. Tests are performed free of charge in most localities by numerous clinics and other facilities, which can be found by calling the local public health department.

Suspicious signs on one's own body or one's partners' include sores, redness, unusual discharge, itchiness or a foul smell in the genital area. Should these be present, avoid sexual relations until they have been checked or at least be sure of protection with a condom and/or diaphragm and spermicides. Although spermicidal jellies, creams and foams do kill some sexually transmitted organisms, oral contraceptives do not (some authorities believe they may even create a favorable environment for gonococcus growth), and use of an IUD may increase the risk of gonorrheal infection. Also, couples who engage in anal sex should be alert for symptoms such as rectal pain and burning, disturbance in bowel function (looseness or painful defecation),

passage of mucus and rectal bleeding. Although the risk of transmitting an STD in sex between women is much lower, it is not nonexistent. Many women who are currently lesbians may have been in the past (or currently are) involved with men and may harbor symptomless STDs, which they can pass on to their partners.

sexual response   A biochemical and physiological process that occurs in both men and women after puberty. Although it presumably has been experienced by countless human beings since human life began on earth, it was not clinically analyzed until the late 19th century, beginning with the work of Henry Havelock Ellis (1859–1939). Great strides were made in the 1940s and 1950s by Alfred C. Kinsey and his associates and in the 1960s by William Masters and Virginia Johnson. It was Masters and Johnson who actually observed many of the couples they studied under laboratory conditions and who discovered that sexual response is divided into four phases: excitement, plateau, orgasm and resolution. There is no real break as a person passes from one phase to another, and each phase varies in duration from occasion to occasion. The same sequence occurs in both men and women, no matter whether they are masturbating or engaging in homosexual or heterosexual relations. There is, however, a considerable difference between men and women in the time it takes to reach orgasm. The average man, proceeding without interruption, ejaculates within three minutes, whereas the average woman, proceeding at her normal pace, takes about 15 minutes to reach orgasm.

The *excitement phase* can be activated by an enormous variety of stimuli—pictures, sounds, colors, music, smells, thoughts, daydreams—all of which can trigger sexual arousal. Direct touching of breasts, nipples, thighs and genitals can be exciting for both the person doing it and the one being touched. The body responds in a variety of ways. Both the heart rate and breathing increase. The skin may flush. The breasts enlarge, and the nipples become erect. Both women and men experience genital vasocongestion (the dilation of arteries in the genital area), causing an ERECTION.

In women the first physical response is usually the secretion of a lubricating fluid by the vaginal lining, which after a few minutes is felt as wetness near the vaginal entrance. The uterus moves upward into the pelvis, in effect lengthening the vagina. In men the penis becomes hard and stiff (erection).

As sexual stimulation continues, the *plateau phase* follows. Here vasocongestion gradually reaches its peak in both men and women. Heart and breathing rates increase still more. Muscle contraction and congestion in the pelvis increase. The CLITORIS becomes very sensitive and retracts (draws back) under its hood. Stimulation of the inner LABIA causes stimulation of the clitoris by moving the hood back and forth over it. The vaginal opening swells, making the actual opening smaller; when the penis finally enters the vagina, this provides a gripping sensation for it. In men the testes become engorged and draw back up to the base of the penis.

The plateau phase finally reaches a peak, resulting in *orgasm*, a sudden, almost seizurelike release of muscle tension and congestion. The muscles of the vaginal opening contract and relax in a rhythmic fashion; in men contractions of the seminal vesicles and prostate gland push the semen into the urethra, where the muscles of the penis forcefully expel it. (See also ORGASM.)

Orgasm is followed by *resolution*. The blood flow is released and the erect tissues lose their stiffness. If there is no further stimulation, the congestion subsides and the body gradually returns to its unaroused state. Men return to a low level of sexual tension rather quickly. While a woman can respond to continued sexual stimulation immediately and have another orgasm soon afterward, a man requires a period for recovery—the refractory period—ranging from a few minutes to hours, depending on the individual and his age. Moreover, women can continue to have orgasm after orgasm. Resolution is accompanied by a sense of relaxation and satisfaction, of general well-being.

The physical changes of sexual response are controlled by the autonomic nervous system and involve involuntary muscles. However, mental processes under conscious control (thoughts, fantasies, feelings) also play a role, making a person receptive to the sexual stimulation that will set the sequence of responses in motion. Moreover, this sequence, once begun, is not inevitable; it can be interrupted at almost any point (by a telephone call, a negative thought such as fear of pregnancy, etc.) so that arousal subsides. Practically the only point of no return is just before ejaculation for the man; once the seminal vesicles and prostate gland propel semen into the urethra, ejaculation cannot be delayed.

Sheehan's disease Necrosis (tissue death) of the anterior lobe of the pituitary gland following a very difficult labor or delivery, involving postpartum hemorrhage and/or shock. It is named for H. L. Sheehan, the physician who first described it. The earliest symptoms are failure to lactate (produce breast milk) and subsequent amenorrhea (no resumption of menstruation). Other signs are shrinking of vaginal tissue and weight gain. Progressively the patient loses her pubic and axillary hair and then begins to lose weight markedly. Undiagnosed, the disease can end in death. The principal treatment is replacement of needed hormones. In mild cases the patient may sometimes become pregnant again, which occasionally results in considerable improvement; a pregnancy apparently stimulates the pituitary gland to grow and function better.

shingles A viral infection of nerve cells that causes painful fluid-filled blisters along the paths of the affected nerves. It is caused by the same virus responsible for chicken pox, *Varicella zoster* (herpes zoster), which is harbored in the nerve cells, dormant for many years. Then, usually after the age of 50, it is reactivated, producing sensitivity or tingling in the affected nerves and sometimes excruciating pain. The first signs usually are itching, burning or pain along one side of the body, often the chest, followed by a rash similar to that of chicken pox. Shingles almost always affects only one side of the body; it is particularly problematic if it affects the skin around the eye. The blisters crust and scab in a few days, and pain and rash usually disappear in a few weeks. However, some individuals continue to have pain in the area for months or even longer, a condition called *postherpetic neuralgia*, which tends to persist particularly in women.

Until recently the only preventive measure was a vaccine against chicken pox, effective only in persons who never had this infectious disease, which can be determined by a blood test. The vaccine is given in two doses, four to eight weeks apart.

In 2006 the FDA approved a vaccine for shingles, which appeared to be effective and safe in patients aged 60 and older, when the likelihood of contracting shingles greatly increases. The government recommends administering the vaccine, Zostavax, routinely from age 60 on. It appears to prevent shingles in half of those who receive it, but is not generally given to those who have had a prior attack of shingles.

The treatment of choice for shingles, other than oral analgesics for the acute pain and cool compresses or lotions such as calamine for the blisters, is an oral antiviral agent such as acyclovir (Zovirax), valacyclovir (Valtrex) or famcylovir (Famvir). Given early, it may lessen the severity of the attack and also decreases the risk of postherpetic neuralgia. Should that condition occur, it is treated like other kinds of CHRONIC PAIN.

shoulder presentation In childbirth, the position of the baby when one of its shoulders is the presenting part, that is, the part that leads the baby's descent into the birth canal. It occurs when the baby lies in *transverse position,* crosswise in the uterus. Shoulder presentation occurs in approximately 1 of every 200 deliveries. The diagnosis is readily made, often just by looking at the mother's abdomen, which appears very wide from side to side. In the course of labor one shoulder generally becomes tightly wedged in the pelvic canal, and often the baby's hand and arm prolapse through the vagina.

The spontaneous birth of a fully developed baby in transverse position is practically impossible, since it cannot emerge unless both its head and trunk enter the pelvis at the same time. Even if the baby can be delivered vaginally, which may be possible with a very small baby and a very large pelvis, the risk is very high (30% of full-term infants

die), chiefly because of the risk of prolapse of the umbilical cord, injury associated with version (turning) and extraction, and lack of oxygen. For a first baby, therefore, if the baby is in transverse lie at the onset of labor a Cesarean section is indicated. External version (turning the baby by manipulating the abdomen from the outside) may be tried late in pregnancy and again early in labor, but often the baby will turn back again. If during early labor the head can be brought down into the pelvis by abdominal manipulation and held there during the next half-dozen contractions, it may remain there, enabling vaginal delivery. If this measure fails or if the membranes ruptured before labor began, a Cesarean may be the only safe procedure.

shrinkage See HEIGHT LOSS.

sickle-cell disease A group of genetic disorders that affect primarily blacks, both men and women, and pose particular health problems for women. They include *sickle-cell anemia, sickle C disease* and *sickle thalassemia,* and they are associated with resistance to malaria, a disease long endemic in those parts of the world where sickle-cell disease is most common. Sickle-cell anemia, the most common of these disorders in North America, affects one in 375 African Americans born in the United States and smaller proportions of children in other ethnic groups. The U.S. Preventive Services Task Force recommends screening for sickle-cell disease in all newborns, since early detection followed by prophylactic oral penicillin substantially reduces the risk of serious infections during the first few years of life. Sickle-cell anemia is characterized by the presence of red blood cells that are sickled (or crescent-shaped) so that they are unable to pass through small arterioles and capillaries (small blood vessels). Accumulations of sickled red blood cells lead to the formation of thrombi (blood clots) and infarcts (tissue that dies because not enough oxygen has reached it), with a potential risk of damage to internal organs, kidney failure, stroke and life-threatening infections. Those sickled cells that can flow through the circulatory system are more fragile than normal red blood cells and break down easily, causing severe anemia. The main symptoms of sickle-cell anemia are extremely painful joints, episodes of acute abdominal pain and ulceration in the lower extremities (legs). The disease usually appears during a baby's first year and is progressive. No cure is yet known, and victims rarely survive beyond the age of 50 (many die earlier). Attacks are treated with fluids, pain relievers, oxygen and sometimes antibiotics. Recently the cancer drug hydroxyurea was approved as a treatment. It does not cure the disease but reduces the excruciating attacks and cuts hospital time, the need for blood transfusions and the occurrence of life-threatening complications such as stroke. However, it could dangerously lower a patient's white blood cell count, raising vulnerability to infection. Another promising approach, at this writing, is transplanting healthy stem cells from the umbilical cord of a newborn baby. In addition, a number of drugs and compounds in trials or about to be tested show some promise in reducing the impact of sickle-cell crises.

Sickle-cell anemia is a recessive gene disease; that is, a person must have two genes for sickle-cell anemia in order to contract the disease. In the United States about 0.3% of blacks have sickle-cell anemia and another 12% have the *sickle-cell trait* (have one gene for the disease). A couple who both have the sickle-cell trait therefore have a 25% chance of producing a child with sickle-cell anemia. For this reason it is highly advisable for all blacks—men and women—to be tested for sickle-cell trait (by means of a simple blood test). Further, women who have sickle-cell disease should never take oral contraceptives, which seem to accelerate their already existing predisposition to form blood clots. They also should never undergo a saline abortion (see under AMNIOINFUSION).

Pregnancy is a serious burden for women with sickle-cell anemia. Usually the anemia becomes worse and the attacks of pain more frequent. Infections and pulmonary (lung) disease are more apt to develop. One-third to one-half of babies conceived by women with the disease die in miscarriage, stillbirth or soon after birth. The greatest danger to the mother is from blood clots, which often occur in the lungs and can be fatal. Even though extreme caution and intensive care may save both mother and baby, most authorities feel that pregnancy in most cases should be avoided, either with stringent birth control measures or sterilization. At the least, tests for sickle-cell trait should be carried out and GENETIC COUNSELING undertaken if the trait is present. If a woman should become pregnant, AMNIOCENTESIS or CHORIONIC VILLUS SAMPLING can reveal if her baby will have sickle-cell disease. If she does bear a child, the baby should be tested at once for the disease. A regimen of penicillin given twice a day, begun at three months and continued for at least five years, appears to give children a much better chance of survival.

side effect   An effect of a medication or medical procedure other than the one for which it was intended. For example, antihistamines—drugs widely used to control allergy—often have the side effect of making one drowsy or sleepy. The severity of some side effects may be such that other drugs must be substituted or all medication must be discontinued.

sigmoidoscopy   See COLONOSCOPY.

sign   Objective evidence of a disease or disorder, such as fever, discoloration or swelling, or the secretion of pus, which can be seen and/or measured by the clinician.

See also SYMPTOM.

silicone implant   See MAMMAPLASTY.

Sims-Huhner test   Also *postcoital test*. Examination of the cervical mucus to determine whether or not it is receptive to sperm. Usually this test is performed only when a couple are having trouble with conception (see INFERTILITY). The test is performed at the expected time of ovulation—some clinicians say just before that time—and the woman is asked to come to the office or clinic within two to 15 hours after intercourse. The cervical mucus is then aspirated with a small suction catheter, the amount measured, the acidity tested, the viscosity, cellularity, ferning, and Spinnbarkeit measured, and the number of actively moving sperm per high-power field counted under the microscope. If there are five or more actively moving sperm per high-power field, the cervical mucus is considered receptive enough to sperm for fertilization to take place. This positive result also implies that the techniques of intercourse used are potentially effective, the mucus is adequate for the transport and preservation of sperm, the ovaries are producing enough estrogen and the male partner probably has a normal sperm count. This test is not, however, a substitute for *semen analysis* (see under SPERM). A negative result—fewer than five active sperm per high-power field—may result from intercourse techniques, OLIGOSPERMIA or AZOOSPERMIA, or poor timing relative to ovulation, since only around this time is the cervical mucus hospitable to sperm (see CERVICAL MUCUS METHOD for explanation). Other possible causes are inadequate estrogen production by the ovaries or a cervical infection.

Sims position   Also *left lateral position.* Lying on the left side during labor, rather than on one's back (see DORSAL LITHOTOMY). This position avoids compression of a large vein (the *vena cava*) when the uterine muscles contract, thereby allowing more oxygen to reach the baby. It also is more comfortable when a woman has BACK LABOR.

sitz bath   A tub filled to the level of 6 inches (15 centimeters) or so with warm water, which is used for soaking. Sitting in a sitz bath for 15 minutes several times a day is a simple and often effective treatment for irritations affecting the genital area, among them cystitis, vaginitis and proctitis. Warm water increases circulation to the affected parts and promotes healing. Some women use HERBAL REMEDIES in the bath water, ginger root (*Zingiber officinale*) to allay itching and comfrey (*Symphytum officinale*) to promote healing.

Sjögren's syndrome   A chronic AUTOIMMUNE DISORDER marked by dryness of the eyes and mouth, caused by destruction of the lymph glands (lacrimal and salivary) that secrete tears and saliva, which are replaced by lymphocytes (immune cells). It may be a primary disease or it may be secondary to other autoimmune disorders, especially rheumatoid arthritis, systemic lupus erythematosus or scleroderma, and in some individuals it is associated with lymphoma (a cancer). Sjögren's, named for the Swedish physician, who first identified it, Henrik Sjögren, affects women 10 times more often than men. Onset is usually between the ages of 45 and 55 but may occur at any age. It is diagnosed by any of several tests: measuring tear production or saliva production, X-rays of salivary glands, a blood test or a lip biopsy. Treatment is directed at relieving symptoms, but no cure is yet available. Eyedrops are used to replace tears, and if those are insufficient, artificial tear inserts or a minor surgical procedure on the ducts may be considered. Diminished saliva is augmented with water and by gum-chewing or sucking, and corticosteroids and immunosuppressive drugs are used during acute flare-ups or when the condition attacks vital organs.

Skene's glands   Also *Skene's ducts, paraurethral ducts.* A pair of glands that run below and parallel to the female URETHRA, opening just below the outer part of the urethral opening. Their function, if any, is not known; some authorities believe they are the female counterpart of the male prostate gland. Their chief importance is the fact that they often harbor the organism causing GONORRHEA, which may be impossible to eradicate without removing these glands. Further, Skene's glands occasionally become infected with other organisms and develop cysts.

skin cancer   See CANCER, SKIN; MELANOMA.

skin changes   Alterations in skin texture, pigmentation and general health that are caused by changes in hormone balance and diet. During puberty many adolescents develop ACNE as a result of increasing androgen (male hormone) levels. For this reason acne is more common and more severe in boys than in girls. During the reproductive years, either pregnancy or use of oral contraceptives, which both involve higher levels of estrogen, can cause changes in pigmentation, such as the giant freckles of CHLOASMA or darkening of the nipples and abdominal midline in PREGNANCY. Oral contraceptives containing a considerable amount of progesterone may cause rashes and/or acne in some women.

During middle age and after menopause, women's skin becomes thinner and loses some of its flexibility and elasticity. The outermost layer of skin, the epidermis, is made up of cells that are being renewed constantly, but with age the renewal process slows down. By the time new skin cells are pushed up toward the surface, they have dried and flattened out. The oil and sweat glands tend to function less vigorously, which can create dry skin, sometimes causing itching and discomfort, as well as making wrinkles and lines more visible. There also may be a change in pigmentation (see LIVER SPOTS), another result of slowed-down cell renewal, as well as the cumulative effect of exposure to sunlight. From middle age on many individuals develop *keratoses,* superficial lesions. One kind, *seborrheic keratoses,* may be round or oval and flesh-colored, brown or black, with a waxy, scaling or crusted surface, and appear anywhere on the body. They are not premalignant and require no treatment unless irritated or itchy. Another kind, *actinic keratoses,* are considered precancerous (see CANCER, SKIN), and most often appear in fair-skinned individuals who have had years of overexposure to sunlight. It is, of course, best to prevent their development by using sunscreens and avoiding overexposure. Even after they develop, a recent study showed that regular use of strong sunscreens for a six-month period actually made many of these lesions fade completely.

Regular use of skin moisturizers and oils, avoiding very dry environments (using humidifiers or placing pans of water in heated or air-conditioned surroundings), avoiding overuse of soap and occasionally taking a steam bath all help make drying skin look smoother and feel better. Currently researchers are experimenting with substances that speed up skin cell renewal, such as low con-

centrations of vitamin A acid. One such product, tretinoin, marketed as Retin-A and Renova, has been found to smooth out fine wrinkles, fade out keratoses, improve skin texture and give a rosy glow to sun-damaged skin. These cosmetic changes have been verified by microscopic evidence showing that Retin-A promotes a major rebuilding of the outer skin layer, the sun-damaged epidermis, by speeding up collagen formation. These improvements appear only after regular use over a period of 6 weeks, with the best effects obtained after 6 to 12 months. Moreover, its use makes the skin extremely sensitive to sun and therefore a strong sunscreen must be used at all times. When the drug is discontinued, its benefits appear to fade away. Another medication is alphahydroxy acid (AHA), a class of compounds, including glycolic acid, that in high concentration are used for chemical peels. They, too, help to smooth dry, scaly skin and increase the density of collagen. Creams sold over the counter contain much less of the acid and do not increase sensitivity to sun; however, their effect on the skin is directly proportional to how strong they are. One study found that using Retin-A at night and a glycolic acid cream during the day yielded greater improvement in skin tone and wrinkling. Increasing research on anti-aging products is being done at this writing.

sleeping pills See INSOMNIA.

smegma A cheesy secretion of certain sebaceous (oil) glands, especially those under the PREPUCE of the penis and clitoris. Accumulated smegma needs to be washed away regularly, particularly in uncircumcised men, as it can be a source of irritation and/or harbor infection-causing bacteria.

smoking, tobacco The habitual use of tobacco in cigars and cigarettes, an acknowledged health hazard, and especially so to women. Smokers who take ORAL CONTRACEPTIVES are at much greater risk for developing heart attacks and stroke than nonsmokers, especially after the age of 30. The rate of MISCARRIAGE among smokers is higher too.

Cigarette smoking during pregnancy poses dangers to the unborn child. The baby's birth weight on the average will be somewhat lower than normal, and the mother has a higher risk of developing hypertension (high blood pressure). Smoking may be linked with other birth defects as well, since nicotine makes the blood vessels constrict, thereby preventing some of the blood-borne oxygen and nutrients from reaching the fetus. Nicotine also is passed on to the baby through the milk of a woman who is breast-feeding. Finally, women smokers are at much greater risk for a heart attack than non-smokers (from 2 to 11 times as great, depending on how much they smoke) and as much at risk as men for higher than normal incidence of emphysema, bronchitis, gum disease, and cancer of the lungs, larynx, oral cavity and esophagus. (For these cancers smoking is considered a major cause.) Smoking also is linked to cancer of the cervix and breast cancer. Moreover, the cancer risks are even higher if heavy smoking is associated with heavy ALCOHOL USE. Smoking is considered a contributory factor to cancers of the bladder, kidneys and pancreas. Recent research shows that cancer risks are high also for passive smokers—women who breathe smoke from others' cigarettes.

Stopping the habit of smoking is not easy. Some find that a nicotine-containing chewing gum helps lessen withdrawal symptoms, as do nicotine skin patches. Others turn to group therapy and support groups of the kind used to control obesity. A U.S. Surgeon General's Report on Smoking indicates that 95% of those who successfully stopped smoking have done so without organized programs, and stopping all at once (so-called cold turkey) appears to be more effective than cutting down gradually.

somatiform disorder Distressing physical symptoms whose medical cause cannot be found or that seem out of proportion to a medical condition. Among them are chest pain, dizziness, constipation, abdominal upset, muscle and skeletal pain and fatigue, and they cause considerable distress and/or interfere with daily functioning. Often there is underlying depression or anxiety, which may respond to counseling, especially cognitive behavior therapy, and medication.

sound An instrument used to determine the length of the uterus prior to inserting an INTRA-UTERINE DEVICE (IUD), performing an endometrial BIOPSY (see def. 8) or some other procedure. The uterus of a nonpregnant woman usually sounds to a depth of 6 to 8 centimeters (2.4 to 3.2 inches).

speculum Also *specula* (pl.). A two-bladed metal or plastic instrument used to examine the inside of the vagina and the cervix. Inserted into the vagina with the blades closed, it is rotated to the proper position and the blades then are opened and locked in place. The blades serve to hold the walls of the vagina apart (they normally are so close together they virtually touch) so that the clinician can examine both them and the cervix. For performing a PAP SMEAR, a narrow spatula and then a cotton swab are inserted between the blades of the speculum to scrape surface cells from the cervix. The speculum is used for most other gynecologic procedures as well, ranging from endometrial biopsy and vacuum curettage to vaginal hysterectomy. Specula come in a number of sizes, including a size for infants.

See also GYNECOLOGIC EXAMINATION.

sperm Also *spermatozoan* (*spermatozoa,* pl.). The male reproductive cell in all animals that reproduce sexually, including human beings. *Spermatogenesis,* the production of sperm, begins at puberty. Stimulated by FSH (follicle-stimulating hormone) and LH (luteinizing hormone), the same pituitary hormones that cause the production of ova (eggs) in women, sperm production takes place in the testes, or male sex glands (see TESTIS). The original sperm cells, or spermatogonia, take about 72 days to develop before they are ejaculated as mature sperm.

A single sperm is a tiny wormlike creature, with an oval head that contains the chromosomes and a long tail whose movements propel it forward. From tip to tail it is about $\frac{1}{600}$ inch (.07 millimeter) long, and 90% of that length is the tail. The size, shape, motility and number of sperm all affect fertility, that is, the ability to fertilize (mate with) an egg. Like the egg, the sperm undergoes meiosis so that it contains only half the number of chromosomes of other cells (23, not 46).

When a man reaches ORGASM, the pelvic muscles expel the sperm from its storage place and it is propelled, along with gland secretions (seminal fluid), through the urethra and out through the opening at the end of the penis. (See PENIS for a more precise description.) Each time this event, called EJACULATION, takes place, as many as 300 million sperm may be set in motion; the average *ejaculate* contains 2 to 5 milliliters (ml) of fluid, with a mean of 40 to 80 million sperm per milliliter. Most of the sperm die within a few hours; only a few reach the fallopian tubes, where they may survive 24 to 48 hours longer. Total survival time of sperm in the female genital tract is thought to be about 96 hours, or four days.

For couples having trouble conceiving, one of the first tests performed is a *semen analysis* to determine if enough normal sperm are being ejaculated. The entire ejaculate must be collected in a clean dry container and taken to the laboratory within one hour of ejaculation. There the total volume and thickness are measured, and a sample is examined under the microscope. The minimum normal values for fertility are:

Total volume, 2 to 5 milliliters with positive fructose (a sugar)
Amount, more than 20 million cells per milliliter
Motility, more than 60% of sperm cells still moving within four hours of ejaculation
Structure, more than 70% of cells having normal shape

A man's sperm count may vary as much as 20% in different samples, and the same specimen may have a counting error of 10%. (See also AZOOSPERMIA; OLIGOSPERMIA.) Sperm also must be able to penetrate the outer layer of the egg in order to effect fertilization, verifiable by an ACROSIN TEST. A similar test is the *two-hour swim-up analysis,* in which a semen specimen is washed with a special saltwater solution (buffer) and the sperm are allowed to swim up for two hours into an overlay of the buffer, which captures the highly motile sperm. The percentage of moving sperm and their motion characteristics (speed, linearity) are measured by a microscope hooked up to a computer. Normal sperm mark-

edly increase their motility after capacitation in preparation for fertilization.

About 4% of all men produce antibodies against their own sperm, a figure that rises to 50 to 60% after vasectomy. Semen analysis reveals this condition. If a couple wishes to conceive, there are several ways to solve the problem: washing the sperm from the semen and inserting it directly into the uterus, steroid therapy or in vitro fertilization.

Occasionally a woman develops antibodies against her partner's sperm, in the same way the body develops antibodies against infectious organisms. Such antibodies appear in the cervical mucus, attach themselves to the sperm and prevent them from moving up into the uterus and tubes. Since normal vaginal secretions are too acid for the alkaline-loving sperm, they soon die there. Antibody development can be a cause of infertility. For couples who want a child, one solution may be for the man to use a CONDOM for a number of months. Without the stimulation of live sperm, antibody production gradually diminishes and the levels of antibodies drop. Conception then may be possible. A blood test, called Duke's test, can determine if antibodies are being produced. If the condition persists, inserting sperm directly into the uterus, steroid therapy to suppress the antibodies or in vitro fertilization may work.

See also INFERTILITY.

sperm bank A registered tissue bank that collects, stores, tests and sells frozen SPERM to be used for ARTIFICIAL INSEMINATION. For men who do not produce enough sperm at one time to fertilize an egg, one solution may be to pool numerous samples of semen and then use this concentrated quantity to achieve conception. U.S. sperm banks maintain exhaustive profiles of donors, so that unrelated donors may be picked for genetic, physical and psychological characteristics. The American Association of Tissue Banks (AATB) provides strict standards for the collection, testing, storage and tracking of semen, and performs on-site inspection. To date only 8 U.S. sperm banks are AATB accredited. Since sperm cannot survive for more than a few hours under ordinary conditions, they are frozen. However, even in normal seminal fluid only one-fourth to one-half of the sperm may be motile (capable of moving) after they are thawed, and sperm from infertile men are even more easily damaged by freezing. (Sometimes no motile sperm at all can be recovered.) For this reason successful artificial insemination may require a donor who can provide a fresh semen specimen. Sometimes frozen sperm from the husband are combined with fresh donor sperm to provide a mixed specimen.

Similar storage for human eggs and human embryos (fertilized eggs) has been used for IN VITRO FERTILIZATION when the original embryo fails to be implanted or to grow. A frozen egg bank has been difficult to establish (eggs do not survive freezing very well) but has become available to a woman with healthy ovaries who is willing to pay the price (it is expensive). The process, similar to IN VITRO FERTILIZATION, involves hormone injections to stimulate the ovaries to produce more than one egg, followed by withdrawal of 12 to 15 eggs through a needle. The eggs are dehydrated so they can be frozen without forming damaging ice crystals. When the woman is ready to use them, they are thawed, rehydrated and reinserted. The pregnancy rate from frozen eggs is only about 20%, but women who are putting off childbearing for various reasons may still wish to undergo the process.

A new way has been found to store and grow a woman's immature eggs that could be used to protect the fertility of women undergoing chemotherapy. Anticancer drugs often destroy the ovary's follicles, where immature eggs remain dormant until they are matured by the body. The new method involves taking pieces of ovary tissue and, by adding artificial growth hormones, growing the eggs within the follicles to an advanced stage. Eventually fully matured eggs from this technique could be used in in vitro fertilization.

Frozen embryos more readily remain viable. Such storage can raise legal problems (of "custody") if the parents should die or, in the case of a frozen embryo, divorce.

See also DONOR EGG; IN VITRO FERTILIZATION.

spermicide A chemical substance used to kill live sperm inside the vagina for purposes of BIRTH CON-TROL. The most common forms are *spermicidal jelly* and *cream,* which are recommended for use with a DIAPHRAGM or CERVICAL CAP but sometimes are used alone or for extra protection with a condom, and *spermicidal foam, foaming tablets* and *suppositories,* generally used alone. Each of these chemical contraceptives contains two components: a relatively inert carrier base and an active spermicidal agent, usually *nonoxynol-9* (an abbreviation for nonylphenoxypolyethoxyethanol). They operate both mechanically, by forming a barrier (a film or coating) over the cervix to delay the movement of sperm, and biochemically, by immobilizing and destroying the sperm they have blocked. The active ingredient in them remains active for six to eight hours.

Creams and jellies used alone are not as effective as foam alone and have a high failure rate. Used with a diaphragm, they are more effective than foam alone. Nevertheless, creams and jellies commonly are sold with a plastic applicator to insert them into the vagina either alone or as a supplement after a diaphragm is already in place (for second intercourse or because the diaphragm was inserted more than two hours before intercourse). If the cream or jelly is used alone, it should be inserted no earlier than 15 minutes before intercourse, with an initial application of *two* full applicators; one additional full applicator should be used for each additional act of intercourse. The stronger, more effective of the creams and jellies tend also to be more irritating, to both vaginal tissue and the penis, than weaker ones.

Foam is a white aerated cream with the consistency of shaving cream. It generally is sold in a can with a plunger-type applicator. Deposited deep inside the vagina, near the cervix, no earlier than 15 minutes (some say 30) before intercourse, it is more effective than either cream or jelly alone but is recommended for use only when the male partner also is using a CONDOM. (Alone it is only 70 to 90% effective.) The can should be thoroughly shaken before use (a total of 20 times is recommended), and the applicator inserted into the vagina as deep as possible. The applicator should be thoroughly washed (but not boiled) after use, and the foam should remain in place for six to eight hours (if it drips, use a sanitary pad).

Foam also comes in the form of a *vaginal suppository, film* or *tablet,* which after it is inserted, dissolves and releases the foam. The suppositories and tablets are inserted high in the vagina, near the cervix. The vaginal contraceptive film is placed on the finger (one sheet at a time) and inserted on or near the cervix. These kinds of foam are approximately as effective as the aerosol foams and therefore should be used with a condom; however, they do not become effective for 10 to 15 minutes after insertion (the time it takes to melt and release foam), which may be a drawback. Also, they remain effective for only an hour.

All of these kinds of spermicide are available in North American drugstores without prescription. Until the late 1970s few brands bore an indication of their *shelf life* (that is, how long the ingredients remain active), which appears to be about three years. It is preferable to buy such products with a clearly marked expiration date on the package, which today is supplied by some, but not all, manufacturers. Most spermicidal jellies, creams and foams have been found to increase protection against gonorrhea, syphilis, chlamydia, trichomonas and bacterial vaginal infections, but the protection they give depends considerably on the meticulousness with which they are used.

sphincter A ringlike muscle that, when contracted, closes a natural opening or passage. Such muscles are particularly important in controlling the passage of urine (*urinary sphincter*—there is one at the upper and the lower ends of the urethra) and of feces (*anal sphincter*). They are found as well in the bile duct, iris of the eye and elsewhere.

spider vein See VARICOSE VEIN.

spina bifida Also *spina bifida operta, cleft spine.* A BIRTH DEFECT in which one or more individual vertebrae fail to close completely. As a result, a sac containing part of the contents of the spinal cord may protrude through the opening, which usually is at the lower end of the cord; it is called a *menin-*

gomyelocele. Muscles and nerves in the legs and lower trunk often are affected. Symptoms usually are present at birth, although in some cases they may develop much later, during the rapid growth spurt of puberty. Among the symptoms are muscle weakness or paralysis, partial or total loss of bladder and bowel control and, in some cases, other deformities resulting from weak muscles. Treatment for the condition depends on its severity; in some cases it is so severe, with the spine virtually completely open, that survival is impossible. In others it may be so mild that there are few obvious signs.

Spina bifida and similar open spinal defects are called *neural tube defects.* They result from a failure of development in the neural tube, which is the embryonic forerunner of the central nervous system, and they occur in nearly 2 of every 1,000 pregnancies in America. Since spina bifida occurs more often in children of parents with this condition, it is advisable for patients to seek GENETIC COUNSELING before undertaking parenthood. The defect may be detected by means of the ALPHA-FETOPROTEIN TEST and also by AMNIOCENTESIS, but only in the case of open lesions.

Women with spina bifida face some special problems. During sexual activity, they may have increased risk of urinary and bowel incontinence during arousal. Genital sensation may be limited or totally absent, and deformities, weakness or paralysis may interfere with intercourse in certain positions. Menstruation and fertility are not affected. Oral contraceptives are contraindicated if there are circulatory problems, and a diaphragm or intrauterine device (IUD) may be difficult to insert if there is pelvic deformity. Pregnancy not only raises the question of passing the defect on to a baby but may, during its course, aggravate back problems, incontinence and urinary tract infections.

The incidence of spina bifida and other neural tube defects may be greatly reduced by routinely giving folic acid (folate) to women who are attempting to conceive for at least one month before conception and then for at least six weeks into the pregnancy. (Also see VITAMIN.) Also, a recent study shows that some women with a particular enzyme deficit may require more vitamin B$_{12}$ as well.

spinal anesthesia   Also *subarachnoid block.* A kind of REGIONAL ANESTHESIA that is administered late in labor as well as being used for Cesarean section and lower abdominal surgery of various kinds. It involves injecting a local anesthetic directly into the spinal cord through a needle inserted between the vertebrae, with the result that all feeling is blocked from the diaphragm to the toes. A variant is *saddle block anesthesia,* which mainly creates numbness in the perineum in the "saddle area" (corresponding to the parts of the body in contact with a saddle, hence "saddle block") and also the legs. In childbirth the anesthetic cannot be given until the cervix has dilated to 5 centimeters or more and the baby has descended well into the birth canal because it both stops contractions and limits the woman's ability to bear down and push the baby out (forceps or a vacuum extractor must be used to deliver the baby). Another drawback is that it can cause severe headache, for as long as four or five days after delivery or surgery if spinal fluid leaks out of the puncture site of the injection. Today this adverse effect usually can be avoided by using a very small-gauge needle to inject the anesthetic. Spinal anesthesia also may cause a sharp drop in the patient's blood pressure as well as nausea and vomiting. Despite these disadvantages it is considered very useful for tubal ligation, appendectomy, Cesarean section and other kinds of lower abdominal surgery, and in childbirth emergencies (fetal distress, hemorrhage in the mother). Some physicians have tried combining low doses of spinal and EPIDURAL ANESTHESIA, affording immediate pain relief from the spinal and lasting relief from the epidural.

Spinnbarkeit   See CERVICAL MUCUS METHOD.

split ejaculation   See OLIGOSPERMIA.

sponge   See CONTRACEPTIVE SPONGE; MENSTRUAL SPONGE.

spotting   See BREAKTHROUGH BLEEDING.

SSRI   Abbreviation for *selective serotonin reuptake inhibitor:* see ANTIDEPRESSANT.

staging   A procedure in which the extent of a progressive disease, usually cancer, is evaluated by means of diagnostic tests (X-ray, blood tests, body scans, urinalysis, etc.). In breast cancer these tests are undertaken after biopsy or mastectomy to ascertain the spread of malignancy beyond the breast. The accompanying charts show the disease stages customarily used for breast cancer, uterine cancer and ovarian cancer. The stage of a cancer determines the nature of the treatment to be used and also gives some idea of the chances of cure and of life expectancy. For this reason accurate staging is of the utmost importance. Many authorities now believe that metastasis (cancer spread) begins much earlier than it can readily be detected and that more sophisticated techniques of examining the tissue, especially the lymph nodes in early breast cancer, will reveal a significant percentage (perhaps 60%) of metastasis. For staging cervical abnormalities, see PAP SMEAR. Also see under CANCER, COLORECTAL, as well as the accompanying charts here.

STAGING BREAST CANCER

STAGE 1: A tumor less than 2 cm in diameter with minor skin involvement, either affixed or not affixed to chest wall, muscle or fascia; axillary nodes not considered to contain growth; no evidence of metastasis

STAGE II: A tumor between 2 cm and 5 cm with possible muscle or chest wall fixation; movable axillary nodes contain cancer; no evidence of distant metastasis; also larger tumor if no axillary nodes involved

STAGE IIIA: A tumor larger than 5 cm with or without fixation or extension to fascia and chest wall; axillary nodes contain cancer and are fixed to one another or other structures; no evidence of distant metastasis

STAGE IIIB: A tumor of any size with metastasis to skin, chest wall or internal mammary lymph nodes

STAGE IV: A tumor of any size with extension to chest wall or skin; supraclavicular or infraclavicular nodes contain cancer, or there is edema of the arm; evidence of distant metastasis

---

STAGING CANCER OF UTERINE (ENDOMETRIAL) CORPUS

STAGE 0: Findings of tissue analysis suspicious but not proven

STAGE I: Cancer is confined to corpus (body) of uterus

    IA: Involves less than half of myometrium

    IB: Involves more than half of myometrium

STAGE II: Cancer found in both corpus and cervix

STAGE III: Cancer has extended outside uterus but not outside pelvis

STAGE IV: Cancer has extended outside pelvis or has obviously involved mucosa of bladder or rectum

STAGING OVARIAN CANCER

STAGE I: Cancer limited to ovaries

    IA: Cancer in one ovary only, no ascites (accumulation of serous fluid)

    IB: Cancer in both ovaries, no ascites present, serous fluid in peritoneal cavity

    IC: Cancer in one or both ovaries, ascites present with malignant cells in fluid

STAGE II: Cancer in one or both ovaries, with pelvic extension

    IIA: Cancer in one or both ovaries, with extension and metastasis to uterus and fallopian tubes

    IIB: Cancer in one or both ovaries, with extension and metastasis to other pelvic tissues

STAGE III: Growth involving one or both ovaries with widespread intraepithelial metastasis to abdomen

STAGE IV: Growth involving one or both ovaries with distant metastasis, outside peritoneal cavity

staining   See BREAKTHROUGH BLEEDING.

statin   A cholesterol-lowering drug that lowers lipids, fats in the blood that can lead to atherosclerosis (see ARTERIOSCLEROSIS). The statins block the synthesis of CHOLESTEROL, thereby increasing the removal of LDL from the bloodstream, and help prevent heart attacks and strokes in individuals at increased risk. Statins lower LDL cholesterol (the kind that helps set the stage for a heart attack or stroke) by 30 to 50% and cut the risk of heart attack, angina, cardiac death and stroke by one-third. They also lower C-reactive protein, an indicator of inflammation that has been linked to heart disease. A preliminary study indicates that they may also help the survival of patients with heart failure who do not have high cholesterol. Like most medications, the statins can give rise to side effects, among them mild constipation, loose stools, bloating, headache, rashes or fatigue. A more serious side effect is liver inflammation, indicated by elevated liver enzymes revealed in a blood test of liver function. When it occurs, the drug is discontinued until liver tests return to normal.

Most statin drugs, including lovastatin (Mevacor), simvastatin (Zocor), fluvastatin (Lescol) and pravastatin (Pravachol), are best taken in the evening, because they are fairly short-acting and the body makes most of its cholesterol in the evening. Lovastatin is better absorbed when taken with food. Atorvastatin (Lipitor) may be taken at any time of day. Also, grapefruit and grapefruit juice interact with all statins except pravastatin, causing blood levels of the drug to rise and hence increasing the risk of side effects. Daily consumption of grapefruit generally has no adverse effects and may result in lower dosages of the statin, but sporadic consumption of grapefruit is not recommended. A recent study showed that atorvastatin is nearly twice as effective in lowering LDL as the other statins.

STD   See SEXUALLY TRANSMITTED DISEASE.

Stein-Leventhal syndrome   See POLYCYSTIC OVARY SYNDROME.

stem cell   An undifferentiated cell that has the potential of becoming one of many kinds of specialized cell. Some stem cells can be triggered to become any kind of cell in the human body; others are already partly differentiated and so can become, for example, any kind of blood cell or nerve cell. Stem cells produce all the cells in the human body. Current research is aimed at directing stem cells to repair or replace damaged cells or tissues in such diseases as Parkinson's, Alzheimer's, diabetes and spinal injury. Currently there are four sources of stem cells: four-to five-day-old embryos produced by IN VITRO FERTILIZATION, miscarried or aborted fetuses, the umbilical cord or placenta after child-birth and bone marrow. The last is the only source currently permitted for stem-cell transplantation into human patients. One's own bone marrow may be used for this purpose; it is then called an *autologous transplant*. Stem cells from bone marrow produce only blood cells and have been used to treat leukemia and other cancers of the blood, sickle-cell anemia and other blood disorders. The other three sources are the subject of controversy.

Current research is directed at finding other sources of stem cells. One promising avenue is using genetically defective fertilized eggs from fertility clinics, which normally are discarded because they stand no chance of implantation and forming a healthy embryo. By removing chromosomes from a single-cell fertilized egg and replacing it with DNA from a skin cell or other mature cell, the modified cell will give rise to stem cells from the resultant embryo.

In November 2007 two sets of researchers independently announced they had succeeded in genetically altering human skin cells into cells that behave like embryonic stem cells. By inserting four genes into the skin cells, the cells regressed to a stem-cell–like state, called induced stem cells. They were believed to be capable of being cultivated into any of the body's 220 cell types, such as heart, liver and blood. However, it would be some time before it was shown conclusively that the new cells have all the capabilities of embryonic stem cells.

See also BONE MARROW TRANSPLANT.

stereotactic biopsy See BIOPSY, def. 5.

sterility The condition of a man who produces very few or no SPERM, so that he cannot impregnate a woman, or a woman who either produces no ova (eggs) or has no uterus in which a fertilized egg can grow. They are then said to be *sterile*. The man's condition, also called *aspermatogenesis*, can be caused by infections such as tuberculosis, mumps (in adults), syphilis and gonorrhea, which inhibit the proper development of sperm, or by tumors, VARICOCELE, structural defects such as uncorrected CRYPTORCHIDISM, congenital disorders such as KLINE-

FELTER SYNDROME, or exposure to radiation, certain drugs and certain industrial chemicals. Prolonged hot baths or other application of heat to the testes may produce temporary sterility (see THERMATIC STERILIZATION), as may any infection associated with a very high fever. Blockage of the vas deferens or other tubes by scar tissue or similar obstruction to the passage of semen from the testes are not, strictly speaking, sterility, since adequate sperm may still be produced but simply do not reach their destination. Aspermatogenesis caused by malfunctioning of the PITUITARY GLAND sometimes can be corrected by administering human pituitary gonadotropin. Also, the administration of a FERTILITY DRUG in small doses for six months to one year sometimes restores sperm production to adequate levels.

For treatment of sterility in women, see INFERTILITY.

sterilization Rendering a person sterile, that is, incapable of reproduction. It may result from an accident, such as overexposure to radioactivity, be the by-product of surgery performed as treatment for some disorder or result from a procedure performed for that very purpose, that is, a form of BIRTH CONTROL. In women sterilization results from a HYSTERECTOMY (removal of the uterus) performed for any reason whatever (although hysterectomies commonly were, and sometimes still are, performed solely to achieve sterility).

The principal form of sterilization for birth control in women is TUBAL LIGATION, which prevents the passage of an egg through the fallopian tubes. In men, it is VASECTOMY, which prevents the passage of sperm through the vas deferens. Two other, more experimental forms of sterilization for men are THERMATIC STERILIZATION and ULTRASOUND (def. 2). Vasectomy is considerably safer and simpler than any form of tubal ligation, but it does not guarantee sterility until all stored sperm have been ejaculated. Three negative sperm counts obtained at monthly intervals are required before one can be sure. Neither tubal ligation or vasectomy is readily or reliably reversible, so neither procedure should be undertaken by anyone unless he or she is quite certain of not wanting any (more) children.

Another form of sterilization for women, which has not yet found wide acceptance, is *bilateral tubal occlusion,* which produces blockage of both fallopian tubes by chemical means. In 2002 Essure, an outpatient method of tubal occlusion, was approved by the F.D.A. Using local anesthetic, the clinician inserts a narrow catheter and releases a small metal spring into each fallopian tube. The hormone-free coil causes inflammation and the formation of scar tissue that blocks the flow of eggs. The principal side effect is one to two days of abdominal cramping.

Voluntary sterilization for the purpose of birth control has long been subject to religious and moral strictures. For years many American hospitals used a "Rule of 120" *age-parity formula* to determine whether a woman might be sterilized. According to this rule, the product of the woman's age and the number of children she had already borne had to be at least 120 before she could be sterilized. Accordingly, neither a 20-year-old woman who had five children (20 × 5 = 100) nor a 35-year-old woman who had three children (35 × 3 = 105) could be sterilized. In 1969 the American College of Obstetricians and Gynecologists deleted the age-parity formula from its manual of standards, but some American physicians and hospitals continued to use it.

Involuntary sterilization, on the other hand, became a political issue. Both mentally retarded and poor women have been sterilized either without their consent or with consent obtained under duress. In some cases women in active labor have been pressed to give written permission for a tubal ligation or hysterectomy immediately following delivery. In 1974 the U.S. Department of Health, Education and Welfare (now the Department of Health and Human Services) issued guidelines emphasizing a woman's right to *informed consent.* They stated that federally funded hospitals must institute a waiting period between the time a woman signs her permission and the time a tubal ligation is performed and that the procedure may be performed only on women who are 21 years old or older. The following year, however, the American Civil Liberties Union found that in a study of 154 teaching hospitals these guidelines were totally ignored in 70% and substantially ignored in another 23%.

See also CASTRATION.

steroid A hormone derived from cholesterol; see HORMONE.

See also ANABOLIC STEROIDS.

sterologist A physician who specializes in helping couples overcome INFERTILITY; the word comes from *sterility.*

stillbirth The delivery of a dead baby. The term usually is reserved for a fetus that is fairly close to term, that is, of 28 weeks' gestation or more, although some authorities put it as early as 20 weeks. In the United States five of every 1,000 babies are stillborn. The most frequent causes are toxemia, Rh antigen factors, anemia, umbilical cord accidents, separation of the placenta and infection. Some cases occur from oxygen deprivation during labor and delivery. Often the precise cause cannot be identified, but the single condition most often associated with stillbirth is failure of the fetus to grow sufficiently. This impairment can result from a problem with the placenta, whereby not enough blood and nutrients reach the fetus; birth defects, chromosomal abnormalities, genetic syndromes or viral infections also might result in impaired growth. The most important way to discover the cause of a stillbirth is a fetal autopsy, a step that grieving parents often prefer not to undertake and which often is not covered by insurance.

Having once experienced a stillbirth, a woman runs the risk of suffering another in a subsequent pregnancy. This risk is anywhere from twofold to tenfold, depending on the cause (if it can be found). Other risk factors for stillbirth are obesity, smoking, an underlying disease like diabetes, hypertension, clotting or a metabolic disorder. Women at risk are advised to count fetal kicks for half an hour twice a day, beginning at 28 weeks of gestation. If the number of kicks decreased significantly, the woman should seek immediate medical care.

See also MISCARRIAGE, def. 5; PREMATURE.

stress incontinence See URINARY INCONTINENCE.

stretch marks See STRIAE.

striae Also *stretch marks*. Pinkish streaks that appear on the abdomen and breasts, and sometimes also on the thighs and buttocks, in the late months of pregnancy. They are not pigment changes but result from decreased elasticity of the skin stretched over the growing uterus and enlarged breasts. At first pale pink and sometimes itchy, they later become white and look like very faint scars. Once they appear, they usually remain for life, although they become much fainter after delivery. About half of all pregnant women develop striae.

stroke See CEREBRAL VASCULAR ACCIDENT.

subcutaneous Under the skin and, therefore, not very deep. For subcutaneous mastectomy, see MASTECTOMY, def. 8.

suction See VACUUM ASPIRATION; for suction by needle, or needle aspiration, see BIOPSY, def. 3.

suicide Taking one's own life. In North America it is estimated that women attempt to commit suicide two or three times more often than men, but more men than women actually succeed in killing themselves. Part of the reason for this disparity is the mode chosen; men tend to use guns, whereas women use poison, most often overdoses of drugs. The peak age for suicide in women is 55 to 65. The most common cause of suicide is DEPRESSION, precipitated by marital or family strife, especially among the young, and by bereavement and physical disability, especially among the elderly. Threats to commit suicide, even if they seem to be an obvious bid for attention or an attempt to manipulate others, should never be ignored because they often are carried out. Crisis centers for potential suicides, which anyone can telephone anonymously for counseling and help, exist in many localities; they usually are listed in telephone directories under such names as "Suicide" and "Help."

superfecundation The fertilization of two eggs within a short period of time (during the same menstrual cycle) but not during the same act of sexual intercourse, resulting in the conception of fraternal twins or some other form of MULTIPLE PREGNANCY.

superfetation Fertilization of two eggs during two successive ovulatory cycles, resulting in MULTIPLE PREGNANCY and birth. It is well recognized in horses and other animals and is believed to occur in human beings as well, although it has never been verified. It requires the occurrence of ovulation *during* the course of (the first) pregnancy.

suppository A medication in the form of a small, solid, bullet-shaped mass that melts readily and is administered by insertion into the vagina or rectum. Suppositories are used for administering medication for local vaginal infections. Some kinds of SPERMICIDE for birth control come in suppository form, but they are considered less reliable than jelly or foam because they do not always melt enough, or in time, for release of the active contraceptive agent. Suppositories made of glycerin and sodium stearate are commonly used to relieve temporary constipation by slightly irritating the mucous membrane of the rectum.

surgery, outpatient Also *ambulatory surgery*. A surgical procedure performed in a hospital or clinic where the patient is not required to stay overnight but goes home on the same day. Among the many types of operation so performed are breast biopsy, hernia repair, tonsillectomy, cataract and hemorrhoid removal, vasectomy, tubal ligation, vacuum aspiration and first-trimester abortion. Depending on the procedure, local, regional or general anesthesia may be used. A patient considering outpatient surgery should make sure that it is preceded by appropriate screening. The clinician should take a careful medical history and perform a physical examination, blood tests, an electrocardiogram in a patient over 40 and a chest X-ray in a patient over 60. Once scheduled, the patient should be advised about any medications that should be taken or avoided before surgery and instructions as to when to stop eating and drinking before surgery (to avoid vomiting and possibly aspirating vomit). Following surgery and a period of recovery of one or more hours, the patient should be escorted home by a responsible adult (relative or friend) who can stay there for a few hours. Patients also should refrain from driving or drinking alcohol for at least 24 hours. Possible complications, which most often arise in the first 48 hours following surgery, include unusual bleeding or pain, nausea and vomiting, fever, light-headedness and shortness of breath, any of which indicate calling the doctor or clinic.

surgery, unnecessary   Treatment of illness, injury or deformity by manual and/or instrumental operations that are not needed in the first place. Estimates by consumer groups, medical groups and others from the early 1960s on say that anywhere from 15 to 30% of surgery performed in the United States each year is unnecessary. Since more women than men consult physicians, are admitted to hospitals and undergo surgery because, unlike men, they frequently see doctors for normal functions (birth control, pregnancy, childbirth, etc.) and also tend to live longer, they are more apt to undergo unnecessary surgery. The single operation most often performed unjustifiably in the United States is HYSTERECTOMY (removal of the uterus). Others are hemorrhoidectomy (removal of a HEMORRHOID), tonsillectomy (removal of the tonsils) and CESAREAN SECTION (surgical delivery of a baby). Some surgery, of course, is not only indicated but lifesaving, and other operations may be urgently required, although they may not need to be done on an emergency basis (see accompanying chart). When, however, any surgery other than emergency surgery is recommended, it is highly advisable to seek a second opinion from a consulting physician, either a specialist in the particular condition or—and some feel preferably—a different kind of specialist. Using a different specialist is based on the theory that gynecologists, surgeons, radiologists and internists, for example, all are trained somewhat differently, so each might bring new information and a fresh viewpoint to the same problem. In the United States, Medicare, Medicaid and many private health insurance

plans, such as Blue Cross and Blue Shield, often not only pay for a second opinion but may require that it be sought, because consultation is far less expensive than surgery.

A set of general rules for avoiding unnecessary surgery and ensuring that one gets the best possible treatment are:

1. Do not go directly to a surgeon but to a general practitioner or internist for initial diagnosis or treatment. Surgeons, trained to operate, are more likely to overlook conservative treatment that might be just as effective.

2. Make sure your surgeon is board-certified (by one of the American or Canadian specialty boards, after a stringent examination), which is an important test of his or her surgical competence, and is a Fellow of the American College of Surgeons (FACS) or, in Canada, the Royal College of Physicians and Surgeons (FRCS), whose membership requirements keep out less competent individuals. (See the Appendix for where to check.)

3. Even if your family doctor and surgeon both recommend surgery, consider getting an independent consultation or opinion before proceeding. The second surgeon should be told that his or her opinion is being sought but that surgery, if decided on, will be performed by someone else, thus removing any financial incentive from the opinion. If the surgery being considered is one of the kinds most often performed (hysterectomy, hemorrhoidectomy, tonsillectomy), get at least two independent opinions.

4. If possible, have surgery performed in an accredited hospital, preferably one that gives staff privileges to both your doctor and your surgeon.

5. Do not insist on surgery; if you shop around for a doctor to perform surgery that is not necessary, you eventually will find one willing to do it.

6. Make sure both your doctor and your surgeon explain the alternatives to surgery and the possible benefits and risks of surgery. Many kinds of postoperative complication may arise, even from simple surgery. The most common seri-

SURGICAL PROCEDURES

Classification	Examples
Emergency (immediate surgery required)	Fractured skull, certain stab or gunshot wounds, extensive burns, urinary obstruction, intestinal obstruction, ruptured appendix or fallopian tube
Urgent (prompt surgery required, within 24 to 48 hours)	Kidney stone, stomach obstruction, abdominal ulcer, bleeding hemorrhoid, twisted ovarian cyst, ectopic pregnancy
Required (surgery within a few weeks or months)	Cataract, spinal fusion, sinus operation, repair of heart or blood vessel defect, removal of very large fibroid
Elective (surgery should be done but no serious problem if it is not)	Simple hemorrhoids, superficial cyst, non-invasive fatty or fibrous tumor, burn scar repair
Optional (surgery advisable but not essential)	Strabismus repair, breast reconstruction, varicose vein stripping, wart removal
Cosmetic (surgery only to improve appearance)	Removal of acne scars, nose reconstruction, breast augmentation, face lift

ous ones are: embolism (blood clot); cardiac arrest; postoperative hemorrhage leading to shock; wound rupture; postoperative infection; pneumonia (once often fatal, now usually controllable with antibiotics).

7. If general anesthesia will be required, make sure it is administered by a physician anesthesiologist or a certified, trained nurse anesthesiologist under the supervision of a physician anesthesiologist; complications and death from anesthesia are one of the most serious risks of surgery.

8. Discuss the fee for surgery with the surgeon and investigate what other costs are involved (assistant's fees, anesthesiologist's fees, hospital fees, special nursing care, your own physician's fees, etc.).

9. Check on your surgeon with other patients and his or her colleagues—ask whom they would select for themselves—and in the *Directory of Medical Specialists,* which lists their schooling, residency and length of practice.

10. Make sure the surgeon you choose is willing to work with your family doctor or internist. Consider using a surgeon who belongs to a group practice, preferably a group with internists, surgeons and other specialists.

11. Consider joining a health maintenance organization (HMO), in which a surgeon's income does not depend on the number of operations performed. One study revealed HMOs perform half as many operations as were performed under health insurance plans that compensated doctors on a per/case basis.

12. Pick a surgeon not too busy to give patients enough time and attention; the best surgeons are busy but they are not rushed, nor do they rush patients through an operation.

13. Remember that the decision to undergo surgery is yours; listen to expert opinion, get as much information as possible, but make your own decisions as to whether or not to go ahead.

See also Resources in the Appendix.

surrogate mother   Also *contract mother, surrogacy.* A woman who agrees to be inseminated with the sperm of the partner of an infertile woman. The surrogate mother carries the baby to term, whereupon it is adopted by the biological father and his partner. The procedure is used by couples who desperately want a baby genetically related to at least one of them (the male partner) and cannot have one of their own because the woman lacks a uterus or ovaries, cannot ovulate, carries a genetic disease or has health problems precluding a pregnancy. The surrogate mother, who is paid all expenses plus a fee, is artificially inseminated. In another kind of arrangement, called *gestational surrogacy,* when a woman ovulates but lacks a uterus or cannot carry a fetus to term, the eggs and sperm of the couple are brought together in a laboratory, and the resulting embryo is implanted in the surrogate mother.

Surrogacy, which is thought to be relatively uncommon, has given rise to serious legal and emotional problems in a number of highly publicized custody cases. In 1988 Michigan became the first state to outlaw the practice entirely, declaring commercial contracts for women to bear children for others void and unenforceable, so that participants in these contracts are punishable as criminals. The issue is controversial; some regard surrogate motherhood as a form of reproductive prostitution, while others see it as a gift a fertile woman can give to an infertile one. In other cases a woman is inseminated with sperm from a homosexual man, bears a child and turns it over to him for upbringing. At this writing some 16 states have enacted laws concerning such issues as whether or not the contract initially signed is legally binding, the parental rights (if any) of the gestational mother and payment for such a service.

symphysis pubis The portion of pubic bone directly underlying the MONS VENERIS. Occasionally obstetricians have performed a *symphisiotomy,* cutting through this section of bone in order to enlarge the space for passage of a baby. Because this surgery involves considerable risk to both mother and baby, it has been largely abandoned in America, where a CESAREAN SECTION is performed instead, but it is still performed elsewhere.

symptom Strictly speaking, subjective evidence of a disease or disorder, which is felt by the patient rather than seen by the clinician. Examples include dizziness, fatigue and pain. However, the term is often loosely used as a synonym for SIGN.

See also SYNDROME.

syndrome A group of symptoms and/or signs that typically occur together in a particular disease or disorder. For example, numbness or paralysis on one side, dizziness and difficulty in speaking constitute the principal symptoms of a cerebral vascular accident, or stroke, and so are sometimes called "stroke syndrome."

syphilis Also *bad blood, lues, pox.* A SEXUALLY TRANSMITTED DISEASE transmitted by sexual intercourse (vaginal, anal, oral) and caused by a microscopic organism, *Treponema pallidum.* The same organism,

a spirochete that burrows through tiny breaks in the skin and mucous membranes, also causes yaws (a skin disease), endemic syphilis and pinta, three disorders that occur mostly in tropical countries. Venereal syphilis, which can be fatal, is transmitted primarily by sexual contact but can also be incurred if fluid from a syphilitic sore or rash gets inside a cut on another person's skin. A fetus inside the womb of an infected mother also can contract the disease. The disease has three stages, *primary, secondary* (subdivided into *early latent* and *late latent*) and *tertiary.* During the primary stage a CHANCRE, a painless ulcerating sore, appears at the point where the organism entered the body, in men usually on the penis and in women on the cervix or inner vaginal walls. It appears 10 to 90 days (three weeks, on the average) after the infectious contact and normally disappears in one to five weeks without treatment. There may also be, at the same time, painless hard swelling of the surrounding lymph nodes, especially in men. It too may disappear spontaneously.

The secondary stage, beginning about six weeks after the chancre appears, is characterized by a generalized non-itchy rash occurring anywhere from the scalp to the soles of the feet. There also may be flulike symptoms, such as sore throat and hoarseness, caused by a rash inside the throat, occasional bone and joint pain, patchy loss of scalp hair and eye inflammation. After some months these symptoms disappear, even without treatment, and the disease enters its latent stage, when it is detectable only by a blood test.

During the primary and secondary stages syphilis is highly infectious (catching), but during the latent stage only the fetus of an infected mother can be infected. The latent stage may last 10 to 15 years. In about one-third of cases the disease then proceeds to the tertiary or late stage, in which it attacks the heart, blood vessels, brain, spinal cord or bone. Heart disease, blindness, loss of muscle coordination, deafness, paralysis, insanity or death may result.

Congenital syphilis is acquired by an unborn baby from its mother. Pregnancy masks syphilis symptoms, making them even more dangerous. Though primary chancres in a pregnant woman may be larger than otherwise, the skin rash of secondary syphilis may be scarcely visible. The syphilis organisms travel from mother to fetus via the placenta.

The placenta is not well enough developed for this transfer until 16 to 18 weeks into the pregnancy, so a syphilis infection detected and treated *before* the fourth month of pregnancy usually will not harm the baby. The more recent the infection in the mother, the more likely it is that the baby will be infected, and the more severe its symptoms. Almost all babies born to women with untreated primary or secondary syphilis develop the disease, and many die either before or soon after birth. However, infants born to women with latent syphilis may either escape infection or develop a case of syphilis that is not immediately life-threatening. All pregnant women in North America must have at least two blood tests for syphilis, the first during the first trimester and the second during the third trimester.

Diagnosing syphilis is not easy, because the symptoms can resemble those of many other disorders. Anyone who develops a sore on the genitals should be examined for syphilis without delay. Fluid from the sore contains the organism, but it is often hard to see under the microscope even with a dark-field test. Blood tests to detect syphilis antibodies are more reliable, and today they are routinely performed on all persons in North America entering a hospital for any reason, giving blood, entering the armed forces or diagnosed as pregnant. Mass testing has uncovered many cases of untreated syphilis in individuals unaware of their infection and has significantly reduced the number of cases in the United States and Canada.

The first blood test for syphilis was developed in 1906 by August von Wasserman. The *Wasserman test* was widely used for half a century but was not wholly accurate. Today there are more than 200 different blood tests for syphilis, of which those most used are the VDRL, RPR, FTA-ABS and MHA-TP. The VDRL (for Venereal Disease Research Laboratory of the U.S. Public Health Service, which developed the test) and RPR (for rapid plasma reagin) are nonspecific tests. They measure levels of a general antibody that appears to fight not only syphilis but several other infections. The other two tests are specifically for syphilis. The FTA-ABS (for fluorescent treponemal antibody absorption test) is regarded as the most accurate test and shows a positive result in anyone who currently has or ever had the disease; however, at least one study indicates that it sometimes fails to give positive results when the organism resides in the patient's ocular fluid. The MHA-TP (microhemagglutination assay for *Treponema pallidum*) also detects the specific antibody for the causative organism.

Treatment for all stages of syphilis consists of antibiotics. The first choice is penicillin by injection, preferably a kind that maintains a constant amount of penicillin in the bloodstream for at least two weeks; slowly excreted, long-lasting forms of penicillin, such as benzathine penicillin or procaine penicillin G with aluminum monostearate (PAM), are preferred. For those allergic to penicillin, doxycycline or tetracycline may be substituted. Treatment of syphilis often results in an uncomfortable reaction, principally a fever and the enlargement of any chancre that is present, but such reactions last only a few hours. After treatment, a series of follow-up tests to make sure the disease is cured must be performed, with blood tests monthly for the first three months and then every third month for a year and every six months for a second year. Intercourse must be avoided for one month after treatment.

Syphilis had become relatively rare in the United States, but recently there have been a rise in cases. In 2006 nearly 10,000 cases of the most contagious forms of the disease were reported. For congenital syphilis, in which infants get the disease from their mothers inside the womb, the rate rose only slightly.

systemic Bodywide, that is, not localized or limited to some particular part of the body or some particular organ. Most of the common childhood diseases, such as measles and chicken pox, are systemic infections (see INFECTION), and most authorities view cancer as a systemic disease.

systemic lupus erythematosus Also *SLE, lupus.* An inflammatory disorder of the body's immune system that affects the connective tissue in numerous parts of the body and afflicts approximately 1 of every 500 American women (and only one-tenth as many men). It is two to three times more common in black women than in whites, and its onset most often occurs between the ages of 20 and 40.

The disease is named for one of its signs, a rash in the shape of a "butterfly" over the nose and cheeks, similar to the facial markings of a wolf (*lupus erythematosus* is Latin for "red wolf"). However, the disease affects not only the skin but also, in different individuals and at different times, all the collagen tissues, including the joints, blood vessels, heart, lungs, brain and, most dangerously, the kidneys. Formerly thought to be an AUTOIMMUNE DISEASE, systemic lupus is now generally described as an "immune complex" disease, in which the patient's antibodies combine with antigens, either foreign or the patient's own, to form complexes that mediate tissue damage. There is a genetic predisposition to the development of systemic lupus, shown by the fact that if one of two identical twins gets the disorder the other twin has a 50 to 60% chance of developing it too, whereas with fraternal twins the second twin has only a 2 to 3% risk.

A person may have systemic lupus without knowing it, and such mild forms require no treatment. Diagnosis is based on a blood test that detects antinuclear antibodies. In patients with more severe cases, usually two or more of the following symptoms are present, although these same symptoms also may appear in mild cases but then are both mild and short-lived: (1) skin rashes or sores, including small ulcers inside the mouth; (2) RAYNAUD'S PHENOMENON, in which the fingers become blue and white after exposure to cold; (3) the characteristic butterfly rash over the cheeks, which often becomes worse after exposure to the sun; (4) painful joints, especially at the fingers, wrists and knees (similar to rheumatoid arthritis); (5) abnormal blood cell count (lowered white cells, red cells or even platelets); (6) inflammation of serous membranes, especially the pericardium (around the heart), peritoneum (around the abdominal cavity) and pleura (around the lungs), often developing into pleurisy; (7) inflammation of the lungs, developing into a mild pneumonia that responds to anti-inflammatory drugs rather than to antibiotics; (8) central nervous system disturbances, sometimes leading to seizures or other problems; (9) kidney disease, a major problem in at least half of systemic lupus patients. Flare-ups interspersed with periods of improvement or remission are typical. In 20% to 30% of patients symptoms remain mild, but in 50% to 75% vital organs are affected.

A number of drugs in common use are capable of inducing a form of systemic lupus, the symptoms of which usually include low-grade fever, skin rash of various kinds, aching muscles and joints, and chest pain (pleurisy). The symptoms usually disappear as soon as the drug is stopped, although laboratory evidence (antibodies) of the disease may persist for months. Among the drugs known to induce systemic lupus are chlorpromazine and some of the phenothiazines (tranquilizers), procainamide (used to regulate heart rhythm), hydrazaline (given for high blood pressure), oral contraceptives, isoniazid (used against tuberculosis) and some others.

Treatment ranges from none for the mildest form of lupus to aspirin and other anti-inflammatory drugs and various steroids, or antimalarial drugs to dampen immune responses. However, long-term steroid treatment may contribute to higher cardiovascular risk. Rapid diagnosis and prompt treatment may help prevent major damage to organs such as the kidneys. Most patients with lupus take at least two drugs, and many take three or four. Birth control pills, containing both estrogen and progestin, have helped some patients. The two most common medications prescribed for lupus are hydroxychloroquine (Plaquenil) and a corticosteroid such as prednisone. Plaquenil was developed to treat malaria and appears to reduce the production of antibodies that cause problems in lupus. Steroids stop the body's immune response and reduce the swelling, tenderness and pain of inflammation. However, they must be given in the lowest effective dose, because they not only cause short-term side effects, such as acne and excessive hair growth, but also long-term side effects such as bone problems, increased risk of infection and cardiovascular disease. In moderate or severe cases immunosuppressive drugs may be used. Originally designed to prevent organ and tissue rejection after transplants, they reduce the immune system's overactivity in lupus and, like steroids, increase risk of infection. The principal immunopressants used are azathioprine (Imuron) and cyclophosphamide (Cytoxan); both have serious side effects.

The newest treatment for severe lupus that cannot be controlled with other therapies is stem cell therapy. The physician collects the patient's own stem cells—immature cells capable of developing into many different cell types—and returns them to the body after a course of high-dose chemotherapy. The chemotherapy eliminates the misguided immune cells causing lupus symptoms, and the stem cells restore them to normal function. Treatment requires a hospital stay of several weeks, and, because of increased risk of infection, prophylactic antibiotics for six months and antiviral drugs for a year after the transplant. The treatment is still experimental, and much further research and testing is required.

Newer treatments still being investigated are agents that suppress immune response more selectively, targeting harmful cells without damaging the rest. Exposure to the sun must be avoided if ultraviolet rays cause a flare-up of symptoms. Some patients become tired very easily and must avoid overexertion. Viral infections may aggravate the symptoms, as may estrogen in the form used in oral contraceptives, which should then be avoided. Pregnancy may trigger a flare-up, but some lupus patients have normal pregnancies and healthy babies. However, there is a higher than average risk of miscarriage and, if the baby is carried to term, a tendency for the disease to flare up again after delivery. Lupus patients also are more apt to develop heart disease, so it is important that they control risk factors such as high cholesterol and high blood pressure.

tachycardia See ARTERY.

tail of Spence An extension of breast tissue toward the axilla (armpit); see BREAST.

tamoxifen See ESTROGEN-RECEPTOR ASSAY; HORMONE THERAPY; SELECTIVE ESTROGEN-RECEPTOR MODULATOR.

tampon An internally worn device of absorbent material intended to soak up menstrual flow. It comes in sizes small enough to permit insertion by most young girls, whose HYMEN as a rule stretches enough to accommodate it. In efforts to improve their product and thus gain a larger share of the market, manufacturers have embellished tampons with various kinds of perfume to mask "natural" odors, various kinds of applicator to make insertion easier, and various sizes and thicknesses to absorb menstrual flow ranging from light to very heavy. Occasionally their efforts have gone astray and their product has become so absorbent, for example, that it is difficult to remove because it expands so much when wet. Also, some women experience considerable vaginal irritation from some kinds of tampon.

In 1980 the use of tampons was linked to the occurrence of a rare but potentially dangerous disease called *toxic shock syndrome,* which affected primarily young women. It is characterized by very rapid onset, and symptoms include high fever, vomiting, diarrhea, dizziness, a sunburnlike rash with peeling (especially on the hands and feet) and a rapid drop in blood pressure, frequently resulting in shock. Most cases seemed to occur in women under the age of 25 and to begin during a menstrual period when tampons were used. It never was determined how tampons contributed to the disease, but manufacturers did respond to public criticism and changed the composition of their product. Also, since 1990 the U.S. Food and Drug Administration has required manufacturers to label their products corresponding to a specific range of absorbency for controlling flow, including an explanation of the range of moisture retention signified. As a result of these measures, the incidence of toxic shock syndrome had dropped markedly in women who are menstruating. (It also can occur with a skin infection, burn, insect bite or surgical wound.) Nevertheless, women still are advised to use regular-size tampons (not "super" or larger), change them frequently and not rely on them exclusively, using external pads at night and for times of light menstrual flow. For women who do develop symptoms of toxic shock syndrome, prompt treatment with antibiotics is essential, along with supportive measures, especially intravenous replacement of fluids and electrolytes. Further, a woman who has had toxic shock syndrome once is at considerable risk—one study says as high as 42%—for developing it again.

Tay-Sachs disease A fatal hereditary disease characterized by the absence of an enzyme, hexosaminidase A, making it impossible for the body to assimilate certain fats. Although a child born with the disorder may seem normal at birth, symptoms appear during the first six months of life, beginning with deterioration of motor ability and voluntary movement. Progressively the child becomes severely retarded and develops blindness, convulsions, and paralysis. Death usually occurs by the age of three or four. No cure is known. A recessive-gene disorder (see BIRTH DEFECTS), Tay-Sachs disease is common among Ashkenazi Jews (from Central and Eastern Europe), among whom an estimated 1 of every 25 persons is a carrier (as opposed to 1 in 300 in other ethnic groups). If both parents are carriers, a fact that can be determined by a simple blood test, there is a 25% risk that any child of theirs will have the disease. Its presence in a fetus can be detected by AMNIOCENTESIS as well as other PRENATAL TESTS. A major international effort at genetic screening, directed at the Ashkenazi Jewish population, has cut the incidence of Tay-Sachs by 95%.

See also GAUCHER'S DISEASE.

temporomandibular joint Also *TMJ, myofascial pain dysfunction, MPD.* A disorder in which muscle spasms and pain affect the hinge joint that connects the lower jaw to the upper jawbone. About 20% of all Americans have this disorder, and women three times as frequently as men. It usually manifests itself between the ages of 20 and 40. Symptoms include an ache in the area of the ear extending to the back of the head and into the face, neck and shoulders; a clicking or popping sound on opening and closing the mouth; pain similar to that of a tooth abscess; difficulty in opening the mouth and chewing; migrainelike headache; a feeling of "plugged" ear or ringing in the ears; and/or tenderness of the jaw muscles. Most often the syndrome is thought to be caused by stress and tension that make an individual clench or grind her teeth. Occasionally the cause is arthritis or malocclusion (poor bite). Treatment includes a soft diet until the severe symptoms subside, applications of moist heat, a muscle relaxant or tranquilizer, analgesics such as aspirin, and a bite plate to be worn while sleeping to prevent grinding. The disorder usually is treated by a dentist rather than a physician.

term See GESTATION.

testes See TESTIS.

testicular feminization See ANDROGEN SENSITIVITY SYNDROME.

testis Also *testicles; testes* (pl.). The male gonad, or sex gland, which is primarily responsible for secreting male sex hormones, or androgens, and for producing the male germ cell, or sperm. There are two testes, one hanging in each side of the SCROTUM, slightly in front of the thighs, behind the penis. Unlike the female gonads, or ovaries, which contain female germ cells at birth, the testes produce sperm only after puberty, but then produce millions every day. Each testis is an oval-shaped structure about 1 ½ inches (3½ centimeters) long and 1 inch (2½ centimeters) thick. It is divided into some 250 compartments, each of which contains several *seminiferous tubules.* Sperm grow and mature within these tubules, and cells between the tubules, called *interstitial cells,* secrete androgens. The seminiferous tubules join together into a dozen or so ducts that form the first part of the *epididymis,* a single tightly coiled duct in which sperm are stored. The cells lining the duct secrete a substance stimulating the development of sperm. Infection and the subsequent formation of scar tissue can block the epididymis, resulting in sterility. Occasionally one or both testes do not descend into the scrotum but remain in the inguinal canal or abdomen, a condition called CRYPTORCHIDISM.

See also PENIS; SPERM.

testosterone The principal male sex hormone, or androgen, produced chiefly by the male gonads, the testes. Its production is controlled in much the same way as the production of estrogen by the ovaries in women, that is, by the pituitary hormones FSH (follicle-stimulating hormone) and LH (luteinizing hormone), which in turn are controlled by the hypothalamus. Before PUBERTY, which in most boys begins between the ages of 10 and 15, the testes secrete only small amounts of testosterone. During puberty this quantity is greatly increased, and it is the substance principally responsible for the appearance of secondary sex characteristics (facial and body hair, bigger muscles, deepening voice, enlarged testes and penis) and the growth spurt characteristic of normal puberty.

In women the ovaries and adrenal glands also are capable of secreting testosterone, but except in diseases such as the adrenogenital syndrome, they do so in very small quantity. After menopause the ovaries produce not only less estrogen but less testosterone. Some women who found their libido lessened considerably at this time appear to have benefited from testosterone injections. In such cases dosage must be carefully monitored so as to avoid such side effects as increased facial hair.

See also ANABOLIC STEROIDS.

test-tube baby   See IN VITRO FERTILIZATION.

thalidomide   A tranquilizer originally made by a West German company and commonly used in the early 1960s, especially in Europe, where it frequently was given to pregnant women. When given early in pregnancy, it was discovered to cause severe malformations in the fetus, especially interfering with the development of normal limbs (arms and legs), so that babies were born with flippers instead of limbs, with hands attached at the shoulder or similar structural abnormalities. The drug was never sold in North America but at least 2½ million "experimental" pills were distributed there, so some American babies were affected. In 1998, however, thalidomide was approved for treatment of skin lesions associated with leprosy. Since the drug is now available in the United States, it is expected that it will be used for such off-label purposes as shrinking tumors in patients with AIDS, treating the potentially fatal side effects of bone marrow surgery, and possibly also for tuberculosis and the blindness resulting from uncontrolled diabetes. (See OFF-LABEL DRUG USE.) Unless used with caution, however, it still causes birth defects and so must be avoided by pregnant women. Consequently researchers are investigating ways to alter the compound so that it continues to fight malignant cells and infection but does not hamper the development of blood vessels (which is how it causes birth defects).

therapeutic touch   A technique of healing that does not involve actually touching the body. Rather, the practitioner holds his or her hands palms down a few inches from the patient, scanning the body from head to toe and sensing so-called blockages or deficits in the patient's energy field. The blockages are opened by using hand motions to transfer energy from practitioner to patient, supposedly promoting healing while reducing pain, anxiety and stress. Created in the early 1970s by a registered nurse, Delores Krieger, therapeutic touch is encouraged by many nurses but is viewed with skepticism by others because there is no valid research supporting its effectiveness.

therapy   Another word for treatment (of any kind). However, it often is used as a synonym for PSYCHOTHERAPY.

See also FEMINIST THERAPY; SEX THERAPY.

thermatic sterilization   Also *thermatic male sterilization, TMS*. A method of using heat to achieve temporary sterility in men. The fact that heat inhibits sperm has been known since ancient times, though it still is not certain whether heat kills sperm or simply slows them down (impairs their motility). In 1921, Martha Voegeli, a Swiss physician working in India, decided to apply this principle as a means of birth control. The procedure she developed requires a man to sit in a bath with water at a temperature of 116 degrees Fahrenheit (47 degrees Celsius) for 45 minutes every day for three weeks; this allegedly renders him sterile for six months, whereupon his fertility is restored. Voegeli claims to have used this method successfully in India for 20 years, from 1930 to 1950. In the 1960s, several American physicians, among them John Rock, who helped develop oral contraceptives, experimented with insulated underwear, which retains body heat, for the same purpose. Apparently this method also was effective, but research results remain too scanty to determine its reliability.

The opposite has also been tried, that is, using a cooling system to overcome male infertility. For this purpose an undergarment that looks like an athletic supporter but is kept damp with distilled water cools the testicles by about 2 degrees (because evaporation carries off heat). Approved by the U.S. Food and Drug Administration in 1985, the device allegedly improves sperm count and quality in 70% of the men who wear it for at least three months.

threatened miscarriage   See MISCARRIAGE, def. 2.

thromboembolism   See EMBOLISM.

thrombophlebitis   See PHLEBITIS.

thrombus   Also *blood clot; thrombi* (pl.). A blood clot that forms within a blood vessel rather than externally. For reasons that are not understood, blood sometimes spontaneously forms such clots. A sizable clot can obstruct the blood vessel in which it formed and, if that vessel is an artery supplying oxygen and vital nutrients to an important organ, such as the heart, lungs or brain, severe or even fatal damage can result. Abnormal clotting within the veins or arteries is called THROMBOSIS; if it occurs in one of the arteries supplying blood to the heart—the *coronary arteries*—it is called a *coronary thrombosis,* and if it affects an artery supplying blood to the brain, it is a *cerebral thrombosis.* The presence of a thrombus in a vein is called *venous thrombosis, thrombophlebitis* or PHLEBITIS.

Although the cause of venous clots is not known, certain factors predispose a person to their formation, among them *stasis,* that is, sluggish blood flow through the veins, which may occur with inactivity, immobilization, obstruction of the blood flow and so on. For this reason they are more likely to form in old age, with long-term bed rest and immediately following surgery and childbirth. Congestive heart failure and shock, estrogen therapy and certain infections and malignancies also increase the likelihood of thrombus formation.

Blood clots frequently occur in the deep veins of the calf muscles, a condition called *deep venous thrombosis.* The typical symptom is a painful swollen leg. Diagnosis is by ultrasound, which can rule out other conditions giving rise to such swelling

and pain. Women are particularly at risk for deep venous thrombosis during pregnancy and for several months following childbirth. It is also a side effect of certain medications, among them birth control pills, estrogen, progesterone, tamoxifen and raloxifene. Also, persons who take frequent long-haul airplane flights can be at risk for clots, a vulnerability that has been given the name *economy-class syndrome.* Leg pain and swelling can show up even two weeks after a long flight. It helps to get up and walk up and down the aisle every hour or so and to do leg-flexing exercises. Some doctors recommend wearing graduated compression support hose on long flights.

Treatment generally involves hospitalization and administration of *anticoagulants,* which reduce the ability of the blood to form clots. One such drug is heparin, administered by injection; another is coumadin, which can be taken orally. Both interfere with the production of essential blood clotting factors and must be used with extreme caution, and never when there is danger of hemorrhage. When the clot does not dissolve, a radiologist may guide a catheter through the blocked vein and apply clot-dissolving drugs directly to the clot or break it up mechanically. Occasionally a clot must be extracted surgically. In some cases the first evidence of a clot is shortness of breath or chest pain, signaling a pulmonary embolism, which can be fatal. Diagnosis here is by a lung X-ray made after the patient either inhales a radioactive aerosol or is injected with a radioactive dye. Treatment is the same for leg-vein clots. In up to 80% of patients, deep venous thrombosis can lead to *post-thrombotic syndrome,* which occurs when a blood clot damages valves in leg veins so that blood flows backward and pools in the legs. Pressure can cause swelling, chronic pain, discoloration and fatigue, and the damage may be permanent.

thyroid   An ENDOCRINE gland consisting of two lobes, one on each side of the trachea (windpipe), joined by a narrow bridge. It produces two hormones, thyroxine (T4) and triiodothyronine (T3), which help regulate growth and METABOLISM and which can be produced only when the body takes in adequate amounts of iodine. Like the hormones involved in the MENSTRUAL CYCLE, the secretion of thyroid hormones involves a stimulating hormone, called *thyroid-stimulating* or *thyrotropic hormone* (TSH), which in turn requires a release factor, called *thyrotropin-releasing hormone* (TRH) or *thyrotropin-releasing factor* (TRF). Also as in the menstrual cycle, these hormones operate by means of a negative feedback mechanism. Increased levels of thyroid hormone suppress TSH release; when hormone levels fall, there is an increase in TRH, triggering TSH production. TRH also stimulates production of prolactin and lactation.

Disorders of the thyroid gland, which occur four to five times more often in women than in men, usually involve either overproduction (*hyperthyroidism*) or underproduction (*hypothyroidism*) of these hormones. The fact that women are more prone to thyroid problems than men, especially at puberty, during pregnancy and at menopause, suggests a possible link between thyroid and ovarian function. The American College of Physicians now recommends a blood test for thyroid disorders at least once every five years for women over the age of 50. The most common tests are for measuring T3 and T4, but these results can be misleading, since their levels may remain normal when TSH is elevated. It is preferable, therefore, also to measure TSH. Not a particularly costly test, it is usually covered by health insurance.

Hypothyroidism is the most common thyroid disorder, occurring in about 1 woman in 10. The drop in thyroid hormone production is gradual, so that one may be scarcely aware of such symptoms as increased sensitivity to cold, constipation, slowing of hair and nail growth, unusual extreme fatigue, and moderate weight gain (10 to 15 pounds). Occasionally it also causes high cholesterol. Also, as the body tries to restore hormone production, the thyroid gland may become enlarged, creating a *goiter*, which appears as a visible swelling at the front of the neck. (See also below.) A less common form of hypothyroidism is caused by *Hashimoto's thyroiditis,* an AUTOIMMUNE DISEASE in which the body produces antibodies against its own thyroid tissue. A hereditary and progressive condition, it surfaces mostly in postmenopausal women, who by then have very low levels of thyroid hormone production. In younger women hypothyroidism also can cause two fertility problems, increased PROLACTIN production and persistent estrogen stimulation. Treatment for hypothyroidism consists of taking a thyroid hormone supplement (usually thyroxine), which generally must be taken for life. Dosage must be carefully calculated since too much can cause heart problems. If thyroxine (T4) alone does not work, sometimes adding T3 is effective. However, thyroid medication robs the body of minerals, so older women who take it may be at greater risk for osteoporosis unless they also take preventive measures.

Myxedema, caused by thyroid hormone deficiency in older children and adults, is marked by personality changes, dry and puffy skin, and edema (fluid retention). It can delay the onset of menstruation in adolescent girls. After puberty it may cause very heavy menstrual bleeding and consequent anemia (occasionally leading to false diagnosis of a uterine tumor), and it usually prevents a woman from becoming pregnant. This condition responds well to the administration of thyroid hormone.

Some kinds of goiter, a condition estimated to be up to five times more common in women than in men, can also be caused by hyperthyroidism. A goiter itself may require no treatment at all unless the enlargement causes uncomfortable pressure on adjacent organs or a tumor is suspected. Treatment is directed at restoring hormone levels to normal by means of drugs that suppress the excess hormone.

The most common form of hyperthyroidism is *Graves' disease,* whose symptoms, in addition to goiter, include nervousness, heat sensitivity, a moderate weight loss despite normal appetite, tremors, increased heart rate and bulging eyes. Women, who are affected seven to nine times as often as men, also may experience menstrual irregularities and impaired fertility. In those with a family history of the disorder, its onset most often occurs between the ages of 20 and 40, sometimes triggered by severe emotional stress or by a hormonal change such as pregnancy. Like Hashimoto's, it is hereditary and is also an autoimmune disorder, but rather than destroying thyroid tissue the antibodies here trigger thyroid enlargement. Treatment involves suppressing the excess hormone production by means of drugs. Because these often have bad side effects, many clinicians prefer to use radioactive iodine, a treatment that has largely replaced partial or total surgical removal of the thyroid gland (*thyroidectomy*). Pregnant patients cannot be given some antithyroid drugs alone because they can affect the fetus, causing thyroid deficiency and possible permanent dwarfism and mental retardation; if they require such medication it must be given together with thyroid hormone in adequate amounts to avoid such damage.

TIA Abbreviation for *transient ischemic attack;* see CEREBRAL VASCULAR ACCIDENT.

tic douloureux Also *trigeminal neuralgia.* Episodes of severe sharp pain in one of the divisions of the trigeminal (fifth cranial) nerve in the upper or lower jaw, usually of brief duration (10 to 15 seconds). It is thought to be caused by a blood vessel pressing against the nerve. This pressure erodes the nerve's protective covering so that it fires off with little or no provocation. It tends to afflict women more than men and women over 50 more than young ones. In young people, it may be an early symptom of MULTIPLE SCLEROSIS, and it may occur in association with that disease during any of its stages. The pain of tic douloureux may be set off by touching a trigger point or by a movement of the jaws, as in chewing, shaving or brushing the teeth. There are no objective signs of the disease, the bouts of acute pain—often many during each day—being the only symptom. Treatment is palliative, usually involving a strong pain reliever (carbamazepine is the one most commonly used). In severe cases, surgery may be considered. Once a last resort, microsurgical techniques have made it more feasible. It consists of a very delicate operation in which the surgeon bores into the back of the skull, moves aside the cerebellum and locates the blood vessel that is pressing against the trigeminal nerve. If a vein, it is cut; if an artery, a tiny pad is placed between it and the nerve. In either case the pressure is removed, relieving the pain.

tipped uterus See RETROVERTED UTERUS.

TMJ See TEMPOROMANDIBULAR JOINT.

toxemia of pregnancy See ECLAMPSIA; PRE-ECLAMPSIA.

toxic shock syndrome Also *TSS.* See TAMPON.

tranquilizers 1. Also *antianxiety drugs.* A class of drugs used to treat anxiety, as well as more serious psychiatric disorders, principally schizophrenia and mania. *Barbiturates,* a group of drugs that are chiefly sedative and sleep producing (such as phenobarbital, pentobarbital and secobarbital, which include Seconal, Nembutal and others), are sometimes described as tranquilizers.

2. minor tranquilizers. Drugs used to treat ANXIETY. They are among the most frequently prescribed drugs in the United States, and many feel they are overprescribed, especially for women. There are two principal kinds, the benzodiazepine compounds (Librium, Valium, Xanax and others), which sedate, relax the muscles and are anticonvulsive as well as combating anxiety, and meprobamate (Equanil, Miltown). Although very effective against anxiety, they also are potentially habit-forming and addictive, so discontinuing the drug abruptly can lead to withdrawal symptoms. They impair alertness, often making one feel drowsy and lethargic, and in large doses cause unsteadiness in stance and gait. They lead to a serious adverse reaction if combined with alcohol, which therefore should be avoided by anyone taking tranquilizers. They probably should not be taken at any time during pregnancy and certainly not during the first three months, since they have been associated with birth defects. They also should be avoided by women who are breast-feeding. As with any strong medication, the risks should be carefully weighed against the benefits. On balance, the minor tranquilizers are considered useful to control distressing symptoms initially but should be used for as brief a time as possible, in conjunction with some kind of psychotherapy that is directed at determining and eliminating the causes of anxiety.

3. major tranquilizers. Also *neuroleptics, antipsychotics.* Drugs used to treat serious psychiatric disorders, principally schizophrenia, acute mania and acute confusional states. They produce a state of emotional calm and virtual indifference, technically called *neurolepsy.* The principal neuroleptics are the phenothiazines, which include chlorpromazine (Thorazine), thioridazine (Mellaril) and trifluoperazine (Stelazine), the butyrophenones, which include haloperidol (Haldol), and various newer drugs. They usually relieve such symptoms as thought disturbances, delusions, hallucinations and agitation, but they are very potent drugs and should not be used by pregnant women.

A number of drugs sometimes called *atypical antipsychotics* have been approved for treating SCHIZOPHRENIA and the manic stages of MANIC-DEPRESSIVE ILLNESS. They also have been used for other conditions, such as dementia, behavioral problems, depression and personality disorders, but they need to be used with care owing to their potency and potentially serious side effects. They include aripiprazole (Abilify), olanzapine (Zyprexa), quetiapine (Saroquel), risperidone (Risperdal) and ziprasidone (Geodon).

trans fat   Also, *trans fatty acids, trans unsaturated fatty acids.* A fat created by hydrogenation used in the manufacture of stick margarines, solid shortenings and numerous cooking oils and prepared foods in order to improve flavor and texture and to preserve freshness. Trans fat both raises LDL and lowers HDL (see CHOLESTEROL), the worst possible effect for risk of heart disease. A new U.S. government ruling requires food manufacturers to label trans fat content of their products in excess of 0.5 grams by January 1, 2006. Ideally, no amount of trans fat should be consumed, but this goal is not entirely realistic, since virtually all packaged and convenience foods contain some. Margarine, fried foods like doughnuts and French fries and some prepared foods contain the most, so it is recommended that they be avoided.

See also DIET.

transient ischemic attack   Also *TIA.*

See also CEREBRAL VASCULAR ACCIDENT.

transition   End of the first stage of labor; see LABOR.

transsexual   A person who undergoes hormone treatment and/or surgery in order to change from his or her biologically determined sex to the opposite sex. Although this change can be accomplished in either direction (from man to woman, or woman to man), in practice it is much easier to change from man to woman, and about 80% of those seeking such a change are men who wish to become women. The penis and testes are removed, and an artificial vagina is constructed. Female sex hormones are given, and sometimes the breasts are surgically enlarged. In changing a woman to a man, both breasts, both ovaries and the uterus are removed. Testes are constructed, and sometimes a penis is made from skin flaps; such a penis is not capable of erection but can be made to function with implants or devices of the kind sometimes used to treat impotent men. Also, male sex hormones are administered. These operations, which are both drastic and irreversible, were devised in the mid-1960s and by the late 1970s some surgeons were already abandoning them in the belief that they did not really change a person's life as much, or as favorably, as had been expected.

Transsexuals believe they are really members of the opposite sex who are trapped in the wrong body—that is, their gender identity does not match their physical identity. After surgery, transsexuals usually fashion new lives for themselves and often try to keep their old identities secret. Many marry and raise adopted children. Frequently, however, they find that their emotional adjustment is no better than before surgery and hormone therapy were undertaken.

Before deciding to undergo a sex change of this kind, anyone considering it is strongly advised to seek counseling from a therapist who specializes in this specific area. At least a year of intensive counseling is recommended, and then most therapists advise the person to live in the desired role for another year before deciding on surgery. (This condition is *required* by the best of the clinics where this treatment is performed.) Many applicants for transsexual surgery do, in the course of these preliminary procedures, change their minds.

Only 10 to 15% of candidates are considered a good risk, according to some psychiatrists working in this field. In the United States about half of the sex-change operations performed are done in university-based programs, which usually require that an individual be successful psychologically, socially and economically in the tested new sex role before surgery is performed.

transvaginal ultrasound   See ULTRASOUND, def. 1.

transverse position   See SHOULDER PRESENTATION.

trapped egg syndrome   See LUTEINIZED UNRUPTURED FOLLICLE.

trichomonas   Also *trich, trichomoniasis.* A vaginal infection caused by a one-celled organism, *Trichomonas vaginalis,* that is extremely common among women but usually only if they are sexually active. Because it can be transmitted sexually, it also is considered a SEXUALLY TRANSMITTED DISEASE, and treatment, to be effective, must be given to both partners. Also, the organism can survive at room temperature for several hours on moist objects and so can be transmitted by a sheet, towel, washcloth or toilet seat used by an infected woman. Trichomonas is one of the most common sexually transmitted infections in the United States, with an estimated 5 million new cases annually.

Trichomonas causes a thin, yellow or greenish, frothy or bubbly discharge, sometimes with a foul odor, as well as itching, soreness and inflammation of the vulva and inside the vagina. Men harbor the organism in their urinary tract and usually have no symptoms at all. In women, however, the organisms also can invade the urinary tract and cause CYSTITIS (def. 1) with symptoms of burning and urinary frequency. Unfortunately, the only invariably effective drug known against trichomonas, metronidazole (Flagyl), taken orally three times a day for 7 days, has side effects, some of them potentially very serious. Further, it should never be used during the first three months of pregnancy or while breast-feeding, and some authorities say never in pregnancy. Side effects include nausea and/or diarrhea, headache, intolerance to alcohol—all alcohol drinks must be avoided while taking this drug and for three days afterward, lest it cause severe allergic reaction—and a lowered white blood cell count. For these reasons the medication should be used with caution, and white blood cell counts should be performed before, during and after treatment. Some authorities believe it is safer to take the drug in a single huge (2,000-milligram) oral dose or in two large doses 12 hours apart rather than for 7 days. The male partner should be treated too. (A female partner need be treated only if she is actually infected.) The drug is also available in vaginal suppository form but is less effective given in this way. For resistant cases, the drug may be repeated or given in higher dosage, and it appears to work best in conjunction with a douche of acetic acid (vinegar works as well). Douches such as Betadine also may help relieve symptoms.

For a mild case, a garlic suppository (peel one clove of garlic, wrap in gauze, insert overnight, change daily) may help relieve irritation. Palliative HERBAL REMEDIES used include douching with a mixture of myrrh (*Commiphora myrrha*) and goldenseal (*Hydrastis canadensis*) twice a day for one to two weeks. However, some authorities believe douching or use of suppositories can drive the infection up higher into the genital tract. All agree, however, that wearing tight pants of any kind should be avoided (if possible, wear no pants at all while at home), as should tampons, vaginal hygiene sprays and sexual intercourse without a condom.

Trichomonas can be severe enough to cause an abnormal PAP SMEAR—on which, however, the organism also can be detected—and it tends to recur. Further, it can encourage the development of venereal warts (see CONDYLOMA ACUMINATA) and YEAST INFECTION. Although trichomonas can cause small red lesions on the cervix, it does not invade the uterus or fallopian tubes, nor does it affect fertility.

See also VAGINITIS.

trigeminal neuralgia   See TIC DOULOUREUX.

triglycerides A kind of lipid, or fat, that is both consumed in the diet and present in the body. The link between them and coronary artery disease is not as a clear as that of CHOLESTEROL. However, their levels are measured because they are used to calculate the LDL in a cholesterol test. High triglyceride levels may be caused by obesity, alcohol abuse, or poorly controlled diabetes, kidney disease or liver disease. Certain medications also may be responsible. A number of individuals have genetic disorders that raise their blood triglyceride levels considerably even though their cholesterol profile is normal, indicating that triglycerides alone may not constitute a risk factor. Because levels vary during the day and rise markedly after a meal, testing should be done only after an 8- or 10-hour fast. Normal triglyceride levels are defined as below 150 mg per deciliter, 150 to 199 mg is borderline, 200 to 499 mg is high and more than that is very high. Lowering triglyceride levels involves the same strategy as lowering cholesterol: a low-fat diet, weight loss, exercise, reducing alcohol intake. If LDL is high, cholesterol-lowering drugs may be prescribed. An increase in the triglyceride level of women in particular seems to increase the risk of coronary artery disease far more than it does in men. At this writing studies of large groups of women are under way.

Two recent studies showed an association between elevated nonfasting triglycerides (tested after a meal) and later problems such as heart attack, stroke and cardiac death, especially in women, suggesting that both fasting and nonfasting levels should be tested.

trimester A three-month period, specifically the three such periods that make up a full-term (nine-month) pregnancy.

triple screen See ALPHA-FETOPROTEIN TEST.

Trisomy 21 See DOWN SYNDROME.

tubal insufflation See RUBIN TEST.

tubal ligation Also *tubal sterilization, tying the tubes.* A deliberate closing of the FALLOPIAN TUBES in order to prevent conception (pregnancy). Tubal ligation can be performed either through an incision in the abdomen or through the vagina, and it has been the principal form of STERILIZATION for women in the Western world since about 1880. Actually, *ligation,* meaning "tying," is a misnomer. Formerly part of each tube was cut off and the cut ends were pinched shut and tied; newer methods use coagulation (cauterization or burning), a laser, or place clips or bands around parts of each tube. All the procedures serve to block the tubes, thereby preventing the passage of sperm upward into the tubes and of eggs downward toward the uterus.

The principal form of *vaginal tubal ligation,* in which a small incision is made in the vagina and the tubes are drawn down through it, is CULDOSCOPY. Vaginal tubal ligation can never be performed immediately after childbirth because the vaginal tissues are still too congested. However, because the uterus is still enlarged, immediately after delivery was at one time considered the ideal time for an abdominal tubal ligation. Today waiting six to eight weeks is considered preferable.

For traditional abdominal tubal ligation, an incision 4 to 5 inches (10 to 12 1/2 centimeters) long is made on the lower abdomen, just above the top of the pubic hair line. The incision may be horizontal (see PFANNENSTIEL INCISION) or vertical. After the abdominal cavity is entered, the tubes are closed off in one of a number of ways: sewed shut with sutures; cut and sutured; cauterized (burned and sealed); or closed with metal or plastic clips or rings.

Abdominal tubal ligation usually is performed under general anesthesia, although occasionally SPINAL or EPIDURAL ANESTHESIA may be used. A hospital stay of several days is required so that the incision can heal. Full recovery takes about six weeks. The principal advantage of abdominal tubal ligation is that the surgeon has adequate access to the tubes to close them off completely, even when there is scar tissue from previous surgery or infection. However, two newer procedures, LAPAROSCOPY ("Band-Aid" surgery) and MINILAPAROTOMY ("minilap"), which are both simpler and less expensive for the patient, have largely replaced the older method. Although usually done under general anesthesia, they are generally performed on an outpatient basis. Still another method of tubal ligation, used less often, is through the uterus, HYSTEROSCOPY. In recent years there has been considerable research into other techniques including the introduction of chemicals such as silver nitrate or zinc chloride into the uterus to block the tubes and the use of silicone plugs for this purpose. To date none of these methods has been clinically endorsed.

The principal complication following tubal ligation is infection. Danger signs are fever; pain not relieved by a mild analgesic such as aspirin, or pain that persists for more than 12 hours; moderate or heavy bleeding from either the incision or the vagina; faintness; chest pain; cough; shortness of breath; or pus from the incision. These symptoms should be reported promptly to the surgeon. Some women should not undergo tubal ligation at all. Among them are women who may be pregnant at the time, have an active pelvic infection, have an abnormal uterine or tubal structure (although even with scarring and adhesions an abdominal procedure may be possible) or have serious medical problems, such as asthma, heart disease, severe obesity or others contraindicating any surgery.

Tubal ligation should be undertaken only by women who are sure they want no more children. Reconstructive surgery to reopen the tubes, called TUBEROPLASTY, has a limited chance of success. Even when it does succeed, it carries a greatly increased risk of tubal pregnancy (ECTOPIC PREGNANCY). The effectiveness of tubal ligation, on the other hand, is quite high. When it does fail and a woman finds she is pregnant, it is due to either incomplete closing of the tubes or, in some cases, ignorance of an already existing pregnancy (one begun just before the surgery). However, over time the risk of failure increases, rising to 1% five years after sterilization and 1.8% after 10 years. Therefore no woman who has had tubal ligation should ignore unexplained bleeding and pain in the lower abdomen, which could signal a pregnancy (especially dangerous if it is an ectopic pregnancy). Women who have undergone tubal ligation are only one-third as likely as other women to develop ovarian cancer, a leading cause of cancer death in American women. The reason is not known.

See also STERILIZATION.

tubal pregnancy   See ECTOPIC PREGNANCY.

tuberoplasty   Also *tuboplasty*. Surgical repair of the FALLOPIAN TUBES to correct blockage resulting either from scar tissue or from TUBAL LIGATION. If previous infections have created enough scar tissue to block the tubes at the end near the fimbriae (and ovaries), thereby preventing the passage of an egg into or through the tubes, a two-stage operation may be performed. First the scar tissue is removed and a small plastic hood is placed over each tube to keep it open. Then, after several months, the plastic tubes are removed. If the surgery succeeds, as it does in about one-fourth of cases, the tubes will remain open. Recently, newer techniques using laser beams rather than surgical instruments have shown great promise. In one procedure the laser is used to destroy the diseased tissue of the tube and cut a hole in the uterus, through which the surgeon then implants a healthy section of the tube.

To repair the tubes after a tubal ligation, because a woman has changed her mind and now wants a child, the two ligated ends of each tube are sewn back together, a delicate procedure best performed with the aid of a microscope (microsurgery); a narrow plastic tube is inserted to keep each tube open until it has healed. Pregnancy following this procedure occurs in fewer than half of cases, and even then there is a high risk (10 to 15%) of ECTOPIC PREGNANCY, with the fertilized egg becoming implanted in the tube instead of the uterus. An alternative procedure is to pull one end of each tube into the uterus and fasten it there, with the fimbriae outside. This method is thought to have a higher rate of success.

To a large extent the success or failure of any repair depends on how the original ligation was accomplished. If the tubes were closed by electrocautery (coagulation or burning), the success rate of repair is only about 10%; if the fimbriae were removed (fimbriectomy), it is near 0%; if a plastic ring (the Falope ring) or titanium and silicone clip (Filshie clip) was used, it may be as high as 50 to 75%. Also, a great deal depends on the skill of the surgeon, so it is advisable to seek one who has had considerable experience with these procedures.

tubes   See FALLOPIAN TUBES.

tumor   Also *neoplasm.* An enlargement caused by the growth of tissue beyond its normal limits. A tumor may be benign (noncancerous), meaning it does not tend to invade other tissues or spread to other parts of the body, or it may be malignant (cancerous; see CANCER). A benign tumor may be solid or contain fluid; of the latter kinds, the most common is the CYST. Among the most common benign solid tumors that affect women is the uterine FIBROID; among the most common malignant ones are the various breast cancers (see CANCER, BREAST).

Turner's syndrome   Also *ovarian dysgenesis.* A congenital condition marked by the absence of ovaries, usually owing to the absence (complete or partial) of one of the two X sex chromosomes. Thus, instead of the normal woman's XX chromosome, there is an XO chromosome (although sometimes the configuration is somewhat different). Turner's syndrome often is not diagnosed until adolescence, when the lack of breast development and menstruation signal that something is wrong. Other signs are very short stature (usually no taller than 4½ feet, or 1.3 meters), a short broad neck and, sometimes, a webbed neck, fingers and toes, a small receding chin and the presence of pigmented moles. There may be associated defects in other organs as well—chiefly the heart, kidneys and ureters, as well as hearing loss. The condition is named for Dr. H. H. Turner, who first described it in 1938. Hormone therapy can establish menstruation and secondary sex characteristics, such as breast development, but it will not spur growth or make childbearing possible (although some women can achieve pregnancy with donor eggs). Turner's syndrome is relatively rare, occurring in about 1 of every 3,000 girls born. Even so, it is the genetic defect most often responsible for female infertility.

twins   See MULTIPLE PREGNANCY.

tylectomy   See MASTECTOMY, def. 7.

ultrasound Also *sonography, B-scan.* **1.** A diagnostic tool in which sound echoes provide a picture of soft-tissue structures inside the body, among them those of the female pelvis. It uses sound waves with frequencies of 2.5 million to 10 million cycles per second to scan the abdomen and pelvic area in linear fashion and then records their reflection (echo) on an oscilloscope screen. The recording is called a *sonogram.* A reflection is recorded whenever the sound waves meet a material of different acoustical density. Hence ultrasound can make an outline of soft-tissue masses in a way that X-rays cannot. A sonogram can show the size of the uterus, the size of a gestational sac or fetus, the position of a fetus, the presence of more than one fetus (twins, triplets, etc.) and some structural defects in the fetus. It also can detect an ectopic pregnancy (outside the uterus) and distinguish between solid tumors and cysts of the ovaries and between some benign (noncancerous) and malignant (cancerous) tumors. Ultrasound has been used to locate pelvic abscesses and wandering intrauterine devices (IUDs), determine whether there is a clot or other solid obstruction in a vein, detect cystic or solid masses in the pelvis and help diagnose cancers of the kidney, pancreas and thyroid. It also may indicate whether a breast lesion detected by mammogram is a solid tumor or a fluid-filled cyst, but it is not reliable alone as a diagnostic tool for this purpose. A newer technique, called high-definition imaging digital ultrasound, is useful for detecting common benign masses in the breast and thus avoiding unnecessary biopsies.

Ultrasound also is extremely useful in guiding needle aspiration for AMNIOCENTESIS and for various other diagnostic and surgical procedures involving the pelvis. With ordinary ultrasound, a transducer, or probe, is passed gently over the skin of the area being investigated.

With *transvaginal sonography* the probe is inserted into the vagina, and a small amount of saline solution may be injected through the cervix to distend the uterus. The images do not differentiate between normal and cancerous tissue, but they are a reliable indication of endometrial hyperplasia (thickening), which can be a precancerous condition. Consequently regular transvaginal ultrasound is now recommended for postmenopausal women taking unopposed estrogen (without added progesterone).

See also CANCER, OVARIAN; *elastography*, under CANCER, BREAST.

2. A means of suppressing sperm formation that still is considered an experimental form of male contraception. The man must sit with his testes resting in a cup filled with water; the water serves as a conductor for high-frequency sound generated by an ultrasound transducer. Experiments on dogs and human beings both indicate that the ultrasound lowers the sperm count considerably, an effect that is believed to be reversible. A major advantage of this means of contraception, should it prove to be reliable, is that ultrasound is quite painless and has no harmful side effects. However, there is no recent or current research on the procedure.

umbilical cord An organ consisting of a semi-transparent, jellylike rope, about 5 centimeters (2 inches) long on the average (but ranging from 5 to 200 centimeters, or 2 to 80 inches, long) that connects mother and fetus through the PLACENTA. It contains two arteries, which transport fetal waste products and deoxygenated blood to the mother, and one vein, which transports blood containing nutrients and oxygen from the mother to the fetus. One of the serious complications of childbirth is a

PROLAPSED CORD, that is, delivery of the cord before the rest of the baby or alongside it. Another is *cord strangulation*, in which the cord becomes twisted around the baby's neck. Both these risks are much greater with abnormal presentation, especially BREECH and SHOULDER PRESENTATION. Another serious problem is compression of the cord; that is, the cord is tightly squeezed during uterine contractions, interrupting the flow of blood through it and hence periodically cutting off the baby's oxygen supply.

Almost immediately after delivery the baby, if normally developed, begins to depend on air for its oxygen supply; the fetal circulation actually changes to allow blood to pass from the right side of the heart through the lungs and from the lungs to the left side of the heart. As soon as the baby is breathing, the cord is no longer needed. The usual procedure for cutting the cord is to apply two clamps to the cord about 2 inches (5 centimeters) from the point where it joins the baby's abdomen, called the *umbilicus* or *navel*. The cord then is cut between the two clamps with sterile scissors, and a sterile tape ligature or clamp is applied about ¾ inch (2 centimeters) from the abdomen. This stump is kept clean and dry with alcohol until it drops off, a week or two later. The umbilical cord is also a source of STEM CELLS.

See also HERNIA, UMBILICAL.

urea A concentrated solution of nitrogen excreted by the kidneys. It is sometimes used in second-trimester abortions, usually in conjunction with prostaglandins; see AMNIOINFUSION.

ureaplasma Also *mycoplasma*. An organism that causes nongonococcal URETHRITIS and, sometimes, bacterial VAGINOSIS; each is considered a SEXUALLY TRANSMITTED DISEASE. The causative organism's full name is *Ureaplasma urealyticum*.

urethra In women, a narrow tube, about 1½ inches (3½ centimeters) long, that lies in front of the lower part of the vagina and conveys urine from the BLADDER to the outside. The upper end opens into the bladder; the lower end opens into the vestibule between the clitoris and the vagina. This lower opening is called the *external urinary meatus* or *urethral orifice*. The urethra is lined with mucous membrane similar to that of the bladder itself. A series of muscle fibers surround the urethra and neck of the bladder, which are maintained in a state of contraction by the sympathetic nervous system. The SPHINCTER muscle of the bladder neck can be relaxed voluntarily in order for urine to be passed. When the urethral or perineal muscles become less elastic, owing to repeated stretching during pregnancy and childbirth or, after menopause, to a decrease in estrogen (which helps maintain elasticity and mucus-producing ability in urethral as well as vaginal tissues), problems with bladder control may develop (see URINARY INCONTINENCE).

One of the most common disorders affecting women is URETHRITIS, inflammation and infection of the urethra. It often accompanies a bladder infection (see CYSTITIS) and, depending on the infecting organism, may be treated in the same way.

urethritis Inflammation and/or infection of the URETHRA, a common disorder in women that often occurs in conjunction with bladder infection and may be treated with the same medications (see also CYSTITIS, def. 1). In the absence of bladder infection, it may be associated with GONORRHEA, TRICHOMONAS, CHLAMYDIA or some other infection of the vagina, or UREAPLASMA. For this reason it is important to find out what organism is responsible and take the appropriate medication to eliminate it (see URINE TEST). Infections not caused by gonococci are called *nonspecific urethritis (NSU)* or *nongonococcal urethritis (NGU)*. Chlamydia is the most common cause but ureaplasma, for which lab tests often are not available, also can be responsible; trichomonas is a less common cause of NGU. Urethritis occasionally is caused by irritation or injury from too vigorous intercourse, by irritation from the rim of a DIAPHRAGM or scratching, or by bacteria from the intestinal tract that enter the urethra after careless (back-to-front) wiping after bowel movements.

Women often have no symptoms of infection. When they do, the most common ones are pain, usually a burning sensation during urination, urinary frequency and also a vaginal discharge, sometimes blood-tinged. Bleeding after sexual intercourse and low abdominal pain also may occur. Men usually do exhibit symptoms, most often mild pain and discomfort in the urethra and a discharge. There also may be urinary frequency and proctitis (inflammation of the rectum). A gonorrhea culture is nearly always indicated for urethritis as well as a urine culture to identify the specific bacteria involved.

Symptoms usually arise two to three weeks after exposure. Undetected, the condition may become worse and lead to complications (see below), so a woman whose partner is diagnosed as having NGU also should be treated for the infection. Usually a broad-spectrum antibiotic such as tetracycline will clear up the condition. During pregnancy erythromycin should be substituted. Sexual intercourse should be avoided until treatment is completed and the symptoms disappear. Further, there should be careful follow-up for three months, since about 20% of patients have relapses that require being treated again.

If neglected, urethritis can lead to serious complications, such as pelvic inflammatory disease and infertility in women, and epididymitis, a painful inflammation of the testes, in men. Also, urethritis appears to be connected with pneumonia and eye infections in babies born of infected mothers and has been suspected as a factor in some infections leading to stillbirth.

In postmenopausal women the shrinking and drying of the labia often leave the urethra more exposed and more prone to infection, occasionally resulting in chronic urethritis (called *senile urethritis*). This condition may be treated with estrogen suppositories into the vagina, a treatment not without risk (see ESTROGEN REPLACEMENT THERAPY).

urethrocele   A bulging of the urethra into the vagina, owing to pelvic relaxation, that is, weakening of the muscles that normally hold the urethra in place. It usually occurs in conjunction with CYSTOCELE and is treated in the same way.

urinalysis   See URINE TEST.

urinary frequency   See FREQUENCY, URINARY.

urinary incontinence   Involuntary release of urine, a condition affecting twice as many women as men, and increasingly so after the age of 50. It is caused by pelvic relaxation, that is, weakening of the pelvic-floor muscles, especially the pubococcygeous muscle, prolapse of the pelvic organs (uterus, bladder) and weakening of the pelvic support structures. It often occurs after childbirth (long labor, rapid delivery, large babies, many pregnancies) or, occasionally, from strenuous physical activity. Sometimes no specific event or activity can be tied to the incontinence. Normally the healthy pubococcygeous muscle encircles the urethra close to where it joins the bladder; it also surrounds and supports the middle third of the vagina and encompasses the rectum just above the anal opening. When this muscle is weakened, the urethra, bladder, rectum and uterus—any or all of these organs—may bulge into the vagina and the bladder neck or urinary sphincter fails to remain closed when additional pressure is placed on it, causing urine to leak. It also may be a consequence of aging, when there is increased probability of involuntary bladder contractions, more nighttime excretion and/or bladder shrinkage.

There are several forms of urinary incontinence. *Stress incontinence* occurs following movements such as coughing, sneezing or exercising, in which the abdomen presses down on the bladder and dysfunction in the bladder outlet allows leakage. *Urge incontinence*, also called *overactive bladder* (OAB), occurs when the bladder spasms instead of relaxing and a person may feel a strong need to urinate but may not be aware of loss of urine at all until she cannot contain leakage in time to reach a toilet. Stress and urge incontinence, or a combination of the two, account for about 85% of all cases of incontinence. *Overflow incontinence* occurs when the distended bladder is unable to empty fully, causing frequent and almost continuous leakage. This type is more common in older men than in women. *Functional incontinence* results from impairment elsewhere in the body, such as a stroke, delirium or temporary impairment from infection or medications.

Most cases of urinary incontinence will respond to treatment, but careful diagnosis is important. It is helpful to keep a voiding chart or diary for about two days before seeing the doctor, keeping track of the time and amounts of liquid intake, normal urination and episodes of incontinence. Primary-care physicians should be able to take care of most cases; if not, they can refer patients to a specialist, preferably a urogynecologist. Urodynamics, a test to measure bladder filling and pressures, is the most common diagnostic test. Mild to moderate stress incontinence often is relieved by KEGEL EXERCISES, which help strengthen the muscles around the urinary sphincter. Women who leak during only a single activity, such as playing tennis, might use a PESSARY, inserted only when needed. For other kinds of incontinence, behavioral techniques may afford relief, for example, going to the toilet on a regular schedule, eliminating certain foods that irritate the bladder (such as caffeine, alcohol, acid juices, spices) or changing the type, dosage or time that necessary medications are taken. Medication, biofeedback and Kegels are the first line of treatment for urge incontinence. A newer noninvasive treatment involves sitting in a chair, fully clothed, as magnetic fields in the chair's seat stimulate the pelvic floor muscles to contract. It is provided in a clinician's office or hospital, usually for two 20–30 minute sessions a week for eight weeks. Called NeoControl Pelvic Floor Therapy, it is not always covered by insurance. Although some medications can help incontinence, they only suppress urine loss without affecting the cause, and often they have severe side effects. However, injections of collagen or carbon-coated beads (Durasphere) into tissue surrounding the urethra effects a bulking action that helps some kinds of stress incontinence. They usually must be repeated to be successful. More severe and chronic stress incontinence may require surgery to correct any underlying physiological conditions. The Burch procedure is used when bladder and urethra are out of their normal position. It involves lifting the wall of the vagina, where the urethra is located, and suturing the vaginal wall to tissue near the pubic bone. Either open abdominal or laparoscopic surgery is used, and reportedly 80 to 85% of cases of urinary incontinence are cured. A more common procedure, used for women with severe stress incontinence caused by weak sphincter muscles, is the sling procedure. A sling, formed from either tissue from the thigh or abdomen or a synthetic material, is placed under the urethra like a hammock, to support and compress it. In still another procedure, called *tension-free transvaginal tape*, a polypropylene or nylon tape is inserted through the vagina to support the bladder neck and urethra. After a few weeks tissue begins to form around the tape, holding it in place. Like the sling procedure, it compresses the urethra closed during movements that increase abdominal pressure (coughing, running, etc.), but no sutures are needed. A new minimally invasive treatment involves inserting two adjustable balloons on either side of the urethra to bolster urethra muscles. At this writing it is being reviewed by the FDA.

Urge incontinence, or overactive bladder (OAB), may be caused by abnormal nerve signals to the bladder that cause it to contract involuntarily so that there is an urge to urinate even if the bladder isn't full. It may also be caused by conditions such as Parkinson's disease, multiple sclerosis and diabetes, which can damage nerves that affect bladder function. Although more than half of all women experience urinary problems after menopause, there is no firm evidence for the influence of hormonal changes. One condition frequently occurring after menopause is *nocturia*, increased frequency of urination at night.

To treat OAB, various medications that try to relax the muscle and prevent abnormal contractions are available but most have noticeable side effects. Anticholinergics cannot be used for this purpose if one has narrow-angle glaucoma. An antidepressant, imipramine, also may help. However, many women cannot tolerate these drugs' side effects (blurred vision, dizziness, dry mouth, constipation). Three newer drugs, solifenacin (Vesicare), trospium (Sanctura), and darifenacin (Enablex), have fewer side effects. An extended oral version of Detrol and a skin patch of oxybutynin (Oxytrol) also are available. These medications may take two to three months to be fully effective. However, oxybutynin is not recommended for women over 65 because it may cause memory impairment. When medications fail, in severe cases a device called InterStim may be surgically implanted to interfere with abnormal nerve signals. Other treatments include stimulating spinal cord nerves to inhibit firing of bladder nerves, and injecting Botox into the bladder. Overflow incontinence may be treated with alpha blockers, drugs used to treat hypertension that affect the same system of nerves that regulates the bladder.

See also URETHROCELE; CYSTOCELE; RECTOCELE; PROLAPSED UTERUS.

urinary infection   See CYSTITIS, def. 1.

urine test   A laboratory test performed on a urine specimen (sample) to determine the presence of blood, protein, sugar, albumin, bacteria and/or other substances. (For urine tests performed to diagnose pregnancy, see PREGNANCY TEST.) A *dipstick urine test,* performed by many clinicians as an office procedure, consists of dipping a strip of chemically treated paper into a urine specimen. By changing color, the paper reveals relative acidity, the presence of blood (hematuria), protein (albumin), bilirubin, sugar and acetone (ketones), which in turn may indicate such disorders as diabetes, kidney or bladder infection or, sometimes, simply contamination of the specimen by menstrual blood or vaginal discharge washed from the vulva. The presence of albumin in a pregnant woman may be a sign of PREECLAMPSIA.

A *urinalysis* is a more complex test but still may be performed in the clinician's office (though more often it is done in a laboratory). It tests both the concentration and the acidity of the urine. Also, the urine is spun in a centrifuge for several minutes to separate solid particles from the liquid. The sediment collected at the bottom is then put on a slide and examined under the microscope for white blood cells and bacteria (present in infection) as well as red blood cells, epithelial cells and any abnormal cell formations (which might indicate kidney disease). If bacteria are present, a *urine culture* may be performed; part of the sample is put in a nutrient (usually a jelly) and incubated (heated) so that the bacteria multiply rapidly. The specific organisms then can be identified more readily, and their susceptibility to various antibiotics can be determined (called a *sensitivity test*).

Still other, more complicated urine tests include the determination of hormone levels, which may require analysis of a woman's entire urinary output over a full day (sometimes called a *24-hour test*).

urostomy   Also *urinary ostomy.* A surgical procedure in which an artificial opening is made to provide for elimination of urine because of the loss of either the bladder or bladder function. It is usually performed because of birth defects, malignancy (cancer), injury or nerve damage. There are several kinds of urostomy. An *ileal conduit* or *ileal bladder,* the most common kind, is performed when the bladder must be removed or bypassed. The conduit is constructed by separating about a 6-inch (15-centimeter) segment of the lower ileum (end of the small intestine) and implanting into it the ureters, which have been detached from the bladder. The rest of the small intestine is then reconnected to the colon. (This procedure may be performed with a segment of the colon, in which case it is called a *uretero-colostomy;* see also COLOSTOMY.) One end of the segment of the ileum is closed; the other end is brought through the abdominal wall to form the *stoma* (external opening), usually on the lower right abdomen. This stoma empties urine only, and an appliance (bag) must be worn at all times to collect urine and control odor. In a *vesicostomy* an opening is made directly in front of the bladder. The opening is sutured to an opening in the abdominal wall, through which urine is eliminated; a bag must be worn to collect urine. A *cutaneous ureterostomy* involves detaching one or both ureters from the bladder and bringing them through the abdominal wall, to empty outside the body; a bag must be worn at all times. A *nephrostomy* connects directly with the kidneys, from which urine drains directly (without passing through ureter or bladder) to the outside through an opening in the back or flank of the body. Either one or both kidneys may be involved. A nephrostomy usually is temporary and is drained by a tube (catheter).

In women urostomy rarely affects sexual function and, when only the bladder is affected, usually does not rule out pregnancy. In men, however, urostomy often affects potency.

uterine monitoring Also, *home uterine monitoring, pregnancy monitoring.* The use of a simple pressure sensor next to the skin to detect and forestall premature labor. The device consists of a belt containing a pressure sensor, which is fastened around the woman's abdomen for two one-hour periods per day. It then can be hooked into a telephone, which sends the two hours of tracing to a clinician. Generally prescribed only for high-risk patients (women with a history of early labor, women experiencing contractions as early as the 24th week or women carrying twins or triplets), the monitor picks up the increase in frequency, length and strength of uterine contractions that marks the beginning of labor. However, the devices are expensive to use and, critics point out, do not necessarily prevent early labor or even unfailingly detect it.

uterine polyp See POLYP, def. 3.

uterine prolapse See PROLAPSED UTERUS.

uterine synechiae Also *uterine adhesions.*
See also ADHESION; ASHERMAN'S SYNDROME.

uterus Also *womb.* A hollow, thick-walled muscular organ that lies in the pelvis of women, behind the bladder and in front of the rectum. It is pear-shaped, with a dome-shaped top, called the *fundus,* and a narrow neck at the bottom, called the CERVIX. The body of the uterus (that is, all but the cervix) is called the *corpus* (Latin for "body"). In adult women who have never borne children, the corpus of the uterus is approximately 8 to 9 centimeters (3 to 3½ inches) long, and 6 centimeters (1¼ inches) at its widest point. Its walls practically touch each other. Childbearing greatly increases the size. After menopause the uterus shrinks considerably, so that cervix and corpus become about equal in length. The muscled walls of the uterus, about 1.1 centimeters (½ inch) thick, called the *myometrium,* make up almost 90% of its size. On the outside they are covered with the *peritoneum,* the membrane that lines the entire pelvic and abdominal cavity. On the

inside they are lined with the ENDOMETRIUM, which varies in thickness during each menstrual cycle, first being built up in preparation for pregnancy and, when no egg is fertilized during a cycle, being shed in menstrual flow, along with some blood from its blood vessels.

The uterus has three openings. At the bottom, the cervix opens into the vagina. Near the fundus, a pair of FALLOPIAN TUBES open into the corpus on either side.

The uterus is partly mobile, that is, the cervix is anchored but the corpus is free to move backward and forward. When a woman is standing her uterus is normally tilted forward at the junction of corpus and cervix, a position called *anteverted.* In about one-fourth of women, however, the uterus is tilted back (see RETROVERTED UTERUS). Anomalies of the uterus are a *septate uterus,* in which a partition of varying thickness extends part or all of the way from fundus to cervix, dividing the corpus into two more or less separate compartments; a *bicornuate uterus,* which consists of two smaller, horn-shaped bodies, each connected to one fallopian tube but sharing a single (although sometimes separate, or divided) cervix; and a *double uterus,* in which there are two separate small bodies, each with its own cervix. These structural anomalies all are relatively rare, are congenital (present from birth) and can interfere with pregnancy and delivery, depending on the extent of abnormality.

The uterus is supported by three sets of strong, supple ligaments and is supplied with a rich network of blood vessels and nerves. Its principal function is to house and nourish a fetus until it is mature enough to be born, an average time span of 38 to 42 weeks. As the fetus grows—or, in the case of multiple pregnancy, two or more fetuses grow—the muscle fibers stretch to accommodate it. Toward the end of a pregnancy the once pear-size organ has grown to 30 centimeters (12 inches) long and increased its weight from 50 grams (2 ounces) to 900 grams (2 pounds). At some point the uterine muscles, which are involuntary, are stimulated to begin contracting, probably by the hormone OXYTOCIN, and it is their work, called LABOR, that pushes the baby down toward the cervix and forces the cervix to widen enough to allow its passage through the vagina. This process is not without discomfort, and indeed each contraction is called a *labor pain*. Oddly, nearly all pain originating in the uterus is perceived in the same way—as a cramp—although differing in duration and severity, whether its cause is the contractions of childbirth, the dilation of the cervix for a D AND C or the shedding of endometrial tissue during a menstrual period. After delivery the uterine muscles and ligaments return to their normal size, the excess tissues being absorbed into the bloodstream and eventually excreted in urine. By the end of a week the uterus weighs 500 grams (1 pound) and, after six weeks, 50 grams (2 ounces). Occasionally the muscles and ligaments weaken as a result of pregnancy and the uterus begins to sag from its normal position (see PROLAPSED UTERUS).

The body of the uterus is subject to a number of disorders and diseases. The development of benign growths such as a FIBROID or POLYPS (def. 3) is very common. More serious conditions are infections, such as PELVIC INFLAMMATORY DISEASE, and endometrial cancer (see CANCER, ENDOMETRIAL). Two of the surgical procedures most frequently performed on women are scraping of the uterine lining for biopsy and/or treatment (see D AND C) and removal of the uterus (see HYSTERECTOMY).

vaccine A preventive medication. The accompanying table shows the recommended schedule for adult immunization as indicated by the U.S. Centers for Disease Control and Prevention.

vacuum aspiration **1.** Also *endometrial aspiration, vacuum curettage, vabra.* The removal of tissue from the uterus by means of suction for diagnostic purposes or, sometimes, to correct menstrual irregularities. It can be performed in a doctor's office or clinic and is used to diagnose ENDOMETRIAL HYPERPLASIA or cancer and to evaluate fertility. In this procedure, a SPECULUM is inserted into the vagina, the cervix is grasped and held in place with a clamp (tenaculum) and a slender plastic tube, or *vacurette,*

RECOMMENDED IMMUNIZATION SCHEDULE FOR ADULTS*	
Vaccine	**Indications**
Tetanus, diphtheria, pertussis (TDP)	All adults. Booster every ten years. Adults with uncertain history of vaccination should receive primary series of three doses (first two, four weeks apart, third, six to 12 months later)
Measles, mumps, rubella (MMR)	Adults born after 1956 who are uncertain of their immune status. Usually one dose; two doses for college students, health care workers, adults recently exposed to measles, and international travelers. Should not be given to pregnant women or women who might become pregnant within next month.
Varicella	Adults aged 19–49 who have not had chickenpox. Two doses four to eight weeks apart. Age 50 and over, only necessary with special risk factors. Should not be given to pregnant women or women who might become pregnant within next month, or individuals infected with HIV.
Human papilloma virus (HPV)	All women from ages 11–12 to 26. Three doses, second two months after first, third six months later.
Influenza	Adults aged 50 and over, younger adults with chronic cardiovascular, pulmonary, liver or immunosuppressive disease or diabetes; health care workers; women pregnant during flu season. One dose annually.
Pneumococcus	Adults aged 65 and over; younger with chronic cardiovascular, pulmonary, kidney, liver or immunosuppressive disease or diabetes. Usually one dose. Some recommend second dose 10 years later.
Hepatitis A	Adults with chronic liver disease or blood clotting disorders; health care workers; travelers to certain countries. Two doses six to 12 months apart.
Hepatitis B	All infants, children and adolescents. Adults on hemodialysis or who have blood clotting disorders; travelers to certain countries. Three doses (second one to two months after first, and third three to four months later).
Meningococcal	College students living in dormitories; adults with no functioning spleen; military recruits; travelers to certain countries. One dose; revaccinate after five years if risk of disease continues.

Adapted from Centers for Disease Control and Prevention

is passed through the cervix into the uterus. The vacurette is attached either to a syringe or a special vacuum pump; when the pump is activated, shreds of tissue are removed from the uterine lining, or endometrium. The vacurette is small enough so that the cervix usually need not be dilated (widened). The procedure takes three to five minutes in all. The woman may feel mild cramping but usually can get up immediately or a few minutes later, take a short rest and go home.

See also BIOPSY, def. 8; MENSTRUAL EXTRACTION.

2. Also *suction abortion, vacuum abortion, early abortion, first-trimester abortion, early uterine evacuation.* The removal of placental and fetal tissue from the uterus by means of suction in order to terminate a pregnancy of 12 weeks or less. It can be performed in a doctor's office, clinic or hospital. The process is essentially the same as in def. 1 (see above) for pregnancies of four to six weeks (counting the first day of the last menstrual period as day 1). However, some clinicians prefer to wait until a patient is at least six weeks pregnant (see MENSTRUAL EXTRACTION, def. 2, for further explanation). For pregnancies of longer duration—7 to 12 weeks—a somewhat larger, nonflexible vacurette (tube) is used, and the cervix must be dilated for its insertion, usually by inserting a series of metal rods of gradually increasing diameter. To avoid the discomfort of such dilatation, most clinicians use a local anesthetic injected in the cervical area (paracervical block); occasionally general anesthesia is used, but it is not advisable unless the procedure is performed in a hospital or surgical clinic. Once inserted, the tip of the vacurette is rotated and moved around the walls of the uterus in order to remove the amniotic sac and also the thickened layer of endometrial tissue formed during the pregnancy. The total amount of tissue and blood removed on the average ranges (depending on the length of pregnancy) from 15 grams (1 ounce) to 150 grams (16 ounces). Some clinicians follow up the suction procedure with an ordinary surgical curette (scraper) to make sure all of the fetal and placental tissue has been removed. The tissue also is carefully examined to document the pregnancy and to rule out HYDATIDIFORM MOLE or some other abnormality, such as an ectopic pregnancy.

Vacuum abortion takes anywhere from 6 to 10 minutes. For most women it is mildly to moderately uncomfortable, beginning with cramping during dilatation of the cervix, cramping and a tugging feeling in the abdomen during the suction process and a few moderate to strong cramps near the end of the procedure, when the uterus finishes contracting. Cramps may last up to 20 minutes or so, sometimes accompanied by nausea.

A wait of an hour or so afterward, in the office or clinic, is normally required, to make sure there is no abnormal bleeding. Some 95% of women experience little or no pain and little bleeding afterward, although light staining often continues for two weeks. Most clinicians prescribe a drug to make sure the uterus contracts to normal size and, sometimes, an antibiotic such as tetracycline for five days to eliminate risk of infection. About 5% of women experience heavy bleeding temporarily and some lower abdominal tenderness, with or without fever. Following abortion, douches, intercourse and the insertion of tampons should be avoided for a week (some clinicians say two weeks). In most women normal menses return within six weeks, but the first period following the procedure may be quite heavy.

Vacuum aspiration was developed in China in the late 1950s. As a method for first-trimester abortion (up to 13 weeks from day 1 of the last menstrual period), it has largely replaced the D AND C in the West. It is easier, cheaper and safer than a D and C. The principal complications, which occur in only a tiny fraction of cases, are infection and incomplete abortion. Fever, severe cramps, back or rectal pain, heavy bleeding and discharge all are symptoms of infection, and any woman experiencing them should contact her clinician at once. Also, if signs of pregnancy persist (such as morning sickness and tender breasts), the woman should see her clinician even before the regular follow-up visit, usually scheduled for two weeks after the procedure, to make sure the curettage was complete and there is no ECTOPIC PREGNANCY (outside the uterus) or a remaining fetus (if there were twins).

Some clinicians will, if the woman wishes, insert an intrauterine device (IUD) at the time of vacuum aspiration. However, many advise against it because it increases bleeding, cramping, pain and the risk of infection, and they therefore suggest waiting until the first menstrual period. Women who use oral contraceptives may begin taking them immediately afterward, since ovulation generally will resume in two or three weeks. Women using a diaphragm should have the size checked during their follow-up visit, lest it has changed.

vacuum extractor   An instrument used in child-birth instead of FORCEPS. One or more round suction cups fit onto the baby's head, and suction is maintained by a pump linked to the extractors by a connecting tube. The instrument's great advantage is that there are no blades grasping the infant's head to add width to an already narrow passage (the mother's pelvis). Its advocates say it causes less damage to both baby and mother, but operators require some training to use it properly. Also, it often leaves a swelling or bruise on the baby's head, which disappears in time. Long used in Europe, South Africa and elsewhere, the vacuum extractor was introduced in the United States around 1974 and has increasingly replaced forceps.

vagina   A canal lined with muscular and membranous tissue that connects a woman's external organs, or vulva, to the uterus. It lies between the bladder and the rectum. In the average adult woman it is 9 to 10 centimeters (3½ to 4 inches) long. At its far end is a cup-shaped area called the *fornix*, into which the CERVIX projects; at the outer end is its external opening, called the *introitus*. In young girls the introitus is partly or completely blocked by the HYMEN. Near the introitus is a muscular SPHINCTER that contracts rhythmically during ORGASM. It is this sphincter that prevents a tampon from falling out. (See illustration under VULVA.)

The pink mucous membrane lining the vaginal walls constantly produces small amounts of mucus, keeping it moist. Except near the introitus, there are relatively few nerve endings, so the vagina is not very sensitive to touch or to pain. The mucous membrane is constantly shedding old cells and replacing them with new ones. This turnover is sometimes noticeable as a slight clear or white discharge. Unless it is irritating or smelly, such a discharge is normal. (See DISCHARGE, VAGINAL.) A

healthy vagina contains numerous microorganisms, among them *lactobacilli*, which break down sugar stored in vaginal cells and produce lactic acid. This acid helps prevent infection by numerous disease-causing organisms and also makes the vagina inhospitable to sperm, which cannot survive in it for more than a few hours.

Under the mucous membrane are layers of muscles, which make the vagina capable of expanding enormously in size in order to allow the passage of a baby.

The vagina has two principal functions. It is the exit passage of the uterus, through which its wastes (endometrial tissue and blood) are expelled as menstrual flow and through which babies emerge into the world. It also is the female organ of sexual intercourse, into which the male inserts his penis. In rare instances a girl is born without a vagina or with one that is closed, a condition called *vaginal atresia*. If the ovaries and uterus are well enough developed for menstruation to occur at puberty, the menstrual flow is then retained, an accumulation that in time becomes painful. In such cases a vaginal passage can be created surgically.

The vagina is subject to a number of common infections, especially YEAST INFECTION and TRICHOMONAS, as well as some of bacterial origin (see VAGINITIS; VAGINOSIS). More serious are the various kinds of SEXUALLY TRANSMITTED DISEASE, transmitted by sexual contact. Cancer originating in the vagina is rare (except in DES daughters; see DIETHYLSTILBESTROL), though it may spread there from the cervix or vulva.

vaginal atrophy   Also *atrophic vaginitis, senile vaginitis, vaginal dryness*. Thinning, drying and loss of elasticity in the tissues lining the walls of the vagina, as well as the urethra, vulva and uterus, which gradually occur in all women to some extent in the years following menopause. Before menopause, estrogen stimulates the endocervical glands to secrete a sticky, thin, clear, alkaline mucus. After menopause, with greatly reduced estrogen production, much less mucus is secreted and the vaginal tissues become thinner, dryer and less elastic. The texture of the vaginal walls changes too, becoming smoother, and their color changes from a deep to a lighter pink. The pubic hair becomes sparser and the labia majora shrink, so that urethra, clitoris and vagina all are more exposed to friction. The vagina gradually shortens and shrinks somewhat, and sometimes the urethral opening is pulled into and becomes part of the outer portion of the vagina. In severe cases these changes not only cause burning, itching and painful vaginal intercourse (DYSPAREUNIA) but can make women more susceptible to urethral inflammation and urinary infections (principally urethritis and cystitis) as well as vaginal infections.

Because these changes are directly related to reduced estrogen production, estrogen in cream or suppository form usually helps restore vaginal tone. These are available in lower dosage than oral estrogen. Premarin and estradiol (Estrace) are available in creams, which are inserted into the vagina daily for two weeks and then once or twice a week. To reduce absorption, fill the standard applicator only one-eighth to one-fourth full. A vaginal tablet that contains 10 mcg of estradiol, Vagifem, is inserted daily for two weeks and then twice a week. The most convenient form of low-dose estrogen is Estring, a silicone-based vaginal ring impregnated with estrogen that fits in the vagina like a diaphragm. It delivers 6 to 9 mcg of estradiol daily for three months and then must be replaced. However, some estrogen from these sources is absorbed into the bloodstream and carries at least some of the same risk as oral ESTROGEN REPLACEMENT THERAPY, which also relieves the condition. Consequently, in assessing the risk versus the benefits, it may be advisable to try other means of dealing with vaginal atrophy. To relieve painful intercourse, use of a water-soluble lubricant such as K-Y jelly often is effective. K-Y jelly or liquid or Vagisil Intimate Lubricant may be used daily and are often effective. They attract moisture to dry vaginal tissues and relieve irritation. Another lubricant for use during sexual activity is Astroglide, which is longer lasting. These products are water-based and contain glycerin and other ingredients. Regular sexual stimulation, either through intercourse or masturbation, helps promote secretion from the vaginal walls and offsets some of the drying. Some women have found that yogurt inserted once a week into the vagina (with an applicator and/or a diaphragm to help keep it in), used either alone or mixed with a vegetable oil such as safflower oil (1 tablespoon yogurt to 1 teaspoon oil), helps prevent drying and also may help restore the normal acid balance in the vagina (see also YEAST INFECTION for further explanation). Another option is Replens, a product that contains pilocarpine; it adheres to vaginal tissues and artificially thickens them to relieve dryness. It is to be used only every other day.

vaginal hygiene   Also *vaginal sprays.*
See HYGIENE.

vaginal infections   See VAGINITIS.

vaginal mycosis   Also *mycotic vaginitis.*
See YEAST INFECTION.

vaginal ultrasound   Also *transvaginal ultrasound.*
See ULTRASOUND, def. 1.

vaginismus   An involuntary spasmodic contraction of the muscles surrounding the vagina. When extreme, it can make it impossible to introduce any object (finger, tampon, penis, speculum) into the vagina. Some degree of vaginismus is not unusual in women for the first few times they engage in vaginal intercourse, especially if they are nervous or tense about coitus or fearful of possible pain caused by penetration of the hymen. Also, if a man tries to insert his penis before a woman is fully aroused, the vaginal entrance may be somewhat constricted. In true vaginismus, however, penetration becomes acutely painful or simply impossible. It nearly always is caused by an unusually strong aversion to any genital contact. Treatment consists of teaching the woman to dilate her own vaginal muscles, first with a fingertip, then a finger, then two fingers, or perhaps with dilators of graduated size, proceeding slowly and in such a way that she can relax and learn to relax those specific muscles.

vaginitis   Also *vulvovaginitis.* A local inflammation that produces severe itching and burning of

COMMON KINDS OF VAGINITIS

Disorder and/ or Infectious agent	Symptoms	How diagnosed	Treatment
Hemophilus vaginalis	Grayish-white, foul-smelling discharge	Wet smear	Antibiotic suppositories or sulfa creams
Herpes infection (Herpes simplex Type II)	Painful itchy blisters and open sores on vulva, sometimes inside vagina	Stained smear as for Pap smear	Acyclovir, wet dressings, anesthetic ointments
Trichomonas (Trichomonas vaginalis)	Yellow or greenish, frothy discharge, offensive odor, itching and soreness on vulva and in vagina	Wet smear	Metronidazole
Yeast infection (Monilia or Candida albicans)	Severe vaginal and vulvar itching, white cheesy discharge with sweetish odor	Wet smear	Antifungal creams or vaginal suppositories; gentian violet; yogurt applied locally

the vulva and often is accompanied by a vaginal discharge. The discharge may be creamy white or white (leukorrhea; see DISCHARGE, VAGINAL) or it may be yellow, watery, or blood-tinged. Causes of vaginitis include an allergic reaction (to soaps, perfumed tampons or pads, synthetic fabric, the partner's seminal fluid), a forgotten tampon or diaphragm, hormonal changes associated with menopause or a skin disorder such as psoriasis. However, in adult women vaginitis is most often the result of infection. Infections can be caused by an overabundance of the same organisms that normally reside in the vagina but have multiplied more than usual, frequently because the vaginal environment has been changed by taking oral contraceptives, hormone therapy, pregnancy, antibiotics, douching or an illness such as diabetes.

The most common kinds of vaginitis are those caused by a yeastlike fungus called *Candida albicans* or *Monilia* and a one-celled parasite named *Trichomonas vaginalis* (see YEAST INFECTION; TRICHOMONAS). Sometimes these two infections occur at the same time. Another organism frequently responsible is the bacterium *Hemophilus vaginalis* (see VAGINOSIS); both it and trichomonas often are transmitted through sexual intercourse and therefore are considered sexually transmitted disorders. Other sexually transmitted infections responsible for vaginitis are HERPES INFECTION, which can create lesions in the cervix,

vagina and vulva, and GONORRHEA. Both cysts and solid tumors can cause vaginitis. Cuts, abrasions or other irritations in the vagina (from childbirth, intercourse, surgery) can become infected, and the presence of a forgotten tampon or diaphragm also can cause infection. In children vaginitis can be induced by a variety of still other organisms, including *Escherichia coli*, normally resident in the gastrointestinal tract, and staphylococcus. Finally, some forms are known as *nonspecific vaginitis (NSV)* or *nongonococcal vaginitis (NGV)* because no particular organism can be identified, although the cause is thought to be bacterial. The organism *Chlamydia trachomatis*, which may cause nonspecific URETHRITIS, is thought to be responsible for some cases of NSV; it responds to antibiotic suppositories (tetracycline or erythromycin; see CHLAMYDIA).

Postmenopausal or *atrophic* (or *senile*) *vaginitis* is caused by a lack of estrogen, which leads to drying of tissues and other changes making the vaginal tissues more susceptible to the above-named infectious organisms (see VAGINAL ATROPHY).

Treatment of vaginitis depends on the cause. Specific drugs and remedies work well for many cases of yeast infection and trichomonas. For nonspecific vaginitis, local applications of antiseptic gels sometimes clear up the condition; oral antibiotics also are used. With any infection it is important to determine the cause, and with some it is necessary to treat the woman's sexual partner as well, to avoid reinfection.

In addition to specific medications, numerous preventive and palliative measures are advised for vaginitis, especially for stubborn cases with a tendency to recur. These include the following:

- Keep up regular washing and gentle drying of the vulva.
- Use all-cotton underpants, which "breathe" better than synthetic fabrics; air has a healing effect, so at home wear no pants.
- After bowel movements, wipe from front to back, so rectal bacteria cannot be transmitted to the vagina.
- Avoid clothing tight in the thighs and crotch.
- Avoid "deodorant" soaps, tampons and sanitary pads, which kill some of the normal organisms and make one more prone to infection by others.
- Avoid dyed (colored) toilet paper and all vaginal sprays.
- In the absence of active infection, use a bland, buffered acid vaginal jelly at bedtime, such as K-Y jelly.
- Try an acid douche, such as 1 to 2 tablespoons white vinegar per quart of warm water, once or twice a week.
- For yeast infections, apply yogurt directly to the vagina, using an applicator or spoon.
- Use a garlic suppository (one peeled clove of garlic, wrapped in a thin layer of clean gauze, dipped in olive oil for easier insertion) overnight, changing daily.
- HERBAL REMEDIES include a douche made by steeping (in water) comfrey leaves (*Symphytum officinale*), goldenseal (*Hydrastis canadensis*), chamomile (*Matricaria chamomilla*) and sage (*Salvia officinalis*).
- To relieve itching, apply a cold compress of milk, yogurt or cottage cheese for 5 to 10 minutes, five or six times a day; or take shallow sitz baths in plain water or in a tea made from sage, nettle (*Urtica dioica*), or chickweed (*Stellaria media*); or wash the area with sassafras bark tea.

See also DISCHARGE, VAGINAL; VAGINOSIS; VULVITIS; WET SMEAR.

vaginosis, bacterial Also *Hemophilus vaginalis, HV, Corynebacterium vaginale, Gardnerella vaginalis.* A form of VAGINITIS marked by a grayish-white or grayish-green, fishy-smelling vaginal discharge. Occasionally there also is some itching and burning, but many women have no symptoms other than the discharge. Caused by bacteria—mainly *Gardnerella vaginalis, Hemophilus vaginalis* (an earlier name for the condition), *Corynebacterium vaginalis, Mycoplasma hominis* or *Mobiluncus*—it tends to affect only the outermost layers of the vaginal surface and therefore causes less inflammation than vaginitis (the "itis" ending signifies inflammation). The smell becomes more intense after coitus (when the discharge is mixed with semen), and indeed, its principal mode of transmission is sexual intercourse, so it is regarded as a SEXUALLY TRANSMITTED DISEASE. It is diagnosed by means of a WET SMEAR and is treated with oral or topical metronidazole (Flagyl) or clindamycin phosphate (Cleocin). These treatments should be avoided during the first months of pregnancy (some say throughout pregnancy) or while breast-feeding. The condition often recurs, so follow-ups may be necessary.

varicocele A varicose vein in the testes (see TESTIS), which allows the blood to pool in the scrotum. This condition, which is a leading cause of INFERTILITY in men (it is found in 40% of all men with fertility problems), can be diagnosed simply by having the man stand and strain the muscles in the lower abdomen while the clinician probes above the testes. The varicocele forms a scrotal swelling that has been described as feeling like a bag of worms. Varicocele, which inhibits sperm production (perhaps because of the heat generated by the swollen area or poor circulation causing toxic buildup), is readily corrected by surgery, which also corrects infertility in more than half of those cases in which semen analysis indicates it to be the cause (see also SPERM).

varicose vein Also *varicosity.* A permanent bulging or swelling in a vein, most commonly in one or more outer veins that run down the leg just under the skin. It can affect both men and women, but in

America 1 in 5 women has one or more varicosities, whereas they are found in only 1 of every 15 men.

For the most part varicose veins are merely unsightly, but they can cause a feeling of heaviness, aching and fatigue in the legs, especially near the end of the day. The ankles may swell and pain may extend down the leg, along the vein. Occasionally the overlying skin becomes scaly and itchy. Other complications are leg cramps (often at night), leg ulcers, PHLEBITIS and blood clots.

The underlying cause of varicosities in veins lies in their structure. Veins are thin-walled blood vessels whose function is to send blood back to the heart and thence to the lungs to be reoxygenated. Since the blood travels in a steady stream in one direction, the veins are lined with one-way valves that ordinarily prevent back flow. As pressure builds behind each valve, it opens, allows blood to pass through and then closes. (Also see VEIN.) In the legs, however, and some other places as well—especially the rectal area (see HEMORRHOID)—pressure may interfere with normal flow and cause the thin walls of veins to become stretched. The valves then do not close properly and blood seeps back, forming small pools that create varicose veins. When the affected part is elevated higher than the heart, the blood returns without help from the valves, and the veins empty, reducing the swelling.

It is not known why some persons develop varicose veins and others do not, but there are several predisposing factors. The disorder tends to run in families, but whether this is due to an inherited weakness in vein walls or valves or whether it reflects a familial pattern of faulty diet or some other factor is not known. High levels of estrogen, especially in pregnancy and sometimes those resulting from oral contraceptives, appear to cause varicose veins. The varicose veins of pregnancy, which can affect the vulva as well, tend to appear in the early months and frequently disappear entirely after delivery. They are caused by the pressure of the uterus on femoral veins and the *vena cava,* causing congestion in the lower extremities that is best relieved by lying on one's side, especially the left side. Standing or sitting in one place for a long time also aggravates varicosities, while walking and other movement that activates the calf muscles helps pump blood up toward the heart

and decreases the blood volume in the legs. Finally, wearing tight boots, garters or girdles, and sitting with the legs crossed, all constrict the leg veins and contribute to varicosities. Diet may play a role, since people with high-fiber diets rarely have varicose veins; presumably a low-fiber diet results in hard stools, and the straining needed for a bowel movement puts enormous pressure on the veins of the legs and rectum. Prolonged sitting on the toilet may further aggravate the problem, since this position cuts off circulation from the rectum.

Preventive measures include a high-fiber diet (high in whole grains, raw fruits and vegetables); avoiding overweight; getting adequate leg exercise (walking, jogging, swimming); moving frequently if confined to sitting or standing positions for long periods (if standing, try shifting one foot onto a low stool for a time, alternating periodically, or shift weight to toes and then back to heels alternately); wearing elastic support hose during pregnancy, especially if either of the woman's parents had varicose veins; avoiding garments tight in the groin and leg areas; and lying on one's side whenever possible. Vulvar varicosities also are relieved by applying ice compresses and, when standing, using support from a sanitary pad.

Treatment for varicose veins other than wearing elastic support hose, which eases the discomfort, consists of either injections or surgery. The injections, called *sclerotherapy,* introduce an irritating substance (usually a strong saline solution) directly into the affected vein, which causes a clot to form and close off that part of the vein. Following injection, the leg is wrapped with compression bandages from the injection site to the toes, and these must remain in place for about three weeks. Oral contraceptives should be avoided for six weeks both before and after treatment, lest they give rise to a blood clot.

Sclerotherapy also can be used to treat so-called *spider veins* (technically called *telangiectases*), which usually cause no symptoms but can be unsightly. Electrocautery is not recommended because it can result in scarring, but newer kinds of laser surgery may be effective.

Surgery, called *stripping the veins,* involves threading a wire through the length of the affected vein (through several incisions made at various points on the leg) and removing the entire vein. It usually is done under general anesthesia and involves little postoperative pain, although elastic support hose must be worn for several weeks afterward to prevent bleeding and allow healing. Although this procedure removes the vein or veins affected, the problem may recur in other veins, which subsequently dilate for the same reasons as those removed did. A less invasive surgical treatment, *ambulatory phlebectomy,* is performed under local anesthesia. The clinician makes small incisions along the length of an abnormal vein and pulls it out bit by bit. It can be used for most large veins. In another version of this procedure, called light-assisted stab phlebectomy, a small fiber with light on it is placed beneath the veins so the varicosities are more easily seen and removed, but it is not yet widely used.

The newest treatment is laser therapy, which uses a focused stream of high-intensity light to destroy tissue. Performed in an office under local anesthesia, the clinician, guided by ultrasound, punctures the vein and inserts a guide wire to the point where blood begins flowing backward. Then he or she inserts a laser fiber, which heats the vein from the inside. The resulting inflammation makes the vein's walls adhere to each other, eventually forming scar tissue. The procedure, called *endovenous laser therapy* (ELVT), takes about three minutes to treat nearly 16 inches of vein. Normal activities can be resumed, but the patient must wear compression stockings for several days. Symptoms may improve in a week or two but changes in appearance take longer. About 5% of patients experience numbness near the knees or ankles, with feeling returning in most within a year. In another 7%, the varicose veins reopen within two years.

Still another new technique is *endoluminal radiofrequency thermal heating* (or *VNUS closure procedure*), which is similar to laser therapy except that the varicose veins are heated with radiofrequency waves. The procedure takes about 20 minutes and may be followed by swelling and pain. In about 10% of patients the varicosities recur.

vas deferens   Also *vasa deferentia* (pl.). One of a pair of straight tubes, about 45 centimeters (18 inches) long, that transport sperm from each TESTIS

to the male urethra (see PENIS). Without them a man is infertile (cannot ejaculate sperm). Surgical severing of both vasa deferentia, called VASECTOMY, is the principal method of male sterilization.

vasectomy   Also *clipping the cords.* Surgically cutting each VAS DEFERENS, the pair of tubes that carry sperm from each testis, in order to render a man sterile. It is the simplest method of STERILIZATION known and has been performed for more than three centuries. The surgery can be performed by a urologist or general surgeon in a clinic, doctor's office or the outpatient department of a hospital, and it takes about 20 minutes. Under local anesthetic a ½-inch (1¼-centimeter) incision is made on either side of the scrotum, over each vas deferens, though some clinicians prefer to make a single incision in the center. Each vas deferens is pulled out through the incision and a segment of it is removed. The loose ends are then closed with a suture of special metal clips or are cauterized electrically (burned shut). The skin is closed with one or two absorbable sutures that dissolve in a week or 10 days.

Following vasectomy, there is a moderate amount of pain on the day of surgery and sometimes also on the next day. Strenuous physical activity should be avoided for about one week. Wearing an athletic supporter helps prevent swelling over the area. Sexual intercourse usually can be resumed seven days after surgery. However, vasectomy is not a reliable means of contraception until the sperm stored in the upper part of the vas deferens and the seminal vesicles is emptied, which normally requires anywhere from 15 to 20 ejaculations. To be absolutely safe, testing of three successive ejaculates should indicate they contain no active sperm.

After vasectomy the testes continue to produce sperm, but at a slower rate, and those that do mature simply disintegrate. The volume of seminal fluid ejaculated changes very little, however, since most of it comes from accessory glands, such as the seminal vesicles and prostate, whose secretions are not cut off. Complications from vasectomy are rare. A man who experiences fever, prolonged or heavy bleeding, or swelling and pain not relieved by applying an ice pack and taking aspirin should contact his surgeon at once, as these may be signs of postoperative infection.

Procedures other than surgery have been used in attempts to close off the vasa deferentia. Among them are the insertion of plugs, valves and clips of various kinds into each vas deferens to serve as a mechanical barrier, and the injection of various substances into the cavity of each vas deferens in order to produce inflammation and scar tissue that will then close it off. None of these methods is considered as satisfactory as the surgical procedure. However, a newer no-scalpel technique developed in China has gained many adherents in North America. With this *no-scalpel vasectomy,* the clinician feels for the vas deferens under the skin of the scrotum, holds it in place with a small clamp, and makes a puncture in the skin. This opening is enlarged slightly so both vas can be cut and tied. The procedure is performed in the doctor's office under local anesthetic, and no stitches are needed.

Vasectomy should not be undertaken unless a man is quite sure he wants no more children. Reversing a vasectomy by repairing the cut ends and rejoining them, a procedure called *vasovasotomy,* is much more difficult and more costly and has less chance of success, although if performed within 10 years of the original surgery it has a 70 to 90% chance of success (after 10 years, only 30%). Occasionally vasectomy occurs accidentally as a complication of traumatic injury, scrotal surgery or lower abdominal surgery such as hernia repair.

Vaseline See LUBRICANT.

vasomotor instability See HOT FLASHES.

VD Abbreviation for *venereal disease.* See SEXUALLY TRANSMITTED DISEASE.

vein One of a system of thin-walled blood vessels that carry blood back to the heart in a steady flow. The veins often are surrounded by muscles. Unlike those of arteries (see ARTERY), the veins' walls are not muscular enough to provide a pumping action to keep blood moving through them, and most of the blood returning to the heart must flow against the force of gravity. At least three factors play a part in maintaining blood flow through the veins. Many veins are provided with one-way valves, which permit the blood to move freely toward the heart but close to prevent movement in the opposite direction. Also, the pressure of blood behind the blood in the veins helps move it along. Finally, the usual activity of the body causes the contraction of muscles, which press against the veins and force blood toward the heart.

The most common diseases affecting the veins are VARICOSE VEINS, in which pressure causes a part of the thin wall to balloon out so that blood can pool there, and PHLEBITIS.

venereal disease See SEXUALLY TRANSMITTED DISEASE.

version Turning, a term used for repositioning a fetus inside the uterus, either by manipulating the mother's abdomen from the outside, before labor has begun (*external version*) or by using either the hands or instruments during labor, while the fetus still is in the uterus but the cervix is completely dilated (*internal version*).

vertex See CEPHALIC PRESENTATION.

vertigo Also *dizziness.* The sensation of having the room spinning about one with, often, loss of balance. The three most common causes of vertigo are benign paroxysmal positional vertigo (BPPV), Meniere's disease and migraine-associated dizziness. The first two are due to problems with the inner ear's vestibular or balance apparatus, and all three affect women more often than men.

BPPV is caused by small crystals in the inner ear becoming displaced and touching sensitive nerve endings. It appears to be induced by a certain head position. It is not known why this occurs, but it can follow a head injury. A simple test for the condition is the Dix-Hallpike maneuver, which involves turning the head down and to one side. If dizziness occurs, along with an eye movement called nystagmus, it is the ear pointing to the floor that has loose crystals. If no symptoms appear, the maneuver is repeated with the head turned to the other side. A treatment called the Canalith Repositioning Procedure consists of positioning the patient so that gravity will move crystals away from nerve endings. It is performed in the doctor's office and takes about ten minutes. If the first treatment is not successful, it is repeated. In about 15% of patients symptoms recur, sometimes as often as once a month, so it is useful for them to learn Canalith Repositioning and do it at home.

Symptoms of Meniere's disease include sudden attacks of severe vertigo, as with BPPV, but also may involve nausea and vomiting, tinnitus (ringing in the ears), progressive deafness and pain or pressure in the affected ear. These symptoms are caused by large amounts of fluid in the inner ear. Again, the ultimate cause is unknown, but the condition seems to run in families and may be linked to allergies. Diagnosis involves a physical examination, tests of hearing and balance and an MRI. The simplest treatment consists of reducing fluid retention by means of a low-salt diet and diuretics and avoidance of caffeine and alcohol, which can affect the vestibular system. If it is not effective, a self-administered Meniett device, which delivers low-pressure air pulses to the inner ear through a tube, may help. If all else fails, surgery may be indicated. In endolymphatic sac decompression, the endolymphatic sac is opened and a shunt inserted to allow fluid to drain into the mastoid space. Another surgical procedure is vestibular neurectomy, which involves severing a nerve in the inner ear. Neither of these procedures impairs hearing. In patients who already have hearing loss, labyrinthectomy, involving partial removal of the inner ear, may be performed.

Migraine-associated dizziness may occur in the absence of a MIGRAINE headache. It occurs when dilated blood vessels in the brain activate the trigeminal nerve, which has nerve endings along these vessels. It is often associated with a long history of motion sickness. In contrast to Meniere's disease, where symptoms usually subside in a matter of hours, migraine-associated dizziness may last longer than 24 hours. Treatment is similar to that for migraine headache.

Another cause of dizziness is labyrinthitis, an inflammation of the inner ear. Often following a cold or other respiratory infection, it may cause nausea and sometimes hearing loss. Symptoms are relieved by medication, but the condition usually cures itself in six to 12 weeks.

vestibule The boat-shaped female genital area surrounded by the LABIA minora (inner lips), extending from the clitoris to the point where the labia majora (outer lips) join. It contains four openings: the urethra, the vagina and the ducts of the two BARTHOLIN'S GLANDS (also called the *vestibular glands*). Under the mucous membrane on each side of the vestibule are the *vestibular bulbs,* two clusters of veins about 3 to 4 centimeters (1.5 inches) long and about 1 centimeter (0.4 inch) wide. During sexual arousal these veins fill with blood, becoming congested and firm to the touch. (Also see illustration under VULVA.)

viable Capable of surviving. The term is usually applied to premature babies; those of less than 24 to 28 weeks' GESTATION rarely are mature enough to survive.

vibrator See ORGASM.

virginity The condition of a woman, called a *virgin,* who has never engaged in vaginal intercourse. In cultures where women are considered the personal property of their husbands, or in patrilineal societies, where property and authority are passed on from a father to his children, virginity is an important concept because it allegedly ensures that the husband is the first person to have vaginal intercourse with his wife and definitely establishes the paternity of her first child. Evidence of virginity traditionally was an intact HYMEN and, physically speaking, a woman is a virgin until her hymen is broken. However, the hymen can be ruptured by many means other than penile penetration, such as a tampon or physical exercise of various kinds, so virginity in this sense has largely lost its meaning. Moreover, a virgin *can* become pregnant, although it does not happen often; sperm deposited on the outer genitals (the vulva) sometimes does move into the vagina and upward to fertilize an egg. In the sense of never having experienced vaginal intercourse, the old meaning of virginity persists, but since the widespread availability of birth control measures has engendered greater sexual freedom (at least in the Western world), the concept has lost much of its former significance.

visualization Also, *guided imagery.* The use of mental imagery to facilitate healing. Combining techniques of meditation and relaxation, it involves picturing an object, scene or process—for example, disease-fighting white blood cells at work—but relaxing and feeling at one with it, so it becomes the only thing one is aware of. Visualization has been used to reduce pain, to lower blood pressure and slow down the pulse and to help in the healing of specific disorders, including cancer. For cancer it is used in conjunction with conventional therapy (drugs, surgery, radiation) but helps relieve the patient's stress and improve his or her attitude toward the disease. Proponents claim that visualization helps strengthen the immune system and thus enhances the body's own disease-fighting mechanisms.

vitamin A group of nutrient chemicals that are considered essential to good health. Chemically they can be divided into two groups: the fat-soluble vitamins, A, D, E and K, which tend to be stored in the body; and the watersoluble vitamins, the B group and C, which except for vitamin B_{12} are not stored in the body and need frequent replenishment. Some vitamins are pro-

PRINCIPAL VITAMINS

Vitamin	Chief food sources	Needed for	Effects of lack, overdose	Recommended daily allowance[a]
A/retinol Beta-carotene	Fish liver oils, liver, egg yolk, butter, cream, green leafy and yellow vegetables	Light reception of retina, functioning of epithelial tissue, helps immune function	*Lack:* night blindness, drying of eye tissue, disease of cornea. *Overdose* (over 3,000 mcg): headache, skin peeling, enlargement of liver and spleen	*W, O, SR:* 700 mcg *P:* 770 mcg *L:* 1,300 mcg
D Calciferol (1 mcg calciferol = 40 I.U. vitamin D)	Fish liver oils, butter, egg yolk, fortified milk and cereals, ultraviolet rays (sunlight)	Calcium and phosphorous absorption, bone calcification	*Lack:* rickets, softening of bone. *Overdose* (over 50 mcg): appetite loss; kidney failure; calcium deposits	*W, P, L:* 5 mcg *O:* 10 mcg [b] *SR:* 15 mcg [b]
E	Vegetable oils, wheat germ, leafy vegetables, egg yolk, margarine, legumes, whole grains, soy beans	Antioxidant protects cells	*Lack:* Breakdown of red blood cells; muscle degeneration. *Overdose* (over 1,000 mg): impaired clotting, easy bruising or bleeding from nose, gums, intestines or kidneys	*W, O, SR, P:* 15 mg *L:* 19 mg
K	Green leafy vegetables, pork, liver, vegetable oils, soybeans	Normal blood clotting	*Lack:* hemorrhage. *Overdose:* kernicterus (nerve disorder); high bilirubin levels in blood	*W, O, SR, P, L:* 90 mcg
B_1 (thiamine)	Dried yeast, whole grains, eggs, enriched cereals, nuts, legumes, potatoes	Carbohydrate metabolism, nerve cell function, heart function	*Lack:* beriberi (disorder affecting heart and nervous system)	*W, O, SR;* 1.1 mg *P, L:* 1.4 mg

Vitamin	Chief food sources	Needed for	Effects of lack, overdose	Recommended daily allowance[a]
B$_2$ (riboflavin)	Milk, cheese, liver, meat, eggs, fish, enriched cereals	Protein metabolism, maintenance of nervous system, healthy skin, hair, muscles, brain	*Lack:* mouth, eye, skin and genital lesions	*A, W, O, SR:* 1.1 mg *P:* 1.4 mg *L:* 1.6 mg
niacin (nicotinic acid, nicotin-amide)	Dried yeast, liver, meat, fish, legumes, wholegrain or enriched cereals	Healthy cell metabolism, monitors cholesterol metabolism, affects metabolic rate and temperature	*Lack:* pellagra (disorder affecting skin, digestive tract, central nervous system) *Overdose* (over 35 mg): liver damage	*W, O, SR:* 14 mg *P:* 18 mg *L:* 17 mg
B$_6$ (pyridoxine)	Dried yeast, liver, organ meats, whole grain cereals, fish, legumes	Healthy cell function and metabolism of amino acids and fatty acids, helps form red blood cells	*Lack:* convulsions in infants: skin and nervous system disorders; mental retardation *Overdose:* over 100 mg	*W:* 1.3 mg *O, SR:* 1.5 mg *P:* 1.9 mg *L:* 2 mg
folic acid (folate)	Fresh green leafy vegetables, fruit, organ meats, liver, enriched breads and cereals	Healthy red blood cells and synthesis of needed compounds; prevent neural tube defects; lowers homocysteine levels	*Lack:* anemia and other blood disorders; infertility; gastrointestinal disorders; may be responsible for eclampsia, miscarriage, abruptio placentae in pregnant women, neural tube defects *Overdose:* over 1,000 mcg	*W, O, SR:* 400 mcg DFE* *P:* 600 mcg DFE* *L:* 500 mcg DFE*
B$_{12}$ (cobalamin)	Liver, beef, pork, organ meats, eggs, milk, milk products, fortified cereals	Healthy red blood cells, nerve cell function, synthesis of DNA, enzyme synthesis	*Lack:* pernicious anemia, other anemias; some psychiatric disorders, dim vision	*W, O, SR:* 2.4 mcg *P:* 2.6 mcg *L:* 2.8 mcg
pantothenic acid	Meat, chicken, milk, eggs, broccoli, whole grains	Metabolism of carbohydrates and fats	*Lack:* neuromotor, cardiovascular and digestive disorders	*W, O, SR:* 5 mg *P:* 6 mg *L:* 7 mg
C (ascorbic acid)	Citrus fruits, tomatoes, potatoes, cabbage, green peppers, broccoli, spinach	Healthy bone and connective tissue, circulatory function, wound healing	*Lack:* scurvy (hemorrhage, loose teeth, gum disease) *Overdose* (over 2,000 mg): stomach upset, diarrhea	*W, O, SR:* 75 mg *P:* 85 mg *L:* 120 mg (Smokers: add 35 mg)
biotin	Liver, kidney, fish, egg yolk, yeast, nuts, legumes	Metabolism of fatty acids, release of energy from carbohydrates	*Lack:* dermatitis, inflamed tongue (glossitis)	*W, O, SR, P:* 30 mcg *L:* 35 mcg

[a] The allowances suggested are based on those recommended by the Food and Nutrition Board, National Academy of Sciences—National Research Council. They are expressed in mg (milligrams) or mcg (micrograms). Where different amounts are recommended for different age groups, the following abbreviations mean: *W* = women aged 19 to 50; *O* = women 51–70; *SR* = over 70; *P* = pregnant women; *L* = breast-feeding women. One microgram (mcg) equals one-millionth of a gram. To convert mcg to International Units (IUs), multiply by 3.3. To convert IUs to mcg, divide by 3.3.

[b] Many authorities now recommend a higher dosage for women over 70, as much as 25 mcg (1000 I.U.)

*DFE = 1 mcg of folate, 0.6 mcg of folic acid in food or supplement, or 0.5 mcg supplemental folic acid taken on empty stomach.

duced in the body. Vitamin D is manufactured in the skin during exposure to sunlight, and vitamin K, biotin and pantothenic acid are made inside the human gut by resident bacteria when certain foods are eaten. Most vitamins, however, must be ingested.

All of the vitamins are needed, although their mode of action is not precisely understood, and all of them are available in a wide variety of ordinary foods. Deficient vitamin intake leads to specific symptoms and diseases.

The B vitamins, especially folic acid (or folate), are important in pregnancy, and pregnant women may need supplements of them. Folic acid and vitamin B$_6$ may reduce the risk of developing heart disease. Vitamin E has been found helpful by some women in relieving the HOT FLASHES of menopause, and is thought to be helpful in preventing heart disease and Alzheimer's, as well as boosting the body's immune system. Vitamin D, which is essential for calcium absorption, is thought to be particularly important for women after menopause to help prevent bone loss (see OSTEOPOROSIS). Another category of vitamins are the so-called *antioxidants*—vitamins E and C, and beta-carotene, a precursor of vitamin A. They neutralize the body's oxygen-free radicals, which are implicated in DNA mutations (which can initiate cancer), atherosclerosis (leading to heart disease), cataract formation and other processes. These vitamins currently are being closely investigated for their disease-fighting ability. Overdoses of certain vitamins, particularly of the fat-soluble ones, especially A and D, also can make a person ill. Nutritionists also recommend upper limits for vitamin B$_6$ (no more than 100 mg a day), folic acid (1,000 mcg) and niacin (35 mg). Recent studies indicate that taking 400 mg or more of vitamin E per day increases the risk of heart disease. See the accompanying table; also see DIET.

vomiting   See NAUSEA; MORNING SICKNESS.

von Willebrand disease   A hereditary platelet disorder that impairs clotting. Its symptoms are extremely heavy menstrual periods (10 pads a day, or more than a super tampon an hour), excessive nosebleeds, easy bruising and bleeding heavily after surgery, including dental work. It is treated by administering factor VIII, a clotting factor, or injecting desmopressin acetate or DDAVP (a synthetic hormone), also available in the form of a nasal spray.

See also HEMOPHILIA.

vulva   Also *pudenda, external genitalia*. The external visible female organs of reproduction, which include the MONS VENERIS (or pubis), LABIA majora and minora (outer and inner lips), CLITORIS, VESTIBULE, opening of the URETHRA, INTROITUS (opening of the vagina), HYMEN and BARTHOLIN'S GLANDS (also called vulvovaginal glands). See also PERINEUM. The vulva is subject to a number of disorders, the most serious of which are cancer and the various infections transmitted by sexual contact (see CANCER, VULVAR; SEXUALLY TRANSMITTED DISEASE).

See also VULVITIS.

vulvar lichen planus   An inflammatory condition that affects the skin, nails, mouth and vagina, most often during perimenopause or postmenopause. It tends to start with itchy portions on the vulva and inside the vagina. Untreated, scarring may develop, causing the labial and clitoral tissues to shrink and the urethral and vaginal openings to narrow. Women then have trouble urinating, pain with intercourse and bleeding after intercourse. The condition is not very common, and the cause is not known. The most successful treatment has been with strong topical corticosteroid medications, such as clobetasol propionate (Temovate), applied twice a day for three months. Others are diflorasone (Maxiflor) and halobetasol (Ultravate). Used together with antifungal or antibacterial agents, the steroid is even more effective. There currently is no cure for the condition, and women therefore will need maintenance therapy.

vulvectomy   See CANCER, VULVAR.

vulvitis   An inflammation or infection of the VULVA. A common cause is *contact dermatitis*, whose chief symptoms are redness, burning or itching, labial swelling and clear blisters that eventually drain and crust over. It can be caused by soap or detergents, bubble bath, condoms, a douche, vaginal foam or other sprays, sanitary napkins or clothing. Vulvitis can result from an allergic reaction to antibiotics or other drugs taken internally. It also may be the result of an infection with PUBIC LICE ("crabs"), a HERPES INFECTION or a vaginal infec-

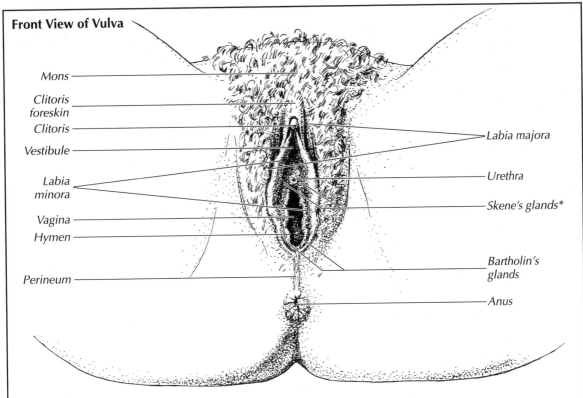

Front View of Vulva

Mons

Clitoris foreskin

Clitoris

Vestibule

Labia minora

Vagina

Hymen

Perineum

Labia majora

Urethra

Skene's glands*

Bartholin's glands

Anus

*The Skene's glands are not visible in this view of the vulva. These glands are attached to the outer wall of the urethra between the urethra itself and the vagina. Small ducts from the Skene's glands empty into the urethra.

© Infobase Publishing

tion or discharge. Treatment is chiefly palliative: sitz baths or compresses to relieve inflammation, antihistamines and topical cortisone creams to relieve itching, and loose clothing (or better, none, since the air helps heal the condition). Meanwhile the cause should be determined and eliminated. Any discharge should be checked for infectious organisms, and any suspicious lesions should be examined to make sure they are not precancerous or malignant (see CANCER, VULVAR). For herbal remedies to relieve itching, see under VAGINITIS.

Other painful conditions of the vulva include vestibulitis (see under BARTHOLIN'S GLANDS), VULVAR LICHEN PLANUS and pudendal neuralgia, which affects the nerves in the vulvar region. The latter may be relieved by low doses of tricyclic antidepressants.

See also VULVODYNIA.

vulvodynia   Chronic burning pain in the vulvar area that is independent of any particular disorder. There appear to be three kinds of vulvodynia: *vulvar vestibulitis,* affecting mainly women in their 30s, with pain at the entrance of the vagina on attempting sexual intercourse or inserting a tampon or other object; *cyclic vulvitis,* which flares up one or two weeks before menstruation and after intercourse; and *essential vulvodynia,* occurring mostly around PERIMENOPAUSE and after menopause, where burning or aching is present most of the time. Some patients with vulvar vestibulitis also have a chronic burning sensation. Recent studies show that about 30% of them have a genetic defect that inhibits blocking an inflammatory substance, interleukin-1. Anti-inflammatory medication, especially the COX-2 inhibitors (see ANALGESIC) may help, though the removal of Vioxx from the market in 2004 sheds some doubt on the safety of these drugs. The pain can be quite severe, enough to impede sitting, walking, wearing tight pants or having sexual intercourse. Diagnosis involves ruling out all possible causes, including infections, cysts and allergic reactions. In most cases vulvodynia is believed to be caused by overactive nerves in the vulvar area. Topical estrogen cream may reduce the pain, and a topical anesthetic such as lidocaine jelly applied before intercourse may relieve discomfort. Sitz baths, wearing all-cotton underwear, and avoiding feminine deodorants may help. Exercises to strengthen pelvic floor muscles and biofeedback to prevent muscle spasm work for some women. Low doses of antidepressants, muscle relaxants or anti-epileptics, all of which inhibit nerve overactivity, also may be helpful. Finally, if conservative measures do not help, women with vulvar vestibulitis have been aided by surgery to remove the involved skin, which, however, involves a lengthy healing period.

warts, vulvo-vaginal, anal See CONDYLOMA ACUMINATA.

water retention See EDEMA.

weight, body Charts for desirable body weight, relative to height and general body frame, are widely available. In most advanced countries of the world where food is available, exceeding one's ideal weight is far more common a problem than underweight. However, research indicates that waist measurement and body-mass index (BMI) are more significant for health risks than weight in pounds (see OBESITY).

Weight loss, unless it can be accounted for by increase in physical activity and decrease in food intake, may be symptomatic of numerous disorders—some of them serious ones—and warrants a thorough physical checkup. More often, however, it is increasing weight that women find troublesome. Except when it is caused by edema (fluid retention), undesired weight gain is nearly always the result of overeating.

See ANOREXIA NERVOSA; BIRTH WEIGHT; CRITICAL WEIGHT; DIET; WEIGHT GAIN.

weight gain 1. premenstrual. Many women regularly gain several pounds during the week preceding their menstrual period. This gain is nearly always the result of fluid retention (sometimes combined with constipation) and somewhat increased appetite, and it disappears during the first few days of menstrual flow. (See also DYSMENORRHEA, def. 5.) The same phenomenon may occur in women taking oral contraceptives; the higher hormone levels seem to cause fluid retention and sometimes increased appetite, manifested in weight gain.

2. in pregnancy. Weight gain is both normal and necessary during pregnancy. From the 1930s to the early 1960s American women frequently were advised to limit their weight gain during pregnancy to 10 to 15 pounds (4½ to 7 kilos), in the belief that it would ease labor and delivery, prevent hypertension and preeclampsia and help maintain an attractive figure. However, some investigators began to observe that the salt-poor, often protein-deficient diets used to restrict weight gain in pregnancy actually could be harmful, producing smaller, less healthy babies and increasing the risk to mothers. Gaining too much endangers both mother and baby, raising the risk of PREMATURE birth, gestational diabetes, preeclampsia and the necessity for Cesarean section. Significant underweight may result in a baby much smaller than it should be, and many such babies never catch up later. Most American clinicians now advise a total weight gain of 28 to 35 pounds if the woman is pregnant with a single fetus and with normal weight at conception, adding a pound a week during the second and third trimesters. Women who are overweight at conception are advised to limit weight gain to 15 to 25 pounds, gaining only two-thirds of a pound each week after the third month. However, even an obese woman should not gain fewer than 15 pounds in all. For women carrying multiple fetuses, a weight gain of 35 to 45 pounds is recommended. (See also BIRTH WEIGHT; DIET.)

3. in menopause. Ideally a woman should weigh the same at menopause (average age, 50) as her ideal weight at the age of 20. Most women, however, tend to weigh considerably more. By the age of 45 metabolism slows down, and only two-thirds the number of calories to maintain the same weight are required. After menopause another portion of the total calorie intake, which formerly supported an active reproductive system, is no longer needed. In young women body fat ranges from 18 to 23% on the average. With age, the amount of muscle tends to decrease and fat accounts for a greater percentage of weight. By age 60 body fat has gradually increased to about 32% in most women. Further, women tend to become less physically active as they get older. Therefore, unless food intake is reduced accordingly, the unneeded calories will turn into extra body fat. Apart from being unattractive, obesity after menopause greatly increases the risk of developing serious disease, specifically arteriosclerosis and coronary heart disease, hypertension (high blood pressure) and diabetes. The moderately active menopausal woman needs approximately 14 calories per pound of body weight per day to *maintain* her weight; any calories in excess will most likely be stored as fat. On the other hand, some authorities regard somewhat increased body fat after menopause as normal compensation for diminished estrogen production by the ovaries, since fat cells produce some estrogen.

See also DIET; OBESITY.

wet smear A simple test of vaginal discharge to determine the cause of a vaginal infection, usually performed in the clinician's office. The clinician places a small specimen of the discharge on a slide, adds a solution of either salt or potassium hydroxide (depending on which organism is suspected) and examines the slide under a microscope. He or she can then see if the organism is *Trichomonas,*

Candida (Monilia) albicans or *Hemophilus vaginalis* (see also TRICHOMONAS; VAGINITIS; VAGINOSIS; YEAST INFECTION). A wet smear cannot, however, rule out GONORRHEA.

wire-localization biopsy See BIOPSY, def. 5.

withdrawal See COITUS INTERRUPTUS.

withdrawal bleeding See ESTROGEN; ESTROGEN REPLACEMENT THERAPY.

womb See UTERUS.

women's doctor See GYNECOLOGIST.

women's health clinic A clinic that provides health care for women. Ideally such a clinic shows particular sensitivity to women's needs. It is directed and staffed mainly by women, is located in a safe and convenient environment and provides health education (in the form of literature, a newsletter, tapes, seminars or other programs). It emphasizes shared decision-making. It offers a multidisciplinary approach, with practitioners in several specialties (not just gynecology), diagnostic tests and alternative treatment (acupuncture, chiropractic and so on).

See also CLINIC; SELF-HELP.

yeast infection   Also *Candida albicans, Monilia albicans, moniliasis, candidiasis, fungus, vaginal thrush, vaginal mycosis, mycotic vaginitis.* One of the most common vaginal infections, caused by a yeastlike fungus called *Candida (Monilia) albicans.* The main symptoms are severe vaginal and vulvar itching and a white, cottage cheese–resembling discharge with a sweetish odor. The organism normally resides in the vagina of most women and gives rise to symptoms only when it multiplies more than usual. Pregnancy and oral contraceptives, which both raise estrogen levels, may cause such an increase, as can an increase in blood sugar, antibiotic therapy, fecal contamination (by wiping from back to front after a bowel movement) or transmission from a sex partner. Some 15 to 25% of women are troubled with yeast infection during pregnancy. An increase in estrogen causes increased glycogen deposits in the walls of the vagina, making a hospitable environment for the fungus to multiply. Diagnosis is by a WET SMEAR, and treatment consists of antifungal creams or suppositories placed in the vagina with an applicator and creams applied to the vulva. The most common creams are nystatin, miconazole (Micatin and Monistat), clotrimazole, econazole and terconazole; in the United States clotrimazole (Lotrimin, Mycelex) and miconazole (Monistat, Micatin) are now available without prescription. Alternatively, propion gel or gentian violet suppositories also may be effective, but these stain clothing. All these medications must be used for at least one to seven days, depending on the strength. Many women use pads during this time, since medication tends to leak from the vagina. Medicated tampons also are available and are less messy. Treatment should continue during a menstrual period, but ordinary tampons should be avoided since they can absorb the medication.

If the vulva are very irritated, a mild steroid cream may be indicated, but used sparingly and only until symptoms subside.

A recent study showed that two-thirds of the women buying over-the-counter vaginal antifungal medications had not accurately diagnosed their conditions. Some had yeast infections but also had other infections that would not respond to antifungal agents, and others had no vaginal infections at all. Also, diagnoses given by clinicians over the phone were often inaccurate. Therefore it is highly advisable to visit a clinician in person.

A remedy found effective by some women is eating yogurt, which suppresses the growth of fungi in the intestinal tract. It also sometimes is effective when applied locally, spooned into the vagina or inserted with an applicator of the kind used for spermicides. Acidophilus capsules inserted as a vaginal suppository may have a similar effect, as may daily douches with diluted yogurt (used for a week). Only "natural," unpasteurized yogurt (made at home or available in health-food stores) can be effective, because it contains live lactobacilli, which help break down the sugar of cervical discharge into lactic acid and therefore help combat the growth of organisms whose growth is encouraged by sugar (see also DÖDERLEIN BACILLI). Ultrapasteurized yogurt does not contain live lactobacilli. However, the effectiveness of yogurt has not been documented sufficiently to recommend it with any certainty; it appears to work for some women and not for others. Also, it is not known whether it is the lactobacilli or the acidity of yogurt that is effective; if it is the latter, vinegar douches are simpler (see below). Other home remedies include applying a poultice of natural (unpasteurized) cottage cheese on a sanitary pad, which also helps relieve itching, and douching once a day with an acidic douche (juice of half a lemon, *or* 2 tablespoons vinegar, *or* 1 teaspoon vitamin C powder, mixed in 1 quart of water), to make the vaginal environment more acid and less hospitable to yeast organisms. Some women find relief by using boric acid (600 milligrains in a size 0 gelatin capsule, or simply filling a capsule of this size with boric acid powder), inserting a capsule once a day for one week, and then twice a week for the next three weeks. Symptoms should improve within four days; if they do not, one's health care provider should be consulted. Some clinicians warn that placing unpasteurized milk products into the vagina puts a woman at risk for becoming a carrier of an organism called *Listeria*, which in pregnancy can infect the fetus, leading to stillbirth, and cause premature labor and meningitis in the mother. Still another home remedy is douching once a day with a solution of 1 teaspoon of 3% hydrogen pyroxide in 6 to 8 ounces of water.

A recent study suggests that at least some cases of recurrent yeast infection are linked to an allergic reaction to the sex partner's seminal fluid. When symptoms flare up soon after intercourse and only one partner experiences them, allergy could be the cause. It is easily treated by using a condom for a time and taking antihistamines until the reaction quiets down.

For severe recurrent chronic infection, a powerful oral antifungal drug, such as fluconazole, may be required, but should not be used by a pregnant or breast-feeding woman. The treatment involves three 150-mg tablets of fluconazole (Diflucan) at 72-hour intervals, followed by 150 mg per week for six months. It greatly reduced the incidence of recurrence but is not a long-term cure.

yogurt   A dairy product that is slightly acidic and, in unpasteurized form, contains live lactobacilli, which are thought to help combat YEAST INFECTION. Yogurt also is an excellent source of dietary calcium.

zygote   Also *fertilized egg*. The single cell that results from the mating of a male germ cell, or sperm, with a female germ cell, or egg (ovum), before it begins to divide (grow). It is not known exactly when the human zygote begins to divide, but it is believed to occur approximately 30 hours after FERTILIZATION, well before IMPLANTATION. Thereafter some authorities call it an EMBRYO, while others use the term "egg" (or "ovum") for four more weeks, until organ development begins.

zygote intrafallopian transfer   Also *ZIFT*. See EMBRYO TRANSFER.

APPENDIX
RESOURCES

Note: Addresses, phone numbers, and Web sites listed are the latest available, but they could change at any time. For further information, check the local yellow pages, or call or write ODPHP National Health Information Center, P.O. Box 23, Washington, DC 20013-1133, (800) 336-4797; (301) 565-4167 in Maryland and metropolitan D.C., and ask this government office to check their database of information resources. Its Web site is http://www.health.gov/nhic. Before contacting these resources, refer to the last paragraph in the Foreword (page viii), which includes some important warnings.

GENERAL HEALTH CARE AND INFORMATION

Black Women's Health Imperative
(202) 548-4000
http://www.blackwomenshealth.org

Food and Drug Administration
Office of Consumer Affairs
(888) 463-6332
http://www.fda.gov

Health Research Group
c/o Public Citizen
(202) 588-1000
http://www.citizen.org

National Health Information Center
(Referral service)
(800) 336-4797
(301) 565-4167 (Maryland and Washington D.C.)
http://www.health.gov/nhic
http://www.healthfinder.gov

National Latina Institute for Reproductive Health
(212) 422-2553
http://www.latinainstitute.org

National Women's Health Information Center
(800) 994-9662 (9 A.M. to 6 P.M.)
http://www.4woman.gov

National Women's Health Network
(202) 347-1140
http://www.nwhn.org

ABORTION

National Abortion Federation
(202) 667-5881
(800) 772-9100 (hotline, Monday to Friday. 8 A.M. to 10 P.M., weekends 9 A.M. to 5 P.M. Eastern Time)
(800) 424-2280 (Canada)
http://www.prochoice.org

ABUSE

See Domestic Abuse

ACUPUNCTURE

American Academy of Medical Acupuncture
(physician acupuncturists)
(800) 521-2262 (for referrals)
http://www.medicalacupuncture.org

American Association of Acupuncture and Oriental Medicine
(651) 631-0204 (Central Time)
http://www.aaaom.edu

AIDS/HIV

AIDS Clinical Trials Information Service
(800) 874-2572

AIDS Treatment Data Network
(212) 260-8868
http://www.ATDN.org

CDC National AIDS Hotline
(800) 232-4636 (24 hours a day, 365 days a year)
(800) 344-7432 (Spanish language, 8 A.M. to 2 P.M. eastern time)
e-mail: cdcinfo@cdc.gov

Teens and AIDS Hotline
(800) 234-8336

ALCOHOLISM

Alcoholics Anonymous World Service Office
(Check phone directory for local offices)
(212) 686-1100
www.alcoholics-anonymous.org

Alcohol and Drug Helpline
(800) 821-4357 (24 hours a day)

Al-Anon Family Group Headquarters
(888) 425-2666 (8 A.M. to 6 P.M. Monday to Friday)
http://www.al-anon.alateen.org

National Institute on Alcohol Abuse and Alcoholism
(301) 443-3860
www.niaaa.nih.gov

National Council on Alcoholism
(800) 622-2255

Women for Sobriety
(215) 536-8026
http://www.womenforsobriety.org

ALTERNATIVE MEDICINE

Alternative Medicine Foundation, Inc.
(301) 340-1960
http://www.amfoundation.org

American Association of Naturopathic Physicians
(866) 538-2267
http://www.naturopathic.org

American Chiropractic Association
(703) 276-8800
http://www.acatoday.com

American Holistic Medical Association
(425) 967-0737; (703) 556-9728
http://www.holisticmedicine.org

American Osteopathic Association
(800) 621-1773 (8:30 A.M. to 4:30 P.M. central time)
http://www.aoa-net.org

National Center for Complementary and Alternative Medicine
(888) 644-6226 (8:30 A.M. to 5 P.M.)
http://www.nccam.nih.gov

National Center for Homeopathy
(703) 548-7790
http://www.homeopathic.org

National College of Naturopathic Medicine
(503) 552-1555
http://www.ncnm.edu

ALZHEIMER'S DISEASE

Alzheimer's Association, Inc.
(800) 272-3900 (24 hours a day, 7 days a week)
http://www.alz.org

Alzheimer's Disease Education and Referral Center
(800) 438-4380 (8:30 A.M. to 5 P.M. Monday to Friday)
http://www.alzheimers.org

ARTHRITIS

American Academy of Physical Medicine and Rehabilitation
(312) 464-9700
www.aapmr.org

The Arthritis Foundation
(800) 283-7800 (9 A.M. to 5 P.M. Monday to Friday)
http://www.arthritis.org

National Institute of Arthritis and Musculoskeletal and Skin Diseases Information Clearinghouse
(877) 226-4267 (8:30 A.M. to 5 P.M.)
http://www.niams.nih.gov

ATRIAL FIBRILLATION

Atrial Fibrillation Foundation
(617) 726-1095
www.affacts.org

AUTOIMMUNE DISORDERS

American Autoimmune Related Diseases Association

(800) 598-4668 (literature requests)
(586) 776-3900 (national office)
http://www.aarda.org

BIRTH CENTERS

American Association of Birth Centers

(215) 234-8068; (866) 542-4784
http://www.birthcenters.org

BIRTH CONTROL

Choice

(215) 985-3300 (hotline in Philadelphia); (800) 848-3367
http://www.choice-phila.org

Planned Parenthood Federation of America

(800) 829-7732 (national office)
(800) 230-7526 (to find nearest local office)
http://www.plannedparenthood.org

BREAST-FEEDING

La Leche League International

(800) 525-3243
http://www.lalecheleague.org

CANCER

African American Breast Cancer Alliance

(612) 825-3675
http://www.aabcainc.org

American Cancer Society

(800) 227-2345 (24 hours, 7 days a week)
http://www.cancer.org

American Society for Colposcopy and Cervical Pathology

(800) 787-7227
http://www.asccp.org

Breast Cancer Action

(877) 278-6772
http://www.bcaction.org

Cancer Care

(800) 813-4673
http://www.cancercare.org

Cancer Hope Network

(877) 467-3638
http://www.cancerhopenetwork.org

Cancer Information Service

(800) 422-6237
http://www.nci.nih.gov

Kidney Cancer Association

(800) 850-9132 (9 A.M. to 5:30 P.M., central time)
http://www.kidneycancerassociation.org

Leukemia and Lymphoma Society

(800) 955-4572
http://www.leukemia-lymphoma.org

National Alliance of Breast Cancer Organizations

http://www.nabco.org

National Bone Marrow Transplant Link

(800) 546-5268
http://www.nbmtlink.org

National Ovarian Cancer Coalition

(888) 682-7426
http://www.ovarian.org

Ovarian Cancer National Alliance

(866) 399-6262
http://www.ovariancancer.org

SHARE—Self-HELP for Women with Breast or Ovarian Cancer

(866) 891-2392 (hotline)
http://www.sharecancersupport.org

Susan G. Komen Breast Cancer Foundation

(800) 462-9273
www.komen.org

Y-ME National Breast Cancer Hotline

(800) 221-2141 (24-hour hotline)
http://www.y-me.org

CEREBRAL VASCULAR ACCIDENT (STROKE)

American Stroke Association

(888) 478-7653 (8:30 A.M. to 5 P.M., Monday to Friday)
http://www.strokeassociation.org

Massachusetts General Hospital Stroke Service
(617) 726-8459
www.massgeneral.org/stopstroke/forpublic.aspx

National Heart, Lung and Blood Institute
(301) 592-8573
http://www.nhlbi.nih.gov

National Stroke Association
(800) 787-6537
http://www.stroke.org

CESAREAN SECTION

Cesarean Support, Education, and Concern
(617) 877-8266
www.childbirth.org

International Cesarean Awareness Network
(800) 686-4226
http://www.ican-online.org

CHILDBIRTH EDUCATION

American Academy of Husband-Coached Childbirth
(800) 422-4784 (9 A.M. to 5 P.M., pacific time)
http://www.bradleybirth.com

American Association of Birth Centers
(215) 234-8068
www.birthcenters.org

International Childbirth Education Association
(952) 854-8660
http://www.icea.org

Lamaze International
(800) 368-4404 (9 A.M. to 5 P.M., Monday to Friday)
http://www.lamaze.org

CHIROPRACTIC

See Alternative Medicine

CHRONIC FATIGUE

American Association of Chronic Fatigue Syndrome
(847) 258-7248
http://www.aacfs.org

CFIDS Association of America, Inc.
(704) 365-2343
http://www.cfids.org

CHRONIC PAIN

American Chronic Pain Association
(800) 533-3231
http://www.theacpa.org

National Chronic Pain Outreach Association
http://www.chronicpain.org

COLITIS AND CROHN'S DISEASE

Crohn's and Colitis Foundation of America
(800) 932-2423 (9 A.M. to 5 P.M.)
http://www.ccfa.org

COSMETIC SURGERY

American Society of Plastic and Reconstructive Surgeons
(888) 475-2784
http://www.plasticsurgery.org

CYSTITIS

Interstitial Cystitis Association
(800) 435-7422
http://www.ichelp.org

DEPRESSION

Depression and Bipolar Support Alliance
(800) 826-3632
http://www.DBSalliance.org

International Foundation for Research and Education on Depression
(410) 268-0044
www.ifred.org

DES (DIETHYLSTILBESTEROL)

DES Action USA
(800) 337-9288
http://www.desaction.org

DIABETES

American Diabetes Association
(800) 342-2383 (8:30 A.M. to 8 P.M., eastern time)
http://www.diabetes.org

DOCTORS AND SURGEONS

American Academy of Family Physicians
www.familydoctor.org

American Board of Medical Specialties
(847) 491-9091 (for information on board-
    certified physicians)
http://www.abms.org

National Association of Women's Health
(312) 786-7468
http://www.nawh.org

DOMESTIC ABUSE

Childhelp USA
(800) 422-4453 (hotline); 24 hours a day, 7 days
    a week
http://www.childhelpusa.org

**Health Resource Center on Domestic
    Violence (Family Violence Prevention)**
(415) 252-8900
http://www.endabuse.org

National Domestic Violence Hotline
(800) 799-7233 (24 hours, 7 days a week)
http://www.ndvh.org

**National Sexual Assault Hotline (part of
    RAINN [Rape, Abuse and Incest, National
    Network])**
(800) 656-4673
(800) 842-4546 (Referrals for facial reconstructive
    surgery for injuries from domestic abuse)
http://www.rainn.org

DOULAS

**Association of Labor Assistants and
    Childbirth Educators**
(617) 441-2500; (888) 222-5223
http://www.alace.org

Dona International
(888) 788-3262
http://www.dona.org

DOWN SYNDROME

National Down Syndrome Congress
(800) 232-6372
http://www.ndsccenter.org

National Down Syndrome Society Hotline
(800) 221-4602
http://www.ndss.org

DRUG ABUSE

Cocaine Anonymous
(310) 559-5833 (Monday to Friday, 9 A.M. to
    5 P.M., pacific time)
http://www.ca.org

Drug and Alcohol Help
(for referrals)
(800) 662-4357

Narcotics Anonymous World Services
(818) 773-9999 (8 A.M. to 5 P.M., Monday to Fri-
    day, pacific time)
http://www.na.org

National Institute on Drug Abuse
(301) 443-1124
(800) 967-5252
http://www.nida.nih.gov

DYSMENORRHEA

Women's Health
(800) 558-7046
http://www.womenshealth.com/hotline

EATING DISORDERS

American Anorexia/Bulimia Association
(212) 501-8351
http://www.njaaba.org

**National Association of Anorexia Nervosa
    and Associated Disorders, Inc.**
(847) 831-3438 (hotline)
http://www.anad.org

National Eating Disorders Association
(800) 931-2237
http://www.nationaleatingdisorders.org

Overeaters Anonymous
World Service Office
(505) 891-2664 (8 A.M. to 4:30 P.M., mountain time)
http://www.oa.org

ENDOMETRIOSIS

Endometriosis Association
(800) 992-3636; (414) 355-2000
http://www.endometriosisassn.org

FIBROMYALGIA

American Fibromyalgia Syndrome Association
(520) 733-1570
http://www.afsafund.org

National Chronic Fatigue Syndrome and Fibromyalgia Association
(816) 737-1343
http://www.ncfsfa.org

National Fibromyalgia Association
(714) 921-0150
http://www.fmaware.org

GAY

See Lesbian

GENETIC DISORDERS

Genetic and Rare Diseases Information Center (National Human Genome Research Institute)
(301) 402-0911
http://www.genome.gov

HAIR LOSS

American Hair Loss Council
(412) 765-3666
http://www.ahlc.org

National Alopecia Areata Foundation
(415) 472-3780 (pacific time)
http://www.naaf.org

HEADACHE

National Headache Foundation
(888) 643-5552
http://www.headaches.org

HEPATITIS

American Liver Foundation Hotline
(800) 465-4837
http://www.liverfoundation.org

Hepatitis Foundation International
(800) 891-0707
http://www.hepatitisfoundation.org

HERPES

Herpes Resource Center
(877) 411-4377
http://www.ashastd.org/hrc

National Herpes Hotline
(919) 361-8488

HOSPICE

Hospice Association of America
(202) 547-7424
http://www.nahc.org

Hospice Education Institute
(800) 331-1620; (207) 255-8800
http://www.hospiceworld.org

National Hospice and Palliative Care Organization
(703) 837-1500
http://www.nhpco.org

HUNTINGTON'S DISEASE

Huntington's Disease Society
(800) 345-4372
http://www.hdsa.org

HYPNOTHERAPY

American Society of Clinical Hypnosis
(630) 980-4740
www.asch.net;info@asch.net

HYSTERECTOMY

HERS Foundation
(888) 750-4377
http://www.hersfoundation.com

IMPOTENCE

Impotence Information Center
(800) 543-9632 (hotline)

INFERTILITY

American Association of Tissue Banks
(703) 827-9582
http://www.aatb.org

American Society for Reproductive Medicine
(205) 978-5000
http://www.asrm.com

RESOLVE
(703) 556-7172
http://www.resolve.org

INSOMNIA

National Sleep Foundation
(202) 347-3471
http://www.sleepfoundation.org

LESBIAN

Gay and Lesbian National Hotline
(888) 843-4564 (4 P.M. to 12 A.M., Monday to
    Friday; Noon to 5 P.M., Saturday)
www.glbtnationalhelpcenter.org

National Gay and Lesbian Task Force
(202) 393-5177
http://www.ngltf.org

**National Latino/a Lesbian, Gay, Bisexual,
    Transgender Organization**
(202) 487-9171
http://www.llego.org

**National Association of Lesbian and Gay
    Addiction Professionals**
(703) 465-0539
http://www.nalgap.org

LUPUS

See Systemic Lupus Erythematosus

LYMPHEDEMA

National Lymphedema Network
(800) 541-3259 (8 A.M. to 5 P.M., pacific time)
http://www.lymphnet.org

MAMMAPLASTY

**American College of Plastic and
    Reconstructive Surgeons**
(888) 272-7711
http://www.plasticsurgeons.org

MASSAGE

American Massage Therapy Association
(877) 905-2700
http://www.amta.org

**National Certification Board for Therapeutic
    Massage and Bodywork**
(800) 296-0664
http://www.ncbtmb.com

MENOPAUSE

North American Menopause Society
(440) 442-7550
www.menopause.org

MIDWIFE

American College of Nurse-Midwives
(240) 485-1800
http://www.acnm.org

Midwives Alliance of North America
(888) 923-6262
http://www.mana.org

MIGRAINE

See Headache

MULTIPLE SCLEROSIS

Multiple Sclerosis Association of America
(800) 532-7667
http://www.msaa.com

Multiple Sclerosis Foundation
(888) 673-6287 (9 A.M. to 7 P.M., Monday to
    Friday)
http://www.msfacts.org

National Multiple Sclerosis Society
(800) 344-4867
http://www.nmss.org

MYASTHENIA GRAVIS

**Myasthenia Gravis Foundation of America,
    Inc.**
(800) 541-5454 (8:45 A.M. to 4:45 P.M., central
    time)
http://www.myasthenia.org

OBESITY

American Obesity Association
(202) 776-7711
www.obesity.org

American Society for Bariatric Surgery
(352) 331-4900
www.asbs.org

Weight-control Information Network
(877) 946-4627 (toll-free)
www.win.niddk.nih.gov

OSTEOPOROSIS

National Osteoporosis Foundation
(800) 223-9994 (24 hours a day)
http://www.nof.org

Osteoporosis and Related Bone Diseases National Resource Center
(800) 624-2663
http://www.osteo.org

OSTOMY

United Ostomy Association
(800) 826-0826
http://www.uoa.org

PHYSICIANS

See Doctors and Surgeons

POLYCYSTIC OVARIES

Polycystic Ovarian Syndrome Association
http://www.pcosupport.org

PREPARED CHILDBIRTH

See Childbirth Education

REFLEX SYMPATHETIC DYSTROPHY

Reflex Sympathetic Dystrophy Syndrome Association
(877) 662-7737
www.rsds.org

REHABILITATION

American Academy of Physical Medicine and Rehabilitation
(312) 464-9700
www.aapmr.org

Commission on Accreditation of Rehabilitation Facilities (CARF)
(888) 281-6531
www.carf.org

RESTLESS LEGS SYNDROME

Restless Legs Syndrome Foundation
(877) 463-6757 (8 A.M. to 5 P.M.)
http://www.rls.org

ROSACEA

Rosacea National Society
(888) 662-5874 (central time)
http://www.rosacea.org

SCLERODERMA

Scleroderma Foundation
(800) 722-4673
http://www.scleroderma.org

SCOLIOSIS

National Scoliosis Foundation
(800) 673-6922
http://www.scoliosis.org

Scoliosis Association
(561) 994-4435
http://www.scoliosis-assoc.org

SELF-HELP

American Self-Help Clearinghouse
(973) 989-1122
http://www.selfhelpgroups.org

National Self-Help Clearinghouse
(212) 817-1822
http://www.selfhelpweb.org

SEX THERAPY

American Association of Sex Educators, Counselors and Therapists
(804) 752-0026
http://www.aasect.org

SEXUALLY TRANSMITTED DISEASE

See also AIDS/HIV, Herpes

American Social Health Association
(919) 361-8400; (800) 227-8922
http://www.asha.org

National Sexually Transmitted Disease Hotline
(800) 227-8922 (24 hours, 7 days a week)
(800) 344-7432 (8 A.M. to 2 A.M., 7 days a week)

SICKLE-CELL DISEASE

Sickle Cell Disease Association of America
(800) 421-8453
http://www.sicklecelldisease.org

SJÖGREN'S SYNDROME

Sjögren's Syndrome Foundation
(800) 475-6473
http://www.sjogrens.org

SPINA BIFIDA

Spina Bifida Association
(800) 621-3141
http://www.sbaa.org

SPERM BANK

See Infertility

STROKE

See Cerebral Vascular Accident

SURGERY

See also Doctors and Surgeons

American College of Surgeons
(800) 621-4111 (central time)
http://www.facs.org

American Society for Laser Medicine and Surgery
(715) 845-9283
http://www.aslms.org

SYSTEMIC LUPUS ERYTHEMATOSUS

Lupus Foundation of America
(800) 558-0121
http://www.lupus.org

SLE Foundation
(800) 745-8787
http://www.lupusny.org

TAY-SACHS DISEASE

See also Genetic Disorders

National Tay-Sachs and Allied Diseases Association
(800) 906-8723
http://www.ntsad.org

THYROID DISEASE

American Thyroid Association
(800) 849-7643 (9 A.M. to 5 P.M., eastern time)
http://www.thyroid.org

Thyroid Foundation of America
(800) 832-8321 (8:30 A.M. to 4 P.M.)
http://www.tsh.org

TURNER SYNDROME

Turner Syndrome Society of the United States
(800) 365-9944 (9 A.M. to 5 P.M., Monday to Friday, central time)
http://www.turnersyndrome.org

URINARY INCONTINENCE

National Association for Continence
(800) 252-3337
http://www.nafc.org

The Simon Foundation
(800) 237-4666
http://www.simonfoundation.org

VULVODYNIA

National Vulvodynia Association
(301) 299-0775
http://www.nva.org

Vulvar Health Awareness Campaign
http://www.vulvarhealth.org

Vulvar Pain Foundation
(336) 226-0704
http://www.vulvarpainfoundation.org

INDEX

This index is designed to be used in conjunction with the many cross-references within the A–Z entries. **Boldface** page numbers indicate main entries in the text. *Italicized* page references (such as *513)* indicate illustrations; the italicized letter *t* following the page locator (such as 56*t)* indicates a table; the letter *f* indicates a footnote to a table.

A

abdominal delivery. *See* Cesarean section
abdominal fat 39
abdominal hysterectomy 232
abdominal tubal ligation 418
abnormal cell division 73
abnormal presentation 1
abortifacient **1–2**, 124
    abortion **2–8**
    amnioinfusion 25–26
    anesthesia 32
    contragestive 124
    counseling 350
    criminal 2
    D and C 136
    dilatation and evacuation 150
    elective 2
    hysterotomy 234
    menstrual extraction 285
    resources 447
    septic abortion 2, 295
    spontaneous 2, 293
    state laws 3–6
    therapeutic 2
    vacuum aspiration 429

abortion pill. *See* contragestive
abruptio placentae 8
abscess **8–9**
    breast abscess 9
    pelvic abscess 8
absolute contraindication 125
abstinence. *See* natural family planning
abuse. *See* domestic abuse
acarbose (Precose) 142
accelerated partial breast irradiation 368
accessory nipple 305
accouchement. *See* labor
Accutane 10
acetaminophen 28
acetylcholine 22
acini 9
acne **9–10**, 393, 405*t*
acquired immunodeficiency syndrome. *See* AIDS
acromegaly **10**, 23
acrosin test 10
ACTH **14**, 230, 300
actinic keratosis **90**, 394
active labor 254, **359**
Actonel. *See* risedronate
acupressure **11**, 206, 274
acupuncture **10–11**
    resources 447
acute 12
acute hydramnios 225
acute pelvic inflammatory disease 328
addiction 12
adenocarcinoma **12**, 73–74, 88, 149
adenofibroma. *See* fibroadenoma
adenohypophysis. *See* anterior pituitary

adenomatous polyps 86
adenomyosis 12–13
adenosarcoma 73–74
adenosis 13
adhesion **13**, 44, 329
adhesive capsulitis. *See* frozen shoulder
adjuvant treatment **13**, 81–82
adnexae 13
adolescence
    acne 9–10
    adolescent nodule 13
    amenorrhea 22–23
    anorexia nervosa 33
    bulimia 69–70
    childbearing 14–15
    critical weight 128
    diet 147
    menarche 279–280
    precocious puberty 346–347
    puberty 362–363
    scoliosis 382, *383*
adolescent nodule 13
adrenalectomy **13**
adrenal glands **13–14**, 20, 130
adrenal hyperplasia. *See* adrenogenital syndrome
adrenal steroid 14
adrenocorticotropic hormone. *See* ACTH
adrenogenital syndrome 14
adult-onset diabetes. *See* Type II diabetes
aerobic exercise 40*t*, **174**
AFP. *See* alpha-fetoprotein test
after-baby blues. *See* postpartum depression
afterbirth. *See* placenta
afterpains **14**, 124
agalactia 14

age, childbearing **14–15**, 15*t*, 154, 154*t*
age-parity formula 402
agoraphobia 15
Ahumada del Castillo syndrome 24
AIC test (for diabetes) 142
AIDS **16–19**, 18*t*, 371, 388–389
    resources 447–448
AIDS-related complex 16
air embolism 164
albumin, urinary 19
albuminuria 19
alcohol abuse 19
Alcoholics Anonymous (AA) 20, 448
alcoholism **19–20**
    resources 448
alcohol use 19–20
aldosterone 20
aldosteronism 20
alendronate (Fosamax) 318
alglucerase 192
allergy 236
allodynia 290
allo-immune disorder 204
alopecia. *See* hair loss
alopecia areata 205
alpha-fetoprotein test (AFP) **20**, 298
alprostadil 237
alternative medicine **20–21**
    acupuncture 10–13
    aromatherapy 38–39
    Ayurveda 47
    biofeedback 52
    cancer 76
    chelation therapy 104
    chiropractic 107–108
    herbal remedies 210–212
    homeopathy 218–219
    hypnotherapy 228–229
    massage therapy 273–274
    naturopathy 303–304
    probiotics 356–357
    therapeutic touch 412
    visualization 438
Alzheimer's disease 21–22
ambulatory phlebectomy 435
ambulatory surgery (*See also* outpatient surgery) 403

amenorrhea **22–24**, 346, 390
amenorrhea-galactorrhea syndrome 24
Amerge 291
American Association of Tissue Banks 396
American ginseng. *See* ginseng
Amitiza (lubiprostone) 249
amniocentesis **24–25**, 355, 377, 392, 398, 411
amniography 25
amnioinfusion 2, **25–26**
amniotic fluid **27**, 225
amniotic sac 27
amniotomy 27
amplified surface microscopy 279
ampulla 333, *332*
Amsler Grid 266
anabolic steroids 27–28
anal canal 28, **36**
anal fissure 28
anal fistula 187
analgesic 28–29, 29*t*
anal intercourse 17,18*t*, **36**
anal sphincter 398
androgen **29–30**, 411–412
androgenetic alopecia 205
androgen insensitivity syndrome 30
andrologist 30
androstenedione 27
anemia **30–31**, 439*t*
anencephaly 304
anesthesia **31–33**
    caudal 94
    epidural 169
    paracervical 326
    pudendal 364
    regional 373
    spinal 399
anesthesiologist 31
aneurysm 96
angina pectoris 33
angiogenesis inhibitors 75
angioplasty 41
angiotensin converting enzyme inhibitors 228
anilingus 36
anorexia nervosa **33**
    resources 451

anoscope 208
anovulation. *See* anovulatory bleeding
anovulatory bleeding **33–34**, 310
anteflexed uterus 34
anterior cruciate ligament 252
anterior pituitary 338
anteverted uterus **34**, 426
antianxiety drugs. *See* tranquilizer
antibody 34
anticancer drugs. *See* chemotherapy
anticoagulants **46**, 413
antidepressants **34–36**, 30, 57, 136
antigen **29**, 212
antigonadotropin. *See* gonadotropin
antimetastatic factors 75
anti-oncogenic factors 75
antioxidant 440
antiperspirant 138
antiphospholipid syndrome 204
antipsychotics 416
anus 28, **36**, *331*, *441*
anxietas tibialis. *See* restless legs syndrome
anxiety **36**, 378
anxiety attack 15, **36**
Apgar score **37**, 37*t*
aphagia 233
aphonia 233
aphrodisiac 37–38
apocrine glands 38
appendectomy **38**, 232, 405*t*
appendicitis 38
apple shape **39**, 308
areola **38**, 305
aromatase inhibitors **82**
aromatherapy 38–39
arteriole 42
arteriosclerosis **39–42**, 40*t*, 41*t*
artery 42
arthritis **42**, 252, 374–377, *375*, 376*t*
    resources 448
arthritis-dermatitis syndrome 199
arthroscopy 252
artificial insemination **42–44**, 152, 246–248, 397

Ascheim-Zondeck test. *See* pregnancy test
ASCUS 325
Asherman's syndrome 44
aspermatogenesis. *See* sterility
aspiration. *See* biopsy; vacuum aspiration
aspirin **28**, 29*t*, 74
asthma 44–45
asymptomatic 45
atheroma 39
atherosclerosis 39
athletic ability, women's 45–46
atrial fibrillation 46
atropic vaginitis. *See* vaginal atrophy
atypical antipsychotics 416
atypical ductal hyperplasia 184
atypical hyperplasia 79
augment anesthesia. *See* anesthesia
aura (migraine) 290
autoimmune disease **39**
    chronic fatigue syndrome 112–113
    fibromyalgia 186–187
    multiple sclerosis 299–300
    myasthenia gravis 300–301
    myositis 301
    rheumatoid arthritis 374–377
    scleroderma 381–382
autologous bone marrow transplant 62
automanipulation. *See* masturbation
AutoNet 325
autonomic hyperreflexia 366
axillary 47
axillary node dissection 276
axillary tail 64
Ayurveda, Ayurvedic medicine 47
azoospermia 47

B

back labor 48
bacterial vaginosis. *See* vaginosis
bad blood. *See* syphilis
bag of waters. *See* amniotic sac

baldness. *See* hair loss
balloon ablation 48
ballottemen *See* quickening
Band-Aid surgery. *See* laparoscopy
barbiturates 415
bariatric surgery **48–49**, 309
barium enema 85
barrier methods (contraception) 49
Bartholin cyst 130–131
Bartholin's glands **49–50**
basal body temperature (BBT) **50**, 51*t*, 302, 321
basal cell carcinoma 90, 90*t*
basal metabolism. *See* metabolism
basic metabolic rate 287
BBT. *See* basal body temperature
beauty parlor stroke syndrome 50–51
bed rest in pregnancy 174
belle indifference, la 233
belly-button operation. *See* laparoscopy
benign 51
benign paroxysmal positional vertigo 436
beriberi 438*t*
beta blocker 120, **227**
beta carotene 438*t*
beta-thalassemia. 57
Bethesda system 325
bicornuate uterus 426
bilateral 51
bilateral tubal occlusion 402
biliary calculi (gallstones) 190
bilirubin. *See* neonatal jaundice
Billings method. *See* cervical mucus method
bimanual pelvic examination. *See* gynecologic examination
binge eating. *See* bulimia
bioassay of HCG 351
biofeedback **52**, 206
biological birth control. *See* natural family planning
biopsy **52–54**, 184, 386
    breast **52–53**, 184
biotin 439*t*
bipolar disorder. *See* manic-depressive illness

Birmingham Hip Resurfacing System 316
birth attendant **54**, 153, 288–290
birth ball 54
birth canal 54
birth center **54**, 352
birth control **54–55**
    barrier methods 49
    cervical cap 98–99, *98*
    cervical mucus method 99–100
    coitus interruptus 116
    condom 117–119
    contraceptive 121–123
    contraceptive sponge 123
    contragestive 134
    diaphragm 144–146
    douching 152
    family planning 177, 302–303
    female condom 118
    intrauterine device (IUD) 244–246
    natural family planning 302–303
    oral contraceptive 312–315
    prophylactic 360
    resources 449
    spermicide 397–398
    sterilization 401–402
    thermatic sterilization 412
birth control pill. *See* oral contraceptive
birth defects **55–57**, 56*t*. *See also* prenatal tests
    age factors 14–15, 15*t*, 154
    Canavan disease 73
    cerebral palsy 95
    congenital infection 120
    cystic fibrosis 132
    Down syndrome 153–154
    erythroblastosis 170
    fragile X syndrome 188
    Gaucher's disease 192
    gene therapy 192–193
    genetic counseling 193
    genetics 194
    genetic testing 195
    hemophilia 207–208
    hermaphroditism 212

Klinefelter syndrome 251–252
muscular dystrophy 300
neural tube defects 304–305
phenylketonuria 336–337
Rett syndrome 374
rubella 378–379
sickle-cell disease 391–392
spina bifida 398–399
Tay-Sachs disease 410–411
thalidomide 412
Turner's syndrome 420
birthing bubble. *See*
decompression bubble
birthing center. *See* birth center
birthing room 57–58
birth stool 58
birth weight 58
birth without violence. *See*
Leboyer method
bisexual 58
bisphosphonates 318–319
blackhead 9
bladder **58–59**, *331, 332*
bladder cancer 78–79
bladder infection. *See* cystitis
blastocyst transfer 247
bleeding, vaginal 59
blepharoplasty 126
bloating. *See* edema
blood chemistry profile 60
blood clot. *See* thrombus
blood count 59, *50t*
blood poisoning. *See* septicemia
blood pressure. *See* hypertension
blood sugar. *See* serum glucose
blood test 59–61
blood urea nitrogen (BUN) 60*t*
bloody show. *See* mucus plug
blowing, blow job. *See* fellatio
board-certified **61**, 404
body mass index (BMI) 40*t*, **308**
body weight. *See* obesity; weight,
body
bonding **61–62**, 378
bone density scan 62, 317, 317*t*
bone loss/resorption. *See*
osteoporosis
bone marrow transplant 62
bone scan. *See* radionuclide
imaging

Botox® **62–63**, 127
botulin toxin 62
BPPV. *See* benign paroxysmal
positional vertigo
brachytherapy **63**, 368
Bradley method **63**, 356
Braxton-Hicks contractions 63
BRCA1, BRCA2 74, **79**
breakthrough bleeding 63–64
breast **64–65**. *See also* entries
beginning with "breast" below
abscess 9
augmentation 269
biopsy 52–53
cancer 79–84
nipple 305
reduction 269
breast abscess 9
breast biopsy 52–53
breast bud 64
breast cancer **79–84**, 80*t*, 81*t*
adrenalectomy 13
biopsy 52–53
cancer in situ 92
hormone therapy 220
inflammatory 87
lumpectomy 276–277
mammaplasty 268–270
mammography 271–273
mastectomy 274–277
Paget's disease 324
radiation therapy 336–337
reconstruction 268–270
self-examination 67, *68*
staging 399*t*
breast cyst. *See* fibrocystic breast
syndrome
breast disease
abscess 9
biopsy 52–53
cancer. *See* breast cancer
cancer in situ 92
cystosarcoma phyllodes 135
ductal papilloma 156
fibroadenoma 183
fibrocystic breast syndrome
184
galactocele 190
lipoma 262
mammary duct ectasia 271

mammary duct fistula 271
mammography 271–273
mastectomy 274–277
mastitis 277
reconstruction 268–270
sclerosing adenosis 382
self-examination 67, *68*
breast-feeding **65–67**
demand feeding 67
lactation 256–257
let-down reflex 261
nipple 305
polygalactia 342
resources 449
breast lumpiness. *See* fibrocystic
breast syndrome
breast reconstruction. *See*
mammoplasty
breast reduction. *See*
mammoplasty
breast self-examination 67, *68*
breast size 64
breech presentation **67–69**, 278
brow presentation 69
bruising 69
B-scan. *See* ultrasound
bubo **69**, 104, 265
buccal smear 57
bulimarexia. *See* bulimia
bulimia **69–70**, 309
resources 451
bunion 70
bunionette 70
Burch procedure 424
burning mouth syndrome 70–71

C

Caesarean. *See* Cesarean section
calcifications, breast 72
calcitonin (Calcimar, Miacalcin)
319
calcium 60*t*, **72–73**, 318
calcium channel blocker 228
calendar method. *See* natural
family planning
calories 147*t*, 147–149, 308
Canalith Repositioning Procedure
437
Canavan disease 73

cancer **73–78**
  adenocarcinoma 12
  adjuvant treatment 13
  adrenalectomy 13
  biopsy 52–54
  bladder 78–79
  breast 79–84
  carcinogen 92
  carcinoma 92
  cervical 84
  chemotherapy 105–107
  choriocarcinoma 111
  colorectal 85–86
  conization 120–121
  DES (diethylstilbestrol) and 149–150
  dysplasia 159–160
  endometrial 86–87
  estrogen-receptor assay 171
  hormone therapy 220–221
  hydatidiform mole 224–225
  hypophysectomy 229–230
  immunotherapy 236
  inflammatory breast 87
  in situ 91–92
  leukoplakia, vulvar 261
  liver 87
  lung 87
  lymphedema 264–265
  malignant 268
  mammography 271–273
  mastectomy 274–276
  melanoma 279
  metastasis 287
  ovarian 88–89
  Paget's disease 324
  pancreas 324–325
  Pap smear 325–326
  pelvic 90
  pelvic exenteration 328
  precancerous lesions 346
  radiation therapy 368–369
  recurrence 372
  remission 372
  sarcoma 380
  screening guidelines 77
  skin 90
  smoking and 394–395
  staging 86, 399–400
  support group 92
  thyroid 91
  tumor 420
  uterine 91
  vaginal 91
  vulvar 91
cancer, breast. *See* breast cancer
cancer in situ **91–92**, 324, 325, 346
cancer stem cell 74
cancer support group 92
cancer survivors 77
Candida albicans. *See* yeast infection
candidiasis. *See* yeast infection
capillary 42
carbon dioxide test. *See* Rubin test
carcinogen 92
carcinoma 92
carcinoma in situ. *See* cancer in situ
carotid endoarterectomy 96
carpal tunnel syndrome 93
castration **93**, 311
cataract 93
cathepsin D 82
catheter, urinary 93–94
catheter ablation 46
CAT scan 88, **94**
caudal anesthesia 94
caul. *See* amniotic sac
cauterization 94
cautery. *See* cauterization
CDKN2A 74
CEA assay 85
celibacy 94–95
cellulite 95
cephalhematoma 95
cephalic presentation 95
cephalopelvic disproportion 359
cerebral embolism 164
cerebral palsy 95–96
cerebral thrombosis 413
cerebral vascular accident (CVA) 96–97
  warning signs 97
certified nurse-midwife (CNM) 289
certified nurse practitioner 306
certified registered nurse anesthetist (CRNA) 307
cervical biopsy 53
cervical canal 101
cervical cancer 12, **84–85**, 325, 369, 381
cervical cap **98–99**, *98*, 122*t*
cervical cyst. *See* Nabothian cyst
cervical erosion. *See* cervicitis
cervical eversion 99
cervical intraepithelial neoplasia (CIN) 99
cervical mucus method 99–100
cervical polyp 343
cervical stenosis 100
cervicitis 100–101
cervix **101**, 117, *145*, *331*, 426
Cesarean section 8, 69 **101–103**, 344–345, 358
  resources 450
CFIDS, CFS. *See* chronic fatigue syndrome
Chadwick's sign 104
chancre **104**, 406
chancroid 104
change of life. *See* menopause
chastity 104
chelation therapy 104
chemo brain 106
chemotherapy 62, **105–107**
chest X-ray 88
Chiari-Frommel syndrome 24
chicken pox 214
childbearing age **14**, 14*t*, 154*t*
childbearing center. *See* birth center
childbed fever. *See* puerperal fever
childbirth. *See* delivery; labor; pregnancy; pregnant patients' rights; prepared childbirth
childbirth education. *See* prepared childbirth
chiropractic 107–108
chlamydia infection **108**, 265, 329, 388, 422, 432
chloasma **108–109**, 349, 394
chloride 292*t*
chocolate cyst. *See* endometrial cyst
cholecystectomy 190
cholescintigraphy 190
cholestasis of pregnancy 250

cholesterol 39, 60*t*, 60–61, **109–111**, 416
cholinesterace inhibitors 22
chondroitin 316
chondromalacia patella 252
choriocarcinoma 111
chorion **111**, 340
chorionic villus sampling (CVS) **111–112**, 356
chromosomal abnormality 15
chromosome **112**, 194, 195, 386
chromosome analysis 193
chromosome defects 56
chromosome test 112
chronic 112
chronic bronchitis. *See* chronic obstructive pulmonary disease
chronic fatigue immune dysfunction syndrome. *See* chronic fatigue syndrome
chronic fatigue syndrome (CFS) 112–113
    resources 450
chronic heartburn. *See* gastric esophageal reflux disorder
chronic hydramnios 225
chronic obstructive pulmonary disease 113
chronic pain **113–114**, 372–373
chronic pelvic infection 328, **329**
chronotherapy 106, **114**
Cialis 238
cilia 176
CIN. *See* cervical intraepithelial neoplasia
circumcision 114–115
clap (slang). *See* gonorrhea
clear-cell adenocarcinoma 12
cleft spine. *See* spina bifida
climacteric. *See* menopause
climax. *See* orgasm
clinic 115
clinical depression 139
clinical nurse specialist (CNS) 307
clipping the cords. *See* vasectomy
clitoridectomy 115
clitoris **115**, 170, 278, *331, 441*
clomiphene citrate 179
clonidine 222
cluster headache 206

CNM. *See* certified nurse-midwife
CNP. *See* certified nurse practitioner
CNS. *See* clinical nurse specialist
coccyx *331*
cock (slang). *See* penis
coitus 116
coitus interruptus **116**, 122*t*
cold knife biopsy. *See* conization
cold sore 213
colon cancer. *See* colorectal cancer
colonoscopy 86, **116**
colorectal cancer **85–86**
colorectal polyps 85–86, **343**
colostomy **116**, 319–320
colostrum 256
colposcope 117
colposcopy 117
colpotomy. *See* culdoscopy
columnar epithelium 99
combination pill 312
combined method. *See* sympto-thermic method
comedo 9
coming. *See* orgasm
Commission for Accreditation of Freestanding Birth Centers 54
complementary medicine 20–21
complete blood count (CBC) 59–61, 59*t*
complete decongestive physiotherapy 264
complex regional pain syndrome. *See* reflex sympathetic dystrophy syndrome
compression fracture 117
compulsive overeating. *See* obesity
computerized axial tomography. *See* CAT scan
Comstock Law 55
condom **117–119**, 122*t*, 389
conduction anesthesia. *See* regional anesthesia
condyloma acuminata 119
cone biopsy. *See* conization
confinement. *See* labor
congenital abnormalities. *See* birth defects
congenital infection 120
congestive 120

congestive dysmenorrhea 157–158
congestive heart failure 120
conization 120–121
conjugated estrogen (Premarin) 172
constipation 121
contact dermatitis 121
contraceptive **121–123**, 122*t*
    barrier methods 49
    birth control 54–55
    cervical cap 98–99, 99, 122*t*
    coitus inerruptus 116, 122*t*
    condom 117–119, 122*t*
    diaphragm 122*t*, 144–146, *145*
    effectiveness of 122*t*
    emergency contraceptive 164–165
    male contraceptive 267–268
    minipill 292
    natural family planning 302–303
    oral contraceptive 312–315
    sponge 122*t*, 123–124
contraceptive sponge 122*t*, **123–124**
contraction, uterine **124**, 254–256
contraction stress test. *See* oxytocin challenge test
contract mother. *See* surrogate mother
contragestive 124
contraindication 125
conversion disorder. *See* hysteria
Cooper's ligaments 64
COPD. *See* chronic obstructive pulmonary disease
copper 292*t*
copulation. *See* coitus
cord bank 62
core needle biopsy 52
corona 332
coronary angiography 40
coronary artery disease. *See* arteriosclerosis
coronary microvascular dysfunction 41
coronary thrombosis 413
corpus, uterine 426

corpus luteum **125–126**
corpus luteum cyst 125
corticotropin-releasing hormone 230
Corynebacterium vaginale 433
cosmetics 126
cosmetic surgery **126–127**, 405*t*
counseling. *See* feminist therapy; genetic counseling; pregnancy counseling; psychotherapy; sex therapy
Cowper's gland *332, 333*
COX–2 inhibitors 29
crabs. *See* pubic lice
cramp 128
cranial arteritis. *See* giant cell arteritis
C-reactive protein **39**, 376
creatinine 60*t*
criminal abortion 2
critical weight 128
CRNA. *See* certified registered nurse anesthetist
Crohn's disease 242
crowning (labor) 255
CRP. *See* C-reactive protein
crush fracture. *See* compression fracture
cryoablation 183
cryoprobe 128
cryosurgery 128–129
cryotherapy. *See* cryosurgery
cryptomenorrhea 23
cryptorchidism **129**, 401
C section. *See* Cesarean section
Ctcolonography. *See* colonoscopy
CT scan. *See* CAT scan
cul-de-sac 129
culdocentesis 129
culdoscopy 129
culture 129
cunnilingus 130
curet (curette) 130
curettage 53,130
curvature of the spine. *See* scoliosis
Cushing's disease 130
Cushing's syndrome 130
CVA. *See* cerebral vascular accident (stroke)

CVS. *See* chorionic villus sampling
cyst 130–132. *See also* fibrocystic breast syndrome
cystectomy 131
cystic disease. *See* fibrocystic breast syndrome
cystic fibrosis **132**, 355
cystitis **132–134**, 393. *See also* urethritis
cystocele 133, **134–135**
cystometrogram 134
cystosarcoma phyllodes 135
cystoscopy 135
cytology 135
cytoplasmic transfer 248

D

Dalkon Shield 246
danazol 136
D and C (dilatation and curettage) **136–137**, 344
    office D and C 54
D and E. *See* dilatation and evacuation
DASH diet 228*t*
deafness 137
decongestive physiotherapy 264
defloration 138
degenerative joint disease. *See* osteoarthritis
delayed puberty 23, **362**
delivery (childbirth) 254
demand feeding 138
Demerol (meperidine) 138
deodorant 138
deoxyribonucleic acid. *See* DNA
Depo-Provera 122*t*, 122, **138**
depression **138–140**, 139*t*, 273
    resources 450
DeQuervain's tendonitis 140–141
dermatomyositis 301
dermoid cyst 131
dermoscope 252
DES. *See* diethylstilbestrol
designer estrogen. *See* selective estrogen-receptor modulator
detoxification. *See* addiction; alcohol use
DI. *See* donor insemination

diabetes 40*t*, **141–144**, 142*t*, 143*t*
diagnosis 144. *See also* diagnostic tests
diagnostic breast ultrasound 272
diagnostic mammogram 272
diagnostic tests and procedures
    acrosin test 10
    alpha-fetoprotein test (AFP) 20
    barium enema 85
    biopsy 52–54
    blood test 59–61
    CAT scan 94
    chorionic villus sampling (CVS) 111–112
    colonoscopy 116
    colposcopy 117
    conization 120–121
    culdoscopy 129
    culture 129–130
    curettage 130
    D and C 136–137
    diagnostic breast ultrasound 272
    diagnostic mammogram 272
    Duke's test 156
    early pregnancy test 161
    genetic testing 195–196
    Gram stain 200
    hysterosalpingography 233–234
    magnetic resonance imager (MRI) 266–267
    mammography 271–273
    Pap smear 325–326
    pregnancy test 350–351
    prenatal tests 355–356
    radioreceptor assay 369–370
    Rubin test 379
    Schiller test 381
    sigmoidoscopy 85
    Sims-Huhner test 392–393
    ultrasound 421
    urine test 425
    wet smear 44
diaphragm 122*t*, **144–146**, *145*, 389, 397
diastolic heart failure 120
diastolic pressure 226
Dick-Read method **146**, 356

diet and nutrition **146–149**, 147*t*, 148*t*
   calcium 60*t*, 72–73
   cancer and 74, 75*t*
   cerebral vascular accident (stroke) and 97
   cholesterol 109–111
   goals for women 147*t*
   hypertension and 227
   migraine and 290
   minerals 291–292
   obesity 308
   vegetarianism 148
   vitamin 438–440
dietary folate equivalent (DFE) 187
diethylstilbestrol (DES) 7, **149–150**
   resources 450
digital mammography 272
digital rectal examination 77*t*
digital tomosynthesis 272
digoxin 104
dilatation and curettage. *See* D and C
dilatation and evacuation (D and E) 26, **150**
discharge, vaginal **150**, 263, 390, 430, 432*t*, 433
discrete 150
disease-modifying antirheumatic drugs. *See* DMARDS
diuretic 151
Dix-Hallpike maneuver 437
dizygotic 297
dizziness. *See* vertigo
DMARDS (disease-modifying antirheumatic drugs) 376–377, 376*t*
DNA (deoxyribonucleic acid) 66, 194, **278**
DNA flow cytometry 82
doctors and surgeons 61, **404**
Döderlein bacilli 151
domestic abuse 151–152
dominant (trait) 57, **194**
dominant-gene defects 57
donor egg **152**, 248
donor insemination (DI). *See* artificial insemination

dopamine 230
Doptone 181
dorsal lithotomy 152
dose. *See* gonorrhea
double-blind study 339
double footling breech 67
double ovulation 321
double uterus 426
douching 122*t*, **152–153**
Douglas cul-de-sac. *See* cul-de-sac
doula 153
dowager's hump 153
Down syndrome 15, 25 **153–154**, 154*t*
drip. *See* gonorrhea
dropped bladder. *See* cystocele
dropping. *See* lightening
dropsy. *See* edema
drug abuse. *See* addiction
drug use and pregnancy 154–155
dry eye 155–156
dry labor 156
dryness, vaginal. *See* vaginal atrophy
dual-energy X-ray absorptiometry 318
dual-photon absorptiometry 318
Duchenne muscular dystrophy 300
ductal cancer in situ 92
ductal lavage 76
ductal papilloma 156
ductless. *See* endocrine
Duke's test 156
duodenal switch 49
dysfunctional bleeding, vaginal 156
dysmenorrhea 158–159
dyspareunia 158–159
dysplasia 159–160
dystocia **160**, 359
dysuria 160

E

early abortion. *See* vacuum aspiration
early labor 359
early pregnancy test 161

early uterine evacuation. *See* vacuum aspiration
easy bruising. *See* bruising
eating. *See* cunnilingus
eating disorders. *See* anorexia; bulimia; obesity
echinacea. *See* herbal remedies 189
eclampsia **161–162**, 347
economy-class syndrome 413
ectasia. *See* mammary duct ectasia
ectopic pregnancy **162**, 380, 405*t*
ectropion. *See* cervical eversion
edema **162–163**, 264–265, 347
effacement 163
effleurage 274
egg. *See* ovum
ejaculate 163, **395–396**
ejaculation **163–164**, 333
ejaculatory duct 332, 333
ejaculatory incompetence. *See* retarded ejaculation
Ekbom syndrome. *See* restless legs syndrome
EK. *See* electrocardiograph
elastography 80
elasticity imaging 80
elective induction of labor 240
elective surgery 405
electrocardiograph (EKG) 40
electrocautery. *See* cauterization
electrodesiccation. *See* cauterization
electrosurgical loop excision. *See* loop electrosurgical excision procedure
elephantiasis 265
elevator (instrument) 292
embolism 164
embolization. *See* uterine artery embolization
embolus 164
embryo **164**, 196
embryo adoption 248
embryoscopy 356
embryo transfer 164
embryo transplant. *See* embryo transfer
emergency contraception 164–165

emergency surgery 405*t*
emmenagogue 1, **165**
emphysema. *See* chronic
    obstructive pulmonary disease
ENCORE 275
endocarditis 295
endocervical 165
endocervical curettage 53
endocervicitis 165
endocervix. *See* cervical canal
endocrine 13, **165**
endocrine manipulation 171
endocrine therapy. *See* hormone
    therapy
endocrinology 165
endogenous depression 139
endoluminal radiofrequency
    thermal heating 435
endolymphatic sac decompression
    437
endometrial ablation. *See*
    endometrial hyperplasia
endometrial aspiration. *See*
    vacuum aspiration
endometrial biopsy 53–54
endometrial cancer **86–87**, 400*t*
endometrial cyst (chocolate cyst)
    167
endometrial hyperplasia **165–
    166**, 346
endometrial polyp 343
endometrial tissue sample 66*t*
endometriosis **166–168**, 330
    resources 451
endometritis **168**, 298
endometrium 168, *165, 331*
endoscope 183
endovenous laser therapy (EVLT)
    435
engagement 168
engorgement, breast. *See under*
    lactation
enzymes 59*t*
ephedra. *See under* herbal
    remedies
epididymis *332,* 333
epidural anesthesia 169
epiluminescence microscopy 252
episiotomy 169–170
Epstein-Barr virus 214

erection **170**, 333
ergot 170
ergotamine tartrate 291
erosion, cervical. *See* cervicitis
ERT. *See* estrogen replacement
    therapy
erythroblastosis (fetalis) 170
erythrocyte sedimentation rate
    376
erythropoietin 31
Esalen 274
escutcheon 296
essential hypertension 226
estradiol 170, 431
Estring 431
estriol 170, 431
estrogen 170–171
estrogen analog. *See* selective
    receptor modulator
estrogen receptor 171
estrogen-receptor assay 171
estrogen replacement therapy
    (ERT) 171–174
estrone 170
Euronie method. *See* prenatal yoga
eversion, cervical. *See* cervical
    eversion
Evista. *See* raloxifene
excise, excision 174
excisional biopsy 52
excitement phase 389
exercise 174–175
exogenous depression 139
expectancy theory 339
extended radical (thorough)
    mastectomy 276
external fetal monitoring 181
external hemorrhoids 208
external os 101
external version **69**, 436
eye disease. *See* cataract; dry eye;
    macular degeneration

F

face lift. *See* cosmetic surgery
face presentation 176
fallen bladder. *See* cystocele
fallen uterus. *See* prolapsed
    uterus

fallopian tubes **176–177**, 233,
    331, 379, 380, 405*t,* 418
false labor 177
false negative/positive (pregnancy
    test) result 351
false pregnancy 177
family planning **177**, 302–303
fasting plasma glucose test 142
fat embolus 164
fatigue 112–113, **177–178**
fat necrosis 178
fecal occult blood test 77*t,* 217
feedback, hormonal **219–220,**
    230
fellatio **178**, 265
female condom 118
Femara. *See* letrozole
FemCap 99
feminine hygiene. *See* hygiene
feminist clinic. *See* self-help
feminist therapy 178–179
fern test. *See* cervical mucus
    method
fertility **179**, 179*t,* 180*t*
fertility awareness. *See* natural
    family planning
fertility drug 179–180
fertility monitor 217
fertility pill. *See* fertility drug
fertility screening 179, 217
fertilization 180–181
fertilized egg. *See* zygote
fetal acoustic stimulator 182
fetal alcohol syndrome 19
fetal cells in maternal blood 181
fetal fibronectin (fFN) 216, **354**
fetal heartbeat 181–182
fetal monitoring 181–182
fetal movement **182–183**, 366–
    367
fetal nuchal translucence. *See*
    nuchal translucency
fetal oxygen monitor 161
fetal placenta 340
fetal reduction 298
fetoscopy 183
fetus 183
fever blister 213
fFN. *See* fetal fibronectin
fiber, dietary 121, **147**, 147*t*

fibrate 111
fibroadenoma 183
fibrocystic breast syndrome 79, **184**
fibrocystic changes. *See* fibrocystic breast syndrome
fibroid **184–185**, *185*, 301, 405*t*
fibromyalgia 186–187
    resources 457–458
fibromyoma. *See* fibroid
fibrosis, cystic. *See* cystic fibrosis
fibrositis. *See* fibromyalgia
fimbriae 176
fimbriectomy 176
fine needle aspiration 52
fissure. *See* anal fissure
fisting 36
fistula **187**, 271
Flagyl (metronidazole) 417
flower of life. *See* ginseng
fluid retention. *See* edema
fluorescent in-situ hybridization 356
fluoride 292
foam, contraceptive. *See* spermicide
foaming suppository tablet 397
focused ultrasound 186
folate. *See* folic acid
Foley catheter 93
folic acid (folate) 30, **187–188**, 398, 439*t*
follicle, ovarian 188
follicle (follicular) cyst 131
follicle-stimulating hormone. *See* FSH
follicular stage **188**, 284
food pyramid 147
forceps 188
foreskin. *See* prepuce
Fosamax. *See* alendronate
fountain of youth root. *See* ginseng
fragile X syndrome 188
frank breech 67
fraternal twins 297–298
French method. *See* coitus interruptus
frequency, urinary 188–189
frigidity 189. *See also* orgasm

frozen egg 397
frozen section 52
frozen shoulder 189
FSH (follicle-stimulating hormone) 179, 180, **189**, 197, 339*t*
full term 196
fulvestrant 82
functional bleeding. *See* dysfunctional bleeding
fundus. *See* uterus
fungus. *See* yeast infection

G
galactocele 190
galactorrhea **190**, 358
gallbladder 190–191
gallstones 190
gamete 194
gamete intrafallopian transfer (GIFT) 191
Gardasil 84, **224**
Gardnerella vaginalis 433
gastric banding 49
gastric bypass 49
gastroesophageal reflux disorder (GERT) 191–192
Gaucher's disease 192
gay 219. *See also* lesbian resources 453
gender identity 192
gene. *See* genetics
gene chip 75
general anesthesia 31
GeneSearch Breast Lymph Node Assay 79
gene therapy 75, **192–193**
genetic code 306
genetic counseling 193
genetic disorders. *See* birth defects
genetic engineering 194
genetics **194–195**
    birth defects 55–57
    chorionic villus sampling 111–112
    chromosome 112
    gene therapy 75, 192–193
    genetic counseling 193

genetic testing 195–196
    nucleic acid 306
    prenatal tests 355–356
genetic testing 195–196
genital herpes. *See* herpes infection
genitalia. *See* genitals
genitals 196, *331, 332*
genital warts. *See* condyloma acuminata
genome 194
gentle birth 259
GERD. *See* gastroesophageal reflux disorder
German measles. *See* rubella
gestation **194**, 352–354
gestational age 352
gestational diabetes 143
gestational surrogacy 405
giant cell arteritis 196–197
GIFT. *See* gamete intrafallopian transfer
ginseng 197
glans 332, *302*
glucometer 217
Glucophage. *See* metformin
glucosamine 316
glucose 60*t*
gluteus free flap 270
glycosuria 141
GnRH (gonadotropin-releasing hormone) 180, **197**
going down. *See* fellatio
goiter 414
gonad 197
gonadotropin 197–198
gonadotropin-releasing hormone. *See* GnRH
gonococcal arthritis 199
gonococcal ophthalmia 199
gonorrhea **197–199**, 388
gonorrhea culture 198
gonorrheal salpingitis 199
gossypol. *See* male contraceptive
gout 199–200
Graafian follicle **200**, 284, 321
Gram stain 200
granny midwife 288
granuloma inguiale 200
granulosa 200

Graves' disease 414–415
gravida 200
group therapy 362
growth and development 200
growth-hormone releasing
    hormone 230
growth spurt 363
guided imagery. See visualization
gynecologic examination **201–
    203**, *201*, 345
gynecologist 201

H

habitual abortion. See habitual
    miscarriage
habitual miscarriage 204–205
hair loss (alopecia) 205
Halo Breast Pap Test System 80
Halsted radical mastectomy 275
hangover headache 206
hardening of the arteries. See
    arteriosclerosis
hard labor 359
Hashimoto's thyroiditis 414
HCG. See human chorionic
    gonadotropin
HDL (high-density lipoproteins)
    109, 110, 111, 110*t*
headache **205–206**, 290–291
    resources 452
health care proxy 206
hearing loss. See deafness
heart attack 39, 40*t*. See also
    arteriosclerosis; heart disease;
    myocardial infarction
heartburn, chronic. See
    gastroesophageal reflux
    disorder
heart disease. See arteriosclerosis;
    atrial fibrillation; mitral valve
    stenosis
heart failure. See congestive heart
    failure
Hegar's sign 207
height loss 207
hematocrit 59*t*
hematuria 207
hemiplegia 96

hemochromatosis 56, **207**
hemoglobin 59*t*
hemophilia 207–208
Hemophilus vaginalis. See vaginosis
hemorrhage, postpartum 345–
    346
hemorrhage, vaginal 208
hemorrhoid 121, **208–209**, 405*t*
hemorrhoidectomy 209, 405*t*
hemorrhoidopexy 209
hepatitis 209–210
HER2 83
HER2/oncogene 83
herbal diuretics 151, 151*t*
herbalism. See herbal remedies
herbal remedies **210–212**, 211*t*
    abortifacient 1
    analgesic 29
    anemia 31
    antidepressant 35
    anxiety 37
    breast-feeding 67
    breast cancer 83
    cystitis 133
    diuretics 151, 151*t*
    dysmenorrhea 157
    dysplasia 160
    emmenagogue 165
    ginseng 197
    headache 206, 290–291
    hemorrhoid 209
    hot flashes 223
    insomnia 243
    irritable bowel syndrome 249
    lactation 256–257
    mastitis 277
    menstrual flow 286
    migraine 291
    pelvic inflammatory disease
        329
    perimenopause 335
    trichomonas 417
Herceptin 83
hereditary acromelagia. See
    restless legs syndrome
hereditary disease. See birth
    defects
heredity. See birth defects;
    chromosome; genetics

hermaphroditism 212
hernia, umbilical 212
herpes infection **212–214**, 432*t*
herpes simplex. *See* herpes
    infection
heterologous insemination
    42–43
heterosexual 214
high blood pressure. *See*
    hypertension
high-density lipoproteins. *See*
    HDL
high forceps 188
high-risk pregnancy 214–215
hip replacement 288
hirsutism 215
histological typing 82
history, medical 201
HIV (human immunodeficiency
    virus) 16–19, **215–216**
HIV antibody test 216
HMG. *See* human menopausal
    gonadotropin
holistic medicine. *See* alternative
    medicine
home birth (home delivery)
    216–217
home medical tests 217–218
homeopathic medicine. *See*
    homeopathy
homeopathy 218–219
homocysteine 22, **219**
homologous insemination 42–43
homosexual **219**, 259–260
honeymoon cystitis 132
hormone **219–220**
    adrenal 13–14
    aldosterone 20
    anabolic steroids 27–28
    androgen 29–30
    danazol 136
    diethylstilbestrol 130–131
    endocrine 165
    estrogen 151–152
    estrogen replacement therapy
        (ERT) 171–174
    FSH 189
    GnRH 197
    hormone therapy 220–221

human chorionic gonadotropin 223
hypothalamus 230
interstitial-cell-stimulating 243
LH 261
oral contraceptive 312–315
oxytocin 322–323
parathyroid 326–327
pituitary 338–339, 339*t*
progesterone 357–358
prolactin 358
selective estrogen-receptor modulator (SERM) 384
steroid 219, 402
testosterone 411–412
thyroid 505–506
hormone, pituitary. *See* pituitary hormones
hormone replacement therapy (HRT). *See* estrogen replacement therapy
hormone therapy 220–221. *See also* estrogen replacement therapy
Horton's disease. *See* giant cell arteritis
hospice 221–222
    resources 452
hospitalist 222
hot flashes (flushes) 222–223
HPV. *See* human papilloma virus
HPV vaccine. *See* Gardasil
HRT. *See* estrogen replacement therapy
HSIL 295
human chorionic gonadotropin (HCG) **223**, 340
human immunodeficiency virus. *See* HIV
human menopausal gonadotropin (HMG) 179, **223**
human papilloma virus (HPV) 84, 119, **223–224**
humpback. *See* kyphosis
Hunner's ulcer 134
Huntington's disease (chorea) 57
    resources 452
husband-coached birth. *See* Bradley method

HV. *See* Hemophilus vaginalis
hyaline membrane disease 25, **224**, 353
Hybrid Capture HPV DNA Assay 326
hydatidiform (hydatid) mole 224–225
hydramnios 225
hydrosalpinx **225**, 328
hydrotherapy 303
hygiene 225–226
hymen **226**, 430, *441*
hymenectomy 226
hymenotomy 226
hyperandrogenism 24
hyperbilirubinemia. *See* neonatal jaundice
hyperemesis gravidarum. *See* morning sickness
hyperglycemia 141
hypermenorrhea **226**, 285
hypermobile testes 129
hyperplasia. *See* endometrial hyperplasia 199
hyperreflexia 366
hypertension 40*t*, **226–228**, 227*t*, 347–348
hypertension headache 206
hypertension prevention 227*t*
hyperthyroidism 414–415
hypnobirth 229
hypnosis 228–229
hypnotherapy 228–229
hypoallergenic 126
hypoglycemia 143, **229**
hypomenorrhea **229**, 285
hypophysectomy 229–230
hypophysis. *See* pituitary gland
hypothalamus 230
hypothyroidism 414
hysterectomy **230–233**, 359, 369, 404
    resources 452
hysteria, conversion 233
hysteria syndrome 233
hysterical neurosis 233
hysterosalpingography 233–234
hysteroscopic myomectomy 301
hysteroscopic resection 185

hysteroscopy 234
hysterosonography 343
hysterotomy 233–234

I
iatrogenic disorder 235
ibuprofen 28, 29
ICSH. *See* interstitital-cell-stimulating hormone
ICSI. *See* intracytoplasmic sperm injection
identical twins 297
idiopathic 235
ileal conduit/bladder 425
ileostomy **235**, 290–291
Imitrex (sumatriptan) 291
immature (infant) 352
immune system. *See* immunity
immunity 235–236
immunization schedule for adults 389
immunocontraception 267
immunotherapy 236
imperforate hymen 226
Implanon 122*t*, 123
implant, breast 269–271
implantation 236–237
implantation bleeding 237
impotence **237–238**, 388
inappropriate lactation. *See* amenorrhea-galactorrhea
incarcerated uterus 374
incest 238
incisional biopsy 52
incompetent cervix (cervical os) 238
incomplete breech 67
incomplete descent (of testes) 129
incomplete miscarriage 294
incontinence. *See* urinary incontinence
incubation period 238
independent midwife 288
indomethacin (Indocin)) 28
induction of labor **238–240**, 239*t*, 322–323
inevitable miscarriage 294

infection **240**, 364–365. *See also* congenital infection, kidney infection; postpartum infection; puerperal fever;sexually transmitted diseases; yeast infection
infertility **240–242**
   acrosin test 10
   artificial insemination 42–44
   azoospermia 47
   basal body temperature 50–51
   donor egg **152**, 248
   embryo transfer 164
   endometriosis 166–168
   fertility 179
   fertility drug 179
   gamete intrafallopian transfer 191
   habitual miscarriage 204–205
   in vitro fertilization 246–248
   miscarriage 293–295
   motility, sperm 296
   necrospermia 304
   oligospermia 310–311
   Rubin test 379
   sperm 395–396
   sperm bank 396–397
   sterility 401
   sterologist 402
   surrogate mother 405–406
infertility resources 452
inflammation 242
inflammatory bowel disease 242
inflammatory breast cancer. *See* cancer, inflammatory breast
informed consent 327
inframammary ridges/folds 64
infusion, herbal 212
inhalation anesthesia 32
inherited disorder. *See* birth defects; congenital infection
injectable contraceptive. *See* Depo-Provera
inpatient 320
insemination 242
in situ. *See* cancer in situ
insomnia 242–243
insufflation. *See* Rubin test
insulin 141

insulin-dependent diabetes 141
intact dilatation and evacuation 150
integrative medicine 15
intercourse, sexual 243
   anal 36
   coitus 116
   oral 315
   sexual response 389–390
interferon 236
interleukin–2 236
intermittent self-catheterization 93
internal (pelvic) examination 202
internal fetal monitoring 181
internal hemorrhoids 208
internal medicine 61*t*
internal os 101
internal version 436
International Units 439*f*
internist 61*t*, 201
interpersonal and social rhythm therapy 246
InterStim 134, 396
interstitial cell 411
interstitial-cell-stimulating hormone 243
interstitial cystitis 133–134
interstitial fibroid 184
interstitial radiation therapy. *See* brachytherapy
intestinal by-pass operation **48**, 309
intimate partner violence (IVP). *See* domestic abuse
intra-amniotic infusion. *See* amnioinfusion
intracytoplasmic sperm injection (ICSI) 247
intraductal papilloma. *See* ductal papilloma
intramural fibroid 184
intra-operative radiotherapy 368
intrauterine device (IUD) 122*t*, **244–246**, 330, 395
intrauterine insemination 42
intrauterine polyp 343
intrauterine pressure catheter 182
intrauterine transfusion 377

introitus **246**, 430
intromission 170
inverted nipple 305
in vitro fertilization **246–248**, 247*t*
in vitro maturation 248
involuntary sterilization 402
involution, uterine 248
iodine 292*t*
iron 292*t*
iron deficiency 30, 31
iron overload 56, **207**
irradiation. *See* radiation therapy
irregular periods 248–249
irritable bowel syndrome 249
ischemia 41
ischial spines 168
isthmus, uterine 207
itching 250
IUD. *See* intrauterine device
IVF. *See* in vitro fertilization
IVM. *See* in vitro maturation

J
jaundice 304
jelly, contraceptive. *See* spermicide
joint replacement 253, **316–317**
juvenile-onset diabetes 141

K
karyotyping 251
kava (Kava-Kava) **37**, 211
Kegel exercises **251**, 359, 424
keratoconjunctivitis sicca. *See* dry eye
keratosis. *See* skin cancer; skin changes
Kerr incision 103
ketoacidosis 143
kicking. *See* fetal movement
kidney infection. *See* pyelonephritis
Klinefelter syndrome 57, **251–252**
kneading 274
knee problems 252–253
knee replacement **252–253**, 316–317
Kock internal reservoir 235

Kotex. *See* sanitary pad
Kronig-Selheim incision 103
K-Y jelly 263
kyphoplasty 318
kyphosis 153, 382

L

labia (majora/minora) 254, *441*
labium. *See* labia
labor **254–256**, *255t*
   amniotomy 27
   anesthesia 32
   back labor 48
   birth attendant 54
   birth ball 54
   birth center 54
   birthing room 57–58
   birth stool 58
   Bradley method 63
   breech presentation 67–69
   brow presentation 69
   cephalic presentation 95
   Cesarean section 101–103
   contraction, uterine 124
   Dick-Read method 146
   dry labor 156
   dystocia 160
   effacement 163
   engagement 168–169
   episiotomy 169–170
   face presentation 176
   false labor 177
   forceps 188
   home birth 216–217
   induction of 238–240
   Leboyer method 259
   midwife 288–290
   mucus plug 297
   obstetrician 309
   oxygen 322
   Pitocin 338
   placenta 339–340
   posterior presentation 343
   postpartum 344–345
   prepared childbirth 356
   prolapsed cord 358
   prolonged labor 359–360
   psychoprophylactic (Lamaze)
     method 360–362

ripe cervix 378
scopolamine 382–384
shoulder presentation 391
Sims position 393
stages of 255t, 361t
umbilical cord 421–422
vacuum extractor 430
version 436
laboratory tests 202–203, 202t
labor coach 360
labor pain. *See* contraction,
   uterine
labyrinthectomy 437
labyrinthitis 396
lactation **256–257**. *See also* breast-
   feeding
   agalactia 14
   amenorrhea-galactorrhea
     syndrome 24
   breast-feeding 65–67
   let-down reflex 261
   polygalactia 342
   prolactin 358
lactation amenorrhea. *See*
   amenorrhea-galactorrhea
lactiferous sinus 305
lactobacilli 430
lactose intolerance 257
La Leche League 65
   resources 449
Lamaze method. *See*
   psychoprophylactic method
laminaria 1, **257**
lanugo 196
laparoscopically assisted vaginal
   hysterectomy 232
laparoscopy 190, **257–259**
laparotomy 259
lapatinib (Tykerb) 83
lap-band surgery 49
large-cell lung cancer 88
laser ablation 369
laser surgery **259**, 275, 395. *See*
   also laser therapy
laser therapy 93, 185, 266, 435.
   See also laser surgery
last menstrual period. *See* LMP
latent phase (labor) 359
laxative 121
lay midwife 288–289

LDL 51t, 94–96
Lea's Shield 99
Leboyer method 259
LEEP. *See* loop electrosurgical
   excision procedure
left lateral position. *See* Sims
   position
leg cramps 128
leg jitters. *See* restless legs
   syndrome
leiomyoma. *See* fibroid
lesbian 259–260
   resources 453
lesion 260–261
let-down reflex **261**, 322
letrozole (Femara) 82
leukemia 73–74
leukoplakia, vulvar 261
leukorrhea. *See* discharge,
   vaginal
Levitra (vardenafil) 238
LGV complement fixation test
   265
LH (luteinizing hormone) 197,
   243, **261**, 339t, 358, 411
libido **261–262**, 388
licensed practical nurse (LPN)
   306
life expectancy 262
light-assisted stab phlebectomy
   435
lightening 262
linea nigra 349
lipoma 262
lipoprotein 109
liposuction 95, **136**
lips, inner/outer. *See* labia
lithotomy. *See* dorsal lithotomy
lithotripsy 190
liver cancer 87
liver disease. *See* hepatitis; cancer,
   liver
liver spots **262–263**, 394
LMP (last menstrual period) 196,
   263
lobular cancer in situ 92
local anesthesia 31–32
local wide excision. *See*
   lumpectomy
lochia 263

loop electrosurgical excision procedure (LEEP) 263
lordosis 382
low blood sugar. *See* hypoglycemia
low-density lipoproteins. *See* LDL
low forceps 188
LPN. *See* licensed practical nurse
LSIL 325
LTH. *See* luteotropic hormone
lubiprostone 249
lubricant 263
Lubrifax 263
lues. *See* syphilis
lumbar epidural bloc. *See* epidural anesthesia
lumpectomy 276–277
Lunelle 123
lung cancer **87**, 394–395
Lupron 180
lupus. *See* systemic lupus erythematorus
luteal phase 284
luteal phase defect 204, **237**
lutein 125
luteinized unruptured follicle 263–264
luteinizing hormone. *See* LH
luteotropic hormone (LTH). *See* prolactin
Lybrel 122
lymph, lymphatic system 264
lymphedema 264–265
lymph nodes 265
lymphocytes 235–236
lymphogranuloma venereum (LGV) 265
lymphoid organs 264
lymphoma 73–74

M

macrocalcifications 72
macronutrients 291
macular degeneration 266
magnesium 292*t*
magnesium sulfate 348
magnetic resonance imager (MRI) 80, **266–267**, 269
maidenhead. *See* hymen
major depression 139

major tranquilizer 416
makeup. *See* cosmetics
male climacteric. *See* male menopause
male contraceptive 267
male erectile dysfunction. *See* impotence
male hormone **29–30**, 136, 411–412
male menopause 268
male sterilization 412–413, **435–436**
malignant 268. *See also* cancer
malignant melanoma. *See* melanoma
mammalgia 268
mammaplasty 268–271
MammaPrint 82
mammary duct ectasia 271
mammary duct fistula 271
mammography 77*t*, **271–273**
Mammotone 53
managed care 328
manic-depressive illness (bipolar illness) 273
manroot. *See* ginseng
Marshall-Marchetti procedure 135
marsupialization **50**, 131
mask of pregnancy. *See* chloasma
massage therapy 273–274
mastectomy 274–277
mastitis 277
masturbation **277–278**, 315
maternal bonding. *See* bonding
maternal placenta 340
maternal serum test. *See* alpha-fetoprotein test
maternity home. *See* birth center
maximal oxygen uptake 45
measles 278
meconium 278–279
medical induction. *See* amnioinfusion
medical massage 274
megaloblastic anemia 31
meiosis 194
melancholia. *See* depression
melanocyte-stimulating hormone 339*t*

melanoma **279**, 279*t*
melasma. *See* chloasma
melatonin 338
membrane rupture. *See* amniotomy
membranes. *See* amniotic sac
menarche 128, **279–280**, 310
Meniere's disease 437
meningomyelocele 398
meniscus 252
menopausal weight gain 443
menopause 280–282
    diet 148
    estrogen replacement therapy (ERT) 171–174
    exercise 174–175
    height loss 207
    hot flashes 222–223
    male 268
    osteoporosis 317–319
    postmenopausal bleeding 344
    skin changes 393–394
    urinary incontinence 423–425
    vaginal atrophy 430
    vitamin 438–439*t*
    weight gain 443
menopause, male. *See* male menopause
menorrhagia. *See* hypermenorrhea
menses. *See* menstruation
menstrual cramps 128, **158–159**
menstrual cup 282
menstrual cycle **282–284**, 283*t*
    premenstrual phase 283*t*
    proliferative phase 283*t*, 359
menstrual extraction 284
menstrual flow **285–286**
    sanitary napkin 380
    scanty flow 381
    tampon 410
menstrual migraine 290
menstrual period. *See* menstrual cycle
menstrual phase 283–284
menstrual regulation. *See* menstrual extraction
menstrual sponge **286–287**, *286*
menstruation. *See* menstrual cycle

mental health
   addiction 12
   agorahobia 15
   alcohol use 19–20
   anorexia nervosa 33
   antidepressants 34–36
   anxiety 36–37
   bulimia 69–70
   depression 138–140
   feminist therapy 178–179
   hysteria, conversion 233
   insomnia 242–243
   manic-depressive illness
      (bipolar illness) 273
   postpartum depression 140
   psychosomatic 362
   psychotherapy 362
   schizophrenia 381
   sex therapy 387–388
   suicide 403
   tranquilizers 415–416
meperidine (Demerol) 138
Meniett device 437
Merci retriever 97
metabolic screening 193
metabolic syndrome **39**, 287
metabolic toxemia of pregnancy.
   See eclampsia; preeclampsia
metabolism 287
metastasis 73, **287**
metformin (Glucophage) **142**, 342
methadone 166
methotrexate **1–2**, 125, 162
metrorrhagia. *See* breakthrough
   bleeding
microcalcifications 72
microgram 439*f*
micromestastases 81
micronutrients 291
Microsort 386–387
microsurgery 287
microvessel disease 41
midcycle 287
midcycle spotting 63
midforceps 188
midwife **288–290**, 289*t*
   resources 453
Mifeprex. *See* mifepristone
mifepristone (RU–486) 1, 2, **124**
migraine 290–291

migraine-associated dizziness 437
Migranal (DHE) 291
milk bank 67
milk cyst. *See* galactocele
milk leg. *See* phlegmasia
mind-body therapies 20
mind visualization. *See*
   visualization
minerals 291–292, 292*t*
minilap, minilaparotomy 292
minipill (progestin-only Pill) 292
minisuction. *See* menstrual
   extraction
minor tranquilizers 415
Mirena 123, 167, **245**
miscarriage 204–205, **293–295**,
   386
misoprostol **124**, 295
missed miscarriage 294–295
mitochondrial disease 56
mitosis194
mitral valve prolapse 295
mitral valve regurgitation 295
Mittelschmerz 295–296
modified radical mastectomy 276
modified rooming-in 378
molar pregnancy. *See* hydatidiform
   mole
Mohs micrographic surgery 90
molecular breast imaging 272
mongolism. *See* Down syndrome
Monilia albicans. *See* yeast
   infection
moniliasis. *See* yeast infection
monoamine oxidase inhibitor 34
monoclonal antibodies 75
mononucleosis 214
monozygotic 297
mons, mons veneris (pubis) 296,
   331, 441
Montgomery's follicles 38
mood elevator. *See* antidepressant
morning-after pill. *See* emergency
   contraception
morning sickness 296
motility, sperm 296
Motrin 28
MRI. *See* magnetic resonance
   imager
MS. *See* multiple sclerosis

mucosa 296
mucous membrane 296–297
mucus method. *See* cervical
   mucus method
mucus plug 297
multifactorial disorder 57
multigravida 297
multipara 297
multiple (sperm) donors 43
multiple pregnancy **297–299**,
   323, 403
multiple punch biopsy 52
multiple sclerosis (MS) 299–300
   resources 453
muscular dystrophy 300
mutant 57, **194**
mutation 194
myasthenia gravis 300–301
Mycoplasma hominis 433
mycotic vaginitis. *See* yeast
   infection
myelin 299
myocardial infarction 39
myofascial pain dysfunction. *See*
   temporomandibular joint
myolysis 185
myoma. *See* fibroid
myomectomy 301
myometrium 426
myositis 301
myxedema 414

N

Nabothian cyst 131
Naprosyn (naproxen) 28, 29*t*
naratriptan (Amerge) 291
narcotic **28**, 138
natural abortion. *See* miscarriage
natural childbirth 160. *See also*
   prepared childbirth
natural family planning 302–303
naturopathy 303–304
nausea 276
nausea gravidarum 296
navel 384
necrospermia 304
needle aspiration **52**, 184
needle biopsy 52
neoadjuvant therapy 81

NeoControl Pelvic Floor Therapy 424
neonatal icterus. *See* neonatal jaundice
neonatal intensive care unit (NICU) 322
neonatal jaundice 304
neoplasm. *See* tumor
nephrostomy 425
nerve compression 274
neural tube defects 20, **304–305**
neurectomy 259
neurohypophysis (posterior pituitary) 338
neurolepsy, neuroleptic 416
neurotransmitter 35
newborn jaundice. *See* neonatal jaundice
NGU. *See* nongonococcal urethritis
NGV. *See* nongonococcal vaginitis
niacin 111, 439t
niacinamide 439t
nicotine 394–395
nicotinic acid 439t
nidation. *See* implantation
nifedepine 268
night sweats 222
nipple 13, 38, 170, 269 270, 271, **305**
nipple banking 271
nit, nits 305, **363–364**
nocturia 189
node 306
nodule. *See* node
nonbenzodiazepines 218
nongonococcal urethritis (NGU) 422
nongonococcal vaginitis (NGV) 432
non-insulin-dependent diabetes 141
nonoxynol 9 397
nonspecific urethritis (NSU) 422
nonspecific vaginitis (NSV) 432
non-steroidal anti-inflammatory drugs. *See* NSAIDs
Non-Stress Test 181
normal diet 146–147
Norplant 122–123

no-scalpel vasectomy 436
nose reconstruction. *See* cosmetic surgery
NP. *See* nurse practitioner
NSAIDs 28–29
NST. *See* non-stress test
NSU. *See* nonspecific urethritis
NSV. *See* nonspecific vaginitis
nuchal translucency-biochemical blood test 154, **306**
nuclear magnetic resonance. *See* magnetic resonance imager
nuclear transfer 248
nucleic acid 306
nullipara 306
nurse 306–307
nurse-midwife 289–290
nurse practitioner 306
nursing. *See* breast-feeding
nutrition. *See* diet; vitamin
nutritional cancer treatment 74, 75t
NuvaRing 122t, 123
nymphomania. *See* libido

O

OAB. *See* overactive bladder
obesity 40t, **308–309**
ob-gyn. *See* obstetrician-gynecologist
obstetrical forceps. *See* forceps
obstetric gestational age 352
obstetrician 309
obstetrician-gynecologist 201
obstetrics 309
occipital nerve stimulation 291
Oncotype DX 82
off-label drug use 310
oligomenorrhea 23, **310**
oligospermia 310–311
omega fatty acids 109
oncogene **74**, 194
one-stage/step approach/ procedure 83, **274**
oophorectomy 89, **311–312**
oophoritis 328
ooplasmic transfer 248
open capsulotomy 270

optional surgery 405t
oral contraceptive 122t, 164–165, 292, **312–315**
oral sex 130, 178, **315**
Oraquick Rapid HIV-1 Antibody test 216
orgasm 115, **315–316**, 390
orgasmic headache 316
Ortho Evra 123
os 101
osteoarthritis 253, **316–317**
osteonecrosis 290
osteopenia 317
osteoporosis 117, 171, 281, **317–319**
    resources 453
ostomy **319–320**
    resources 454
otosclerosis 137
outpatient **320**, 367–368
outpatient surgery 403–404
ova. *See* ovum
ovarian ablation 220
ovarian cancer **88–89**, 311, 400t
ovarian cyst **131–132**, 321
ovarian dysgenesis. *See* Turner's syndrome
ovarian follicle 188
ovariectomy. *See* oophorectomy
ovary 311–312, **320–321**, 331
overactive bladder 423–424
overflow incontinence 423
oviducts. *See* Fallopian tubes
ovo-lacto vegetarians149
ovulation 284, **321–322**
    basal body temperature 50–51, 51t
    menstrual cycle 282–284, 283t
    Mittelschmerz 295–296
    ovarian follicle 188
ovulation method. *See* cervical mucus method
ovum 322
oxybutinin (Oxytrol) 424
oxygen in childbirth 322
oxytocin (Pitocin) 230, 239, **322–323**, 339
oxytocin challenge test 181
Oxytrol 396

P

Paclitoxel. *See* taxol
Paget's disease 324
pain
 chronic 113–114
 pelvic 330–331
 resources 450
painkiller. *See* analgesic
palpate 324
palpitations 324
pancreas 324–325
pancreatic cancer 324–325
pancreatitis 324
panic disorder. *See* anxiety
pantothenic acid 439*t*
Papanicolaou smear. *See* Pap
 smear
papilloma virus (HPV). *See* human
 papilloma virus
PapNet 325
Pap smear/test 84, 202, **325–326**
paracervical anesthesia (block)
 326
paralysis 233, **326, 366**
paraplegia 326
parathyroid 326–327
paraurethral ducts. *See* Skene's
 glands
parental bonding. *See* bonding
paresis 233
partial-birth abortion 150
Partial-Birth Abortion Ban Act
 132
partial breast irradiation 368
partial hysterectomy 230
partial mastectomy 276
partial zona dissection 247
parturition 327
patella 252, 254
patient advocate 327
patients' rights **327–328**, 351–
 352
pear shape **39**, 308
pediatric gestational age 352
pedicle *185*
pediculosis pubis. *See* pubic lice
pelvic abscess **8**, 328
pelvic cancer 90
pelvic cavity. *See* pelvis
pelvic congestion syndrome 120

pelvic contraction 359
pelvic examination 77*t*, *201, 202*
pelvic exenteration 328
pelvic floor exercise. *See* Kegel
 exercises
pelvic floor tension myalgia 330
pelvic inflammatory disease (PID)
 318–330
pelvic organ prolapse 325
pelvic pain 330–331
pelvis *331*, 331–332
penile implant 238
penis **332–333**, *332*
 circumcision 114–115
 ejaculation 163–164
 erection 170
 implant 238
 impotence 237–238
peptides 333
percutaneous umbilical blood
 sampling (PUBS) 333
perforated uterus 137, **245**
Pergonal **180**, 200 333
perimenopause 333–335
perinatology 335
perineal massage 335
perineum 203–204, **335**, *441*
period, menstrual. *See* menstrual
 flow
periodic abstinence. *See* natural
 family planning
peripheral dual energy X-ray
 absorptiometry 317
peritoneum 426
peritonitis 38
permanent colostomy 116
permanent section 52
persistent sexual arousal
 syndrome 335–336
pessary 336
PET scan 336
Pfannenstiel incision 336
P53 gene 74
phagocytes 236
phallus. *See* penis
phenylketonuria (PKU) 55,
 336–337
phlebitis **337**, 413
phlegmasia 337
phobia 36

phosphorus 292*t*
photodynamic therapy 87, **266**
phototherapy **140**, 304
physical examination. *See*
 gynecological examination
Physician Data Query 76
physiologic jaundice. *See* neonatal
 jaundice
phytoestrogen 173
pica 337
PID. *See* pelvic inflammatory
 disease
PIF. *See* prolactin inhibiting factor
piles. *See* hemorrhoid
Pill, the. *See* oral contraceptive
pineal body (gland) 338
piriformis syndrome 338
pit. *See* Pitocin
Pitocin 338
pituitary gland 338–339, 339*t*
pituitary hormones 339*t*
PKU. *See* phenylketonuria
placebo 339
placenta **339–340**, 344
placental insufficiency. *See*
 postmature
placenta previa 340–341
Plan B (emergency contraceptive)
 164–165
plasma cell mastitis. *See* mammary
 duct ectasia
plateau phase 390
platelet 59*t*
PMR. *See* polymyalgia rheumatica
PMS. *See* congestive
 dysmenorrhea
polycystic ovary syndrome 23,
 341–342
polygalactia 342
polygenic disorder. *See*
 multifactorial disorder
polyhydramnios. *See* hydramnios
polymenorrhea 342
polymyalgia rheumatica 342–343
polymyositis 301
polyovulation 297
polyp 85, 86, **342**
polypeptide hormones 219
positron emission tomography. *See*
 PET scan

postcoital test. *See* Sims-Huhner test
posterior pituitary 338
posterior presentation 343–344
postherpetic neuralgia 393
postmature 194, **344**
postmenopausal bleeding 344
post-oral contraceptive amenorrhea. *See* post-Pill amenorrhea
postovulatory phase 284
postpartum 140, **344–345**, 364–365
postpartum depression 140
postpartum examination 345
postpartum hemorrhage 345–346
postpartum infection. *See* puerperal fever
post-Pill amenorrhea 346
post-thrombotic syndrome 413
post-traumatic stress disorder **37**, 372
potassium 292t
potency 237–238
pox. *See* syphilis
PPNG (penicillin-producing Neisseria gonorrhoeae) 199
precancerous lesions 159–160, **346**, 394
precision biopsy 53
precocious puberty 346–347
preconception care 347
preconception counseling. *See* pregnancy counseling
Precose. *See* acarbose
prediabetic 141
preeclampsia 161, **347–348**
preemie. *See* premature
pregnancy **348–350**
  counseling 350
  diabetes and 143–144
  diet 147–148
  drug use and 154–155
  ectopic 162
  exercise 154–155
  fetal movement 182–183
  miscarriage 293–295
  patients' rights 351–352
  prenatal care 354–355
  prenatal tests 355–356
  weight gain 443

pregnancy counseling 350
pregnancy-induced hypertension. *See* preeclampsia
pregnancy monitoring. *See* uterine monitoring
pregnancy test 217, **350–351**
pregnant patients' rights 351–352
prehypertension 227, 227t
preimplantation genetic diagnosis (PGD) 247, **355**
Premarin. *See* conjugated estrogen
premature **352–354**, 353t
premature ejaculation 163–164
premature menopause 280
premenstrual dysphoric disorder (PMDD) 157–158, **354**
premenstrual syndrome (PMS). *See* congestive dysmenorrhea
premenstrual tension. *See* congestive dysmenorrhea
premenstrual weight gain 443
premonitory stage 290
Prempro 173
prenatal care 354–355
prenatal perineal massage 335
prenatal tests **355–356**
  alpha-fetoprotein test 20
  amniocentesis 24–25
  chorionic villus sampling 111–112
  fetoscopy 183
  nuchal-translucency biochemical blood test 306
  percutaneous umbilical blood sampling 333
prenatal treatment 57, **377**
prenatal yoga 356
preovulatory phase 284
prepared childbirth **356**, 360–362, 361t
prepuce (foreskin) 114–115, **324**, 332
presacral and uterosacral neurectomy 168
presbycusis 137
presenile dementia 21
preterm labor. *See* premature
Preven 164–165

primary amenorrhea 22–23
primary dysmenorrhea 156
primary hypertension 226
primary infertility 240
primigravida 356
primipara 356
probiotics 249, **356–357**
prodromal 255
Progestasert 173
progesterone 357–358
progesterone withdrawal test 357
progestin 357, 358
progestogen 357
prognosis 358
prolactin 24, 339t, **358**
prolactin-inhibiting factor (PIF), **24**, 230, 358
prolapse 358
prolapsed cord 358
prolapsed uterus 336, **358–359**
proliferative stage (phase) 188, *283*, **284**, 359
prolonged labor 359–360
Prometrium 342
promiscuous. *See* libido
prophylactic 360
propranolol 291
prostaglandins 1, 156, **360**
prostaglandin abortion 26
prostate *332*, 333
Protectaid 123
protein 60t, 147, 147t
protein hormones 219
proteinuria 348
proton pump inhibitors 170
proton therapy 369
Prozac (fluoxetine) **35**, 223
pruritus. *See* itching
pseudocyesis. *See* false pregnancy
pseudohermaphroditism 190
pseudolumps 184
psoriasis 39
psychogenic 360
psychoprophylactic (Lamaze) method 356, **360–362**, 361t
psychosomatic 362
psychotherapy 178–179, **362**, 387–388
pubertal failure 363

puberty 362–363
    acne 9–10
    adolescent nodule 13
    precocious puberty 346–347
pubic bone *331*
pubic hair 363
pubic lice 363
pubic mound. *See* mons veneris
pubis. *See* mons veneris
pubococcygeous 364
PUBS. *See* percutaneous umbilical
    blood sampling
pudenda. *See* vulva
pudendal anesthesia (nerve block)
    364
puerperal fever (sepsis) 364–365
puerperium 365
pulling out. *See* coitus interruptus
pulmonary cancer. *See* lung cancer
pulmonary edema 163
pulmonary embolism 164
pulse 42
punch biopsy 52
purpura simplex. *See* bruising
purulent 365
pus 365
pustule. *See* acne
pyelonephritis 365
pyosalpinx 328
pyridoxine (vitamin B6) 439*t*

Q

quadrantectomy 276
quadriplegia 366
quadruple screen 154
quantitative computerized
    tomography 318
quickening 366–367
quintuplets 297

R

rabbit test 351
radiation absorbed dose (rad) 271
radiation therapy 368–369
radical hysterectomy 232, **369**
radical mastectomy 275, 276
radical trachelectomy 84
radiofrequency ablation **186**, 369

radioimmunoassay. *See*
    radioreceptor assay
radioimmunotherapies 105
radionuclide imaging 369
radioreceptor assay 369–370
radiotherapy. *See* radiation
    therapy
raloxifene (Evista) 221, **318**
range of motion 274
rape 370–372
rape crisis center 370
Raynaud's phenomenon 372
reactive depression 139
reactive hypoglycemia 229
Reality Vaginal Pouch 118
recessive **57**, 194
recessive-gene disorder **57**, 194
recombinant DNA research 194
rectal cancer. *See* colorectal cancer
rectal examination 202
rectocele 372
rectouterine pouch. *See* cul-de-sac
rectovaginal examination 202
rectovaginal fistula 187
rectum *331*
recurrence 372
reflexology 274
reflex sympathetic dystrophy
    syndrome (RSD) 372–373
reflux esophagitis 191
refractory period 315
regional anesthesia 31, **371**
    caudal 94
    epidural 169
    paracervical 326
    pudendal 364
    spinal 399
registered nurse (RN) 306
rehabilitation massage 274
relative contraindication 125
remission 73, **372**
repeat Cesarean 102
resolution 390
respiratory distress syndrome. *See*
    hyaline membrane disease
restless legs syndrome 373
retarded ejaculation 163
Retin-A (tretinoin) 10, **394**
retracted nipple 305
retroflexed uterus 373

retrograde ejaculation 163
retrolental fibroplasia 373–374
retroverted uterus 374
Rett syndrome 374
rheumatic fever 42
rheumatism 374
rheumatoid arthritis 374–377,
    375
rheumatoid factor 376
Rh factor 377–378
Rh incompatibility 377
Rh-negative 377
Rhogam 377
Rh-positive 377
rhythm method. *See* natural
    family planning
riboflavin 439*t*
ribonucleic acid. *See* RNA
rickets 438*t*
rimming. *See* anilingus
ripe cervix 378
risedronate (Actonel) 318
rizatriptan (Maxalt) 291
RN. *See* registered nurse
RNA (ribonucleic acid) 306
Roe v. Wade 2
rooming-in 378
rosacea 378
Roux-en-Y. *See under* bariatric
    surgery
RU–486 (mifepristone) 1, **124**
rubber. *See* condom
rubella (German measles) 378–
    379
rubeola. *See* measles
Rubin test 379

S

SAD. *See* seasonal affective
    disorder
saddle block anesthesia. *See* spinal
    anesthesia
safe *See* condom
safe period 302
safe sex 18*t*
saline abortion 26
saline implant 269
saliva test 322
salpingectomy 380

salpingitis 177, 328, **380**
sanitary napkin (pad) 380
sarcoma 380
scabies 380
scanning. *See* CAT scan; magnetic
    resonance imager (MRI);
    radionuclide imaging
scanty flow 285, **381**
scar tissue. *See* adhesion
Schiller test 381
schizophrenia 381
scintimammography 272
scleroderma 381–382
    resources 454
sclerosing adenosis 382
sclerotherapy 434
scoliosis 382–383, *383*
scopolamine 382–384
screening guidelines (for cancer)
    77t
scrotum *332*, 384
scurvy 439t
seasonal affective disorder (SAD)
    140
Seasonique (Seasonale) 122
sebaceous cyst 130
seborrheic keratosis 384
secondary amenorrhea 23–24
secondary areola 38
secondary dysmenorrhea 156
secondary hypertension 226, **228**
secondary infertility 240
secondary sex characteristics 363,
    384
second opinion 404
secretory phase 284, **384**
sedimentation rate 61
segmental mastectomy 276
selective estrogen-receptor
    modulator (SERM) 220, **384**
selective reduction 247
selective serotonin reuptake
    inhibitor (SSRI) 34–35
selenium 292t
self-help 384–385
    resources 454
semen 333, **385**
semen analysis 393, **396**
seminal fluid 333
seminal vesicle *332*, 333

seminiferous tubule 333, *332*
senile urethritis 423
senile vaginitis. *See* vaginal atrophy
sensitivity test 425
sensorineural hearing loss 137
sentinel-node biopsy 81, **386**
septate uterus 426
septic abortion 2, **386**
septicemia **199**, 328
septic miscarriage 295
serial induction 239
SERM. *See* selective estrogen-
    receptor modulator
serologic test 60
serotonin reuptake inhibitors. *See*
    selective serotonin reuptake
    inhibitor
serotonin poisoning 386
serotonin syndrome 386
sertraline hydrochloride. *See* Zoloft
serum cholesterol 61
serum glucose 61
serum potassium 61
serum triglycerides 612
sex, determination of 386–387
sex chromosome 112, **195**
sex drive. *See* libido
sex-linked recessive gene disorder
    57, **195**
sex-linked trait 57, 195
sex therapy 387–388
    resources 454
sexual dysfunction 388
sexual intercourse. *See*
    intercourse, sexual
sexually transmitted disease (STD)
    388–389
    AIDS 16–19
    bubo 69
    chancre 104
    chancroid 104
    chlamydia 108
    condyloma acuminata 119
    gonorrhea 197–199
    granuloma inguiale 200
    hepatitis 209–210
    herpes infection 212–214
    lymphogranuloma venereum
        265
    pubic lice 363–364

scabies 380
syphilis 170–171
trichomonas 417, 432t
ureaplasma 422
vaginitis 431–433
sexual response 389–390
    anal 36
    clitoris 115
    coitus 116
    erection 170
    intercourse 243
    oral 315
    orgasm 315–316
Sheehan's disease 390
shelf life, spermicide's 398
shiatsu 274
shingles 214, **390–391**
shoulder presentation 391
show. *See* mucus plug
shrinkage. *See* height loss
Siamese twins 297
sick headache. *See* migraine
sickle-cell anemia 391
sickle-cell disease 391–392
    resources 454
sickle-cell trait 392
sickle thalassemia 391
side effect 392
sigmoid colostomy 117
sigmoidoscopy 77t, 85
sign 392
SIL (squamous intraepithelial
    lesions). *See* dysplasia
silicone implant 269
simple mastectomy 276
Sims-Huhner test 392–393
Sims position 393
single-embryo transfer 247
single footling breech 67
single-gene defects 57
single-photon absorptiometry
    317
sitz bath 393
Sjögren's syndrome 393
Skene's glands **393**, *441*
skin cancer **90**, 279
skin care 393–394
skin changes 393–394
    acne 9–10
    cancer 90, 279

chloasma 108–109
   liver spots 262–263
   striae (stretch marks) 403
SLE. *See* systemic lupus
   erythematosus
sleeping pills 218
sleeplessness. *See* insomnia
sling procedure 424
small-cell lung cancer 88
smart drug 75
smegma 332, **394**
smoking, tobacco 87, **394–395**
social phobia 36
sodium 292*t*
soft chancre. *See* chancroid
somatiform disorder 395
somatostatin 230
sonogram 421
sonography. *See* ultrasound
sonohysterography 137
sound, uterine 245, **395**
spasmodic dysmenorrhea 156–
   157
speculum 244, **395**
sperm 296, 310–311, 333, **395–
   396**, 401
sperm antibodies 156, **396**
spermatogenesis 395
spermatozoan. *See* sperm
sperm bank 396–397
sperm count 396
sperm defects **310–311**, 396
sperm donor 361
spermicide 122*t*, 397–398
sperm motility. *See* motility, sperm
sphincter 398
sphygmomanometer 226
spider vein 434
spina bifida 398–399
spinal anesthesia 399
Spinnbarkeit 99
spiral-computed CAT scan 75
spirometry 113
split ejaculation 311
spontaneous abortion. *See*
   miscarriage
sports massage 274
spotting. *See* breakthrough bleeding
squamous cell carcinoma (lung)
   88; (skin) 90

squamous intraepithelial lesions.
   See dysplasia
squamous epithelium 99
squeeze technique 163–164
Stage 0 91, **400**, 400*t*
staging (cancer) 74, **399–400**,
   399*t*, 400*t*
staining. *See* breakthrough bleeding
stasis 413
statin 111, **400–401**
STD. *See* sexually transmitted
   disease
Stein-Leventhal syndrome. *See*
   polycystic ovary syndrome
stem cell 62, 74, 372, **400–401**,
   409
stereotactic biopsy 53
sterility 401
sterilization 401–402
   castration 93
   tubal ligation 418
   vasectomy 435
steroid 27–28, 219, **402**
sterologist 241, **402**
stillbirth 402
St. John's wort 35, **212**
stoma **319**, 425
straight. *See* homosexual
stress incontinence 423–424
stress test 175
stretch marks. *See* striae
striae 403
stripping the membranes 239
stripping varicose veins 405*t*,
   434–435
stroke. *See* cerebral vascular
   accident
Strontium 290
subarachnoid block. *See* spinal
   anesthesia
subcutaneous 403
subcutaneous mastectomy 277
subfertility. *See* oligospermia
submucosal fibroid 184, *185*
submucous fibroid 184, *185*
subserosal fibroid 184, *185*
subserous fibroid 184, *185*
subtotal hysterectomy 230
suction abortion. *See* vacuum
   aspiration

sugar. *See* glucose
sugar diabetes. *See* diabetes
suicide 403
sumatriptan 291
sunscreen 90
superfecundation 403
superfetation 403
support group **92**, 385
suppository 403
suppressor gene 74
suppurative mastitis 277
supracervical hysterectomy 230
surfactant 224
surgery 403–405
   cosmetic 126–127
   hysterectomy 230–234
   outpatient, 403–404
   unnecessary 404–405, 405*t*
surgical biopsy 52
surrogate mother 405–406
Swedish massage 274
symphisis pubis 406
symptom 406
sympto-thermic method 51, **303**
Synarel (nafarelin) 186
syndrome 406
Syndrome X 41
synechia. *See* adhesion
synovitis 374
syphilis 406–407
systemic 407
systemic adjuvant therapy 81
systemic embolism 164
systemic sclerosis. *See* scleroderma
systemic lupus erythematosus
   407–409
systolic heart failure 120
systolic pressure 22

T

tachycardia **42**, 324
tai chi 175
tail of Spence 64
tamoxifen 82, **220–221**
tampon 410
tapotement 274
targeted therapies/drugs **75**, 105
Taxol 106
Taxotere 82–83

Tay-Sachs disease 57, **410–411**
Tazorac 10
telangiectasis. *See* spider vein
temperature method. *See* basal body temperature
temporal arteries 196–197
temporal arteritis. *See* giant cell arteritis
temporary colostomy 116
temporomandibular joint 411
tenaculum 136
tendinitis 252–253
tension-free transvaginal tape 425
tension headache 206
teratogens 56
term. *See* gestation
testes. *See* testis
testicle. *See* testis
testicular feminization. *See* androgen insensitivity
testis *332*, 411
testis determining factor 386
testosterone 29, 281, **411–412**
test-tube baby. *See* in vitro fertilization
thalassemia 391
thalidomide 412
tecae interna 200
therapeutic abortion 2
therapeutic touch 412
therapy 412. *See also* chemotherapy; psychotherapy
    adjuvant 13
    feminist 178–179
    gene therapy 192
    hormone therapy 220–221
    massage therapy 273–274
Thermage 127
thermatic sterilization 412–413
thiamine 438*t*
thinning, hair 205
ThinPrep smear 325
threatened miscarriage 294
three-day measles. *See* rubella
thromboembolism 164
thrombophlebitis 413
thrombosis 413
thrombus 413
thyroid 413–415

thyroid cancer 91
thyroidectomy 415
thyroid-stimulating hormone (thyrotropin) 339*t*, 414
thyrotropin-releasing hormone 230, **414**
TIA. *See* transient ischemic attack
tic douloureux 415
tipped uterus (womb). *See* retroverted uterus
tissue plasminogen activator (TPA) 97
TMJ. *See* temporomandibular joint
tonsillectomy 403
topical anesthesia 31
total cryptorchidism 129
total hysterectomy 230
total knee replacement 252–253
total mastectomy 276
toxemia of pregnancy. *See* eclampsia; preeclampsia
toxic alopecia 205
toxic facelift. *See* Botox
toxic metabolic headache 206
toxic shock syndrome 410
TPA. *See* tissue plasminogen activator
trachelectomy. *See* radical trachelectomy
TRAM. *See* trans rectus abdominal muscle flap
tranquilizers 415–416
transcranial magnetic stimulation (TMS) 291
transcutaneous electrical nerve stimulation **113**, 134
trans fat 110, **416**
trans fatty acids. *See* trans fat
transformation zone 117
transfusion syndrome 298
transient ischemic attack (TIA) 96
transition (labor) 255*t*, 256, **359**, 361*t*
trans rectus abdominal muscle flap (TRAM) 270
transsexual 416–417
transvaginal sonography 89, 137, **421**
transverse colostomy 117

transverse position. *See* shoulder presentation
trapped egg syndrome. *See* luteinized unruptured follicle
tretinoin. *See* Retin-A
trichomonas **417**, 432, 432*t*
tricyclic antidepressant 34
trigeminal neuralgia. *See* tic douloureux
trigger point therapy 331
triglycerides 110*t*, **418**
trimester 317–318, **418**
triple screen 20, **154**
triplets 297
trisomy 13 56
trisomy 18 56
trisomy 21 56, **154**
trocar 258
Tro-car biopsy 52
Tru-cut biopsy 52
tubal insufflation. *See* Rubin test
tubal ligation 122*t*, 129, 258, 292, **418–419**
tubal pregnancy. *See* ectopic pregnancy
tubal sterilization. *See* tubal ligation
tubercles of Montgomery 38
tuberoplasty (tuboplasty) 419
tumor 73, 262, 380, **420**
tumorectomy, tumor excision. *See* lumpectomy
Turner's syndrome 420
24-hour test (urinary) 425
twins **297–299**, 321–322, 403
two-hour swim-up analysis 396
two-stage (two-step) procedure **83**, 274
tying the tubes. *See* tubal ligation
tylectomy. *See* lumpectomy
Tylenol (acetaminophen) 28, 29*t*
Type I diabetes 141
Type II diabetes 141
Type III (gestational) diabetes 143

U

ulcerative colitis 235, **242**
ulcus molle. *See* chancroid
ultrasonic liposuction 126

ultrasound 25, 89, 137, 273, 298, 340, **421**
ultrasound densitometry 318
umbilical cord 358, **421–422**
umbilical hernia. *See* hernia, umbilical
umbilicus. *See* navel
undescended testes. *See* cryptorchidism
unopposed estrogen 172
Urban operation 276
urea 422
urea abortion 26
ureaplasma 422
ureter *332*
uretero-colostomy 425
urethra *331, 332,* 422, *441*
urethritis 422–423
urethrocele 423
urge incontinence 424
uric acid 60*t*
urinalysis 425
urinary bladder. *See* bladder
urinary catheter. *See* catheter, urinary
urinary frequency. *See* frequency, urinary
urinary incontinence 358–359, **423–425**
urinary infection. *See* cystitis; pyelonephritis
urinary ostomy. *See* urostomy
urinary screening 193
urinary sphincter 398
urinary tract infection. *See* cystitits; pyelonephritis
urine culture 425
urine test 202, **425**
urogynecologist 424
urostomy 425
uterine artery embolization 186
uterine biopsy. *See* endometrial biopsy
uterine cancer **91**, 400*t*
uterine contraction. *See* contraction, uterine
uterine decensus. *See* prolapsed uterus
uterine dysfunction 359
uterine fibroid embolization 186

uterine inertia 359
uterine involution. *See* involution
uterine monitoring 426
uterine polyp 165, **343**
uterine suspension **168**, 259, 374
uterine synechiae. *See* Asherman's syndrome
uterus *201, 331,* **426–427**. *See also under* uterine (above)
    anteflexed 34
    anteverted 34
    perforated 245
    prolapsed 358–359
    retroflexed 373
    retroverted 374
UVA 90
UVB 90

V

vabra. *See* vacuum aspiration
vaccine 428
vacurette 428
vacuum abortion. *See* vacuum aspiration
vacuum aspiration 1, 2, 53, **428–430**
vacuum curettage. *See* vacuum aspiration
vacuum extractor 430
vagina 144–146, *145, 185, 331,* **430**, *441*
vaginal atresia 430
vaginal atrophy 281, **430–431**
vaginal birth after Cesarean (VBAC) 102
vaginal bleeding. *See* bleeding, vaginal
vaginal cancer 12, **91**, 130–131
vaginal discharge. *See* discharge, vaginal
vaginal dryness. *See* vaginal atrophy
vaginal fistula 187
vaginal hysterectomy 231
vaginal mycosis. *See* yeast infection
vaginal thrush. *See* yeast infection
vaginal tubal ligation 418
vaginismus 431

vaginitis 431–433, 432*t*
vaginosis, bacterial 433
varicocele 433
varicose vein (varicosity) 349, 405*t*, **433–435**
vas deferens *332, 333,* **435**
vasectomy 122*t*, 435–436
Vaseline 263
vasocongestion 389
vasomotor instability. *See* hot flashes
vasopressin 230
vasovasotomy 436
VBAC. *See* vaginal birth after Cesarean
VD (venereal disease). *See* sexually transmitted disease
vector 191
vegans 149
vegetarianism 149
vein 433–435, **436**. *See also* vena cava
vena cava 152, **182**, 393
venereal disease. *See* sexually transmitted disease
venereal warts. *See* condyloma acuminata
venous thrombosis 413
ventricular fibrillation 46
vernix caseosa 196
version 436
vertebroplasty 318
vertex presentation 95
vertical sleeve gastrectomy 49
vertigo 436–437
vesicostomy 425
vesicovaginal fistula 187
vestibular bulbs 437
vestibular glands. *See* Bartholin's gland
vestibular neurectomy 437
vestibule 437, *441*
viable 437
Viagra 132, **237–238**, 388
vibration massage 274
VIN. *See* vulvar intraepithelial neoplasia
violence against women. *See* domestic abuse; rape
virginity 437–438

virilism. *See* adrenogenital syndrome
virotherapy 75
virtual colonoscopy. *See* colonoscopy
visiting nurse 307
visualization 438
vitamin **438–440**, 438–439*t*
vitamin A **438**, 438*t*, 440
vitamin B group 440
vitamin B₁ 438*t*
vitamin B₂ 439*t*
vitamin B₆ 439*t*, 440
vitamin B₁₂ 438, 439*t*
vitamin C 439*t*
vitamin D 438*t*, 438, 440
vitamin E 438*t*,, 438, 440
vitamin K 438*t*, 439
VNUS closure procedure 435
voluntary sterilization 402
von Willebrand disease 440
vulva 53, **440**, *441*
vulvar biopsy 53
vulvar cancer 91
vulvar intraepithelial neoplasia 91
vulvar lichen planus 440
vulvar vestibulitis 441
vulvitis 440–441
vulvodynia 441–442
vulvovaginal glands. *See* Bartholin's glands
vulvovaginitis. *See* vaginitis

W

waist-to-hip ratio 40, 40*t*, **308**
warts. *See* condyloma acuminata
Wasserman test 407
water pill. *See* diuretic
water retention. *See* edema
waters. *See* amniotic fluid
wedge excision. *See* lumpectomy
weight, body 308, **443**
weight gain 443
Wertheim procedure 232, **369**
wet nurse 56, 57
wet smear 432*t*, **442**
white blood cell count 59*t*
whitehead 9
white leg. *See* phlegmasia
winter blues. *See* seasonal affective disorder
wire-localization biopsy 53
withdrawal bleeding 173
withdrawal method. *See* coitus interruptus
womb. *See* uterus
womb room 322
women's doctor. *See* gynecologist
women's health clinic 444

XYZ

X-linked (trait) 57, **195**
yeast infection 431–433, 432*t*, **445–446**
yogurt 446
ZIFT. *See* zygote intrafallopian transfer
zinc 292*t*
zoledronic acid (Zometa) 82, 319
Zoloft (sertraline hydrochloride) 37
Zometa 82, 319
Zomig (zolmitriptan) 291
zona pellucida 181
zygote 164, **446**
zygote intrafallopian transfer (ZIFT) **164**, 191